William H. Bush

UROLOGIC IMAGING AND INTERVENTIONAL TECHNIQUES

UROLOGIC IMAGING AND INTERVENTIONAL TECHNIQUES

EDITED BY

William H. Bush, M.D.
Department of Radiology
Virginia Mason Clinic
Seattle, Washington

With 32 contributors

Urban & Schwarzenberg · Baltimore–Munich

Urban & Schwarzenberg, Inc.
7 E. Redwood Street
Baltimore, Maryland 21202
USA

Urban & Schwarzenberg GmbH
Pettenkoferstrasse 18
D-8000 München 2
West Germany

Printed in Germany

Notices

The Editor, Authors, and the Publisher of this work have made every effort to ensure that the drug dosage schedules herein are accurate and in accord with the standards accepted at the time of publication. The reader is strongly advised, however, to check the product information sheet included in the package of each drug he or she plans to administer to be certain that changes have not been made in the recommended dose or in the contraindications for administration.

The Publishers have made an extensive effort to trace original copyright holders for permission to use borrowed material. If any have been overlooked, it will be corrected at the first reprint.

Library of Congress Cataloging-in-Publication Data

Urologic imaging and interventional techniques.
Includes bibliographies and index.
1. Genitourinary organs--Imaging. 2. Genitourinary organs--Diseases--Diagnosis. 3. Genitourinary organs--Interventional radiology. I. Bush, William H.
[DNLM: 1. Diagnostic Imaging. 2. Urologic Diseases--diagnosis. WJ 141 U775]
RC874.U74 1989 616.6'0757 88-26164
ISBN 0-8067-2551-6

Sponsoring Editor: Charles W. Mitchell
Manuscript Editor and Proofreader: Molly Ruzicka
Production Coordination: Charles W. Mitchell and Kathleen D. Courtney
Indexer: Deborah K. Tourtlotte
Printer: Kastner & Callwey, Munich

ISBN 0-8067-2551-6 Baltimore

ISBN 3-541-72551-6 Munich

DEDICATION

Hans Rudolph Feindt

During life and work, each of us encounters many individuals; from some encounters, we take away a little, from some nothing. However, if we are fortunate, we may have a rare and special experience that remains with us forever. Dr. Hans Rudolph Feindt was such an influence on me and many others.

A unique person, Dr. Feindt was inquisitive, insatiable in his desire to explore and experience life, demanding of his colleagues and of himself. An awareness and a drive pervaded his work in radiology and his approach to life. He set high goals for himself even in his younger years, and demanded that his coworkers and residents-in-training do the same. He considered himself to be a physician for his patients, a teacher and nurturer of young radiologists, and last, but not least, an organizer, coordinator, and politician for a large radiology department in the immense city hospital of Hamburg, Federal Republic of Germany.

For some, these characteristics made him intolerant and intolerable. However, for many of us, this drive and zeal set an example, altering our perceptions of medicine, radiology, and life itself. He fought for and fostered a strong, growing radiology department, the Albers-Schönberg-Institut at the Allgemeines Krankenhaus St. Georg in Hamburg. His death at age 68 created an acute sense of loss among those of us who had worked and lived with him. We his friends, in Germany and throughout the world, his students, and his patients will not forget this wonderfully complex man and his impact on our lives.

WHB

FOREWORD

New and exciting developments in radiology and urology have made the subspecialty of uroradiology one of the most, if not *the* most, rapidly growing disciplines in medical imaging. Advances in diagnostic imaging and interventional techniques have found a receptive audience of urologists and radiologists worldwide. Nearly every innovation in these areas has been eagerly incorporated into the everyday practice of clinical urology. Such enormous strides have, naturally, resulted in a number of textbooks that chronicle the growth and development in the field.

While some of these publications detail the diagnostic principles of uroradiology and others exhaustively review the interventional techniques intrinsic to its practice, there has long been a need for a work incorporating the two philosophies. I believe that with the appearance of *Urologic Imaging and Interventional Techniques* this need has been met. Not only has the editor managed to combine the features of both diagnostic and interventional uroradiology into one book, but he has, equally importantly, accomplished this in a clear and concise fashion while still providing a panoramic view of the subject.

William H. Bush is eminently qualified to edit a textbook such as this. He has an extensive background in all of the facets of uroradiology. Not only has he practiced the specialty for many years, but he is an esteemed teacher, and his countless written contributions, based on original innovative concepts, have made him a leader in the field. For this book he has assembled a coterie of outstanding contributors – each an authority in his or her own right – to provide timely and thorough reviews of the major topics in uroradiology today.

This worthwhile book should appeal to all those seeking a one-volume state-of-the-art review of uroradiology. Its compact format makes it convenient to use, and it will prove an ideal text to bridge the gap between the introductory and encyclopedic publications on the subject.

Howard M. Pollack, M.D.
Hospital of the University of Pennsylvania
Philadelphia

PREFACE

Urologic Imaging and Interventional Techniques is written for practicing urologists and general diagnostic radiologists. It also provides a primer for residents who want to know more about uroradiology. It offers varied information to each reader: to some, an overview of current uroradiological practice; to others, in-depth instruction.

As editor, my goal was to assemble experts in the specialties of radiology, urology, and internal medicine for the purpose of providing readers a concise overview of their area of expertise as well as specific recommendations and suggestions: a "how I do it" approach to uroradiology. I have avoided inundating the reader with innumerable diagnostic variations or therapeutic options, or an undue number of references.

The book is organized into two major sections: imaging and intervention. The chapters on imaging cover each of the primary modalities in radiology, including excretory urography, ultrasonography, nuclear medicine, computed tomography, and magnetic resonance imaging. In addition, there are specific chapters on radiation, contrast media, lymphography, angiography, and neonatal and pediatric uroradiology. Two chapters summarize an integrated approach to imaging of the upper urinary tract and the lower urinary tract, respectively.

The section on intervention addresses percutaneous access to the kidney and treatment options now available – nephrostomy, stents, endopyelotomy – the field of endourology. Renal calculus disease is covered in more detail, including a chapter on medical evaluation of patients with kidney stone disease. Percutaneous balloon catheter angioplasty is discussed, following a background chapter on renovascular hypertension. Current concepts on embolotherapy for the genitourinary system conclude this section.

Conceptually, this textbook should offer urologists and radiologists a resource of practical pointers and information to aid their clinical practice.

William H. Bush, M.D.

CONTENTS

CONTRIBUTORS

Edward A. Benson, M.D.
Section of Endocrinology and Diabetes
Virginia Mason Clinic and Medical Center
Clinical Assistant Professor of Medicine
University of Washington School of Medicine
Seattle, WA

George E. Brannen, M.D., F.A.C.S.
Section of Urology
Director of Renal Transplantation
Virginia Mason Clinic and Medical Center
Clinical Associate Professor of Urology
University of Washington School of Medicine
Seattle, WA

Patrick J. Bryan, M.B., F.R.C.R.
Associate Professor of Radiology
Director, Division of Ultrasound
Case Western Reserve University School
of Medicine/University Hospitals of Cleveland
Cleveland, OH

William H. Bush, M.D.
Head, Uroradiology
Virginia Mason Clinic and Medical Center
Clinical Associate Professor of Radiology
University of Washington School of Medicine
Seattle, WA

Harold E. Butler, M.D.
Assistant Professor of Radiology
Case Western Reserve University School
of Medicine/University Hospitals of Cleveland
Cleveland, OH

Prof. Dr. Christian G. Chaussy
Department of Urology
Krankenhaus Harlaching
Munich, Federal Republic of Germany

Pauline K. Chu, M.D.
Assistant Professor of Radiology
Loma Linda University School of Medicine
Loma Linda, CA

Richard H. Cohan, M.D.
Assistant Professor of Radiology
Duke University Medical Center
Durham, NC

Robert D. Crane, M.D.
Section Head, Computed Tomography/Magnetic Resonance Imaging
Virginia Mason Clinic and Medical Center
Clinical Assistant Professor of Radiology
University of Washington School of Medicine
Seattle, WA

Eva V. Dubovsky, M.D., Ph.D.
Professor and Director
Division of Nuclear Medicine
University of Alabama Hospital
Nuclear Medicine Service
Birmingham Veterans Administration Medical Center
Birmingham, AL

N. Reed Dunnick, M.D.
Professor of Radiology
Director, Division of Diagnostic Imaging
Duke University Medical Center
Durham, NC

Jack S. Elder, M.D.
Director of Pediatric Urology
Rainbow Babies and Children's Hospital
Associate Professor of Surgery and Pediatrics
Case Western Reserve University School
of Medicine
Cleveland, OH

Robert K. Feldman, M.D.
Interventional Radiology
Virginia Mason Clinic and Medical Center
Seattle, WA

Peggy J. Fritzsche, M.D.
Director of Uroradiology
Loma Linda University Medical Center
Professor of Radiology
Loma Linda University School of Medicine
Loma Linda, CA

Robert P. Gibbons, M.D.
Section of Urology
Director, Center for Kidney Stone Treatment
Virginia Mason Clinic and Medical Center
Clinical Professor of Urology
University of Washington School of Medicine
Seattle, WA

Prof. Dr. Dieter Jocham
Department of Urology
Klinikum Grosshadern
University of Munich (LMU)
Munich, Federal Republic of Germany

Douglas Jones, B.Sc.
Director, Northwest Medical Physics Center
Lynnwood, WA

Reiley Kidd, M.D.
Chief, Department of Radiology
Virginia Mason Clinic and Medical Center
Seattle, WA

Thomas J. Kofler, M.D.
Director, Interventional Radiology
Swedish Hospital Medical Center
Seattle, WA

Andrew J. LeRoy, M.D.
Consultant in Diagnostic Radiology
Mayo Clinic
Associate Professor of Radiology
Mayo Graduate School of Medicine
Rochester, MN

Gregory P. Lewis, M.D.
Diagnostic and Interventional Radiology
Virginia Mason Clinic and Medical Center
Seattle, WA

Joseph P. LiPuma, M.D.
Associate Professor of Radiology
Section Head, Angiography and Interventional Radiology
Case Western Reserve University School of Medicine/University Hospitals of Cleveland
Cleveland, OH

William M. Marks, M.D.
Diagnostic Radiology
Virginia Mason Clinic and Medical Center*
Diagnostic Radiology
Providence Hospital and Medical Center
Seattle, WA

Timothy P. Maroney, M.D.
Clinical Assistant Professor of Radiology
University of California, San Francisco*
San Francisco, CA

Department of Radiology
John Muir Hospital
Walnut Creek, CA

Linda D. Mulder, M.D.
Radiology Resident
Department of Radiation Sciences
Loma Linda University Medical Center
Loma Linda, CA

Matthew D. Rifkin, M.D.
Director, Division of Magnetic Resonance Imaging
Department of Radiology
Thomas Jefferson University Hospital
Professor of Radiology and Urology
Jefferson Medical College
Thomas Jefferson University
Philadelphia, PA

Henrietta Kotlus Rosenberg, M.D.
Senior Radiologist and Director
Division of Ultrasound
The Children's Hospital of Philadelphia
Professor of Radiology
University of Pennsylvania School of Medicine
Philadelphia, PA

Prof. Dr. Egbert Schmiedt
Director, Department of Urology
Klinikum Grosshadern
University of Munich (LMU)
Munich, Federal Republic of Germany

Robert F. Spataro, M.D.
Associate Professor of Radiology
University of Rochester Medical Center*
Radiology Department
The Genesee Hospital
Rochester, NY

John Stassi, M.D.
Department of Radiology
Thomas Jefferson University Hospital*
Philadelphia, PA

Pick, Levine & Stassi, Radiology Associates
Havertown, PA

Charles J. Tegtmeyer, M.D.
Director, Division of Angiography, Interventional Radiology, and Special Procedures
University of Virginia Health Sciences Center
Professor of Radiology
Professor of Anatomy
University of Virginia School of Medicine
Charlottesville, VA

John R. Thornbury, M.D.
Professor of Radiology
Clinical Sciences Center
University of Wisconsin
Madison, WI

Robert L. Wilburn, M.D.
Section of Nephrology
Virginia Mason Clinic and Medical Center
Seattle, WA

* Contributor has subsequently relocated to second affiliation listed

ACKNOWLEDGMENTS

This book is the culmination of the efforts of many individuals, to whom I wish to express my gratitude. My idea for a concise, reasonably priced book on uroradiology was encouraged initially by Charles Mitchell, editor at Urban & Schwarzenberg, who has remained a strong supporter of this endeavor.

Because of the enthusiastic involvement of my two friends and editorial consultants in Seattle, Mary Wieckowicz and Mary Hill, this book has been accomplished in a timely fashion. Their critical review of each chapter and thoughtful suggestions helped immeasurably to clarify the text. Their experience and indefatigable effort were invaluable to me.

To my colleagues in the radiology department at Virginia Mason Clinic, I wish to extend thanks for their assistance with the book and their tolerance during the writing of it; to my colleagues in urology, particularly Drs. George Brannen and Robert Gibbons, thank you for your support, encouragement, and cooperation in all of the new techniques and procedures we have undertaken; this book is a result of the outstanding relationships between our sections of urology, nephrology, and radiology.

A special thank you to Mary Schoenmakers who handled the extensive correspondence and assisted with manuscript preparation.

And to the spouses of all of the contributors to this book, I wish to express my gratitude for your tolerance and for the encouragement you have given all of us; these thoughts go especially to my wife, Janet, and to my two young daughters, Anne and Jane.

CHAPTER

1

Contrast Media Comparison: Ionic and Nonionic

Robert F. Spataro

Conventional ionic contrast media are termed ratio 1.5 agents because three iodine atoms are supplied by the two particles of contrast media as they ionize in solution (Table 1–1). High concentrations are necessary to deliver enough iodine for contrast enhancement, making the osmolality of conventional agents four to seven times that of human plasma (Table 1–2). This hyperosmolality and the chemical properties of the agents cause substantial adverse effects.

Nonionic contrast media were introduced in the late 1960s (Almen 1969, 1980). These monoacidic monomers are based on benzoic acid derivatives similar to conventional ionic contrast, but contain no groups that will ionize in solution, and are thus completely nonionic. In solution, these agents provide three iodine atoms and only one uncharged particle (ratio 3 agents).

Metrizamide (Amipaque), the first nonionic agent, was used mainly for myelography. It has

Table 1–1 Generalized Contrast Media Structures

	Number of Iodine Atoms	Number of Particles in Solution	Ratio of Iodine to Particles in Solution
Ionic Monoacidic Monomer			
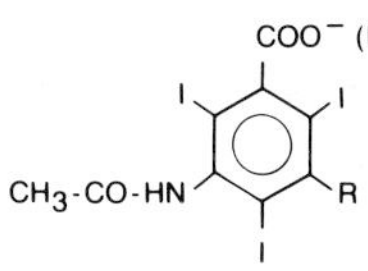 Hypaque, Renografin (diatrizoate); Conray (iothalamate); Metrizoate	3	2	1.5
Ionic Monoacidic Dimer			
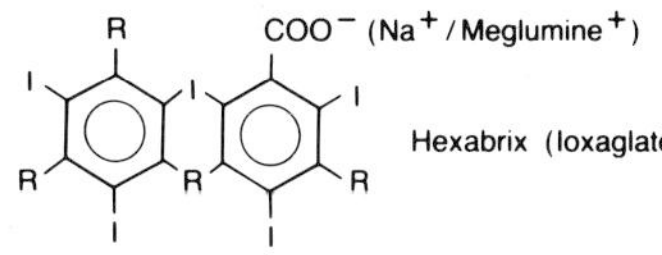 Hexabrix (Ioxaglate)	6	2	3
Nonionic Monomer			
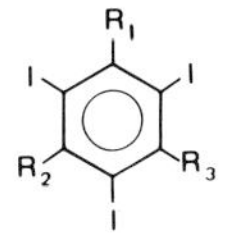 Isovue (iopamidol); Omnipaque (iohexol); Amipaque (metrizamide); Ioversol; Iopromide	3	1	3
Nonionic Dimer			
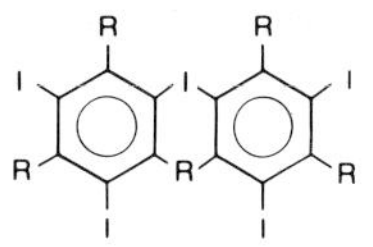 Iotrol	6	1	6

Note: Generalized contrast media structures are shown for currently available approved contrast media and for contrast media in the process of FDA approval. The differences between conventional ionic monoacidic contrast media, ionic monoacidic dimers, nonionic monomers, and nonionic dimers are illustrated, and the ratio of iodine atoms to particles in solution is shown, comparing ratio 1.5, ratio 3, and ratio 6 contrast structures.
Source: Adapted, by permission, from Spataro RF: Newer contrast agents for urography. *Radiol. Clin. North Am.* 22:365–379, 1984.

Table 1–2 Physical Properties of Contrast Media

Contrast Media	Iodine Content (mgl/ml)	Osmolality (mOsm/kg H_2O)	Molecular Weight	Viscosity 37° (mPas)
Hypaque 50% (Sodium diatrizoate)	300	1500	614	2.5
Conray (Methylglucamine iothalamate)	282	1217	614	4.0
Renografin 60 (Sodium/Methylglucamine diatrizoate)	288	1511	614	3.9
Isopaque 280 (Methylglucamine calcium metrizoate)	280	1500	628	4.0
Conray 400 (Sodium iothalamate)	400	1965	614	4.5
Amipaque (Metrizamide)	280	450	789	5.0
Isovue (Iopamidol)	300	616	777	4.5
Iopromide	300	607	791	4.8
Omnipaque (Iohexol)	300	620	821	4.8
Ioversol (MP-328)	320	716	807	6.0
Hexabrix (Sodium/methylglucamine ioxaglate)	320	580	1269	7.5
Iotrol	300	300	1626	9.1
Human blood plasma		300		

Source: Adapted, by permission, from Spataro RF: Newer contrast agents for urography. *Radiol. Clin. North Am.* 22: 365–379, 1984.

been replaced by the less expensive iohexol (Omnipaque) and iopamidol (Isovue) (Bryan et al. 1982; Hammeke et al. 1985). Unlike metrizamide, these newer agents are stable premixed solutions, and are less costly and less toxic. New nonionic agents being tested and awaiting U.S. Food and Drug Administration (FDA) approval are ioversol (MP-328) and iopromide.

Another type of low-osmolality agent is ioxaglate (Hexabrix), a monoacidic ionic dimer. Six iodine atoms are present on two joined benzoic acid rings; the agent ionizes to two particles in solution, making it a ratio 3 agent (Table 1–1). This compound has an osmolality of approximately 600 mOsm/kg H_2O, which is only twice the osmolality of human plasma and less than half that of conventional ionic monoacidic monomers. The osmolality of iohexol and iopamidol is somewhat greater than that of ioxaglate (616 mosm/kg and 672 mOsm/kg, respectively), and less than half that of the conventional ionic agents. Ioxaglate is, however, still an ionic compound and dissociates in solution to produce an anion and a cation.

Reviews of the properties and effects of conventional and new low-osmolality agents show the nonionic monomers to be clearly superior to ratio 1.5 ionic agents and apparently superior to the ionic ratio 3 low-osmolality agent ioxaglate (Dawson 1984, 1985; Spataro 1984).

Types of Adverse Effects

Hemodynamic and Cardiac

Conventional ionic contrast media increase serum osmolality, cause a rapid influx of water from the interstitial to the intravascular space, increase circulatory blood volume about 15%, and decrease hematocrit correspondingly. These changes cause tachycardia and substantially increased cardiac output. A transient decrease in systemic blood pressure is most common, but occasionally there is a blood pressure increase, often associated with nausea and vomiting (Fischer et al. 1984). The agents decrease peripheral vascular resistance, cause vasodilation, and increase blood flow, manifesting to the patient as flushing. Pulmonary arterial pressure becomes transiently elevated with the intravenous injection of ionic agents. Venous and arterial pain and local and systemic sensation of heat are also due to hyperosmolality. Conventional contrast media also deform red blood cells, increase cell rigidity, and cause vascular endothelial damage. All of these effects are substantially reduced with low-osmolality contrast media.

Direct myocardial effects are prominent with intracoronary and intraaortic injections, but similar changes of lesser magnitude occur after intravenous injections. The risk of ventricular fibrillation is higher with ratio 1.5 agents than with ratio 3 agents. Electrocardiographic changes frequently occur during coronary arteriography (Berg et al. 1973). Up to 8% of patients may demonstrate some electrocardiogram (ECG) abnormality after intravenous injection. Minor abnormalities include premature atrial contractions and single premature ventricular contractions (PVC), whereas major changes include bigeminy PVC, ventricular tachycardia, and T-wave depression (Wolf 1980). Conventional agents cause direct depression of cardiac contractile function, due to the cation content. Most of the adverse cardiac electrophysiologic effects seem related to hyperosmolality, calcium binding, and the sodium/calcium ratio. They are significantly reduced with ratio 3 low-osmolality agents (Heron et al. 1984; Higgins 1984).

Neurotoxicity

Increased blood brain barrier permeability is seen after intravascular injection of ionic agents, an effect largely dependent on osmolality. Less penetration occurs with ioxaglate, iopamidol, and iohexol (Drayer et al. 1984).

Ionic agents injected into the intrathecal space cause cerebral edema, petechial hemorrhages, and marked seizure activity. These effects occur with both conventional ionic agents and the low-osmolar ionic dimer ioxaglate; these ionic agents cannot be used for myelography or ventriculography. Nonionic agents are significantly less toxic to brain cells and are used for myelography. The new nonionic agents should be inherently safer for intravascular as well as intrathecal use. Some studies postulate that central nervous system toxicity, particularly in the limbic system, may be a mechanism for severe adverse reactions in many patients. If this theory is correct, nonionic contrast agents may be safer because of their low neurotoxicity.

Thrombophlebitis

Contrast media may induce thrombophlebitis following phlebography or intravenous injections for urography or computed tomography (CT). The incidence after phlebography with conventional ratio 1.5 hyperosmolar contrast agents may be as high as 30% and is most likely due to venous endothelial damage from both hyperosmolality and direct chemotoxicity. Dilution of conventional hyperosmolar contrast agents reduces the osmolality and incidence of thrombophlebitis. Clinical studies show that ioxaglate and metrizamide reduce contrast-induced thrombophlebitis to less than 5%; the other low-osmolality agents are expected to have a similar effect (Thomas et al. 1983).

Bronchospasm

Subclinical bronchospasm, as measured by pulmonary function testing, is usually seen in patients receiving intravenous doses of conventional hyperosmolar contrast media. However, patients receiving hyperosmolar injections of saline and dextrose do not manifest bronchospasm. The adverse effect of contrast media on pulmonary air flow is not due to hyperosmolality alone, but apparently to a direct chemotoxic effect on the tracheobronchial tree (Littner et al. 1977). Iopamidol, iohexol, and ioxaglate all show less adverse change in pulmonary air flow than conventional agents (Dawson 1984).

Anaphylactoid Reactions

The effects of contrast media on enzyme inhibition, complement activation, histamine release, coagulation, and protein binding are an indication of contrast chemotoxicity and generally relate to safety.

Protein-binding affinity measured by an equilibrium dialysis technique appears to correlate well with contrast media toxicity. Protein binding of iohexol and iopamidol is significantly lower than with iothalamate; ioxaglate has an intermediate amount of protein binding. The amount of protein binding correlates well with lethal dose (LD_{50}) studies in animals (Dawson 1985).

Conventional ionic agents inhibit platelet responses, increase thrombin time, and have adverse effects on coagulation, whereas nonionic agents do this to a lesser extent, with ioxaglate being intermediate in its effect (Rao et al. 1985; Stormorken et al. 1986). These effects on coagulation also have implications concerning clot formation on catheters during arteriography.

Since complement activation has been postulated as a mechanism for at least some types of serious adverse contrast reactions, the degree of complement activation may indicate a safety factor (Lasser et al. 1979). Complement activation by measurement of C_{3a}, anaphylatoxin release, has been shown to occur with both ionic and nonionic agents, but quantitative evaluation is not yet available (Dawson et al. 1983). Histamine release has also been implicated as a mediator of both minor and major adverse contrast reactions. All low-osmolality agents release less histamine from basophils than conventional contrast media.

Enzyme inhibition by radiographic contrast media, particularly inhibition of acetylcholinesterase, is postulated as a mediator of some adverse reactions. Cholinergic effects may produce symptoms such as vasodilation and flushing, anxiety, sweating, bronchospasm, nausea and vomiting, and skin reactions including urticaria. These symptoms are common with conventional contrast agents that inhibit acetylcholinesterase.

The nonionic agents iopamidol and iohexol have less inhibiting effects on the enzyme acetylcholinesterase; ioxaglate has more enzyme inhibition than nonionic contrast media. This difference, as well as an increased release of histamine by ioxaglate, may account for its higher incidence of nausea, vomiting, and urticarial reactions (Dawson, Edgerton 1983; Manhire et al. 1984; Spataro et al. 1987).

Contrast-Induced Renal Failure

The incidence of contrast-induced renal failure is extremely low in healthy outpatients and very low in hospitalized patients without underlying renal disease (Harkonen, Kjellstrand 1981). However, the incidence of contrast nephropathy becomes significant in patients with preexisting renal insufficiency or diabetes mellitus and renal insufficiency. Those patients have a 50% or higher incidence of renal deterioration after contrast media administration. Although this is reversible in most cases, it may not be in diabetic patients with underlying renal disease. Dehydration, multiple myeloma, other nephrotoxic drugs, and vascular disease also increase the risk of contrast nephropathy. Preliminary experimental evidence suggests that newer contrast media may be less nephrotoxic than conventional agents, but clinical studies have failed to support this in patients with impaired renal function.

Renal damage is indicated by proteinuria (albuminuria). Transient proteinuria may be seen after arteriography and urography in humans and animals. The amount of proteinuria with conventional contrast media and with metrizamide is significant. In animals, iohexol, iopamidol, and ioxaglate produce significantly less proteinuria than conventional agents or metrizamide, suggesting this to be an agent-specific effect (Speck et al. 1983).

Comparative experiments in rabbits have shown that to produce renal insufficiency a higher dose of iohexol is necessary, compared to diatrizoate. At high doses, a larger percentage of animals will develop renal insufficiency with a conventional agent than with iohexol (Golman, Almen 1985). In high-dose urography in patients with renal failure, renal function tends to deteriorate with both iohexol and metrizoate; no difference in clinical nephrotoxicity was noted with the nonionic contrast agent (Smith et al. 1985).

Table 1–3 Incidence of Adverse Reactions with Ionic Contrast Media

Reactions	Rate (%)
All adverse reactions to contrast media Includes minor reactions that require no treatment, such as nausea, vomiting, limited urticaria, mild rash, lightheadedness, and mild dyspnea	1/20 (5)
Intermediate reactions Includes extensive urticaria, facial edema, bronchospasm, laryngeal edema, dyspnea, rigors, mild chest pain, and hypotension; these often require treatment but not hospitalization and are not considered life-threatening	1/100 (1)
Severe reactions Includes laryngeal edema, pulmonary edema, refractory hypotension, circulatory collapse, severe angina, myocardial infarction, cardiac arrhythmias, convulsions, coma, and respiratory and cardiac arrest; these reactions require hospitalization and are considered life-threatening	1/2,000 (0.05)
Cardiac arrest	1/6,000 (0.017)
Death	1/40,000 (0.0025)

Source: Adapted, by permission, from Spataro RF: Newer contrast agents for urography *Radiol. Clin. North Am.* 22:365–379, 1984.

Frequency and Severity of Adverse Effects

The incidence of all adverse reactions to conventional contrast media is approximately 5%, but the great majority of reactions are minor (Table 1–3; Ansell et al. 1980; Hobbs 1981; Shehadi, Toniolo 1980). Reactions that may require treatment but not hospitalization occur in approximately 1% of patients receiving intravascular contrast. Severe, potentially life-threatening reactions occur in approximately 1 of 2,000 patients (0.05%). Cardiac arrest occurs in 1 of 6,000 cases, and 1 of 40,000 patients may die.

Limited data are available to assess adverse reactions and fatalities associated with the new low-osmolar nonionic agents. In a study of over 50,660 patients injected with iohexol, the overall rate of adverse reaction was 2.1%; approximately 1.2% of these were considered mild and 0.9% moderate. Six of the 50,660 patients were classified as having severe reactions, a rate of approximately 1 per 8,500 examinations, or 0.012%, which is 4 times better than the results with conventional ionic contrast (Dahlstrom et al. 1985; McClennan 1986; Schrott et al. 1986). A death rate of 7 patients in 2 million examinations with nonionic contrast has been reported in Europe (Grainger 1984).

Twenty-eight deaths have been reported with ioxaglate in approximately 3 million patients, a death rate of 1 per 100,000 examinations. These early studies show that the overall rate of adverse reactions to low-osmolality contrast media injections has been reduced. And, more importantly, the incidence of moderate, severe, and fatal reactions has been significantly reduced, particularly with nonionic agents.

Acute intravenous median lethal dose (LD_{50}) studies in mice show that the new low-osmolality contrast media are significantly less toxic than currently used contrast agents (Table 1–4). Conventional contrast agents show an LD_{50} of approximately 7–10 g I/kg; ioxaglate has an LD_{50} of 12–15 g I/kg (a 1.5–2 times better safety factor); and iopamidol and iohexol have an LD_{50} of approximately 20–25 g I/kg (a 3–4 times better safety factor). The new nonionic agents ioversol (MP328) and iopromide have LD_{50} values similar to the other nonionic agents.

Table 1–4 Acute Intravenous Toxicity (LD_{50}) of Contrast Media in Mice

Iothalamate	(Conray)	$LD_{50} \cong$ 9–10 g I/kg[a]
Diatrizoate	(Hypaque) (Renografin)	$LD_{50} \cong$ 7–10 g I/kg[bc]
Metrizoate		(same as above)
Metrizamide	(Amipaque)	$LD_{50} \cong$ 17.5–18.7 g I/kg[a]
Iohexol	(Omnipaque)	$LD_{50} \cong$ 23–25 g I/kg[d]
Iopromide		$LD_{50} \cong$ 16.5 g I/kg[e]
Iopamidol	(Isovue)	$LD_{50} \cong$ 20–23.6 g I/kg[c]
Ioversol	(MP-328)	$LD_{50} \cong$ 20 g I/kg[b]
Ioxaglate	(Hexabrix)	$LD_{50} >$ 12.8 g I/kg[b]; $LD_{50} \cong$ 15 g I/kg[f]

[a] Salverson S: Acute toxicity of metrizamide. Acta Radiol. 335(Suppl.): 5–13, 1973.
[b] Mallinckrodt, Inc., St. Louis, MO 63134.
[c] E. R. Squibb and Sons, Inc., Princeton, NJ.
[d] Salveson S: Acute intravenous toxicity of iohexol in the mouse and in the rat. Acta Radiol. 362(Suppl.): 73–75, 1980.
[e] Schering AG, Federal Republic of Germany.
[f] Sovak M, et al: Combined methods for assessment of neurotoxicity. Testing of new nonionic radiographic media. Invest. Radiol. 15:S248–S253, 1980.

Source: Adapted, by permission, from Spataro RF: Newer contrast agents for urography. Radiol. Clin. North Am. 22:365–379, 1984.
Note: The relative acute intravenous toxicity of contrast media in mice is illustrated. The LD_{50} of conventional ionic ratio 1.5 contrast media such as iothalamate, diatrizoate, and metrizoate is in the range of 7–10 g of iodine per kg. The LD_{50} of the monoacidic dimer ioxaglate, a ratio 3 contrast agent, lies between 12.8 and 15 g of iodine per kg. The LD_{50} of nonionic contrast media such as iopromide, metrizamide, iohexol, iopamidol, and ioversol lies between 16.5 and 25 g of iodine per kg. Since differences in LD_{50} doses show significant variation in different laboratories, with different strains of mice and different injection rates, small variations in LD_{50} doses may not be significant. However, it is clear that the LD_{50} doses of ratio 3 nonionic contrast media are at least twice that of conventional ratio 1.5 ionic contrast media; that of the monoacidic dimer ioxaglate is intermediate.

Since all the new low-osmolality contrast agents, particularly the nonionic agents, have significantly lower acute intravenous toxicity in animals, they will, in this author's opinion, also show a similar safety factor in humans.

Diagnostic Quality

Excretory Urography

Especially in high-dose urography, conventional contrast agents provide the parenchymal nephrogram density and urinary opacification to make an accurate diagnosis. Many authors have reported that a dose of 300 mg I/kg body weight (1 ml contrast medium/kg; 0.5 ml contrast medium/lb) may be an ideal dose for excretory urography. This is based on the fact that urinary iodine concentration rises only slightly after a dose of 300 mg I/kg is injected. However, urinary iodine concentration is not the only factor involved. Experimental evidence has shown that although urinary iodine concentration with conventional contrast media peaks between 300–600 mg I/kg with only small differences between doses, the total urinary iodine excretion rate (iodine concentration times urine volume) increases significantly with increasing doses. The maximum iodine excretion rate may peak at as high as 600 mg I/kg or higher (Dure-Smith et al. 1971).

Based on experimental work and clinical experience, the author believes that the optimum dose for urography with conventional ratio 1.5 agents is 450 mg I/kg (1.5 ml contrast medium/kg; 0.7 ml contrast medium/lb) in adults. This is the usual dose in clinical practice at the University of Rochester Medical Center, which equates to approximately 100 ml of conventional contrast media in the average patient. This dose provides consistently good diagnostic quality with no significant change in side effects from lower doses.

Low-osmolality ratio 3 agents provide better diagnostic quality and better patient safety and tolerance for excretory urography (Robey et al. 1984; Spataro 1984; Spataro et al. 1987; Winfield et al. 1983). In experimental work, ioxoglate, iopamidol, and iohexol have been shown to give twice the iodine concentration in the urine as do conventional agents at the same injected dose (Evill, Benness 1978; Sjoberg et al. 1980; Spataro et al. 1982; Wilcox et al. 1983). Ioxaglate gave higher blood and urinary iodine concentrations than nonionic low-osmolality agents. The higher urinary iodine concentrations with ioxaglate may be due to reabsorption of sodium ions and water, which increases tubular concentrations, a mechanism not available with nonionic agents.

All patient trials using low-osmolality contrast media have shown better patient tolerance and fewer adverse side effects than those with conventional ratio 1.5 agents (Dawson et al. 1984; Levorstad et al. 1983; McClennan et al. 1986; Robey et al. 1984; Spataro et al. 1987; Spataro et al. in preparation; Thompson et al. 1984; Winfield et al. 1983; Wolf et al. 1983). Nonionic agents have a lower incidence of flushing, heat, nausea and vomiting, tachycardia, hypotension, lightheadedness, pain in the injection arm, and skin reactions (urticaria). Ioxaglate has fewer adverse side effects, but a similar incidence of nausea, vomiting, and urticaria as conventional contrast media and a higher incidence of adverse reactions than nonionic agents.

In clinical trials of 50 ml total doses, low-osmolality contrast media give equivalent or better quality excretory urograms than similar or sometimes even higher doses of conventional agents. In every clinical trial, denser opacification of the collecting system and bladder has been reported with all low-osmolality contrast agents. Less distention and filling of the renal pelvis, ureters, and bladder have also occurred. Overall, the quality of the urograms has been about equal.

In clinical trials of 100 ml total doses, or when using compression, low-osmolality contrast agents of all types give higher urinary iodine concentrations; denser opacification of the calices, renal pelves, ureters, and bladder; and diagnostically superior excretory urograms (Spataro et al. 1987; Spataro et al., in preparation). A less significant improvement in nephrogram density has also been observed. Thus low-osmolality contrast agents, particularly nonionic agents, appear to have significant advantages in excretory urography.

Computed Tomography

Because of the excellent contrast resolution of computed tomography, high iodine concentrations are not so essential as in arteriography, venography, and urography. Renal cortical enhancement is not significantly different using a hyperosmolar or low-osmolar contrast agent, but renal medullary and renal parenchymal (medullary plus cortical enhancement) is greater with low-osmolar contrast media (Spataro et al. 1984; Wilson, Evill 1981).

Iodine concentrations in the excreted urine and the renal pelvis, ureter, and bladder are significantly higher with low-osmolar agents. This is an advantage in intravenous excretory urography, but has few advantages for contrast-enhanced CT. Low-osmolar contrast agents may have a slight advantage in dynamic CT scanning and in patients with impaired renal function when higher concentrations of iodine may be helpful. The higher concentration of contrast in the collecting structures is sometimes a disadvantage because more artifacts may be seen.

Renal Angiography

Angiography with equal concentrations of conventional ratio 1.5 agents and new low-osmolality ratio 3 agents produces similar results. However, angiography with low-osmolality agents causes less dramatic changes in renal hemodynamics (Morris et al. 1978). Because iohexol, iopamidol, and ioxaglate cause less proteinuria, reduced alteration in renal blood flow, and decreased urinary enzyme excretion, less renal toxicity is anticipated. Because the nonionic agents inhibit coagulation minimally, their use in arteriography must be modulated by meticulous catheter technique and, in some cases, heparinization of the solution or the patient.

Clinical Implications

In two separate studies, patients who had adverse contrast media reactions with conventional ionic agents were given nonionic agents. The patients had virtually no adverse reactions (Holtas 1984; Rapaport et al. 1983). In Rapaport's group, 3 of 6 patients had experienced serious life-threatening reactions with conventional contrast; other reactions were intermediate and minor. Of 5 patients who had been given steroid premedication, 1 patient with a cerebral arteriovenous malformation had a grand mal seizure. In Holtas's study, 2 of 17 patients had had serious prior reactions with conventional ionic agents, and the rest had minor or intermediate reactions; by using nonionic contrast media, even without steroid premedication, no significant adverse reactions occurred. There is, thus, early clinical evidence that nonionic agents may offer a significant safety advantage, specifically in patients with prior adverse reactions.

Since nonionic contrast media cost 10 to 20 times as much as conventional agents, there is a problem of how to introduce these expensive new drugs into daily radiologic practice (Fischer et al. 1986; Grainger 1984; McClennan 1987; White, Halden 1986; Wolf 1986). Current practice in the United States is to mainly use low-osmolality agents for patients at high risk for adverse reactions, including patients less than 1 year old or very old, debilitated patients, and those with previous significant adverse reactions, allergies, asthma, severe cardiovascular disease, or renal failure, especially diabetic nephropathy. Low-osmolality contrast media should also be used in painful peripheral and other arteriography. Further clinical trials are needed to confirm that low-osmolality contrast agents can significantly lower morbidity and mortality.

References

Almen T: Contrast agent design: Some aspects of the synthesis of water soluble contrast agents of low osmolality. *J. Theor. Biol.* 24:216–226, 1969.

Almen T: New media. Experience from 10 years of development of water soluble nonionic contrast media. *Invest. Radiol.* 15(Suppl.):S283–288, 1980.

Ansell G, Tweedie MCK, West CR, et al.: The current status of reactions to intravenous contrast media. *Invest. Radiol.* 15(Suppl.):S32–39, 1980.

Berg GR, Hutter AM, Pfister RC: Electrocardiographic abnormalities associated with intravenous urography. *N. Engl. J. Med.* 289:87–88, 1973.

Bryan RN, Centeno RS, Hershkowitz N, et al.: Neurotoxicity of iohexol: A new nonionic contrast medium. *Radiology* 145:379–382, 1982.

Dahlstrom K, Shaw DD, Claus W, et al.: Summary of U.S. and European intravascular experience with iohexol based on the clinical trial program. *Invest. Radiol.* 20(Suppl.):S117–S121, 1985.

Dawson P: New contrast agents. Chemistry and pharmacology. *Invest. Radiol.* 19(Suppl.):S293–S300, 1984.

Dawson P: Chemotoxicity of contrast media and clinical adverse effects: A review. *Invest. Radiol.* 20(Suppl.): S84–S91, 1985.

Dawson P, Edgerton D: Contrast media and enzyme inhibition. I cholinesterase. *Br. J. Radiol.* 56:653–656, 1983.

Dawson P, Heron C, Marshal J: Intravenous urography with low-osmolality contrast agents: Theoretical consideration and clinical findings. *Clin. Radiol.* 35:173–175, 1984.

Dawson P, Turner MW, Bradshaw A, et al.: Complement activation and generation of C_{3a} anaphylatoxin by radiological contrast agents. *Br. J. Radiol.* 56:447–448, 1983.

Drayer BP, Velaj R, Bird R, et al.: Comparative safety of intracarotid iopamidol, iothalamate meglumine, and diatrizoate meglumine for cerebral angiography. *Invest. Radiol.* 19(Suppl.):S212–S218, 1984.

Dure-Smith P, Simenhoff M, Zimskind PD, et al.: The bolus effect in excretory urography. *Radiology* 101:29–34, 1971.

Evill CA, Benness GT: Urographic excretion studies: Preliminary results with six-iodine, singly ionizing sodium salt P-286. *Invest. Radiol.* 13:325–327, 1978.

Fischer HW, Katzberg RW, Morris TW, et al.: Systemic response to excretory urography. *Radiology* 151:31–33, 1984.

Fischer HW, Spataro RF, Rosenberg PM: Medical and economic considerations in using a new contrast medium. *Arch. Intern. Med.* 146:1717–1721, 1986.

Golman K, Almen T: Contrast media-induced nephrotoxicity. Survey and present state. *Invest. Radiol.* 2(Suppl.):S92–S97, 1985.

Grainger RG: The clinical and financial implications of the low-osmolar radiological contrast media. *Clin. Radiol.* 35:251–252, 1984.

Grainger RG: The clinical and financial implications of the low-osmolar radiological contrast media. Further correspondence. *Clin. Radiol.* 35:422, 1984.

Hammeke TA, Grogan JP, Haughton VM, et al.: Evaluation of myelographic contrast-medium tolerance with psychometric testing. *AJNR* 6:343–348, 1985.

Harkonen S, Kjellstrand C: Contrast nephropathy. *Am. J. Nephrol.* 1:69–77, 1981.

Heron CW, Underwood SR, Dawson P: Electrocardiographic changes during intravenous urography: A study with sodium iothalamate and iohexol. *Clin. Radiol.* 35:137–141, 1984.

Higgins CB: Contrast media in the cardiovascular system. *In* Sovak M (ed.): *Radiocontrast Agents.* Berlin, New York, Springer-Verlag, 1984, pp. 193–251.

Hobbs BB: Adverse reactions to intravenous contrast agents in Ontario, 1975–1979. *J. Can. Assoc. Radiol.* 31:8–10, 1981.

Holtas S: Iohexol in patients with previous adverse reactions to contrast media. *Invest. Radiol.* 19:563–565, 1984.

Kumar S, Hull JD, Lathi S, et al.: Low incidence of renal failure after angiography. *Arch. Intern. Med.* 141: 1268–1270, 1981.

Lasser EC, Slivka J, Lang JH, et al.: Complement and coagulations: Causative considerations in contrast catastrophies. *Am. J. Roentgenol.* 132:171–176, 1979.

Levorstad K, Kolbenstvedt A, Loyning EW: Iohexol compared with metrizoate in urography. *Acta Radiol.* (Diagn.) 24:337–341, 1983.

Littner MR, Rosenfield AT, Ulreich S, et al.: Evaluation of bronchospasm during excretory orography. *Radiology* 124:17–21, 1977.

Manhire AR, Dawson P, Dennet R: Contrast agent induced emesis. *Clin. Radiol.* 35:369–370, 1984.

McClennan BL: Contrast reactions: The "new" low osmolar contrast media. – The Society of Uroradiology 7th Annual Postgraduate Course Uroradiology '86 Book of Papers. May 1986, pp. 23–25.

McClennan BL: Low-osmolality contrast media: Premises and promises. *Radiology* 162:1–8, 1987.

McClennan BL, Ling D, Rholl KS, et al.: Urography with a low osmolality contrast agent. Comparison of Hexabrix with Conray 325. *Invest. Radiol.* 21:144–150, 1986.

Morris TW, Katzberg RW, Fischer HW: A comparison of the hemodynamic responses to metrizamide and meglumine/sodium diatrizoate in canine renal angiography. *Invest. Radiol.* 13:74–78, 1978.

Rao AK, Rao VM, Willis J, et al.: Inhibition of platelet function by contrast media: Iopamidol and ioxaglate versus iothalamate. *Radiology* 156:311–313, 1985.

Rapaport S, Bookstein JJ, Higgins CB, et al.: Experience with metrizamide in patients with previous severe anaphylactoid reactions to ionic contrast agents. *Radiology* 143:321–325, 1983.

Robey G, Reilly BJ, Carusi PA, et al.: Pediatric urography: Comparison of metrizamide and methylglucamine diatrizoate. *Radiology* 150:61–63, 1984.

Schrott KM, Behrends B, Kaufmann J, et al.: Iohexol in excretory urography. *Fortschritte der Medizin* 104: 153–156, 1986.

Shehadi HW, Toniolo G: Adverse reactions to contrast media. *Radiology* 137:299–302, 1980.

Sjoberg S, Almen T, Golman K: Excretion of urographic contrast media for urography. *Acta Radiol.* 362 (Suppl.):93–98, 1980.

Smith H-J, Levorstad K, Berg K, et al.: High-dose urography in patients with renal failure. *Acta Radiol.* (Diagn.) 26:213–220, 1985.

Spataro RF: Newer contrast agents for urography. *Radiol. Clin. North Am.* 22:365–379, 1984.

Spataro RF, Fischer HW, Boylan L: Urography with low-osmolality contrast media: Comparative urinary excretion of iopamidol, Hexabrix, and diatrizoate. *Invest. Radiol.* 17:494–500, 1982.

Spataro RF, Fischer HW, Katzberg RW, et al.: Comparison of nonionic contrast media and conventional hyperosmolar contrast media in high-dose clinical urography. In preparation.

Spataro RF, Fischer HW, Kormano M: Clinical comparison of Hexabrix, iopamidol, and Urografin 60 in whole body computed tomography. *Invest. Radiol.* 19(Suppl.): S372–S375, 1984.

Spataro RF, Katzberg RW, Fischer HW, et al.: High-dose clinical urography with the low-osmolality contrast agent Hexabrix: Comparison with a conventional contrast agent. *Radiology* 162:9–14, 1987.

Spataro RF, Katzberg RW, Fischer HW, et al.: Urography with the new nonionic contrast medium ioversol. In preparation.

Speck U, Press WR, Mützel W: Albuminuria following renal arteriography with various ionic and nonionic contrast agents in the rat. *In* Taenzer V, Zeitler E (eds.): *Contrast Media.* Stuttgart–New York, Thieme–Stratton, 1983, pp. 25–29.

Stormorken H, Skalpe IO, Testart MC: Effect of various contrast media on coagulation, fibrinolysis, and platelet function. An in vitro and in vivo study. *Invest. Radiol.* 21:348–354, 1986.

Thomas ML, Briggs GM, Kuan BB: Contrast agent-induced thrombophlebitis following leg phlebography: Meglumine ioxaglate versus meglumine iothalamate. *Radiology* 147:399–400, 1983.

Thompson WM, Foster WL, Halvorsen RA, et al.: Iopamidol: New, nonionic contrast agent for excretory urography. *Am. J. Roentgenol.* 142:329–332, 1984.

White RI, Jr., Halden WJ, Jr.: Liquid gold: Low-osmolality contrast media. *Radiology* 159:559–560, 1986.

Wilcox J, Evill CA, Sage MR, et al.: Urographic excretion studies with nonionic contrast agents. Iopamidol vs. iothalamate. *Invest. Radiol.* 18:207–210, 1983.

Wilson BC, Evill CA: Correlation of computed tomography and nephrography in quantitative comparison of urographic contrast agents. *Radiology* 140:127–134, 1981.

Winfield AC, Dray RJ, Kirchner JK, Jr., et al.: Iohexol for excretory urography: A comparative study. *Am. J. Roentgenol.* 141:571–573, 1983.

Wolf GL: The fibrillatory propensities of contrast agents. *Invest. Radiol.* 15(Suppl.):S208–S214, 1980.

Wolf GL: Safer, more expensive iodinated contrast agents: How do we decide? *Radiology* 159:557–558, 1986.

Wolf K-J, Steidle B, Skutta T, et al.: Iopromide. Clinical experience with a new non-ionic contrast medium. *Acta Radiol. (Diagn.)* 24:55–62, 1983.

Suggested Reading

Amiel M. (ed.): *Contrast Media in Radiology.* Berlin, Heidelberg, New York, Springer-Verlag, 1982.

Contrast material symposium. *Invest. Radiol.* 19(4, Suppl.):S99–S156, 1984.

Iopamidol: Intravascular and intrathecal applications. Worldwide symposium. *Invest. Radiol.* 19(5, Suppl.):S157–S288, 1984.

Ioxaglic acid: A new low osmolality contrast medium. Symposium proceedings. *Invest. Radiol.* 19(6, Suppl.): S289–S392, 1984.

Sovak M (ed.): Radiocontrast agents. *Handbook Exp. Pharm.* (Springer-Verlag, New York, Heidelberg) 73, 1985.

A worldwide clinical assessment of a new nonionic contrast medium: Iohexol. *Invest. Radiol.* 20(Suppl.):S1–S122, 1985.

CHAPTER

2

Management of Adverse Effects of Contrast Media

William H. Bush

The indications for radiographic contrast media have increased substantially with the advent of computed tomography (CT) and digital subtraction angiography. Examinations requiring contrast media are often requested by clinical specialists unfamiliar with the types of adverse effects of contrast. In addition, certain groups are at higher risk for severe adverse reactions. By understanding these risks and the effect of contrast media on the kidney, the radiologist can tailor an examination to the clinical setting, or, alternatively, can choose a diagnostic method that avoids use of contrast.

Conventional contrast agents in common use are ionic solutions of triiodinated benzoic acid that have a side chain to which sodium or some other cation is attached. These agents are freely filtered by the glomerulus in the kidney and are neither secreted nor absorbed by the tubule.

Newer nonionic and low-osmolar contrast agents have fewer side effects and lower toxicity (Spataro 1984). Less histamine is released, inhibition of acetylcholinesterase is reduced, and there is less activation of complement. Clinically, bronchospasm is minimized, there are fewer electrocardiographic changes, and the incidence of nausea, vomiting, and vascular pain is reduced. Life-threatening adverse reactions are reduced substantially but not eliminated.

Types of Adverse Effects

The adverse effects of currently used ionic contrast media can be divided into four major categories: 1) the vasomotor effect, 2) the anaphylactoid (allergiclike) reaction, 3) the vagal reaction, and 4) acute renal failure. The patient experiencing an anaphylactoid reaction presents with different clinical signs and requires entirely different treatment than the person with a vagal reaction. Contrast-induced renal failure can usually be avoided if the clinician, urologist, or radiologist learns to identify patients at high risk and chooses alternate examination methods.

Vasomotor Effect

The vasomotor effect, due to changes induced by the hyperosmolarity of the contrast, is a common event following injection of ionic contrast agents. Symptoms of warmth, a "metallic" taste, a vague "tingling" sensation, and slight nausea are so frequent with conventional ionic agents that they are an accepted part of high-dose urography or bolus-type injection for computed tomography, and are experienced by up to 50% of patients.

These effects can be mitigated by a slower injection rate. Since the so-called hypertensive urogram is a poor screening test for renovascular hypertension, a large rapid bolus injection of contrast is not necessary in urography. Even a good "dynamic" CT scan can be obtained with a moderate injection rate (e.g., 20–30 ml/min). In addition, vascular discomfort is reduced if the contrast media is warmed before it is injected. All of these vasomotor effects are nearly eliminated with the newer low-osmolar agents (Spataro 1984).

Vasomotor symptoms are almost always self-limited and require no treatment except reassuring the patient that the unpleasantness will subside.

Anaphylactoid Reaction

Minor anaphylactoid reactions such as mild flushing, erythema, and scattered urticaria are relatively common with conventional ionic contrast agents. Previously termed a hypersensitivity or allergic reaction, this reaction does not fulfill the criteria of a true anaphylaxis. There are only isolated reports of true antibody reactivity to contrast, and most investigators have not been able to confirm a true allergic reaction; hence, the term *anaphylactoid*. Five percent to 6% of patients experience a reaction to contrast media, the majority being of a minor nature (Shehadi 1982). Moderate anaphylactoid reactions occur in less than 2% of examinations, and severe life-threatening reactions occur at a rate of 1 to 2 per 1,000 examinations. Mortality rates range from 1:10,000 to 1:75,000 examinations (Hartman et al. 1982).

There is no agreement on the etiology of the anaphylactoid reaction. Several inciting factors may exist, any of which can potentially trigger a reaction. The final determinant is the individual patient's reactivity. Stress and fear seem to heighten the chance of contrast reactions (Lalli 1974). Histamine is suggested as an important component of the reaction pathway, since the clinical signs and symptoms of an anaphylactoid reaction can be reproduced by an intravenous injection of histamine. Complement activation, coagulation system activation, prekallikrein transformation, and generation of bradykinin initiated by contrast contact with the vascular endothelium may be factors (Lasser 1987). The central nervous system may be the common initiator or a mediator of these adverse reactions (Lalli 1980). Susceptible individuals may be more sensitive to levels that are innocuous to most patients.

Patients with a history of atopy are at higher risk for an anaphylactoid reaction (Ansell et al. 1980). Whereas the rate of moderate reactions in an unselected group of patients is less than 2%, the rate is 3%–4% in patients with a history of atopy (Witten et al. 1973). Similarly, patients who give a history of "shellfish allergy" also have a somewhat higher rate of contrast reactions. Whether the causative factor is the carrier protein, the iodine, the charged ionic solution, the high osmolarity, or a combination of these, is uncertain. There is no correlation between the anaphylactoid reaction and an "allergy" to topical iodine (e.g., Betadine) manifested as contact dermatitis.

Nonfatal anaphylactoid reactions to ionic contrast agents are more common in the 20- to 29-year-old age group, and overall, reactions are less frequent in children and the elderly. However, fatal reactions are more common in patients over age 50, with cardiovascular collapse often a major component of this reaction in the older age group. An equal distribution of reactions is seen between the sexes. The reaction rate is higher with intravenous compared to intraarterial administration, although a higher percentage of reactions by the intraarterial group are of a serious, life-threatening nature.

Patients who have had one anaphylactoid reaction are at high risk for a second reaction (Siegle, Lieberman 1978). In the Mayo Clinic series, this repeat reaction happened to nearly one-third of patients with previous reactions; however, this retrospective study may have included vagal-type reactions (Witten et al. 1973). The data from Shehadi and McClennan show a 19% rate of recurrent, severe reactions (McClennan 1987). Unlike a true anaphylaxis, the repeat reaction rate is neither consistent nor predictable. The severity of the second reaction is usually not worse than earlier reactions.

A mild anaphylactoid reaction of slight nasal stuffiness, mild transitory itching, or scattered urticaria without respiratory symptoms usually requires no treatment. Reassurance is important. An antihistamine may be given (e.g., diphenhydramine, 25–50 mg orally). However, antihistamines do not have a major role in the treatment of major reactions and may exacerbate hypotension.

An accelerating anaphylactoid reaction of laryngospasm, bronchospasm, angioedema, hypotension, and tachycardia requires prompt treatment, including maintaining airway patency, giving supplementary oxygen, and establishing a route for the administration of intravenous fluids and adrenergic drugs. Therefore, the initial intravenous route for contrast administration should be maintained throughout the examination, until the potential for nearly all reactions has passed. In the series reported by Shehadi, all fatal reactions began within 15 min of injection (Shehadi 1985). Simple measures must not be forgotten, such as releasing any compression placed on the abdomen for urography, and elevating the patient's legs to improve central vascular volume.

Some patients will have a reaction dominated

by a profound hypotension, associated with moderate respiratory symptoms and tachycardia; this latter sign differentiates this reaction from the vagal reaction of hypotension and bradycardia. The marked hypotension is treated most effectively with the rapid infusion of large volumes of intravenous fluids such as isotonic saline or lactated Ringer's solution. With a hand pump, up to 200 ml/min may be administered through a 19-gauge needle, and rapid infusion of up to 3 L may be necessary (Van Sonnenberg et al. 1987).

Anaphylactoid reactions manifesting both respiratory and cardiovascular signs and symptoms should be treated with intravenous fluids and with adrenergic drugs, primarily because they act on the heart, the peripheral vascular system, and the major airways. Epinephrine is the preferred adrenergic drug for treating anaphylactoid reactions (Barach et al. 1984). These drugs generally have both alpha- and beta-stimulating properties. Alpha-adrenergic (alpha-agonist) effects primarily cause vasoconstriction. Beta-adrenergic drugs increase strength (ionotropic) and rate (chronotropic) of contraction of the heart, but also increase frequency of ventricular arrhythmias. The beta-adrenergic (beta-agonist) effects peripherally cause smooth muscle relaxation, arteriolar vasodilation, and, of importance, bronchiolar relaxation (Smith, Corbascio 1970). In the cellular energy cycle, the beta-adrenergic effect raises the level of adenosine monophosphate (AMP), which allows less release of reactive mediators like histamine and the more potent leukotrienes. Administered early during the reaction and given at low doses, epinephrine is very effective in reversing a potentially life-threatening reaction.

For a moderate anaphylactoid reaction, when peripheral circulation still remains adequate and profound hypotension has not developed, 0.1 ml (0.1 mg) of 1:1,000 epinephrine is given subcutaneously. If a marked allergiclike reaction is developing and a more rapid effect is essential, intravenous epinephrine should be used; this will also eliminate the problem of poor peripheral absorption. A low dose of epinephrine given at a slow infusion rate (10 μg/min) is recommended, as beta receptor sites respond at lower doses, and slower infusion rates affect beta receptors preferentially. Thus, bronchodilation and a moderate increase in systolic pressure occurs, and severe hypertensive effects are minimized.

A recommended initial intravenous dose in adults is 10 μg/min. One-tenth milliliter (0.1 mg) of 1:1,000 epinephrine provides 100 μg; this is diluted to 10 ml with normal saline and injected slowly over 10 min. A prepared solution of 1:10,000 is also available, providing 100 μg/ml. Infusion can be continued by adding 1 ml (1 mg) of 1:1,000 epinephrine to 250 ml of 5% dextrose water; this provides 4 μg/ml, and the infusion is given at 1–4 μg/min. In children, an infusion rate of 0.1 μg/kg/min is recommended (Barach et al. 1984).

Epinephrine must be used cautiously in elderly patients or if hypoxia is present, as the combination can cause severe cardiac arrhythmias. In addition, patients who are receiving beta-blocking drugs such as propranolol (Inderal) may not respond effectively to epinephrine, since beta-agonist effects are blocked and the amount of cyclic AMP does not increase. In fact, cyclic AMP may decrease, owing to unopposed alpha-agonist effects, and, as a result, mediator release may increase. Epinephrine, because of its alpha and beta effects, should be avoided if possible in such patients. Other patients who have been on long-term adrenergic medications (such as for asthma) may be "desensitized" to beta-agonist effects and may require higher doses of epinephrine.

The H_1 antagonist, diphenhydramine (Benadryl), is used commonly in addition to epinephrine to treat anaphylactoid reactions. The dose is 25–50 mg intravenously. The exact mechanism of effect is unclear; diphenhydramine likely inactivates unbound circulating histamine, but it seems to have little effect on the clinical manifestations of a reaction already in progress. Presumably, this is because diphenhydramine does not inactivate or block the effects of leukotrienes, and the bronchoconstrictor effect of the leukotrienes is many times greater than that caused by histamine. Diphenhydramine should not be used in place of epinephrine. Cimetidine (Tagamet), an H_2 antagonist, has been suggested to complete the antihistamine effect. The usual dose is 300 mg. Since unopposed H_1 effect on the coronary arteries is vasoconstriction, an H_1 blocker (e.g., Benadryl) should be combined with the H_2 blocker (cimetidine) for patients with coronary artery disease. Further complicating the concept of using cimetidine is that histamine itself seems to act through the H_2 receptor to block further histamine release; therefore, blocking the H_2 receptor with cimetidine may well be counterproductive in mitigating histamine release.

Corticosteroids are helpful in severe anaphylaxis-like reactions, even though the mechanism of action remains undefined (Lasser et al. 1977). The primary effect likely relates to the stabilizing effect of corticosteroids on the cell membrane, thereby preventing generation of arachidonic acid and potent leukotrienes, prostaglandins, and platelet-activating factor (Zipser, Laffi 1985). High doses of corticosteroids (such as 200–1,000 mg hydrocortisone) are given intravenously. Corticosteroids can also be continued as an intravenous drip solution (300–500 mg hydrocortisone in a 250-ml solution administered at 60 ml/hr).

Sometimes bronchospasm is the only manifestation of the reaction to contrast media, or epinephrine alone is insufficient to relieve the bronchospasm of a severe anaphylactoid reaction. Inhaled bronchial dilators such as albuterol (Proventil), metaproterenol (Alupent), and terbutaline (Brethaire) are recommended, as they are potent selective beta-2 adrenergic stimulators. When inhaled, large amounts of medication can be administered to airway tissue before systemic effects occur. The Alupent inhaler, for example, is easily administered as two inhalations. Since the duration of effect is up to 5 hr, a dose should not be repeated for 4–6 hr. In a difficult situation when adequate distribution with the inhaler fails, one ampule (1 ml; 1 mg) of terbutaline, for example, can be diluted with 1 ml saline and administered by a vaporizer for rapid effect. Prior to the availability of inhaled beta-2 adrenergic drugs, the treatment for bronchospasm unrelieved by epinephrine was intravenous aminophylline. Small doses must be administered slowly to minimize a hypotensive effect. The suggested dose is 250 mg; a 10-ml solution of 25 mg/ml is given slowly at the rate of 1 ml/min, monitoring respiration and blood pressure. However, either metaproterenol or terbutaline is preferable, and the inhaled or vaporized route is recommended.

Vagal Reaction

The patient with a vagal reaction gradually becomes confused, apprehensive, and diaphoretic. The patient has a combination of hypotension and prominent sinus bradycardia. Untreated, the reaction can progress over 5–15 min to unresponsiveness and cardiac arrest.

Etiology of the vagal reaction is unknown. Not only is it observed after injections of contrast, but it also is seen with other procedures using needles and with common duct manipulation, proctoscopy, and barium enema examination. A mild form is frequently observed by anesthesiologists in the induction room, suggesting that this reaction is accentuated or even elicited by anxiety.

Manifestations of increased vagal tone on the heart include depressed sinoatrial and atrioventricular node activity, and inhibition of the atrioventricular conduction system; peripherally, there is vasodilation (Stanley, Pfister 1976).

The combination of prominent sinus bradycardia (<50) and hypotension (systolic pressure <80) identify the vagal reaction. Recognition of the bradycardia associated with a hypotensive adverse reaction is essential because treatment is specific and different from that for the anaphylactoid reaction. Treatment involves increasing intravascular fluid volume and reversing the bradycardia. Elevation of the patient's legs and the rapid administration of intravenous fluids accomplish the former; intravenous atropine corrects the bradycardia (Fischer, Colgan 1976; Stanley, Pfister 1976). The atropine should be given in large doses (0.8–1.0 mg), because small doses may accentuate cardiac arrhythmias (Fischer, Colgan 1976). Therefore, it is recommended that 1 mg be given intravenously initially, followed in 3–5 min by another 0.8–1 mg if bradycardia persists. The pulse rate determines further therapy; if bradycardia persists, an additional dose of atropine is given to a total of 3 mg in adults. Despite resolution of the bradycardia, hypotension may persist, requiring further intravenous fluids.

Atropine blocks the vagal cardiac slowing but does not correct peripheral vasodilation. Ephedrine, on the other hand, has both beta- and alpha-adrenergic effects. It directly stimulates the heart, producing tachycardia, increased stroke volume, and increased cardiac output, and it also causes peripheral vasoconstriction (Smith 1979). A dose of 10 mg intravenously is suggested. Unfortunately, ephedrine does not consistently give a satisfactory pressor response, and tachyphylaxis occurs with repeated doses. An excess can cause hypertension and tachycardia (Smith 1979).

Intravenous fluids and atropine are the best treatment for a vagal reaction. The fluids fill the dilated vascular space and atropine corrects the bradycardia.

Combined Reactions

As previously stated, treatment of the anaphylactoid and vagal reactions is drug-specific. Some crossover effect, however, seems to occur between antihistamines and atropine. Diphenhydramine (Benadryl) has a mild atropinelike effect at usual doses; atropine has a mild antihistaminic effect, but only at higher doses. The effect of antihistamines is not adequate to treat the vagus reaction specifically; it may, however, explain some therapeutic responses in treating unspecified contrast reactions. In the rare circumstance that anaphylactoid and vagal reactions occur simultaneously, ephedrine (10 mg intravenously) and aggressive intravenous fluid therapy are recommended; inhaled beta-adrenergic drugs can be added to the regimen. Intravenous fluids are the cornerstone of the treatment of reactions to contrast media.

If a severe vagal or anaphylactoid reaction has progressed to cardiovascular collapse and ventricular fibrillation or cardiac arrest, standard cardiopulmonary resuscitative measures must be employed. An airway must be established, ventilation initiated, cardiac massage quickly started, and intravenous fluid access established. Cardiac monitoring is then obtained, as defibrillation may be necessary. Although a severe reaction is uncommon, adequate resuscitative skills and equipment must be available and should make death a rare event.

Renal Failure

The mechanism of contrast-induced acute renal failure has not been established, although possibilities include tubular toxicities, acute tubular necrosis, tubular obstruction by Tamm-Horsfall protein, renal ischemia due to vasoconstriction and increased blood viscosity, and immunologic injury. Contrast-induced renal failure is encountered in the clinical settings of small vessel renal disease, diabetic nephropathy, myeloma, extracellular volume depletion, low cardiac output, advanced age (likely involving many of the preceding factors), hyperuricemia, sickle cell anemia, preeclampsia, hypertension, and concomitant administration of nephrotoxic drugs (Byrd, Sherman 1979). A large dose of contrast compounds the risks.

The patient with normal renal function is at minimal risk for contrast-induced renal failure. Less than 1% of patients with a normal serum creatinine will show dysfunction after receiving contrast (Van Zee et al. 1978). Ionic contrast media has a uricosuric effect, but this poses no problem if renal function is normal. However, contrast media can exacerbate nephrotoxicity and renal failure in the patient receiving aminoglycoside drugs such as gentamicin, kanamycin, streptomycin, and tobramycin.

Renal function deteriorates fairly rapidly in contrast-induced renal failure. Oliguria, defined as urine volume less than 400 ml/day, is frequent but not invariable. A mild decrease in urine output may not be immediately evident clinically; therefore, renal status should be monitored by serum creatinine determination.

Diabetic patients with normal renal function (serum creatinine $\leq$1.5 mg/dl) are not at increased risk for contrast-induced renal failure (Berkseth, Kjellstrand 1984; Van Zee et al. 1978). The risk of developing renal insufficiency with contrast media correlates directly with the degree of preexisting renal impairment. Harkonen and Kjellstrand (1977) found an increase in serum creatinine (defined as a rise of 1 mg/dl over baseline) in only 4% of diabetics who had an initial creatinine of less than 2 mg/dl. However, serum creatinine increased after contrast administration in 75% of patients who had a prestudy creatinine of greater than 2 mg/dl; for 45% of these patients, the rise was not completely reversible.

Major risk factors in diabetic patients receiving ionic contrast agents by intravenous or intraarterial routes are: 1) diabetic nephropathy (small vessel renal disease), especially associated with type I or juvenile diabetes; 2) serum creatinine greater than 1.5 mg/dl; 3) anemia with hemoglobin less than 8 g/dl; 4) hypertension; and 5) extracellular volume depletion (Berkseth, Kjellstrand 1984; Weinrauch et al. 1977).

Minimizing Adverse Effects of Contrast

Patients at higher risk for an anaphylactoid reaction are those who have previously experienced such a reaction, as well as those with a strong history of allergy, asthma, or atopy (eczema). Anxious patients should probably also be added to the higher risk group. Patients with renal insufficiency, especially with serum creatinine over 2 mg/dl, are at risk for contrast-induced renal failure. Diabetic patients with signs of renal insufficiency and a creatinine level of over 1.5 ml/dl are at high risk; 90% of cases of contrast-induced nephropathy occur in patients with preexisting renal insufficiency, and over 50% involve patients with diabetes mellitus.

Alternative Studies

The kidney can be imaged well with ultrasound. Computed tomography without contrast provides excellent pararenal anatomy, but is less specific than ultrasound in detecting small renal tumors; however, CT even without contrast is specific for renal angiomyolipoma. Radionuclide scanning with ^{99m}Tc-DMSA clearly defines normal parenchyma and will confirm the presence of a column of Bertin causing a renal pseudotumor. Similarly, assessment of renal perfusion and excretion can be obtained with radionuclide scanning using hippuran ^{131}I, hippuran ^{123}I, ^{99m}Tc-DPTA, or ^{99m}Tc-GHA.

Magnetic resonance (MR) imaging requires no contrast media or radiation. Although still very costly, it is the best imaging procedure for the central nervous system and neck; for these patients, the problems inherent in contrast media are resolved. MR imaging is becoming the procedure of choice for musculoskeletal, vascular, and pelvic abnormalities; because quality images are possible in multiple planes, MR will replace CT for imaging tumors of the pelvis. MR and CT are equivalent in imaging the adrenal and kidney; since venous invasion is better defined on MR, it is likely to replace CT for the preoperative staging of renal carcinoma.

The renal collecting system can be clearly imaged by retrograde ureteropyelography, optimally with fluoroscopic monitoring of filming; absorption of contrast has not been a problem. However, the test cannot be used indiscriminately, as an anaphylactoid reaction has been recorded with retrograde pyelography and also during contrast cystography (Johenning 1980).

Use of Nonionic Agents

The sensation of heat and other unpleasant chemotoxic-type side effects are infrequent with the newer low-osmolar contrast agents such as iopamidol (Isovue), iohexol (Omnipaque), and ioxaglate (Hexabrix). These new agents bind calcium to a lesser extent, have less severe cardiac effects, and cause fewer arrhythmias. They reduce side effects in patients undergoing coronary and cerebral angiography. The nonionic agents iopamidol and iohexol seem to offer advantages over the low-osmolar, ionic dimer ioxaglate, in reducing the number of serious anaphylactoid reactions to contrast; however, a life-threatening reaction can still occur (Rapaport et al. 1982). The high cost of the newer nonionic agents will, for the time being, limit their use to patients who have substantial risk for adverse reactions to contrast media.

Whereas conventional ionic contrast media causes a decrease in renal blood flow, this occurs to a lesser degree with nonionic agents. There is also less proteinuria, although enzymuria persists. However, adverse renal effects seem to be caused more by a yet-undefined chemotoxic effect rather than by hyperosmolarity and may be specific for each contrast agent (Speck et al. 1983).

Premedication

For the patient who has previously reacted to contrast, alternative diagnostic methods that do not require contrast are preferred, such as ultrasonography or MR imaging. However, if the alternatives do not provide adequate information, premedication of the patient before the contrast procedure will reduce the severity of a reaction. Zweiman et al. (1975) showed only a 9% reaction rate after pretreatment of reactive patients with steroids. Kelly et al. (1978) found a 5% reaction rate after pretreatment of high-risk patients with steroids plus antihistamines. The suggested pretreatment regimen was 50 mg Benadryl 1 hr before the examination and 150 mg prednisone given in three divided doses of 50 mg every 6 hr beginning 13 hr before the examination; no severe reactions occurred in this pretreated patient group.

Subsequently, patients have been reported who have had a severe anaphylactoid reaction despite pretreatment with steroids and antihistamines and even with the H_2 histamine blocker cimetidine. Interestingly, histamine itself inhibits release of histamine from human basophils and mast cells through the H_2 receptor, by increasing levels of cellular cyclic AMP; blocking this H_2 receptor with cimetidine may actually increase histamine release.

In a large prospective study, Lasser and colleagues showed that a two-dose corticosteroid regimen (32 mg of methylprednisolone given orally 12 hr before and then 2 hr before contrast administration) reduced significantly the incidence of anaphylactoid reactions (Bettman 1987, Lasser et al. 1987). Overall, pretreatment, particularly with steroids, does help, but is not absolutely protective. Pretreatment is also still suggested when using nonionic contrast for patients who have had a prior serious anaphylactoid reaction.

Pretesting

Pretesting with small amounts of contrast to identify potential contrast reactors has generally been abandoned because of unreliability. A highly diluted, graduated method of intravenous injections of contrast has been suggested, but its use has not been widely supported. Pretesting by identifying conversion of prekallikrein to kallikrein has been proposed for higher-risk patients (Lasser et al. 1981).

Mitigating Renal Failure

Routine urography no longer requires dehydration or purgatives to achieve good visualization. Therefore, patients with renal insufficiency should be adequately hydrated, even though not all studies support a direct causative relationship between dehydration and acute renal failure (Berkseth, Kjellstrand 1984).

Hydration during and after a contrast study may reduce the incidence and severity of contrast-induced renal failure in patients with renal insufficiency. Contrast-induced renal failure during angiography occurred less often in diabetic patients given intravenous saline during the examination (Eisenberg et al. 1981). In addition to hydration and volume expansion (1.5 to 2.5 L) before and during contrast administration, the use of mannitol is now recommended in specific cases. A suggested dose is 50 g in 180 ml of 5% dextrose solution given within 45 min of contrast (Mission, Cutler 1985). Furosemide (Lasix) has been suggested for this role, but evidence of specific protection is minimal, and its use is not advised (Table 2–1).

Informed Consent

Most radiologists do not obtain informed consent for routine contrast use (Spring et al. 1984). Lalli suggests that obtaining consent in routine urography may increase the patient's anxiety and

Table 2–1 Adverse Effects of Contrast Media

Effect	Major Symptoms	Primary Treatment
Vasomotor effect	Warmth Nausea Emesis	Reassurance
Anaphylactoid reaction	Urticaria Bronchospasm Hypotension	Adrenergics (IV epinephrine) Inhaled beta-2 adrenergics (albuterol, metaproterenol, or terbutaline) IV fluids
Vagal reaction	Hypotension Bradycardia	IV fluids IV atropine
Nephrotoxicity	Acute renal failure	Avoidance (other tests) Hydration Diuretics (mannitol)

thereby lower the "threshold" for adverse reactions (Lalli 1974). In a subsequent large multiinstitutional patient survey, Spring found that 90% of patients preferred receiving information about the procedure and possible risks (Winfield et al. 1986). At Seattle's Virginia Mason Medical Center, we have begun using a signed consent form for all patients that includes an explanation of why conventional ionic contrast, rather than nonionic, is being used for low-risk patients.

Conclusion

Adverse effects from currently used conventional ionic contrast material include the vasomotor effect, anaphylactoid (allergic-like) or vagal (bradycardia and hypotension) reactions, and renal failure. Each effect likely has more than one etiology, and certain patients are at higher risk for developing the reactions. The urologist and radiologist must be able to differentiate between clinical manifestations of the anaphylactoid reaction and the vagal (bradycardia and hypotension) reaction. Specific treatment for the anaphylactoid reaction is epinephrine; specific medication for the vagal reaction is atropine.

Alternate diagnostic modalities should be considered for high-risk patient groups. Newer nonionic contrast material is available to mitigate reactions in such patients. For patients at high risk for an anaphylactoid reaction, even if nonionic contrast media is being used, premedication is recommended using a combination of prednisone and antihistamines. For patients at high risk for contrast-induced renal failure, and who yet require a contrast examination, hydration, diuretics, and nonionic agents are recommended.

References

Ansell G, Tweedie MCK, Weset CR, Evans DAP, Couch L: The current status of reactions to intravenous contrast media. *Invest. Radiol.* 15(Suppl., 6): S32–39, 1980.

Barach EM, Nowak RM, Tennyson GL, Tomlanovich MC: Epinephrine for treatment of anaphylactic shock. *J.A.M.A.* 251(10): 2118–2122, 1984.

Berkseth RO, Kjellstrand CM: Radiologic contrast-induced nephropathy. *Med. Clin. North Am.* 68(2): 351–370, 1984.

Bettman MA: Radiographic contrast agents – A perspective. *N. Engl. J. Med.* 317: 891–893, 1987.

Byrd L, Sherman RL: Radiocontrast-induced acute renal failure: A clinical and pathophysiologic review. *Medicine* 58: 270–279, 1979.

Eisenberg RL, Bank WO, Hedgcock MW: Renal failure after major angiography can be avoided with hydration. *Am. J. Roentgenol.* 136: 859–861, 1981.

Fischer HW, Colgan FJ: Causes of contrast media reactions. *Radiology* 121: 223, 1976.

Harkonen S, Kjellstrand CM: Exacerbation of diabetic renal failure following intravenous pyelography. *Am. J. Med.* 63: 939–946, 1977.

Hartman GW, Hattery RR, Witten DM, Williamson B: Mortality during excretory urography: Mayo Clinic experience. *Am. J. Roentgenol.* 139: 919–922, 1982.

Johenning PW: Reactions to contrast material during retrograde pyelography. *Urology* 16: 442–444, 1980.

Kelly JF, Patterson R, Lieberman P, Mathison DA, Stevenson DD: Radiographic contrast media studies in high-risk patients. *J. Allergy Clin. Immunol.* 62: 181–184, 1978.

Lalli AF: Urographic contrast media reactions and anxiety. *Radiology* 112: 267–271, 1974.

Lalli AF: Contrast media reactions: Data analysis and hypothesis. *Radiology* 134: 1–12, 1980.

Lasser EC: A coherent biochemical basis for increased reactivity to contrast material in allergic patients. *Am. J. Roentgenol.* 149: 1281–1285, 1987.

Lasser EC, Berry CC, Talner LB, Santini LC, Lang EK, Gerber FH, Stolberg HO: Pretreatment with corticosteroids to alleviate reactions to intravenous contrast material. *N. Engl. J. Med.* 317: 845–849, 1987.

Lasser EC, Lang JH, Lynn SG, Hamblin AE, Howard MM: Prekallikrein-kallikrein conversion rate as a prediction of contrast media catastrophies. *Radiology* 140: 11–16, 1981.

Lasser EC, Lang J, Sovak M, Kolb W, Lyon S, Hamlin AE: Steroids: Theoretical and experimental basis for utilization in prevention of contrast media reactions. *Radiology* 125: 1–9, 1977.

McClennan BL: Low-osmolality contrast media: Premises and promises. *Radiology* 162: 1–8, 1987.

Mission RT, Cutler RE: Radiocontrast-induced renal failure. *West. J. Med.* 142: 647–664, 1985.

Rapaport S, Bookstein JJ, Higgins CB, Carey PH, Sovak M, Lasser EC: Experience with metrizamide in patients with previous severe anaphylactoid reactions to ionic contrast agents. *Radiology* 143: 321–325, 1982.

Shehadi WH: Contrast media reactions: Occurrence, recurrence, and distribution patterns. *Radiology* 143: 11–17, 1982.

Shehadi WH: Death following intravascular administration of contrast media. *Acta Radiol. Diag.* 26: 457–461, 1985.

Siegle RL, Lieberman P: A review of untoward reactions to iodinated contrast material. *J. Urol.* 119: 581–587, 1978.

Smith NT, Corbascio AN: The use and misuse of pressor agents. *Anesthesiology* 33: 58–101, 1970.

Smith RB: Cardia arrest or bradycardia following venipuncture (letter). *J.A.M.A.* 242: 142, 1979.

Spataro RF: Newer contrast agents for urography. *Radiol. Clin. North Am.* 22(2):365–380, 1984.

Speck U, Press WR, Mutzel W: Albuminuria following renal arteriography with various ionic and nonionic contrast agents in the rat. *In* Taenzer V, Zeitler E (eds.): *Contrast Media.* Stuttgart–New York, Thieme, 1983.

Spring DB, Akin JR, Margulis AR: Informed consent for intravenous contrast-enhanced radiography: A national survey of practice and opinion. *Radiology* 152:609–613, 1984.

Spring DB, Tennenhouse DJ, Akin JR, Margulis AR: Radiologists and informed consent lawsuits. *Radiology* 156:245–249, 1985.

Stanley RJ, Pfister RC: Bradycardia and hypotension following use of intravenous contrast media. *Radiology* 121:5–7, 1976.

Van Sonnenberg E, Courtney CC, Pfister RC: Life-threatening hypotensive reactions to contrast media administration: Comparison of pharmacologic and fluid therapy. *Radiology* 162:15–19, 1987.

Van Zee BE, Hoy EW, Talley TE, Jaenike JR: Renal injury associated with intravenous pyelography in nondiabetic and diabetic patients. *Ann. Intern. Med.* 89:51–54, 1978.

Weinrauch LA, Healy RW, Leland OS, Goldstein HH, Kassissich SD, Libertino JA, Takacs FI, D'Elia JA: Coronary angiography and acute renal failure in diabetic azotemic nephropathy. *Ann. Intern. Med.* 86:56–59, 1977.

Winfield AC, Ford CV, James AE, Heller RM, Lamballe AK: Response of patients to informed consent for excretory urography. *Urol. Radiol.* 8:35–39, 1986.

Witten DM, Hirsch FD, Hartman GW: Acute reactions to urographic medium. *Am. J. Roentgenol.* 119:832–840, 1973.

Zipser RD, Laffi G: Prostaglandins, thromboxanes, and leukotrienes in clinical medicine. *West. J. Med.* 143:485–497, 1985.

Zweiman B, Mishkin MM, Hildreth EA: An approach to the performance of contrast studies in contrast material reactive patients. *Ann. Intern. Med.* 83:159–162, 1975.

Suggested Reading

Anderson RJ: Radiocontrast nephrotoxicity (editorial). *West. J. Med.* 142:685, 1985.

Anto HR, Chou SY, Porush JG, Shapiro WB: Infusion intravenous pyelography and renal function: Effects of hypertonic mannitol in patients with chronic renal failure. *Arch. Intern. Med.* 141:1652–1656, 1981.

Dure-Smith P: Fluid restriction before excretory urography. *Radiology* 118:487–489, 1976.

Eisenberg RL, Bank WO, Hedgcock MW: Renal failure after major angiography. *Am. J. Med.* 68:43–46, 1980.

Greenberger PA, Patterson R, Simon R, Lieberman P, Wallace W: Pretreatment of high-risk patients requiring radiographic contrast media studies. *J. Allergy Clin. Immunol.* 67:185–187, 1981.

Harkonen S, Kjellstrand C: Contrast nephropathy. *Am. J. Nephrol.* 1:69–77, 1981.

Lasser EC: Basic mechanisms of contrast media reactions. *Radiology* 91:63–65, 1968.

Schatz M, Patterson R, O'Rourke J, Nickelsen J, Northrup C: The administration of radiographic contrast media to patients with a history of previous reaction. *J. Allergy Clin. Immunol.* 55:358–366, 1975.

Seaman WB (ed.): *Prevention and Management of Adverse Reactions to Intravascular Contrast Media.* Chicago, American College of Radiology, 1977.

Teruel JL, Marcen R, Onaindia JM, Serrano A, Querade C, Ortune J: Renal function impairment caused by intravenous urography. *Arch. Intern. Med.* 141:1271–1274, 1981.

Van Arsdel PP: The complex world of adverse reactions. *Am. J. Roentgenol.* 132:309–310, 1970.

CHAPTER

3

The Excretory Urogram (IVP)

John R. Thornbury and William H. Bush

The intravenous pyelogram (IVP) was first described in a landmark article in the *Journal of the American Medical Association* over 60 years ago (Osborne et al. 1923). With the introduction of diatrizoate-based radiopaque contrast material in the 1950s, excretory urography became the initial diagnostic imaging examination of the urinary tract and retroperitoneum. This inexpensive examination could be performed in outpatient and inpatient settings with minimum risk. Furthermore, it provided abundant and easily interpreted information about normal and pathological anatomy.

IVP was the examination of choice until the mid-1970s, when computed tomography (CT) and ultrasound (US) provided more specific information for many clinical situations. However, the IVP is an important diagnostic test that should be retained as the primary screening imaging modality for the patient with urinary tract disease (Fig. 3–1). Although specific applications have changed somewhat, the effectiveness of the IVP requires not only technical knowledge but also the ability to triage patients at high risk for adverse effects of its use. This requires close communication between the clinician and the radiologist. The current clinical selection criteria for the IVP are effective, and present use seems appropriate (Doubilet et al. 1985).

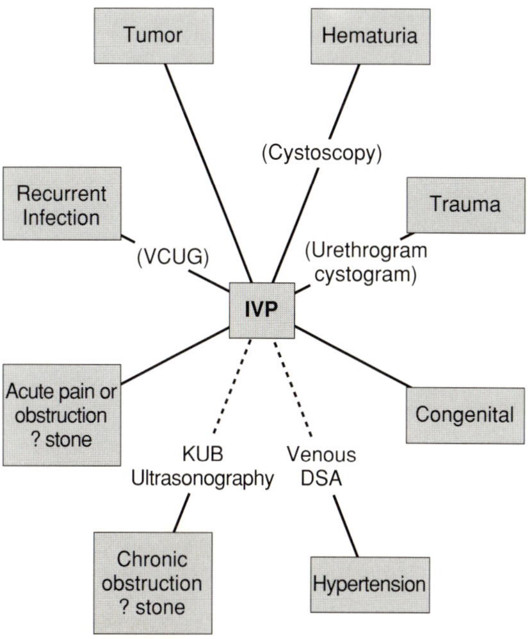

3–1 Illustration of central role of excretory urogram in evaluation of patient with urinary tract disease.

Technique

Radiographic contrast material is filtered by the glomerulus. A rapid bolus injection increases plasma concentration and results in a high-quality nephrogram (Cattell et al. 1967). Contrast agents offering different iodine concentrations and combinations of sodium and methylglucamine salts are available (Benness 1970; Mission, Butler 1984). Experience over the past 25 years has revealed that increased amounts of contrast material can be safely administered. The usual dose (if renal function is normal) is in the range of 400 mg of iodine/kg of body weight (Benness, Evill 1983; Mission, Butler 1984). The authors' usual dose for excretory urography is 100 ml of methylglucamine iothalamate (282 mg I/ml).

Early investigations indicated that better urograms were obtained if patients were dehydrated; however, later studies showed that with higher doses of contrast agents, dehydration was not necessary (Dure-Smith 1976). Furthermore, dehydration increases the risk of contrast-induced renal failure, particularly when there is compromised renal function (Mission, Butler, 1984; Teruel et al. 1981). A potent sequence of dehydrating purgatives should also be avoided. Attempts to thoroughly cleanse the bowel may create gas, which further compromises the urogram. Use of nephrotomography decreases the need for a clean colon. In the authors' practice, the patient is given two Dulcolax tablets during the afternoon of the day before the examination and is encouraged to eat normally and to maintain usual fluid intake throughout the day. A light breakfast or lunch and modest fluid intake are allowed on the day of the examination.

Filming

Some radiologists advocate limiting the number of films taken before and following contrast injection, so as to reduce the radiation dose to the patient. Others advise maximizing the information obtainable with the first examination, which requires more filming, particularly tomography and oblique films. The authors believe nephrotomography to specifically define the kidneys is critical to optimal excretory urography. Although renal imaging is improved by oblique films of the kidneys, nephrotomography provides the best definition of renal margins and caliceal anatomy.

The authors' usual examination begins with a scout film of the abdomen (KUB). Tomograms prior to contrast injection are added if renal calculi are to be excluded. Contrast is then injected as an intravenous bolus. A nephrotomogram is obtained 1 min after the start of injection; it is taken at the conclusion of contrast injection if the injection was done slowly through a small needle. At 3 min a plain film of the kidney region is obtained and abdominal compression is applied for improved collecting system distension (Fig. 3–2). However,

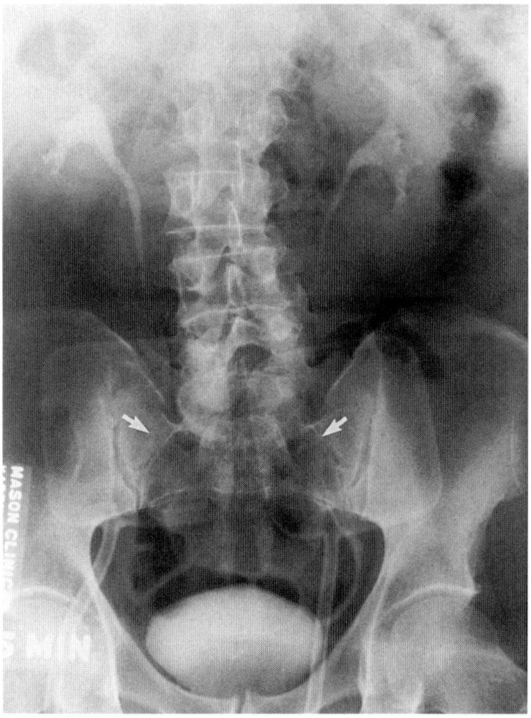

3–2 Film from urogram illustrating correct position of compression devices to provide ureteral distention. Devices must be placed so that the ureter is compressed as it crosses over iliac vessels (arrows). Position of iliac vessels can be estimated by drawing a line from L4 to medial aspect of femoral head.

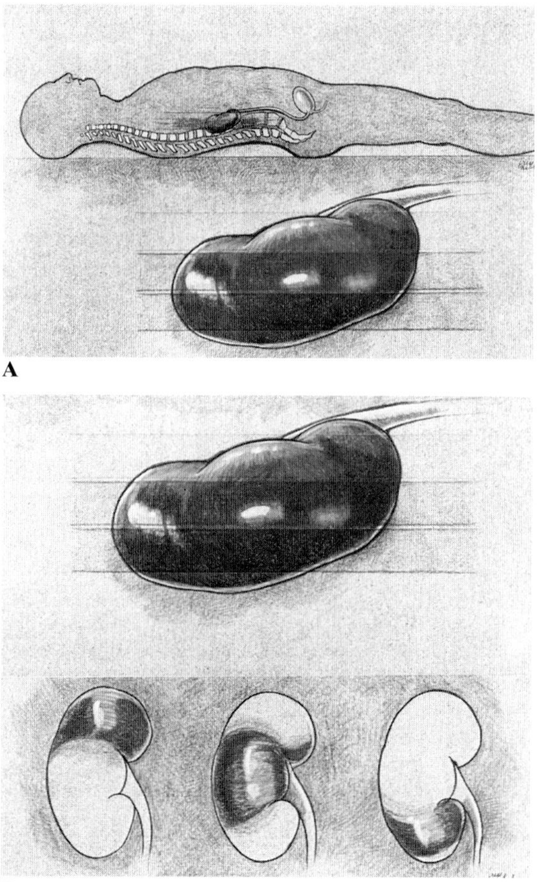

A

B

3–3 (A, B) Multiple tomograms are necessary in most patients to image completely the kidneys. Because upper pole of kidney is more posterior in the body, the lowest nephrotomogram will define upper pole but not mid and lower sections of kidney. Adjacent, more anterior nephrotomograms, are necessary to completely define kidney. (Reprinted with permission from Bush WH, Gibbons RP: *A Case for the IVP, AUA Update Series.* © 1986, American Urological Association Office of Education, Bellaire, TX.)

abdominal compression is not used if: 1) there is a clinical question of an obstructing renal calculus, 2) the patient has acute abdominal pain or possibly an abdominal aortic aneurysm, or 3) there has been recent abdominal surgery.

At 10 min following the injection, three tomograms of the kidneys are obtained. Compression is then released, and an immediate plain film of the entire abdomen is obtained to show the filled ureters. Oblique films can also be taken at this time. If there is incomplete ureteral filling, a prone radiograph is done. A postvoid film of the bladder is usually obtained. If there is a question of ureteral obstruction, delayed films are obtained. Tailored urography using this sequence of films has worked optimally for the authors but is not, by any means, the only way to perform the urographic examination.

In most patients, the kidneys are rotated obliquely and the lower pole of the kidney is situated more anteriorly (Fig. 3–3). Therefore, three or four adjacent 1.5-cm-thick tomograms are necessary to completely image both the upper and lower poles of the kidney. A midlevel can be estimated by using one-half the distance from the table top to the anterior abdominal wall (McDonnell 1972). The location of the kidney related to body size has been reviewed by Rhodes et al. (1987). An additional anterior tomogram may be necessary to image the lower pole. Tomography with the patient in an oblique position can be done to specifically define the anterior and posterior margins of the kidney.

Decision Process

Many algorithms describe the use of imaging examinations for urinary tract assessment. The basic rule is two-part:

1. Choose the examination that provides the most timely and useful information with the least cost and least risk to the patient.
2. Do not request any imaging examination if there is little, or no, predictable effect on treatment options.

Physicians (including urologists and radiologists) must be familiar with the advantages of CT, ultrasound, and IVP in particular clinical problem settings. The physician's own personally reviewed experience is valuable in this regard. For example, Lang et al. (1985) described the comparable results of using excretory urography, CT, radionuclide renography, and angiography in renal trauma patients. The ability to predict the presence or absence of each type of injury provides information about how often diagnostic predictions are right or wrong; and if wrong, what proportion are false positive (overcall) and false negative (undercall).

Concern over adverse reaction to the contrast material also influences choice of diagnostic tests. The adverse clinical effects of intravenous contrast media are divided into four groups: the mild reaction, such as hives or nausea or vomiting; the life-threatening cardiovascular or respiratory reaction; the vagal reaction; and the contrast-induced acute renal failure. Since certain patients are at higher risk for these adverse reactions, the clinician must take this into account when considering use of urography. If reaction risk is not acceptable, the clinician can turn to diagnostic imaging methods such as ultrasound that do not require contrast media. Newer nonionic contrast agents appear to have lower rates of adverse reactions, particularly in high-risk groups of patients such as previous reactors or severe asthmatics.

Risks, cost, pain, and anxiety about not having a firm diagnosis are other factors in physicians' decision making. New emphasis on informed consent mandates that the patient participate with the physician in decisions about diagnostic testing and treatment.

Special Situations

If the patient is hypotensive, normal excretion of contrast media by the kidneys will not be achieved, and useful information, particularly about the collecting systems and ureters, will be limited. Likewise, if evidence from prior clinical examination and laboratory tests in the emergency room indicates modest to severe renal insufficiency, contrast use is contraindicated. If mild to moderate insufficiency is present (serum creatinine in the range of 2.0–3.5 mg/dl), risk of contrast-induced nephrotoxicity from urography must be balanced against the possibility of gaining useful information from ultrasonography or noncontrast CT.

Usually a large dose of intravenous contrast, 36–40 g of iodine, is needed to opacify the collecting system and ureter. Emergency patients have not had any bowel preparation and often have been receiving intravenous fluids or blood.

Injured patients commonly have excessive intestinal fluid and gas. These shadows often obscure renal and psoas outlines and cause confusing opacities that mimic calculi in the renal or ureteral region. Oblique films or tomograms prior to contrast injection will help sort out densities, confirm or refute calculi, and make renal margins more apparent. Tomography that includes all of the parenchyma and margins of both kidneys should be obtained immediately after injection to optimize visualization of the renal parenchyma at the height of contrast opacification. This will highlight renal margin defects and inhomogeneity of the nephrogram due to injured tissue.

Normally, the intense early nephrogram opacification will fade by 3–5 min after the start of contrast injection. Contrast will then first appear in the minor calices at about 3 min and will opacify the urine in the collecting system by 5 min and the ureters by 10 min; ureter opacification should be symmetrical. The bladder urine will be partly opacified by 15 min; if opacification or filling is delayed, then additional films at intervals appropriate to the emergency circumstances will be needed. If the opacification sequence is normal, an abdominal film at 15 min will usually complete the examination.

Monitoring of the films is important so that the examination can be modified according to the imaging findings. Modification may include additional views, special positioning, or even repeat tomography in situations where renal structures are only faintly visualized. Consultation by the radiologist with the managing physician will enhance the diagnostic information.

Renal Trauma

Despite the urgency in the emergency situations, it is important to follow basic principles of excretory urography to avoid errors in treatment decisions. These basics are:

1. The patient must have a reasonably normal blood pressure and renal function.
2. Adequate dose of intravenous contrast media is required.
3. Good-quality films must be obtained, and tomography should be included.
4. Films must be monitored for possible modifications.

The basic treatment decision is surgical versus nonsurgical management. For conservative management to be a reasonable choice, the patient must be clinically stable, the presence of normal or reasonably normal renal function must be established, and the type and extent of upper tract injury must be identified with high certainty. The question of preexisting upper tract pathology and the rare possibility of unilateral renal agenesis or gross positional anomalies of the kidney must be considered.

In the large series of 388 renal trauma patients reported by Lang et al. (1985), 31% proved to have "no discernible injury," and 26% had only renal contusion. Overall, 22% required surgical exploration, whereas 78% had nonsurgical management. McAninch and Federle (1982) estimated that about 75%–80% of all patients with renal trauma have minor isolated renal injury. For such minor trauma patients, they recommended that excretory urography be the initial imaging examination (Fig. 3–4). For patients suspected of having major renal injury or trauma to multiple organs, dynamic CT scanning is recommended as the initial imaging examination.

Dynamic CT scanning offers the most comprehensive information for making the choice between operative and nonoperative management (Lang et al. 1985; McAninch, Federle 1982). These criteria include the amount of nonviable renal tissue, extent of perirenal hemorrhage, extravasation of urine, and status of the renal pedicle. While excretory urography can provide clues, CT provides precise anatomic information about all of these items except arterial anatomy of the renal pedicle. Renal arteriography is required for this assessment, particularly when dynamic CT findings or clinical findings increase the suspicion of severe pedicle arterial injury.

How reliable is excretory urography when its result is "no discernible injury," that is, when the urogram is "normal"? Lang et al. (1985) found that in 88% of patients who ultimately proved to have no discernible renal injury, the urogram was normal. In the remaining 12%, the urogram showed abnormal contrast excretion features without other anatomic deformity (Fig. 3–4). In these cases, further imaging examinations (dynamic CT scan or arteriography) indicated no renal injury.

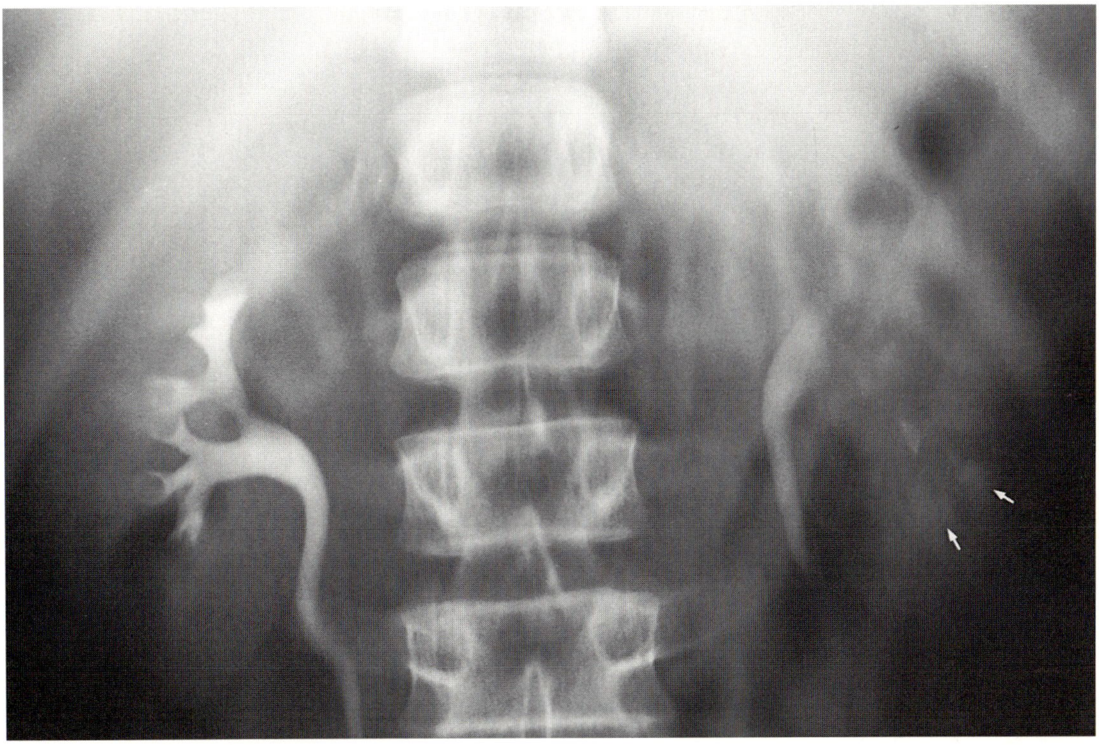

3–4 Urogram showing decreased excretion from left kidney with a compressed, "spidery" collecting system as a result of renal contusion. There is minimal extravasation in medullary region of lower pole (arrows).

Table 3–1 is adapted from that paper and describes the basic urographic imaging features that are helpful in predicting the type of injury in the specific patient. When the urographic findings indicate that a type of injury does not fit with the clinical findings, or the imaging information is of limited quality due to the condition of the patient, one must assume that a more serious type of injury is actually present. The most appropriate next examination must then be selected, most commonly CT or angiography (Fig. 3–5). It should not be necessary to go beyond excretory urography often.

An excretory urogram may not always be mandatory. Clinical suspicion for renal injury is an indication for urography, regardless of whether microscopic hematuria is present. If clinical suspicion or gross hematuria had been used as the indication for IVP rather than microscopic hematuria alone, 75% of patients would not have needed an IVP (Guice et al. 1983).

Table 3–1 Urographic Findings in Renal Trauma

Type of Injury	Excretory Urography
Contusion	Decreased contrast excretion
Parenchymal tear	Cortical defect
Acute hematoma:	
Intra- and/or subcapsular	Defect in margin and/or parenchyma
Peri- and/or pararenal	Displaced kidney
Infarct	Partial or total lack of contrast excretion
Penetrating injury to collecting system	Extravasation of contrast material
Arterial injury:	
Renal artery severed or thrombosed	Lack of contrast excretion
Subintimal flap	Decreased excretion
Arteriovenous fistula	Decreased excretion

Source: Adapted from Lang et al. (1985).

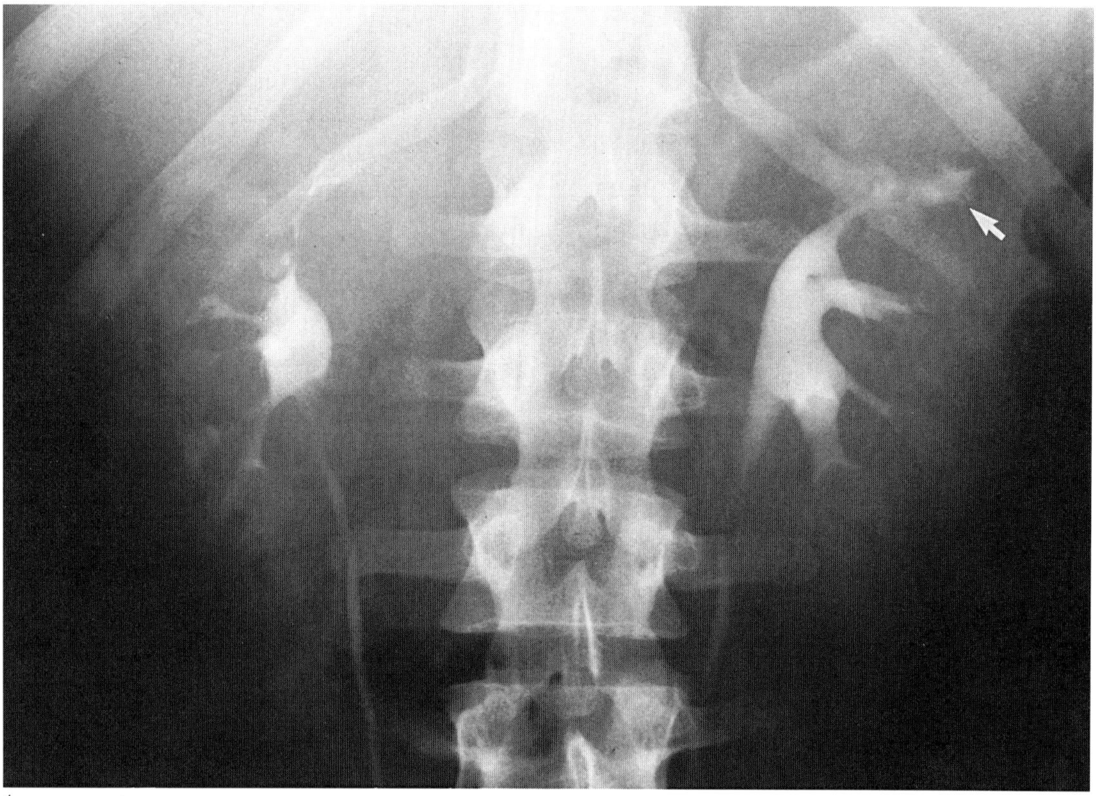

A

3–5 Renal fracture suspected by findings on tomography done during urography. **(A)** Ten-min film of IVP shows extravasation in upper pole (arrow). **(B)** Tomography more clearly defines injury (arrows) and shows defects in paren-

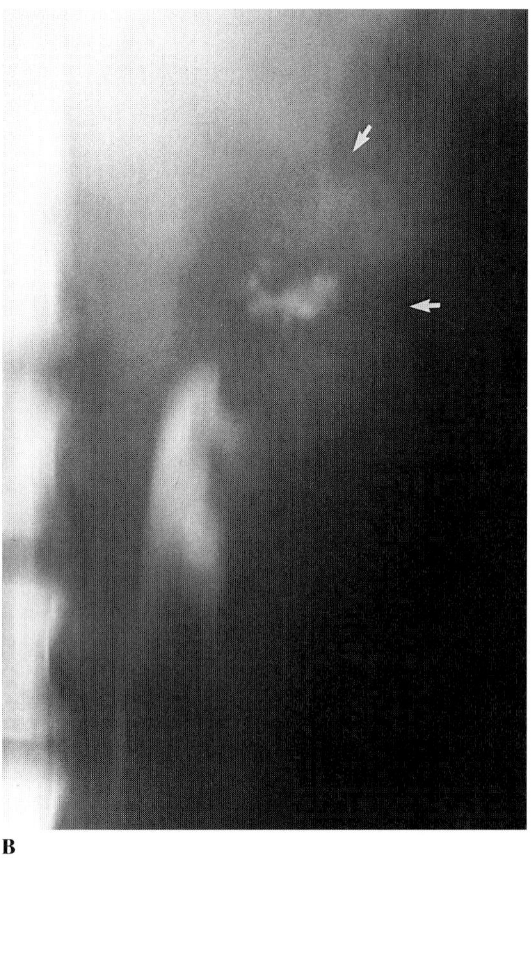

B

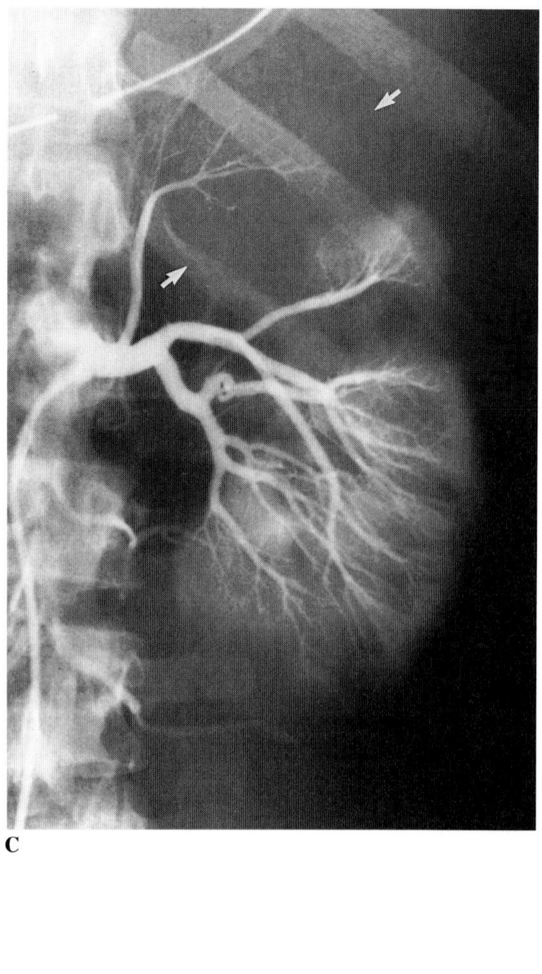

C

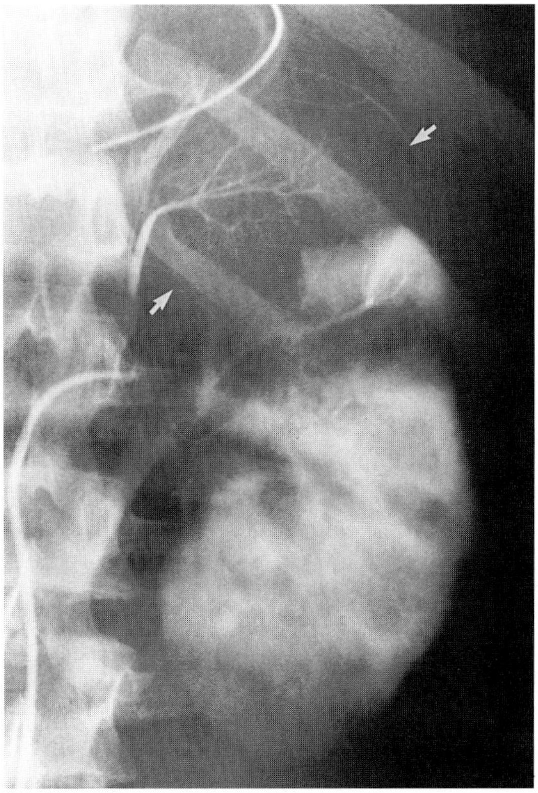

D

chymal opacification. Arterial **(C)** and parenchymal **(D)** phases of angiogram confirm fractures of upper kidney and hematoma in upper pole (arrows).

Nontraumatic Hematuria

Excretory urography is the best initial imaging method for patients with hematuria. Tailored urography will demonstrate renal size and margins, caliceal and renal pelvic anatomy, and most of both ureters. Optimum imaging of the kidneys must include tomography or detailed oblique films. The blind spot of the kidney on urography is the anterior aspect of the kidney (Fig. 3–6). A small tumor located in this position usually will be missed unless detailed anteroposterior tomography, oblique filming, or oblique tomography is done. It must be kept in mind that excretory urography has very low sensitivity for detecting pathology in the bladder that causes hematuria. Recognizing these limitations, evaluation of the patient with hematuria, and an apparently normal excretory urogram, should be followed by cystoscopy and renal ultrasonography or CT.

Renal ultrasonography is the suggested second imaging modality for a renal mass discovered on the IVP when further evaluation is necessary. Most masses will be benign cysts, and ultrasonography can confirm this accurately. When a cyst is not confirmed, CT scanning should follow for evaluation and staging of the now-suspected renal neoplasm; CT evaluates not only the opposite kidney but the paraaortic nodal regions and the liver for metastases. Magnetic resonance (MR) imaging is currently under evaluation. Preliminary results suggest MRI may be comparable to CT in depicting and characterizing solid and cystic masses of the kidney. MRI does have the advantage of readily differentiating vascular structures from nodal metastases and is more sensitive in determining whether the renal vein is free of tumor thrombus (Hricak et al. 1983). Renal arteriography is selectively used to confirm malignant neovascularity in diagnostic problem cases or to occasionally provide an anatomic guide of the vascular system and the tumor for the urological surgeon.

Urinary Infection

Routine use of excretory urography is not recommended for the usual uncomplicated lower urinary tract infection; however, for persistent, recurrent, or unusual types of infections, urography provides the best imaging method. Voiding cystourethrography (radionuclide or radiopaque contrast media) is commonly used to evaluate children for vesicoureteral reflux and bladder emptying problems. However, in the absence of reflux, renal ultrasonography, rather than excretory urography, is recommended (Leonidas et al. 1985). If reflux is present or if the ultrasonography is suspicious or abnormal, excretory urography should be performed.

Upper Urinary Tract Obstruction

Ultrasonography is a good screening test with an 85% accuracy for detecting hydronephrosis (Della-Palina et al. 1983). When ultrasonography is positive, excretory urography is required for determination of renal parenchymal status and the site and nature of the obstruction. However, the urogram is more sensitive than ultrasonography for diagnosing acute hydronephrosis and forniceal rupture, and for detecting ureteral or renal calculi (Laing et al. 1985) (Fig. 3–7). From 70%–90% of

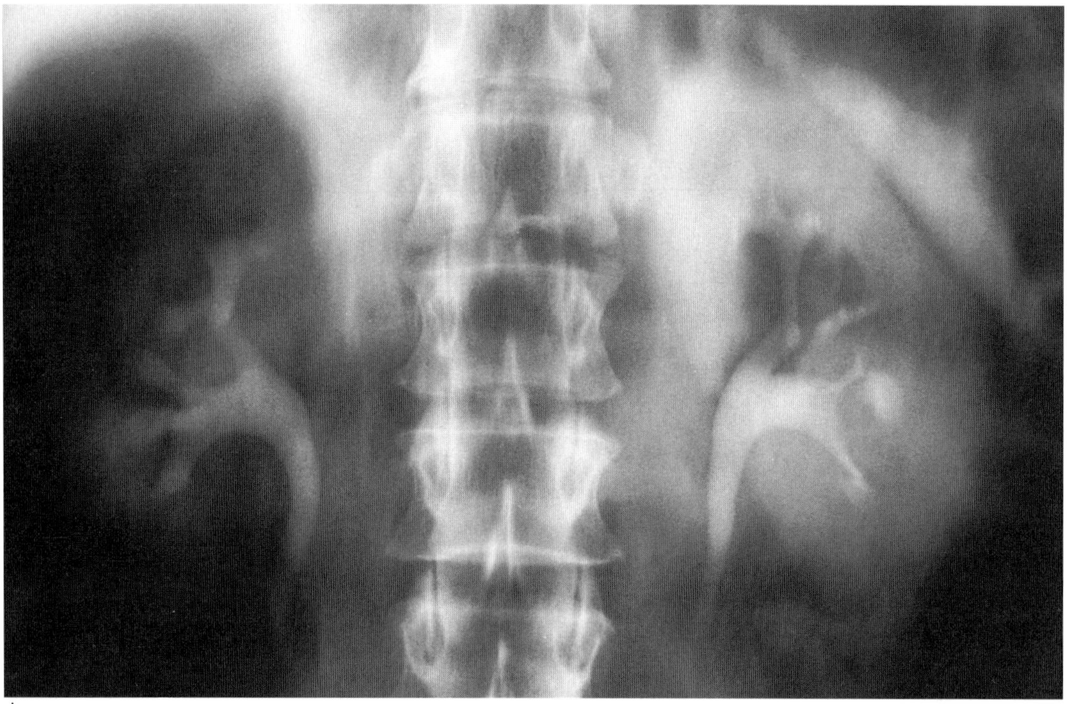

A

3–6 An anterior renal mass not evident on the urogram. A mass located directly anteriorly or a small mass directly posteriorly will be missed with frontal filming, even with good tomography; oblique filming is then helpful. **(A)** Frontal tomogram through anterior half of kidneys is normal. **(B)** CT scan clearly showing this mass (arrows), a low-grade neoplasm of the distal renal tubular cell. A = aorta; D = duodenum and pancreas; V = inferior vena cava.

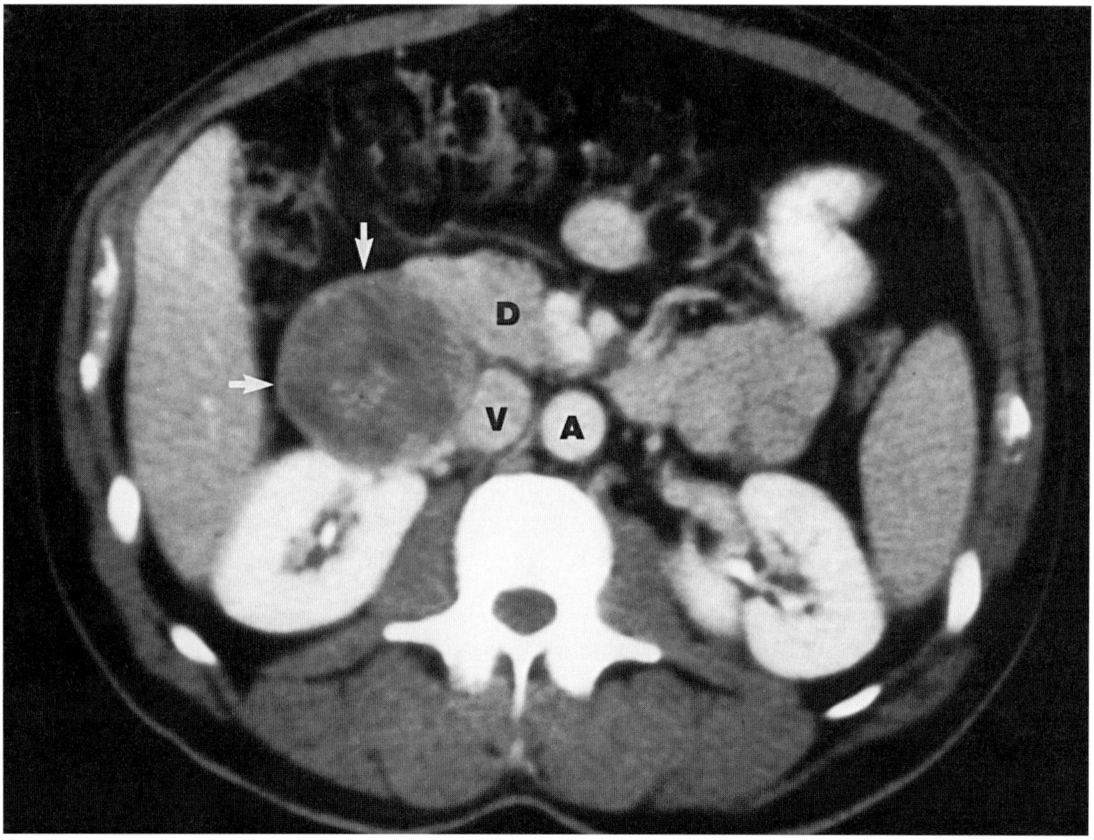

B

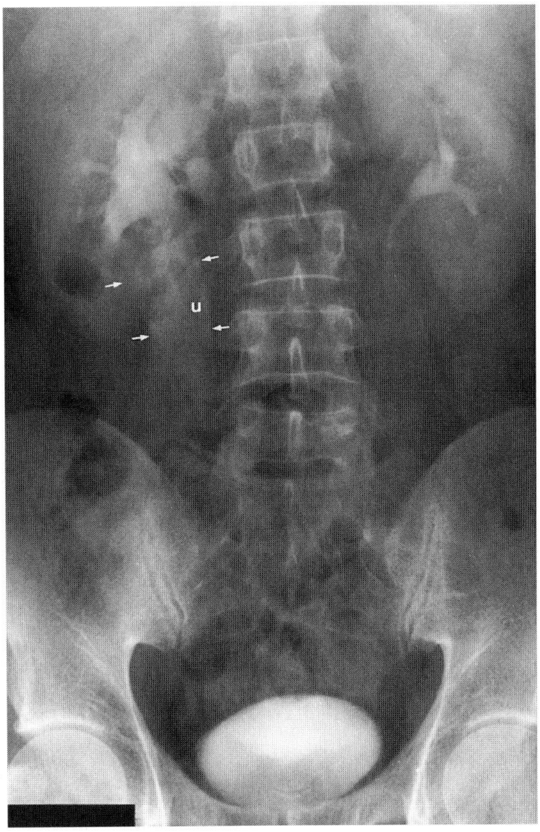

3–7 Excretory urogram showing effects of acute obstruction of right ureter by calculus; note only minimal dilatation of calices. Forniceal leak and extravasation toward renal hilum have allowed decompression of collecting system. In acute obstruction, the calices as imaged by ultrasonography may be normal. In chronic obstruction, ultrasonic findings are usually characteristic. U = urine-filled, unopacified ureter. Small urinoma outlined by arrows.

ureteral calculi are radiopaque and will be seen on the plain film of the abdomen. If chronic pain or symptoms of urinary obstruction are present, a plain film plus ultrasonography may be used instead of the IVP (Thornbury, Parker 1982). When ureteral obstruction is present but no opaque calculus is seen on the plain film, CT should be considered for detecting a low-density or nonopaque calculus.

Hypertension

Excretory urography (including the "hypertensive" variation) is a nondiscriminatory test for renovascular hypertension (Thornbury et al. 1982). Renal arteriography, rather than urography, is the primary imaging choice for evaluating adult patients for renovascular hypertension. However, its use should be reserved for patients whose hypertension is not controlled by antihypertensive medication, that is, for patients with moderate to severe hypertension (diastolic BP 105 mm Hg or over) and who are judged likely to benefit from surgery or angioplasty (Thornbury et al. 1984). In some patients, outpatient intravenous digital subtraction arteriography or outpatient arterial DSA is recommended for diagnosing renovascular hypertension (Hillman et al. 1982).

Summary

The choice of imaging examination should be based on clinical assessment of the patient and requires that the physician hypothesize a differential diagnosis and estimate the most likely of one or two diagnoses. This prior diagnostic weighting coupled with knowledge from the literature and the physician's own experience should allow the appropriate decision on whether or not urography should be used.

References

Benness GT: Urographic contrast agents: A comparison of sodium and methylglucamine salts. *Clin. Radiol.* 21:150–156, 1970.

Benness GT, Evill CA: Urographic physiology and contrast materials. *In* Friedland GW, Filly RA, Goris ML, et al. (eds.): *Uroradiography: An Integrated Approach.* New York, Churchill Livingstone, 1983, pp. 155–156.

Bush WH: Risk factors and clinical considerations in the management of contrast-induced adverse reactions. *In* Parvez Z, Moncada R, Sovak M (eds.): *Contrast Media: Biological Effects and Clinical Applications,* Vol. 2, Boca Raton, FL CRC Press, 1987, pp. 397–419.

Cattell WR, Fry IK, Spencer AG, et al.: Excretion urography. I: Factors affecting the excretion of Hypaque. *Br. J. Radiol.* 40:561–580, 1967.

Della-Palina L, Bazzocchi M, Pozzi-Mucelli RS, et al.: Ultrasonography in the diagnosis of hydronephrosis in patients with normal renal function. *Urol. Radiol.* 5:221–226, 1983.

Doubilet P, McNeil BJ, VanHouten FX, et al.: Excretory urography in current practice: Evidence against overutilization. *Radiology* 154:607–611, 1985.

Dure-Smith P: Fluid restriction before excretory urography. *Radiology* 118:487–489, 1976.

Guice K, Oldham K, Eide B, Johansen K: Hematuria after blunt trauma: When is pyelography useful? *J. Trauma* 23:305–311, 1983.

Hillman BJ, Ovitt TW, Capp MP, et al.: Renal digital subtraction angiography: 100 cases. *Radiology* 145: 643–646, 1982.

Hricak H, Crooks L, Sheldon P, et al.: NMR imaging of the kidney. *Radiology* 146:425–432, 1983.

Laing FC, Jeffrey RB, Wing VW: Ultrasound versus excretory urography in evaluating acute flank pain. *Radiology* 154:613–616, 1985.

Lang EK, Sullivan J, Frentz G: Renal trauma: Radiological studies. Comparison of urography, computed tomography, angiography, and radionuclide studies. *Radiology* 154:1–6, 1985.

Leonidas JC, McCauley RGK, Klauber GC, Fretzayas AM: Sonography as a substitute for excretory urography in children with urinary tract infection. *Am. J. Roentgenol.* 144:815–819, 1985.

McAninch JW, Federle MP: Evaluation of renal injuries with computerized tomography. *J. Urol.* 128:456–460, 1982.

McDonnell F: Measurement of the normal position of the kidney in relation to the coronal planes of the body: A study of 35 adults. *J. Can. Assoc. Radiol.* 23:241–244, 1972.

Mission RT, Butler RE: Radiocontrast-induced renal failure. *West. J. Med.* 142:657–664, 1984.

Osborne ED, Sutherland CG, Scholl AJ, Rowntree LG: Roentgenography of urinary tract during excretion of sodium iodide. *J.A.M.A.* 80:368–373, 1923.

Rhodes RA, Fried AM, Lorman JG, Kryscio RJ: Tomographic levels for intravenous urography: CT determined guidelines. *Radiology* 163:673–675, 1987.

Spataro RF: Newer contrast agents for urography. *Radiol. Clin. North Am.* 22(2):365–380, 1984.

Teruel JL, Marcen R, Onaindia JM, et al.: Renal function impairment caused by intravenous urography. *Arch. Intern. Med.* 141:1271–1274, 1981.

Thornbury JR, Parker TW: Ureteral calculi. *Semin. Roentgenol.* 17:133–139, 1982.

Thornbury JR, Stanley JC, Fryback DG: Hypertensive urogram: A nondiscriminatory test for renovascular hypertension. *Am. J. Roentgenol.* 138:43–49, 1982.

Thornbury JR, Stanley JC, Fryback DG: Optimizing workup of adult hypertensive patients for renal artery stenosis. *Radiol. Clin. North Am.* 22:333–339, 1984.

CHAPTER

4

Ultrasonography of the Urinary System

William M. Marks

The use of ultrasonography in recent years has contributed to the declining need for the intravenous urogram. Ultrasonography is safe for young or pregnant patients because it requires no radiation. It can often be used for those who are allergic to iodinated contrast material, can be done at the patient's bedside, and is less expensive than most other imaging tests. In general, ultrasonography is an anatomically sensitive, although not tissue-specific, modality that relies greatly on the skill of the examiner.

In ultrasound, an acoustic wave is generated by the application of electrical energy to a crystal in the ultrasound transducer. This transducer acts as both an emitter and receiver of the sound waves, functioning in the latter role 99% of the time. The acoustic wave is transmitted to the tissues by a coupling medium, such as gel or mineral oil, between the transducer and the skin. The wave propagates through tissue and is reflected back at the interface of tissues of different acoustical properties. The ultrasound pulse may completely pass through a substance such as a fluid; be partially transmitted and reflected by it, as with renal and hepatic parenchyma; or be totally reflected by it without any significant transmission, as in bone and areas of gas. The reflected wave travels back to the transducer, is converted into electrical energy, amplified, and processed to produce an image.

Transducer technology has advanced rapidly in recent years with substantial improvement in image quality. Although high-frequency transducers improve resolution, penetration generally declines. The appropriate transducer for an exam has a focal zone that covers the region of interest, allowing for optimal lateral resolution. Kidneys are satisfactorily imaged in most patients with 3- to 5-MHz transducers, which have a long internal focus. In children, better resolution can be obtained with 5-MHz transducers. Higher-frequency transducers, to 10 MHz, provide better images of superficial structures such as testicles.

Real-time sonography is preferred to static imaging in most institutions, because examinations can be performed faster and, in general, yield better quality images. Motion, such as peristalsis, can be identified with this method. Static images remain useful when an anatomic site or pathologic mass cannot be seen in a single image or when relationships to surrounding organs are needed.

Evaluation of the Normal Kidney

The right kidney is best evaluated with the patient supine or in the left decubitus position; and the left kidney, with the patient in the right decubitus position or supine while scanning from the flank. Either kidney may also be scanned with the patient prone. Both kidneys should be scanned along the longitudinal and transverse axes.

Renal size can be determined by ultrasonography, although this may be technically difficult in some patients, owing to overlying ribs, obesity, or minimal differentiation between echogenic retroperitoneal nonrenal tissue and echogenic kidneys. The normal adult right kidney measures 10.74 cm in mean length (S.D. ± 1.35 cm), and the left 11.10 cm (S.D. ± 1.15 cm) in mean length (Brandt et al. 1982). These are anatomically accurate numbers, although slightly smaller than measurements on intravenous urograms, since the kidney is magnified on the urogram because of its separation from the film by retroperitoneal and back tissues. In larger patients, this effect is in-

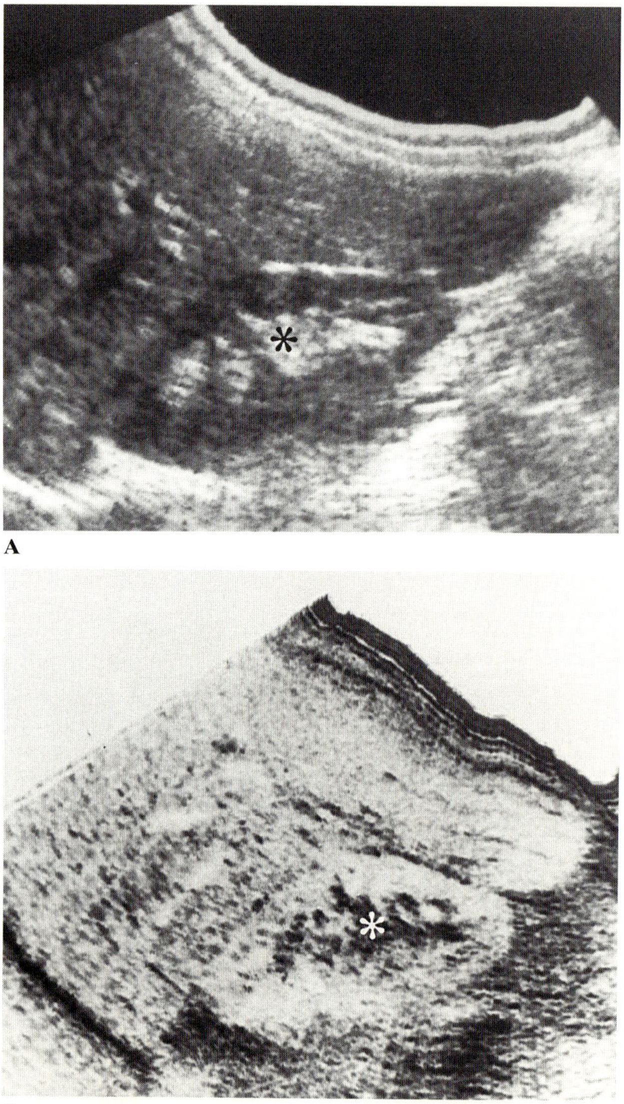

A

B

4–1 Normal right kidney demonstrated by two conventionally available formats: **(A)** white echoes on black background and **(B)** black echoes on white background. Renal cortex is less echogenic than liver. Central echoes (*) arise from interfaces with collecting system, vascular structures, and fatty tissue.

creased. This depth factor of magnification does not occur with ultrasound.

The normal liver and pancreas generate higher amplitude echoes than the normal kidney. The spleen and kidney have approximately the same echogenicity. Centrally, the kidney has bright echoes, representing reflections from renal collecting structures, arteries, veins, and sinus fat (Fig. 4–1).

When a kidney is not identified in its usual location in the renal fossa, an ectopic location should be sought. Pelvic and horseshoe kidneys are usually easily identified with ultrasound. A functional test with a radionuclide agent may be necessary to determine if functional renal tissue is present across the midline of a fused or horseshoe kidney.

Sonographic Distinction of Cystic and Solid Renal Masses

As the acoustic beam passes through the fluid of a simple cyst, no significant reflections or interactions occur and, thus, no echoes are produced. Conversely, the tissue adjacent to the cyst produces multiple reflections or echoes as the sound passes through it. Behind the posterior margin of the cyst, more echoes are present than at a similar level of adjacent solid tissue, since the sound beam that passed through the cyst fluid has not been attenuated or diminished in strength. This effect of posterior acoustical enhancement, or relative increased intensity of echoes seen behind the cyst, is an excellent distinguishing sonographic feature of solid and cystic masses.

Artifactual echoes may be created within any cystic structure by the sonographic technique. These are usually due to variations of the time-gain compensation curve or reverberation echoes (Fig. 4–2). Therefore, presence or lack of internal echoes should not be the sole criterion to distinguish solid from cystic lesions.

The characteristics of the wall or margin of a cystic mass help distinguish simple cysts from necrotic tumors or abscesses. A simple renal cyst has a thin, well-defined smooth margin, while the walls of more ominous pathologic masses are thicker, irregular, and less defined.

Another distinguishing feature between cystic and solid masses is the presence of a refractive shadow (Fig. 4–3) adjacent to the cyst. Snell's law of refraction explains the bending or refraction of sound beams passing through substances of different acoustical velocities (Sommer et al. 1979). Refractive shadows can occur at the margin of pathologic and normal cystic structures, including simple or complicated cysts, abscesses, gallbladder, and vascular structures.

Cystic Masses

Cysts are common in patients over 50 and are usually asymptomatic. On ultrasound, these benign masses demonstrate posterior acoustical enhancement, smooth wall margins, spherical or ovoid shape, and absence of internal echoes (Fig. 4–2). When all of these criteria are met, sonographic accuracy is 98%. In a series of 182 biopsy-proven masses, Pollack and colleagues (1982) found that no mass rigidly meeting these criteria proved to be a neoplasm.

Cystic masses sometimes do not meet these criteria. Most often such a mass represents a simple cyst complicated by infection or hemorrhage (Fig. 4–4); however, a cystic or necrotic hypernephroma or an abscess cannot then be excluded. There are differing opinions as to management of these atypical cystic masses. When the cystic mass has irregular, thickened walls or thick internal septations, computed tomography or fine-needle aspiration is usually performed. A benign simple cyst may have a thin solitary septation within it. If this is the only variance from a classic cyst, it is often followed sonographically to assure stability. Interpretation should be made in conjunction with other tests and clinical findings.

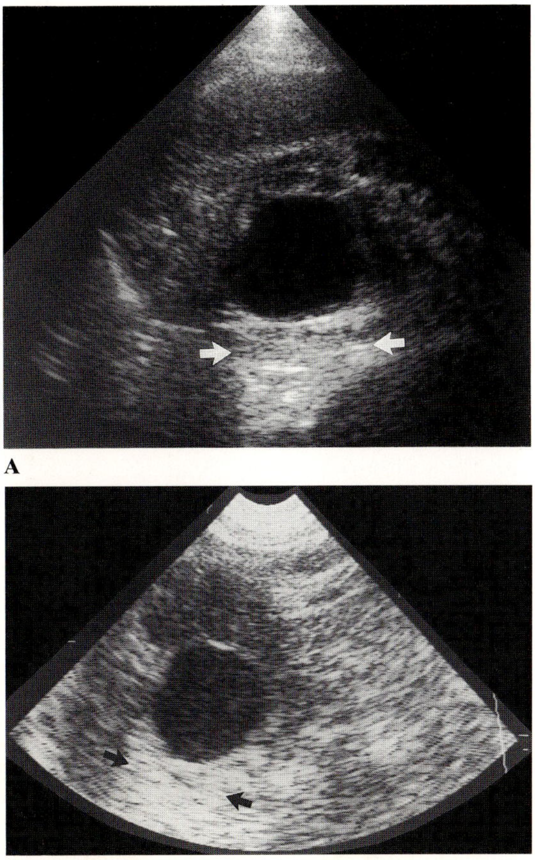

A

B

4–2 **(A)** Typical anechoic renal cyst demonstrating posterior acoustical enhancement (arrows). **(B)** Same renal cyst scanned at different gain setting with multiple low-level internal echoes and good sound transmission (arrows).

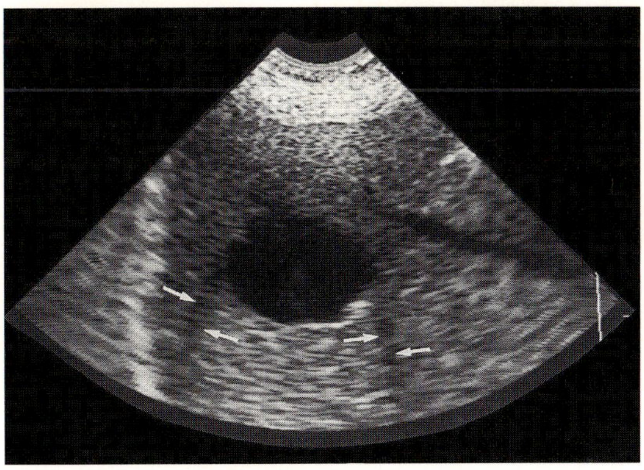

4–3 Refractive shadows (arrows) characteristically arise from lateral margins of a cystic mass.

In addition, obstruction of an upper or lower pole moiety in a duplicated collecting system, a large caliceal diverticulum, and hydrocalycosis may all closely resemble the simple renal cyst.

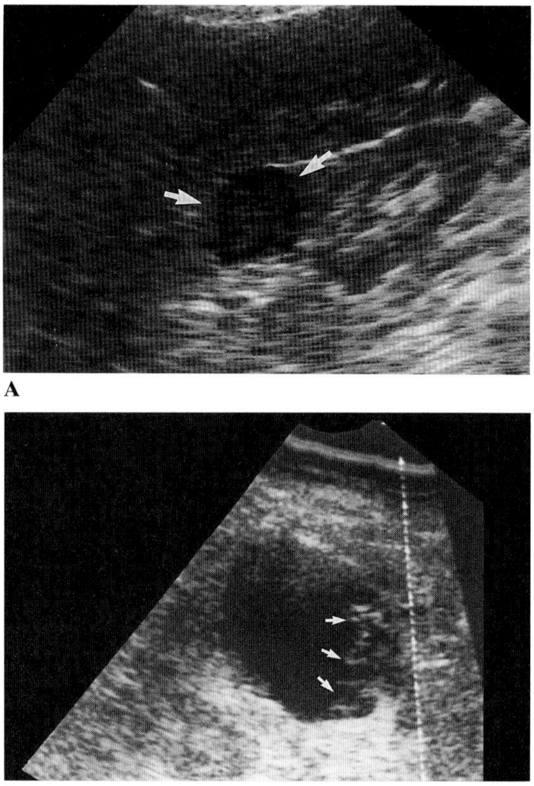

4–4 Atypical renal cysts. **(A)** Hemorrhagic cyst (arrows) filled with low-level echoes. **(B)** Wall irregularity (arrows) in infected cyst. Either appearance could also represent hypernephroma or abscess. (Courtesy L. Mack, Seattle, WA.)

Solid Masses

The ability of ultrasound to differentiate histology based on the appearance of a solid mass is much less specific. Solid neoplasms can usually be detected if 2 cm or larger; these typically generate multiple internal echoes, demonstrate poor transmission of sound, and are less well defined than cysts. With high-resolution ultrasound equipment, the echogenicity or acoustical impedance of the mass is usually the limiting factor. Masses with the same echogenicity as the renal parenchyma will be detected only if they deform the kidney.

Hypernephromas account for over 90% of primary renal malignancies and are the most common solid mass in adults. Hypernephromas are usually hypoechoic, but sometimes nearly isoechoic or hyperechoic (Fig. 4–5). Invasion of the renal veins and inferior vena cava by tumor thrombus may also be seen (Fig. 4–6). Computed tomography is currently the preferred staging method (Cronan et al. 1982; Levine et al. 1980).

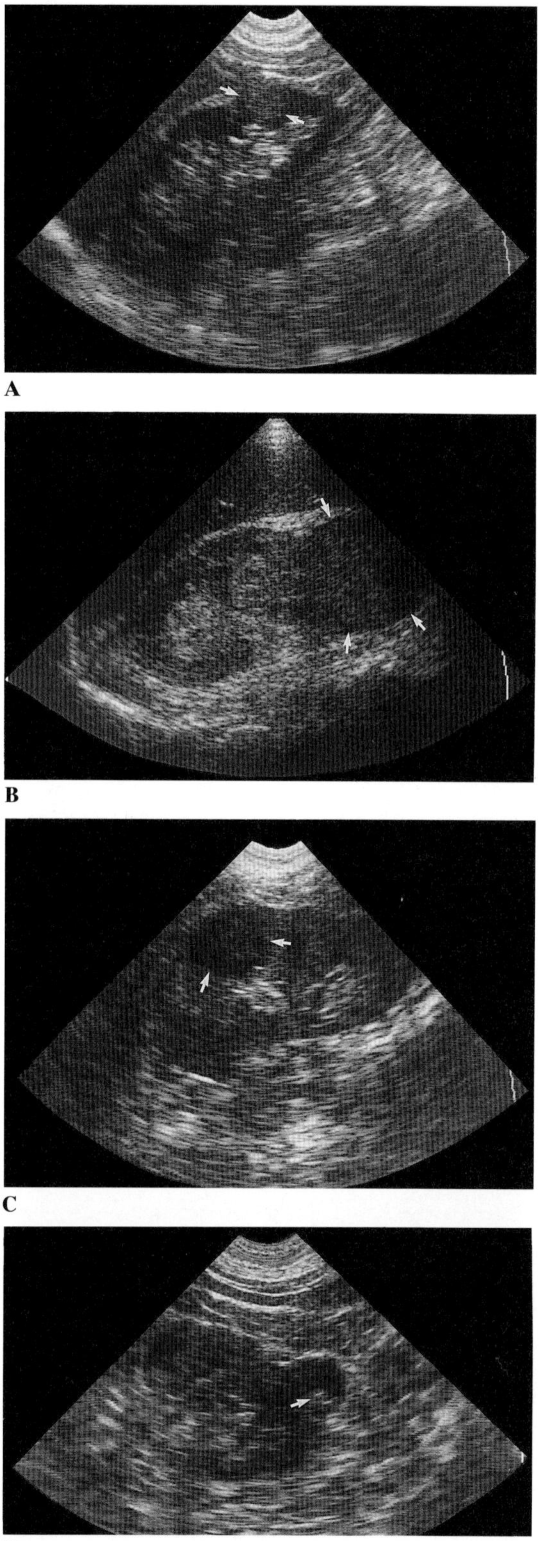

4–5 Hypernephromas may be **(A)** more echogenic than normal renal cortex (arrow); **(B)** the same echogenicity as renal cortex (arrows); or **(C)** less echogenic (arrows). **(D)** Wall nodularity (arrow) is demonstrated in small cystic tumor.

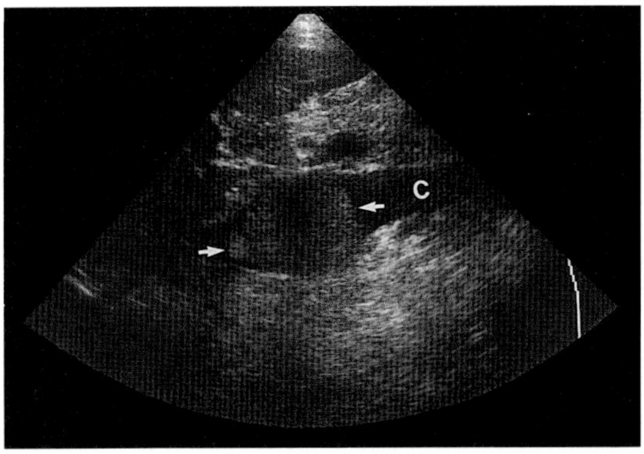

4–6 Longitudinal scan shows thrombus (arrows) within inferior vena cava (C) in patient with large hypernephroma (Fig. 4–5 B). Patient's head is to left, feet to right.

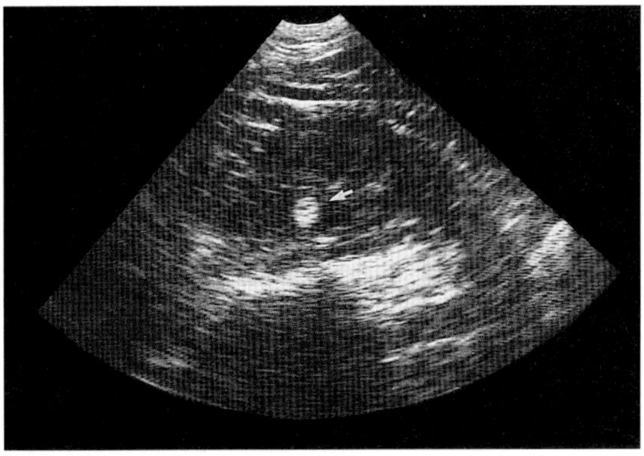

4–7 **(A)** Typical angiomyolipoma appears as a small, discrete focus of increased echogenicity (arrow). **(B)** Computed tomography confirms diagnosis, demonstrating small fat-containing mass (arrow).

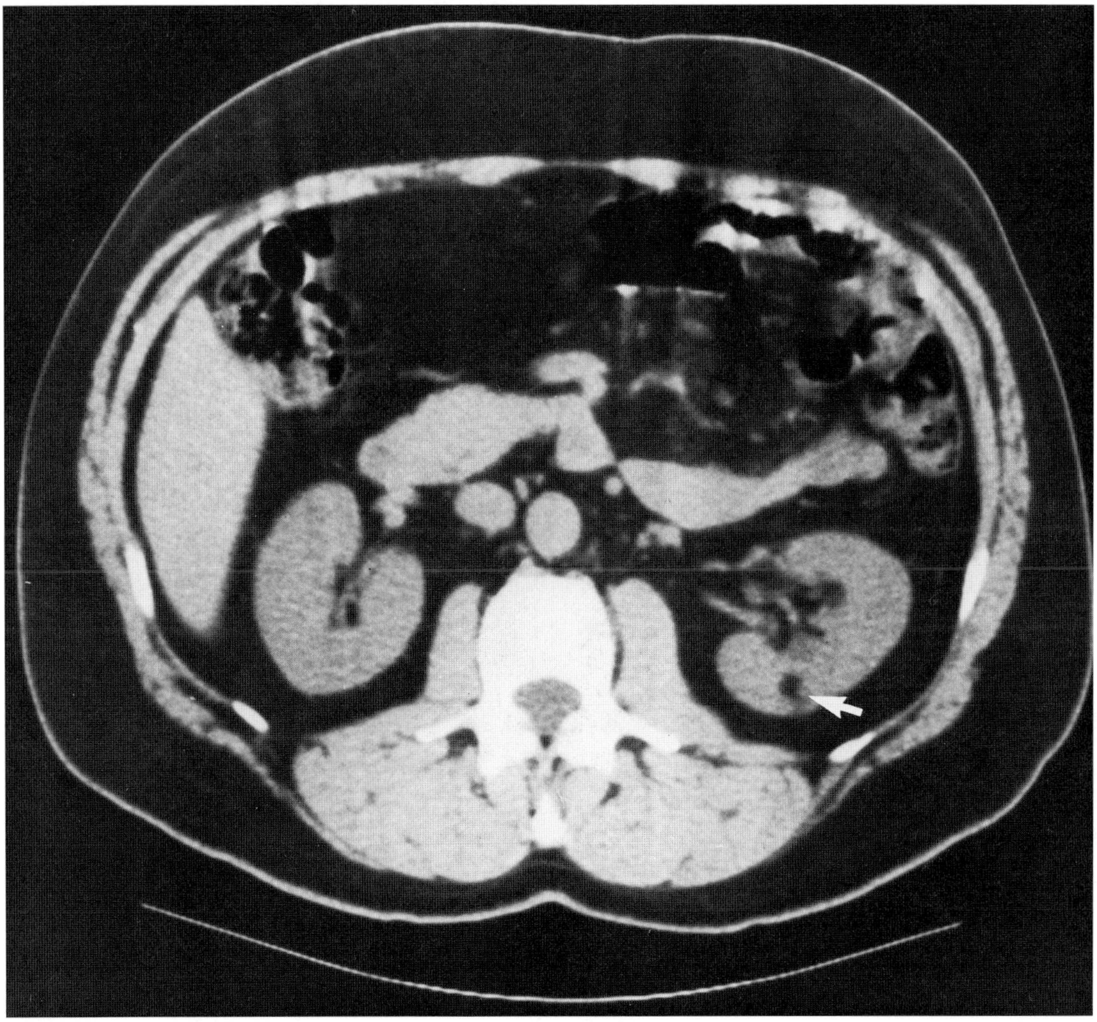

4–7B

Angiomyolipoma usually has a high fat content and typically appears as a well-defined hyperechoic mass on ultrasound (Fig. 4–7). Oncocytomas may have a hypoechoic central scar. Renal lymphoma presents as a renal mass 80% of the time, but it can present as diffuse renal enlargement.

Not all solid parenchymal masses are neoplastic. Persistence of fetal lobe configuration and excessive prominence of a normal cortical column, also termed a column of Bertin, can produce a mass effect on urography and displace the pelvicaliceal complex on ultrasound; however, this area shows normal parenchymal echoes and does not distort the normal external renal contour. In a series of 22 cases of large columns of Bertin (Lafortune et al. 1986), the most common location was the junction between the upper and middle third of the left kidney.

Evaluation of Renal Failure

There are three causes for renal failure: renal artery thrombosis (prerenal failure), intrinsic renal disease, and obstructive uropathy. Renal size, echogenicity, and presence or absence of hydronephrosis can usually be determined by ultrasonography. As intrinsic renal disease progresses to chronic renal failure, the cortical echogenicity increases and becomes greater than the liver. Renal length decreases, and the cortex thins with loss of the corticomedullary definition.

Prerenal Failure

Renal arterial thrombosis presents with acute renal failure. Occasionally, echogenic material may be detected within a renal artery, and a Doppler study shows no flow. However, normal renal vessels are often difficult to study with either real-time or Doppler analysis because of kidney location deep in the body. Transplant kidneys, on the other hand, can be studied readily with these methods because of the superficial position of the allograft. Acute sonographic changes include increased renal size and decreased echogenicity secondary to edema. Focal areas of infarction may present initially as hypoechoic masses and later as echogenic or atrophic regions in the renal cortex secondary to fatty infiltration, fibrosis, or scarring. As renal thrombosis becomes chronic, cortical echogenicity increases and size decreases.

Intrinsic Renal Disease

Acute tubular necrosis often results in normal-appearing kidneys, although, at times, the medullary pyramids are prominent. Acute glomerulonephritis and other autoimmune processes may result in renal enlargement initially, but chronically the kidneys are small and echogenic. Chronic pyelonephritis is usually a focal process resulting in cortical scars over an enlarged distorted calix. In papillary necrosis, a sloughed papilla creates an anechoic space adjacent to the renal sinus, which may be confused with a caliceal diverticulum or hydronephrosis.

Adult autosomal dominant polycystic kidney disease and medullary cystic disease are two diseases frequently complicated by renal failure. In adult polycystic renal disease, ultrasound may be useful to confirm the diagnosis, to follow the anatomic progression of disease, to detect extrarenal abdominal cysts, and to screen family members. However, a patient should not be given this diagnosis solely on the basis of an ultrasound exam demonstrating only several renal cysts bilaterally, as these can occur unassociated with polycystic disease and without serious sequelae. In the appropriate clinical setting, the detection of cystic changes within the renal medulla should suggest medullary cystic disease.

Obstructive Uropathy

Five percent of cases of renal failure are caused by obstruction of the collecting system. Ultrasonography should be used to rapidly exclude or confirm the presence of obstruction in the azotemic patient, obviating the need for intravenous contrast media. As the upper collecting system fills with fluid, it displaces the normal central echoes with anechoic fluid (Fig. 4–8). The fluid-filled calices can be sonographically followed into the dilated renal pelvis and proximal ureter. Ultrasonography may reveal lymphadenopathy, retroperitoneal fibrosis, aneurysm, or pelvic mass as a cause of the obstruction. Often, however, overlying bowel gas interrupts sound wave transmission over the ureter, and the cause of obstruction will not be evident from the sonogram alone.

The sensitivity of ultrasound for detecting hydronephrosis approaches 100%. The rare false-negative cases include instances of retroperitoneal fibrosis when the renal pelvis cannot dilate or when a staghorn calculus fills the collecting system and acoustical shadowing from the calculus obscures the dilation. Laing and colleagues (1985) reported that ultrasound is not as sensitive as urography in

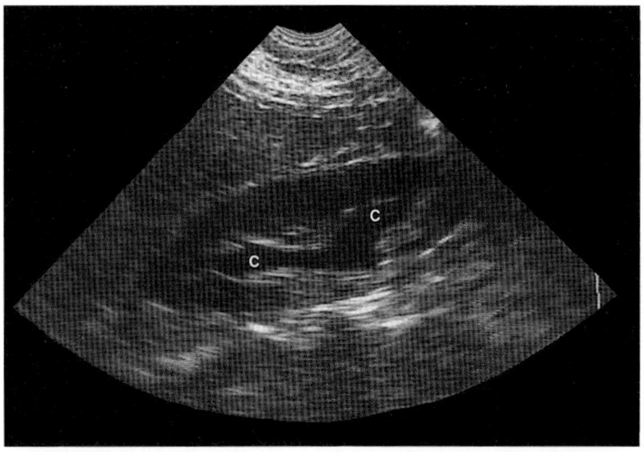

A

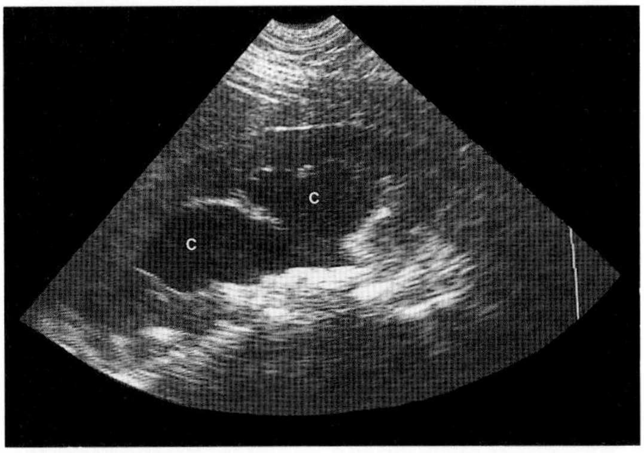

B

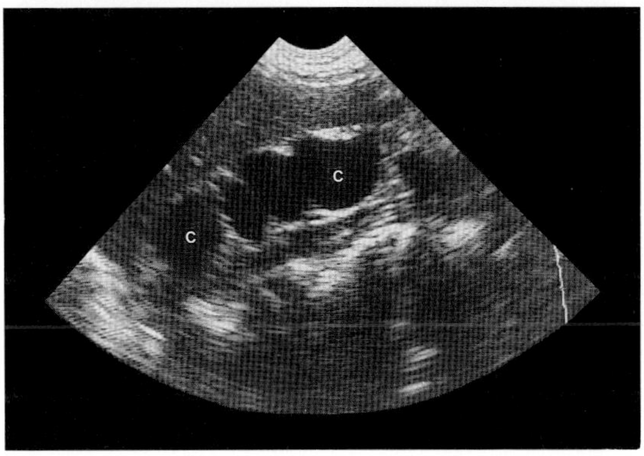

C

4–8 **(A)** Mild, **(B)** moderate, and **(C)** severe hydronephrosis show progressive distension of fluid-filled collecting system **(C)** and splaying of central echo complex.

detecting hydronephrosis caused by acute ureteral obstruction with a calculus. For fluid-depleted patients, the urographic contrast media acts as a fluid load to the kidney and collecting system, emphasizing the dilation. In these patients, sensitivity of the ultrasound exam is improved by adequate oral hydration beforehand, intravenously if necessary (Erwin et al. 1984, 1985).

Optimal hydration also results in a full bladder – assuming complete bilateral obstruction is not complete – through which a distal ureteral or ureterovesical junction stone may be identified

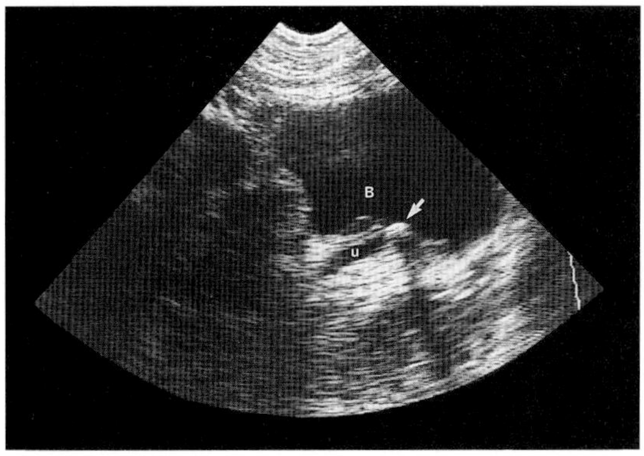

4–9 Oblique scan through urinary bladder (B) shows dilated ureter (U) and shadowing from calculus, obstructing ureterovesical junction (arrow).

(Fig. 4–9). A major disadvantage of sonography versus urography is failure to visualize much of the ureter and the site of obstruction, due to overlying bowel gas.

The specificity of sonographic findings of hydronephrosis is 90%–93%, with false-positive results ranging from 8%–26% (Amis et al. 1982). Many anatomic and physiologic causes of dilation may mimic hydronephrosis, including: a prominent extrarenal pelvis; a distended urinary bladder with prominent calices, which revert to normal following voiding; congenital megacalices; and caliceal diverticula. Ultrasound scans should be obtained after voiding, because a distended bladder can cause upper tract dilatation that can be misinterpreted as hydronephrosis.

Pyelonephritis, papillary necrosis, or diuresis from overhydration, medications, or diabetes insipidus may have a similar appearance to hydronephrosis. Vesicoureteral reflux may also result in a false-positive diagnosis of hydronephrosis. With careful observation, sinus lipomatosis, peripelvic cysts, and central tumors (Fig. 4–10) can be distinguished.

Nonvisualized Kidney on Excretory Urography

Multicystic dysplastic kidney, xanthogranulomatous pyelonephritis (Fig. 4–11), and infiltrative processes such as lymphoma, transitional cell carcinoma, or amyloidosis are examples of parenchymal lesions that may result in a unilateral nonfunctioning kidney.

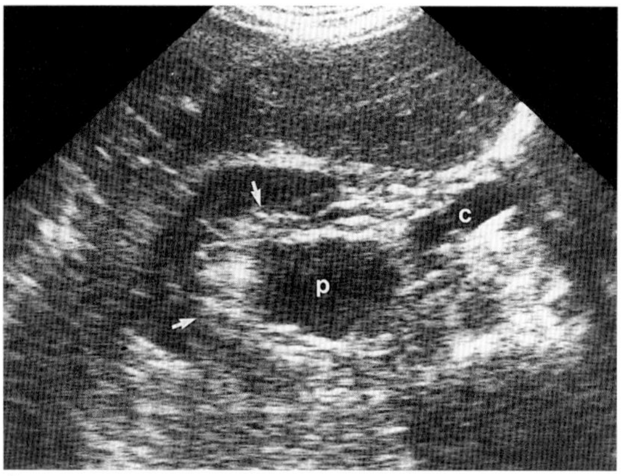

A

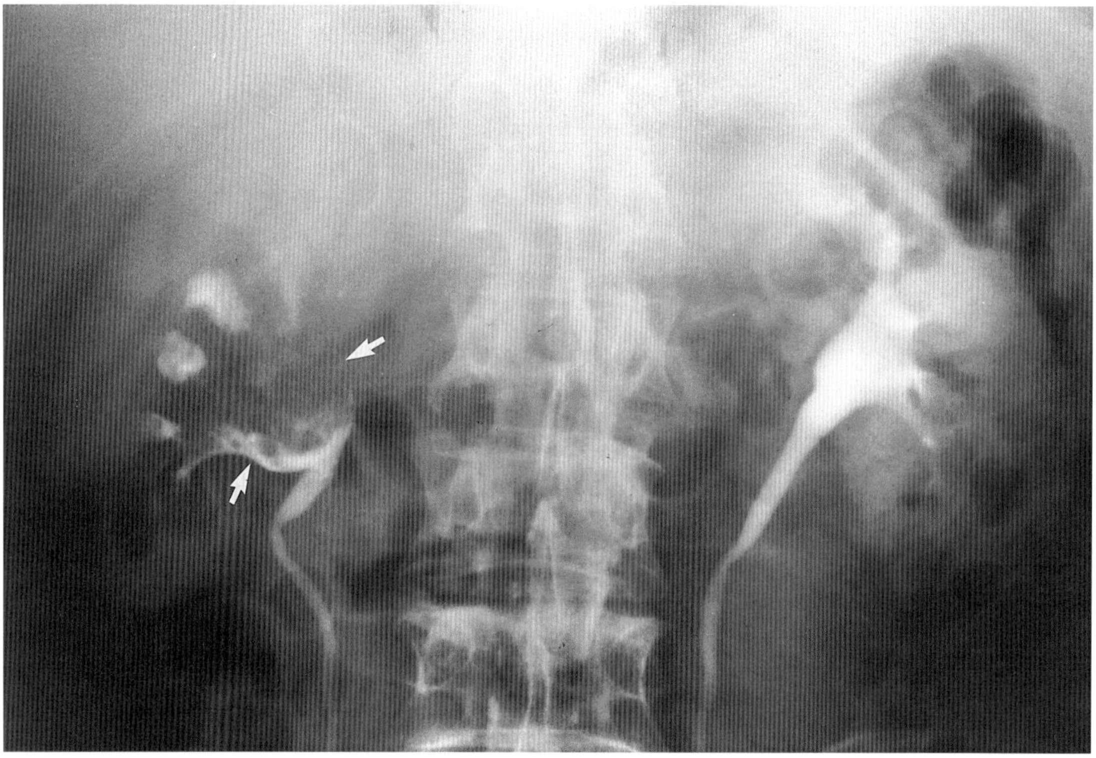

B

4–10 Potential false-positive for hydronephrosis due to large transitional cell tumor in renal pelvis. **(A)** Transverse scan at level of right renal hilum with spreading of central echoes (arrows). Note less acoustical enhancement present behind renal pelvis (P) than posterior to adjacent fluid-filled inferior vena cava (C). **(B)** Renal pelvis of right kidney is filled with transitional cell tumor on urogram (arrows). (Courtesy S. Teefey, Seattle, WA.)

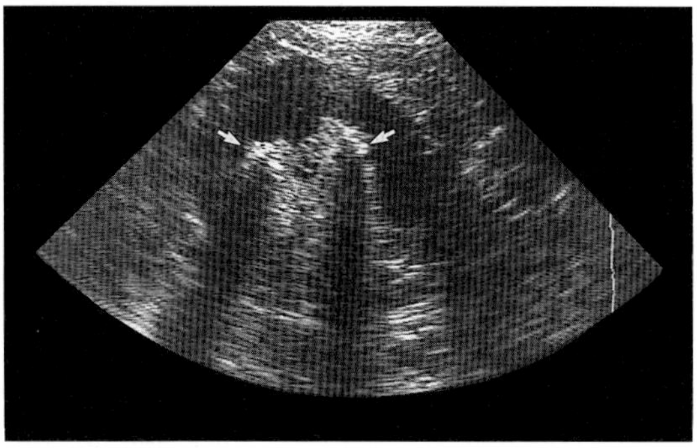

4–11 Prominent central calculi (arrows) demonstrate acoustical shadowing in patient with xanthogranulomatous pyelonephritis and nonvisualized kidney on urogram.

Ultrasonography is an excellent technique to investigate the patient in whom one kidney is poorly visualized on the excretory urogram. The sonogram should be interpreted in conjunction with the urogram. A hydronephrotic nonfunctioning kidney can be distinguished from other conditions that produce a hypofunctioning kidney. However, a small kidney may be difficult to image because of its size. Increased echogenicity may also make it hard to distinguish the kidney from surrounding retroperitoneal structures. When the kidney is not seen in the renal fossa, an ectopic location should be considered.

Renal Infection

Acute pyelonephritis may cause no sonographic change or may result in diffuse enlargement with a heterogenous parenchymal pattern. Focal, hypoechoic, solid-appearing masses that disrupt the corticomedullary junction may be seen in acute bacterial nephritis (Fig. 4–12). These masses have a nonspecific sonographic appearance, but the clinical situation should suggest the diagnosis. Ultrasound may be useful in monitoring treatment. If the mass persists and becomes more sonolucent with better defined margins, an abscess is likely to develop, and percutaneous aspiration and drainage can be performed with ultrasound guidance.

Renal abscess is differentiated from a simple cyst by the presence of a thicker, more irregular wall. Internal echoes are more prevalent, and there may be acoustical shadowing from small gas bubbles. However, sonographic transmission may be similar to that seen with a simple cyst. On sonographic criteria alone, a renal abscess cannot be distinguished from a cystic tumor or hemorrhagic cyst; fine-needle aspiration for gram stain and culture is essential. Needle tract seeding of infection or tumor is not a problem with fine-needle techniques.

Ultrasonography is useful in detecting perinephric abscesses. The sonographic appearance of an irregular sonolucent or hypoechoic mass, adjacent to or partially surrounding the kidney, with posterior acoustical enhancement, suggests the diagnosis. Gas within an abscess may produce extreme echogenicity and even obscure coexisting fluid or the adjacent kidney. Perinephric hemato-

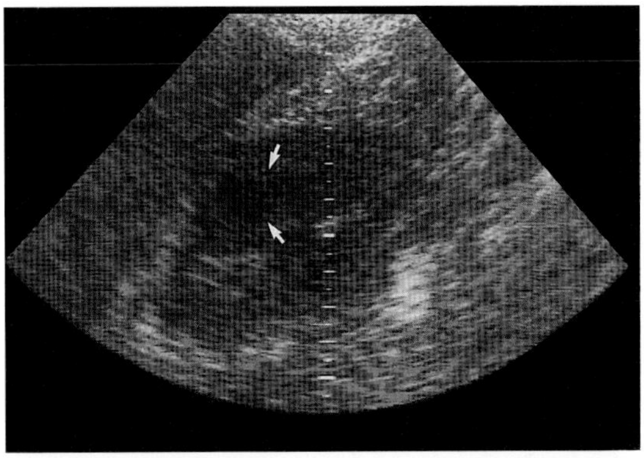

4–12 (A) Subtle area of decreased echogenicity is seen in the renal cortex (arrows) due to localized nephritis (lobar nephronia). **(B)** Abnormality is better defined as low attenuation region by computed tomography (arrow). (Courtesy L. Mack, Seattle, WA.)

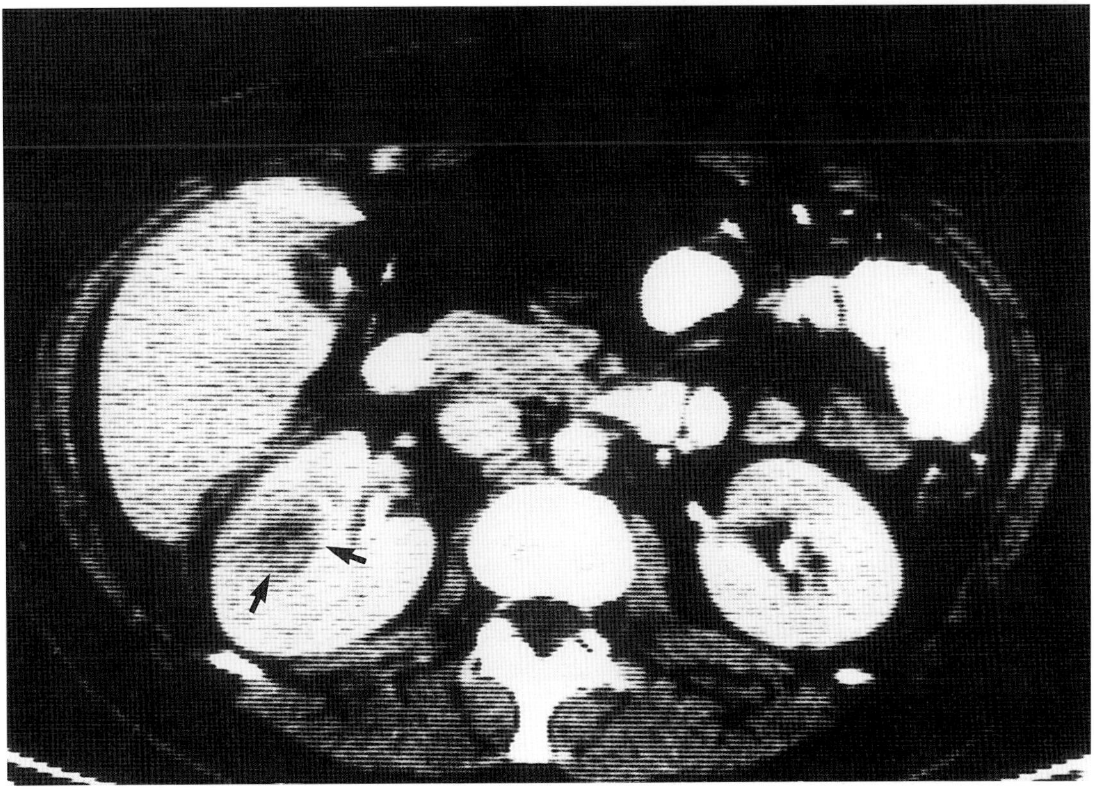

ma (Fig. 4–13) and urinoma may have a similar appearance, although urinoma tends to be more inferomedial to the kidney. Computed tomography is generally the preferred procedure for defining pararenal processes.

Renal Stones

Renal calculi can be diagnosed by the presence of high amplitude echoes with posterior acoustic shadowing (Fig. 4–14). The ability of sonography to detect stones depends on their size and position, and a calculus medially located in the renal pelvis or at the ureteropelvic junction may be missed. Opaque and nonopaque stones are detected with equal accuracy, but small stones are not seen so well as large ones. In patients allergic to contrast media or who have compromised renal function, sonography can be a primary imaging test.

Using a 7-MHz real-time transducer and a water bath, renal stones as small as 2 mm have been detected in vitro (Stafford et al. 1981). The error rate was 16.6%. Most errors are false-negative, because of small stone size and lack of acoustical shadowing. Intrarenal gas can cause false-positive signs (Fig. 4–15); however, larger amounts of gas should be detected on plain films. Computed tomography without intravenous contrast is generally the most effective test for detecting nonopaque renal calculi.

Echogenic renal pyramids in adults are diagnostic of medullary nephrocalcinosis, even when no calcifications are seen on plain films. In infantile polycystic disease, the medulla may also have increased echogenicity due to extensive tubular ectasia. Cortical calcification may be seen after cortical necrosis.

Sonography facilitates intraoperative removal of renal stones and can detect stones 2 mm or greater in size. The transducer is placed in a sterile plastic sleeve or surgical glove; a gel within the sleeve eliminates air bubbles between transducer and covering. The kidney is then irrigated in sterile saline to produce good contact during the study.

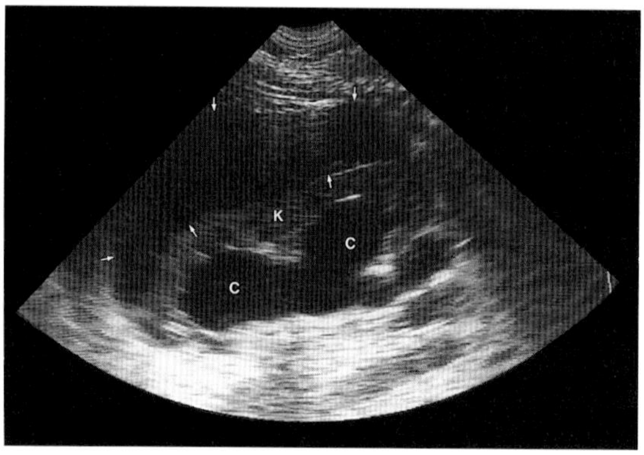

4–13 Perinephric hematoma (arrows) was a complication of extracorporeal shock wave lithotripsy. Stone fragments within the ureter produced the hydronephrosis. K = kidney; C = dilated calices.

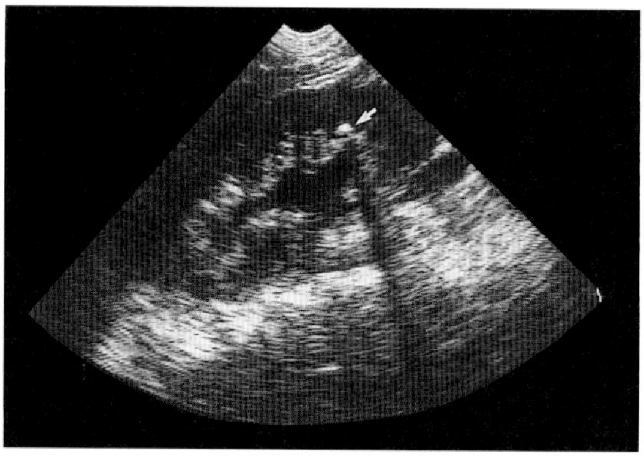

4–14 Typical renal calculus seen as high amplitude echo (arrow) with posterior acoustical shadowing.

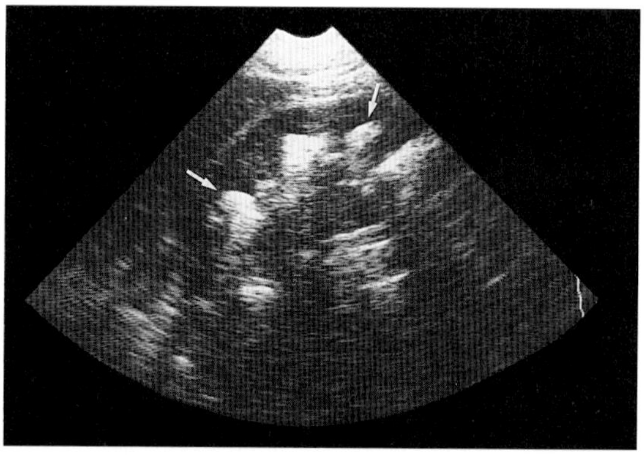

4–15 Potential false-positive scan for renal calculi. Intrarenal gas collections cause areas of intense echogenicity (arrows). No shadowing is present in this case, but can occur with larger accumulations.

Renal Transplant

With ureteral obstruction, marked distension of the transplant collecting system is uncommon because of postoperative fibrosis and scarring; conversely, the collecting system of a renal transplant may be more prominent than a normal kidney in the absence of obstruction, and it is more influenced by bladder distension than the normal system. Postvoid scans should be obtained to see if pelvicaliceal dilatation improves. A radionuclide scan, intravenous urogram, or retrograde study may be necessary for confirmation. If no imaging test offers a definitive answer, trial placement of a ureteral stent may be required.

Fluid collections around the transplant can be detected with ultrasound but usually require clinical correlation, percutaneous aspiration, or additional studies to distinguish the types. Lymphoceles and urinomas are usually simple fluid collections with thin, well-defined wall margins and few, if any, septations. A radionuclide study will confirm a urinoma by demonstrating activity in the space. Hematoma and abscess are more complex masses with thick, irregular walls and internal septations.

Ultrasonography has been used to help detect acute rejection or to distinguish it from acute tubular necrosis. In acute tubular necrosis, the transplant typically appears normal. In severe acute rejection, the ultrasound is generally abnormal and may show progressive renal enlargement, indistinctness of the corticomedullary junction, enlarged hypoechoic medullary pyramids, perivascular edema, and increased cortical echogenicity. However, drug toxicity and glomerulonephritis can produce similar findings. Ultrasound cannot reliably differentiate acute rejection from cyclosporine toxicity (Linkowski et al. 1987). Current reports suggest that duplex sonography will be valuable in detecting acute rejection (Rigsby et al. 1986), in addition to evaluating arterial and venous patency.

Urinary Bladder and Urethra

The wall of the normal urinary bladder is 3 mm–6 mm thick. Because an underfilled bladder may appear falsely thickened, ultrasound of this region should be done on a full bladder. Thickening of the wall by inflammation, infection, or neoplasm may be identified by sonography. Focal sessile and polypoid masses protruding into the bladder lumen may be seen (Fig. 4–16). Biopsy is required to distinguish neoplastic from inflammatory processes. Intravesical lesions that move when the patient shifts position include calculi, blood clots, and fungus balls. Calculi can be distinguished by their accompanying acoustical shadow. Bladder diverticula and ureteroceles can be definitively identified (Fig. 4–17).

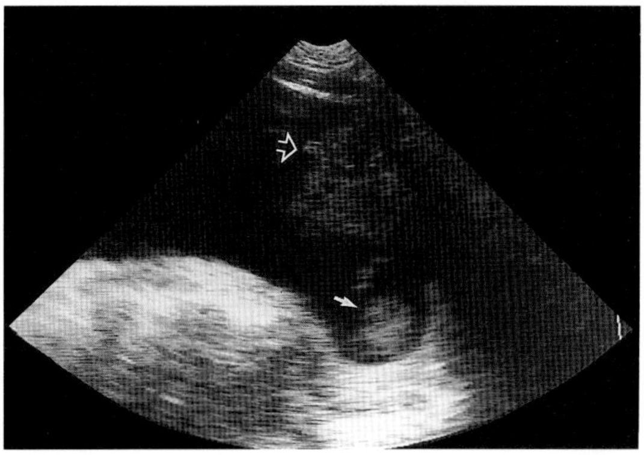

4–16 Longitudinal scan demonstrates frondlike projections (open arrow) from papillary tumor extending into the bladder. Small intravesical blood clot (arrow) caused urinary retention.

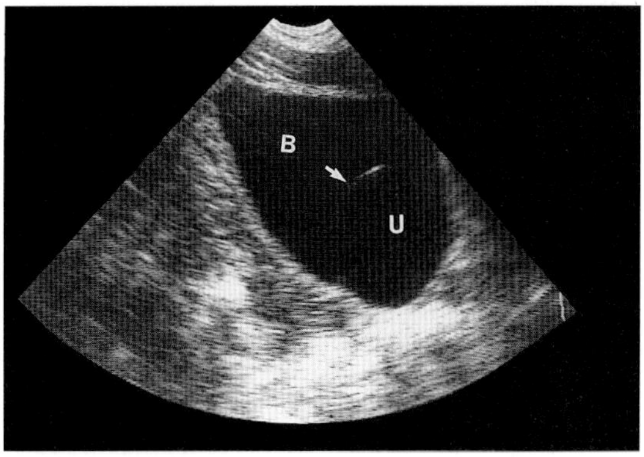

4–17 Oblique scan shows the thin-wall (arrow) of a ureterocele (U) protruding into the bladder (B).

Ultrasound can be used to estimate bladder volume and postvoid residuals. Although there are inaccuracies in the methods for calculating these volumes, the results are clinically helpful. Sonography has been used to evaluate stress incontinence. In neuromuscular bladder dysfunction, Shapeero and colleagues (1983) reported that transrectal real-time voiding cystourethrosonography was superior to radiographic voiding cystourography and reduced the number of urodynamic studies needed.

The urethra is better studied with transrectal or transvaginal sonography than with a transabdominal approach. The latter method can distinguish dilation of the bladder neck and prostatic urethra from posterior urethral valves. Urethral diverticula have been demonstrated in men and women.

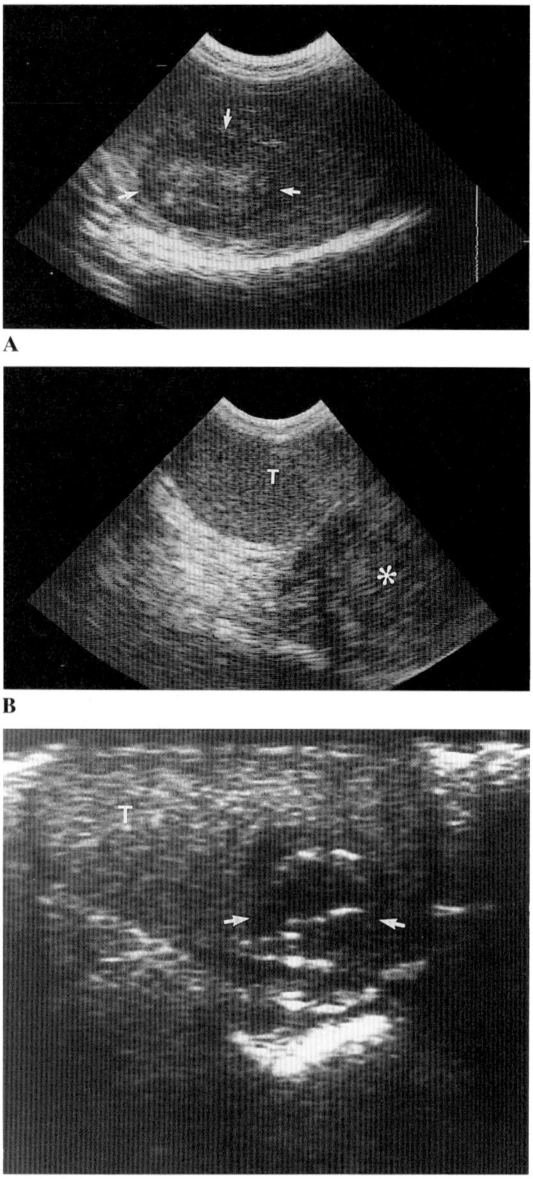

4–18 Spectrum of testicular lesions. **(A)** Well-marginated slightly hyperechoic seminoma (arrows) is distinguished from normal homogeneous testicle. **(B)** Hypoechoic anaplastic carcinoma diffusely involves left testicle (*); opposite, normal right testicle (T) for comparison. **(C)** Discrete complex intratesticular mass (arrows) was an epidermal inclusion cyst. T = normal area of testicle.

Scrotum

Ultrasonography can reveal the cause of scrotal swelling or pain. Differentiation between testicular and extratesticular pathology can be made in nearly all cases (Carroll, Gross 1983). In patients with an unknown primary tumor or testicular tumor in a metastatic site, the clinical exam may be normal, yet ultrasound can reveal a small nonpalpable testicular neoplasm. A normal testicular ultrasound is highly reliable.

The most common sonographic feature of a testicular neoplasm is the presence of a focal testicular mass. Most tumors are predominantly hypoechoic, but a hyperechoic or mixed pattern may be found (Fig. 4–18). A diffuse alteration of the normal homogeneous parenchymal pattern may also occur. Bright echogenic foci without associated masses may be found in regressed tumor (Grantham et al. 1985). Therefore, the sonogram is highly sensitive, but not specific (Fig. 4–18C). Biopsy is necessary to distinguish malignant from benign conditions.

Sonography is often helpful in nonmalignant conditions. In a study by Wolverson and colleagues (1983) of 20 patients with undescended testes, sensitivity was 88%, specificity 100%, and accuracy 91%. The authors concluded that computed tomography should be reserved for cases of negative or equivocal ultrasound. Magnetic resonance imaging is able to define the normal iliac and femoral vessels, and is therefore better for evaluating the undescended testicle than computed tomography. Angiography is rarely required.

Ultrasound may be helpful in defining small varicoceles; large varicoceles are usually apparent from physical examination. During the Valsalva maneuver or with the patient in the upright position, pampiniform plexus veins may dilate more than the normal 1-mm to 2-mm diameter.

Conclusion

Sonography provides a fast, safe, and cost-effective method for evaluating much of the urinary system. It provides anatomically accurate information, but in many instances it is not pathologically specific. Advances in sonographic technology indicate greater future usefulness for this technique.

References

Amis ES, Cronan JJ, Pfister RC, Voder IC: Ultrasonic inaccuracies in diagnosing renal obstruction. *Urology* 19:101–105, 1982.

Brandt TD, Neiman HL, Dragowski MJ, Bulawa W, Claykamp G: Ultrasound assessment of normal renal dimensions. *J. Ultrasound Med.* 1:49–52, 1982.

Carroll BA, Gross DM: High-frequency scrotal sonography. *Am. J. Roentgenol.* 140:511–515, 1983.

Cronan JJ, Zeman RK, Rosenfield AT: Comparison of computerized tomography, ultrasound, and angiography in staging renal cell carcinoma. *J. Urol.* 127:712–714, 1982.

Erwin BC, Carroll BA, Sommer FG: Renal colic: The role of ultrasound in initial evaluation. *Radiology* 152:147–150, 1984.

Erwin BC, Carroll BA, Sommer FG: US in the evaluation of acute flank pain. *Radiology* 157:554, 1985.

Grantham JG, Charboneau JW, James FM, Kirschling RJ, Kvols LK, Segura JW, Wold LE: Testicular neoplasms: 29 tumors studied by high-resolution US. *Radiology* 157:775–780, 1985.

Lafortune M, Constantin A, Breton G, Valle C: Sonography of the hypertrophied column of Bertin. *Am. J. Roentgenol.* 146:53–56, 1986.

Laing FC, Jeffrey RB, Wing VW: Ultrasonography versus excretory urography in evaluating acute flank pain. *Radiology* 154:613–616, 1985.

Levine E, Maklad NF, Rosenthal SJ, Kyo RL, Weigel J: *Urology* 16:317–322, 1980.

Linkowski GD, Warvariv V, Filly R, Vincent F: Sonography in the diagnosis of acute renal allograft rejection and cyclosporine nephrotoxicity. *Am. J. Roentgenol.* 148:291–295, 1987.

Pollack HM, Banner MP, Arger PH, Peters J, Mulhern CB, Coleman BG: The accuracy of gray scale renal ultrasonography in differentiating cystic neoplasms from benign cysts. *Radiology* 143:741–745, 1982.

Rigsby CM, Taylor KJW, Wattin G, Burns PN, Bia M, Princenthal RA, Kashgarian M, Flye MW: Renal allografts in acute rejection. Evaluation using duplex sonography. *Radiology* 158:375–378, 1986.

Shapeero LG, Friedland GW, Perkash I: Transrectal sonographic voiding cystourethrography. Studies in neuromuscular bladder dysfunction. *Am. J. Roentgenol.* 141:83–90, 1983.

Sommer FG, Filly RA, Minton MJ: Acoustic shadowing due to refractive and reflective effects. *Am. J. Roentgenol.* 132:973–977, 1979.

Stafford SJ, Jenkins JM, Staab EV, Boyce I, Fried FA: Ultrasonic detection of renal calculi: Accuracy tested in an in vitro porcine kidney model. *J. Clin. Ultrasound* 9:359–363, 1981.

Wolverson MK, Houttuin E, Heiberg E, Sundaram M, Shields JB: Comparison of computed tomography with high-resolution real-time ultrasound in the location of the impalpable undescended testicle. *Radiology* 146:133–136, 1983.

Suggested Reading

Amis ES, Hartman DS: Renal ultrasonography, 1984: A practical overview. *Radiol. Clin. North Am.* 22:315–332, 1984.

Bosniak MA: The current radiological approach to renal cysts. *Radiology* 158:1–10, 1986.

Charboneau JW, Hattery RR, Ernst EC, James EM, Williamson B, Hartman G: Spectrum of sonographic findings in 125 renal masses other than benign simple cyst. *Am. J. Roentgenol.* 140:87–94, 1983.

Ellenbogen PH, Scheible FW, Talner LB, Leopold GR: Sensitivity of gray scale ultrasound in detecting urinary tract obstruction. *Am. J. Roentgenol.* 130:731–733, 1978.

Lee JKT, McClennan BL, Meison GL, Stanley RJ: Acute focal bacterial nephritis: Emphasis on gray scale sonography and computed tomography. *Am. J. Roentgenol.* 135:87–92, 1980.

McClennan BL: Current approaches to the azotemic patient. *Radiol. Clin. North Am.* 17:197–211, 1979.

Orgaz RE, Gomez AZ, Ramirez CT, Torres JL: Applications of bladder ultrasonography. Bladder content and residue. *Urology* 125:174–176, 1981.

Resnick MI, Sanders RC: *Ultrasound in Urology.* Baltimore, Williams & Wilkins, 1979.

Rifkin MD: Ultrasonography of the lower genitourinary tract. *Urol. Clin. North Am.* 12:645–656, 1985.

Rifkin MD, Kurtz AB, Pasto ME, Goldberg BB: Diagnostic capabilities of high-resolution scrotal ultrasonography: Prospective evaluation. *J. Ultrasound Med.* 4:13–19, 1985.

Rosenberg ER, Korobkin M, Foster W, Silverman PM, Bowie JD, Dunnick NR: The significance of septations in a renal cyst. *Am. J. Roentgenol.* 144:593–595, 1985.

Scheible W, Talner LB: Gray scale ultrasound in the genitourinary tract. A review of clinical applications. *Radiol. Clin. North Am.* 17:281–300, 1979.

Tackett RE, Ling D, Catalona WJ, Melson GL: High resolution sonography in diagnosing testicular neoplasms: Clinical significance of false-positive scans. *J. Urol.* 135:494–496, 1986.

CHAPTER

5

Radionuclide Testing of the Urinary System

Eva V. Dubovsky

The radiopharmaceuticals that measure effective renal plasma flow (ERPF), glomerular filtration rate (GFR), transit times, and bladder kinetics are as important as the imaging of urological systems or organs. With recent progress in structural imaging by ultrasound, computed tomography (CT), and magnetic resonance (MR), the role of nephrologic nuclear medicine clearly lies in quantitative functional evaluation of the urinary tract.

Renal radiopharmaceuticals contain small amounts of chemical carriers and radioactive tracers that result in less radiation exposure than standard radiographic examinations. In addition, there are no osmotic or ionic changes and few pharmacologic effects or allergic reactions. This lack of side effects is especially important in renal transplantation, pediatric, and end-stage renal disease patients.

Radiopharmaceuticals

The disappearance of selected radiopharmaceuticals from the blood and their localization and appearance in the kidney and urine can provide a quantitative index of renal function. These agents can be used for kidney and bladder imaging if a suitable gamma ray emitting isotope is used as a label (Table 5–1).

Drugs are excreted from the kidneys by two mechanisms – glomerular filtration and tubular secretion. Chelates, such as ethylenediaminetetraacetic acid (EDTA) or diethylenetriaminepentaacetic acid (DTPA), are excreted only by glomerular filtration. Orthoiodohippurate (OIH), excreted by filtration in the glomeruli and secretion in the proximal convoluted tubules, is almost completely eliminated from the plasma, and thus can be used to measure renal plasma flow. The ability of a radiopharmaceutical to measure GFR depends on the state in which it exists in the plasma, since only the fraction unbound to proteins or red cells can be filtered. A third group of agents, such as dimercaptosuccinic acid (DMSA) and glucoheptonate (GH), is bound to the renal parenchyma. All of these agents concentrate to varying degrees in the cortex and localize in the cells of the proximal and distal tubules.

Radiopharmaceutical selection therefore depends on the clinical problem. After intravenous bolus injection, all radiopharmaceuticals are carried in the bloodstream to the kidneys and, during their first pass, provide information about regional perfusion. In this capacity, the usefulness of each material depends only on the quantity and type of radioactive label, since information improves as the number of detected gamma rays

Table 5–1 Abbreviation Key

Radiopharmaceuticals:	
^{51}Cr-EDTA	Chromium-ethylenediaminetetra-acidic acid
^{67}Ga-Citrate	Gallium citrate
^{131}I-OIH	Iodine-Orthoiodohippurate
^{111}In-WBC	Indium-labeled white blood cells
^{99m}Tc-DMSA	Technetium-dimercaptosuccinic acid
^{99m}Tc-DTPA	Technetium-diethylenetriaminepenta-acidic acid
^{99m}Tc-GH	Technetium-glucoheptonate
^{99m}Tc-MAG$_3$	Technetium-mercaptoacetyltriglycine
^{99m}Tc-Sulfur Colloid	Technetium-sulfur colloid
Nonradio-pharmaceuticals:	
EI	Excretory index
ERPF	Effective renal plasma flow
GFR	Glomerular filtration rate
PAH	Para-aminohippuric acid
SPECT	Single proton emission computed tomography

Table 5–2 Renal Radiopharmaceuticals: Recommended Doses and Dosimetry

Radiopharmaceutical	Recommended Dose (MBq)[a]	% Dose in Kidneys	Radiation Absorbed Dose (mGy)		
			Kidney[b]	Bladder[c]	WB[d]
^{99m}Tc-DTPA	370–740	8	4.4	56	1.8
^{99m}Tc-GH	370–740	12	40[d]	160	1.4
^{99m}Tc-DMSA	180q	42	38[e]	15	0.8
^{131}I-OIH	11.1[f]	N/A	0.28	13.5	0.054
^{123}I-OIH[g]	37	N/A	0.21	9.5	0.08

[a] MBq, mega becquerel.
[b] Radiation dose using maximum recommended dose in a standard man with normal function.
[c] Radiation absorbed dose to the bladder wall when bladder is empty before test and patient does not void for 4 hr.
[d] WB, whole body.
[e] Renal cortex.
[f] 5.5 MBq per kidney.
[g] If no contaminants are present.

increases. Within the first minute, the agent is well mixed with plasma. Its fate then depends on the mode in which the kidney extracts the nonradioactive carrier from the blood, regardless of which radionuclide is used as a tracer. If the carrier is rapidly excreted, the material will be more suitable for functional studies and evaluation of the collecting system. If the carrier is retained in the tubular cells, the material will provide information about the renal cortex.

In recent years, ^{131}I or ^{123}I-labeled OIH, ^{99m}Tc-DTPA, ^{99m}Tc-GH, and ^{99m}Tc-DMSA have been the most frequently used radiopharmaceuticals. Mercaptoacetylglycylglycylglycine (^{99m}Tc-MAG$_3$) is one of several new agents being tested as possible replacements for iodine-labeled agents (Chervu, Blaufox 1982; Taylor et al. 1986).

^{131}I-OIH

Most of the OIH entering the kidney is extracted from the plasma by filtration and secretion during a single pass; therefore, the rate of its extraction is a measure of ERPF (Dubovsky, Russell 1982). About two-thirds of the OIH is reversibly bound to plasma proteins; the unbound fraction is filtered. The remainder is carried through the efferent arterioles to the peritubular capillaries, from which it is rapidly extracted by the tubular cells. OIH extraction and excretion are faster than that of any other agent. Within 1 min, 18% of the injected dose is localized in the kidneys; at 3 to 5 min, peak concentration (about 25% of the dose) is reached. The normal mean parenchymal transit time of hippurate in well-hydrated subjects is 2.2 min; 40% to 50% accumulates in the urine within 15 min, 70% within 30 min, and over 80% in 60 min. Excretion via the hepatobiliary pathway, which is negligible (2%) in normal subjects, becomes more prominent in patients with chronic renal failure, appearing as increased liver uptake.

Desirable biological properties of OIH, unfortunately, are counterbalanced by physical properties of the labeling agent. The relatively high-energy gamma rays of ^{131}I are not imaged efficiently by a scintillation camera, and its beta particles are responsible for a high radiation absorbed dose, thus limiting the permissible dosage. In patients with normal renal function, the radiation dose from 300 μCi (11.0 MBq) of ^{131}I-OIH is approximately 0.3 mGy to the kidneys, 0.06 mGy to the whole body, 0.12 mGy to the testes, 0.2 mGy to the ovaries, and 6.4 mGy, 10 mGy, and 13.5 mGy to the bladder wall at 2 hr, 3 hr, and 4 hr, respectively (Tables 5–2, 5–3).

A significant reduction in the radiation absorbed dose to the bladder can be achieved by studying the patient with 50 ml to 150 ml of urine in the bladder at the time of OIH administration and immediately emptying the bladder when the test is completed. In diseased kidneys, the radiation absorbed dose will depend on the percentage removed from the circulation and the resident time in the kidney parenchyma or collecting system.

Table 5–3 Radiation Quantities and Units

1 Gy (gray)	= 100 rad
1 rad	= 10 mGy
1 mGy	= 100 mrad
1 Sv (sievert)	= 100 rem
1 rem	= 10 mSv
1 mSv	= 100 mrem
1 Bq (becquerel)	= 1 disintegration per sec
1 Ci (curie)	= 3.7×10^{10} disintegrations per sec
1 Ci	= 3.7×10^{10} Bq
1 mCi	= 37 MBq (mega becquerel)
1 MBq	= 0.027 mCi

OIH is commercially available with less than 2% free iodide; large amounts of free iodide introduce an error in measurement of ERPF, since the iodide is cleared from the blood at a different rate than OIH. In addition, the radiation absorbed dose to the thyroid gland may become very high. The newer ^{123}I-OIH provides an ideal imaging energy and more favorable dosimetry.

^{99m}Tc-DTPA

The biological behavior of ^{99m}Tc-DTPA closely resembles that of the radiographic contrast agents diatrizoate and iothalamate, other chelates (EDTA), and inulin. ^{99m}Tc-DTPA is removed from circulation by glomerular filtration. Renal peak concentration is reached in 3 min to 5 min, and mean intraparenchymal transit time is about 3 min, at which time the anatomy of the kidneys is best defined. The high concentration of ^{99m}Tc-DTPA in the urine (50% at 2 hr, 95% at 24 hr) is helpful in assessing the pelvocaliceal system (Arnold et al. 1975).

Radiation absorbed dose is approximately 6 μGy/MBq to the kidneys, less than 3.5 μGy/MBq to the gonads, and 20 μGy/MBq to the whole body. However, the bladder wall can receive as much as 0.076 mGy/MBq (60 mGy/740 MBq), if the bladder is not emptied immediately after completion of the test (Tables 5–2 and 5–3).

^{99m}Tc-DMSA

Most of the injected DMSA is bound to plasma proteins. Its blood clearance is slow, renal uptake high (25% at 1 hr, 40% at 6 hr), and urinary excretion low (10% at 1 hr, 40% at 24 hr). Excellent detail of the cortex is obtained by imaging at 3–6 hr. Liver uptake is relatively high in patients with renal insufficiency, and 24-hr delayed scintigrams may be necessary. High uptake and prolonged time in the renal parenchyma are responsible for the relatively high radiation absorbed dose to the kidneys (0.2 mGy/MBq) (Atkins, Thomas 1985; Table 5–2).

^{99m}Tc-GH

Glucoheptonate forms a stable complex with technetium that disappears rapidly from the blood and appears in the urine at approximately the same rate as agents that measure GFR. ^{99m}Tc-GH is suited for perfusion studies and evaluation of the collecting system early after injection and can demonstrate cortical morphology on delayed views, as with ^{99m}Tc-DMSA. Approximately 12% of the dose accumulates in the renal cortex at 3 hr.

The absorbed radiation dose to the renal parenchyma is much lower with GH than DMSA because of the former's lower concentration in the renal cortex; this permits use of a higher dose (550–740 MBq) (Tables 5–2, 5–3).

^{99m}Tc-MAG$_3$

^{99m}Tc-MAG$_3$, a new technetium labeled analog of OIH, has recently become available. Its advantages include short biological T-½, excellent imaging properties, and low radiation absorbed dose. The ^{99m}Tc-MAG$_3$ images are superior to those obtained with OIH, and the time-activity curves differ only in minor detail. Bolus perfusion images can be obtained, as with other Tc-labeled agents. Although plasma clearance of ^{99m}Tc-MAG$_3$ is lower than that of OIH, the two are strongly correlated, so that it can be used for quantitation of renal function.

Secondary Radiopharmaceuticals

Some radiopharmaceuticals, normally used for imaging other organs, provide useful information about the kidneys. On bone scintigrams, over 30% of the injected dose of ^{99m}Tc-labeled phosphates is excreted in the urine within 3 hr. Early postinjection images can detect renal lesions and evaluate differential renal function. Space-occupying lesions (tumors, cysts, and abscesses) generally appear as areas of reduced uptake. Diffusely increased renal uptake can be found in radiation nephritis, after amphotericin or cancer chemotherapy, and in heterotopic calcifications and iron overload states. Retention of activity in the collecting system usually indicates obstruction (Fig. 5–1), but can be due to extrarenal pelvis, atonic system, reflux, or congenital megaureter.

^{67}Ga-citrate imaging may also demonstrate renal disease, since 30% of the ^{67}Ga dose is excreted in the urine during the first 24-hr period. Persistent uptake in the kidneys after 48 hr is strong evidence of renal disease, such as pyelonephritis, interstitial nephritis, lymphoma, infected polycystic kidneys,

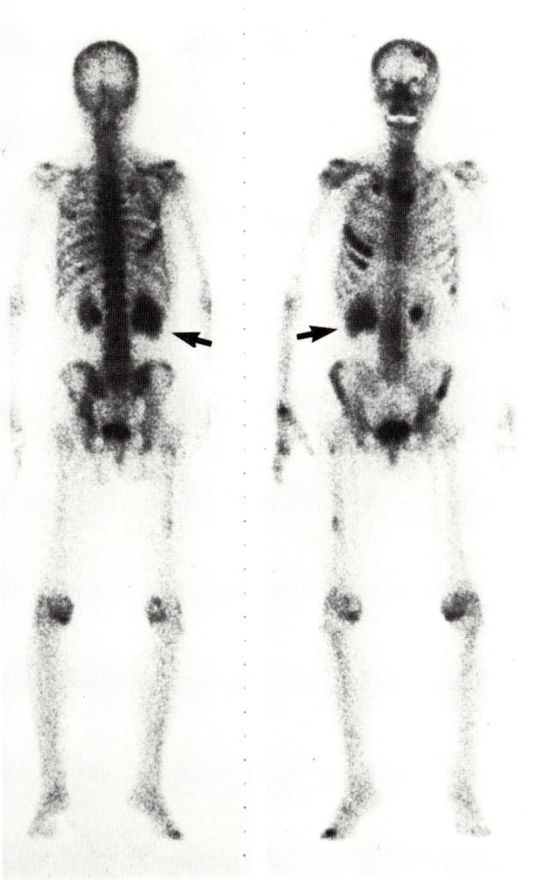

5–1 Bone scintigram (740 MBq ^{99m}Tc-MDP) demonstrating widespread metastatic disease from prostate carcinoma. Bone scan also demonstrates right hydronephrosis (arrow).

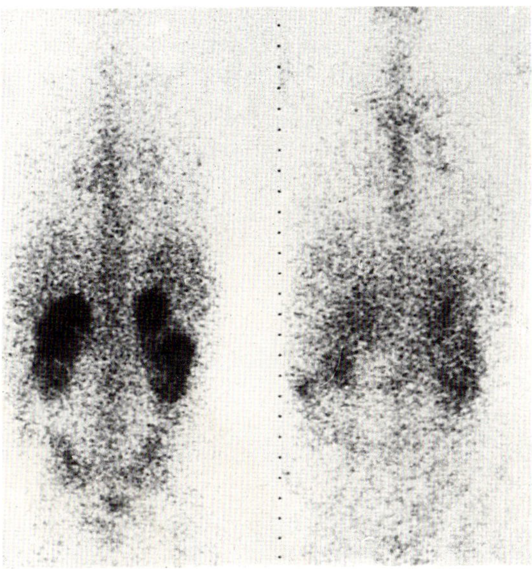

5–2 ^{67}Gallium citrate (180 MBq) scintigram in patient with lymphoma primarily involving kidneys. Additional abnormal findings are present in both perihilar regions.

or amyloidosis (Fig. 5–2). ^{67}Ga scintigrams also demonstrate renal metastases from ^{67}Ga-concentrating tumors, such as melanoma. Striking uptake is occasionally seen in hypernephroma, but not consistently enough to be useful in evaluating renal tumors.

Technical Aspects of Renal Imaging

Instrumentation

A low-energy, all-purpose, parallel-hole collimator is usually used with Tc-labeled agents. Resolution of static images with DMSA or GH may be improved using high-resolution or pinhole collimators. ^{123}I and ^{131}I both require a medium- or high-energy collimator. If the available camera has only a small field of view, it may be necessary to use a diverging collimator.

Patients are examined in the supine position with the detector beneath the table. A sitting or standing position is also used for evaluation of renal hypertension. An anterior view is obtained in patients with renal transplant or horseshoe kidney, and for study of bladder function.

Scintiangiography

Scintiangiography (perfusion, flow study, first transit) is commonly performed as a first phase of DTPA or GH imaging, and rapid sequence images are obtained while the agent is confined to the intravascular space. Scintiangiography detects whether the blood supply to the kidneys has been impaired or completely blocked and also provides information about symmetry of perfusion (Fig. 5–3).

Structural Imaging

At present, static scintigraphy of renal parenchyma has only a limited role in determining size, shape, and position of the kidneys and in following infectious processes.

^{99m}Tc-DMSA is recommended for static imaging. Administration of 180 MBq allows an early blood pool image, and, after 90 to 120 min, high-quality static images. Efficient accumulation of DMSA in the renal cortex and its negligible urinary excretion are useful in identifying abnormally situated kidneys, such as pelvic and horseshoe

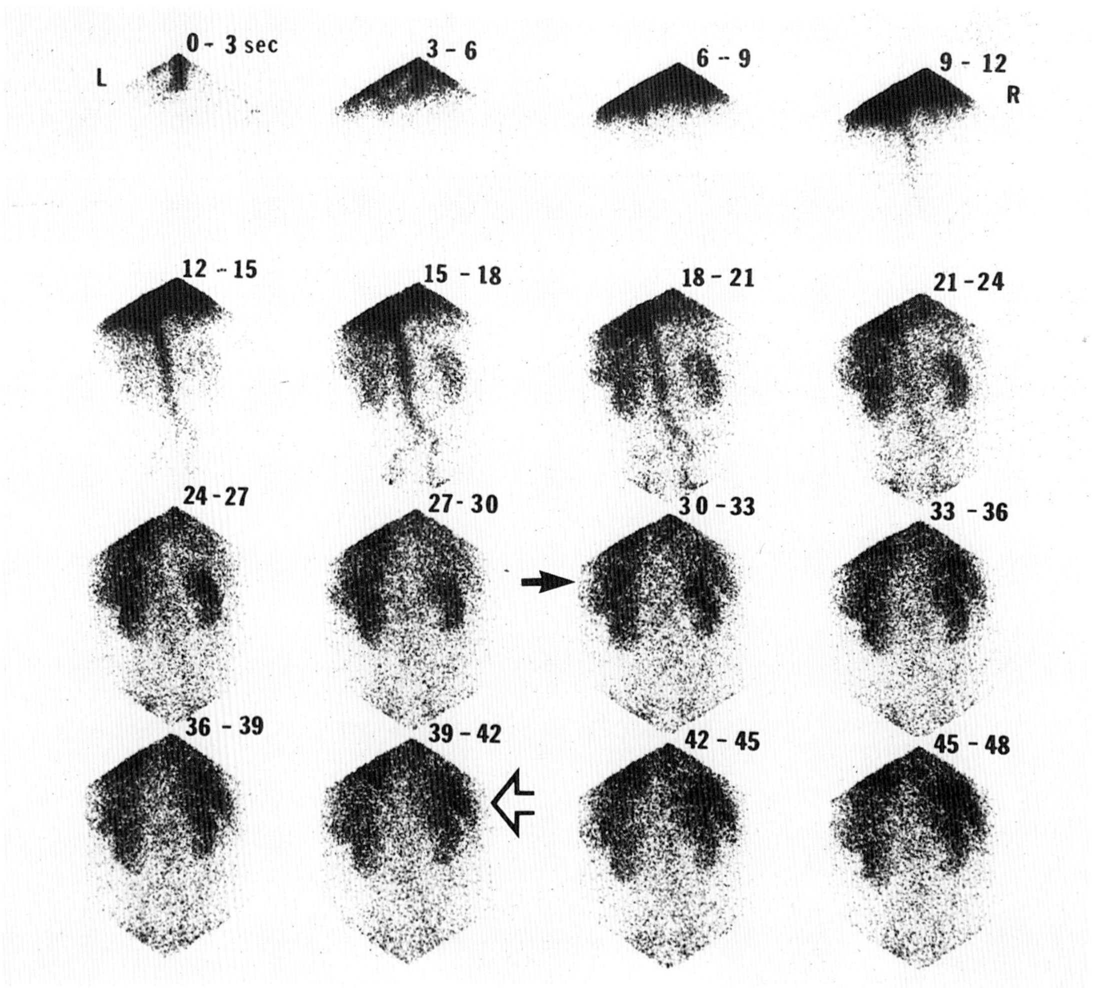

5–3 Normal renal scintiangiogram (740 MBq ^{99m}Tc-DTPA) performed as posterior view, demonstrating symmetric flow to both kidneys. Note normal prominent vascular pool in spleen (arrow) and liver (open arrow).

kidneys or crossed renal ectopia. In addition, the "cortical pseudotumor," such as dromedary hump, fetal lobulation, lobular compensatory hypertrophy, and prominent column of Bertin, can be accurately distinguished from true pathology such as cyst, tumor, abscess, infarct, or hemorrhage due to trauma (Older et al. 1980).

Since uptake of DMSA by the renal tissue is determined by blood flow and number of functioning nephrons, it will also yield information on the presence of parenchymal renal disease in general and its distribution throughout the cortex in particular. To avoid false-negative interpretation, posterior oblique views should be obtained routinely. Lateral views, anterior views, and single photon emission computed tomography (SPECT) have been helpful for more anteriorly located lesions.

^{99m}Tc-GH can be used for the same indications as DMSA. Lower cortical uptake is compensated for by a higher permissible dosage. GH is a multipurpose renal radiopharmaceutical because, in addition to high-resolution static scintigrams obtained 90 min to 120 min after injection, it permits excellent evaluation of the collecting system and high-quality scintiangiography. Another advantage of GH over DMSA is its stability and availability.

Dynamic Renal Imaging

Dynamic imaging with ^{99m}Tc-GH, ^{99m}Tc-DTPA, and ^{99m}Tc-MAG$_3$ after the scintiangiogram is currently the best method for evaluating the collecting system. Dynamic scintigrams obtained for 30 min have been recommended for

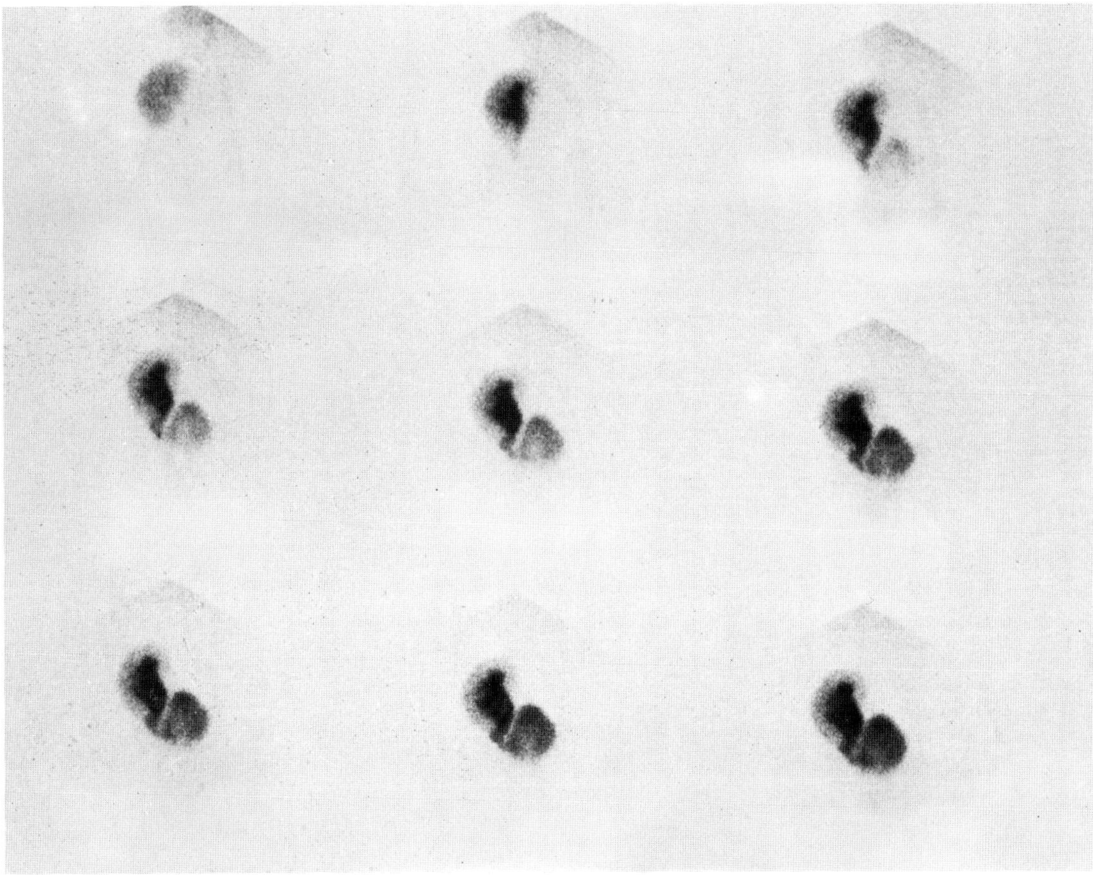

5–4 Dynamic scintigram of transplanted kidney performed with 180 MBq of ^{99m}Tc-GH, demonstrating normal perfusion of graft with mild obstructive pattern due to incomplete obstruction at ureterovesical junction caused by edema. (Time in minutes.)

evaluation of obstructive patterns and posttraumatic complications, such as urine leaks or surgical complications in renal transplantation (Fig. 5–4).

Since the low permissible dosage of ^{131}I-OIH prevents scintiangiographic sequence, the usual imaging procedure consists of 2- to 3-min frames recorded for 30 min as a posterior view. The procedure provides information on renal function and the collecting system, rather than structural detail. ^{123}I-OIH can be used with improved resolution, compared to ^{131}I-OIH.

Time-Activity Curves (Radionuclide Renography)

Camera renograms have the advantage over probe curves of more precise region-of-interest selection and background subtraction with computer processing (Taplin et al. 1963). ^{131}I-OIH is the most commonly used tracer for renography.

The renogram is a graphic expression of changes in activity counts over the kidneys in time. Radioactivity in the kidney rises rapidly during the first minute after administration of OIH, because the radionuclide is highly concentrated in the plasma. It is immediately filtered and secreted by the tubular cells. In the next few minutes, the hippurate leaves the intravascular space and is partially distributed in the extracellular space, thus decreasing plasma concentration and contributing to a slower rise of the curve. After approximately 2.5 min, activity begins accumulating in the calices and renal pelvis. The curve reaches maximum between 3 min and 5 min, after which it begins to decline due to a decrease in the amount of plasma OIH presented to the kidney. The fraction of total activity entering the kidney at any time is a function of renal blood flow and is constant. The slope of the time-activity curve reflects renal plasma flow only during the first few minutes, whereas the remainder of the curve is influenced by many factors. The patient's state of hydration plays a major role, even in the normal subject. Dehydration, especially when paired with extrarenal pelvis, may mimic obstruction (Fig. 5–5).

Variation in kidney size, position, and, most importantly, depth of the kidney, affect the renogram. The lower pole of an inferiorly located kidney is tilted anteriorly, resulting in distortion of the camera image. Such a kidney not only appears smaller, but gamma ray absorption by the more deeply situated tissue is greater and is seen as reduced height of the respective time-activity curve.

Generation of renograms involves two important steps: the selection of the renal region-of-interest and the selection of the nonrenal area best representing the background. In patients with poorly functioning kidneys, OIH is cleared from the circulation very slowly, the renal parenchyma is visualized late in the study, background activity is high, and delineation of the right kidney tissue is further complicated by presence of liver activity. This becomes especially crucial in patients with asymmetric renal uptake, because the first portion of the renographic curve is used to estimate the differential function.

Quantitation of Renal Function

Nuclear medicine provides noninvasive quantitation of renal function that is accurate, simple, reproducible, does not require urine collection, and can be performed on an outpatient basis.

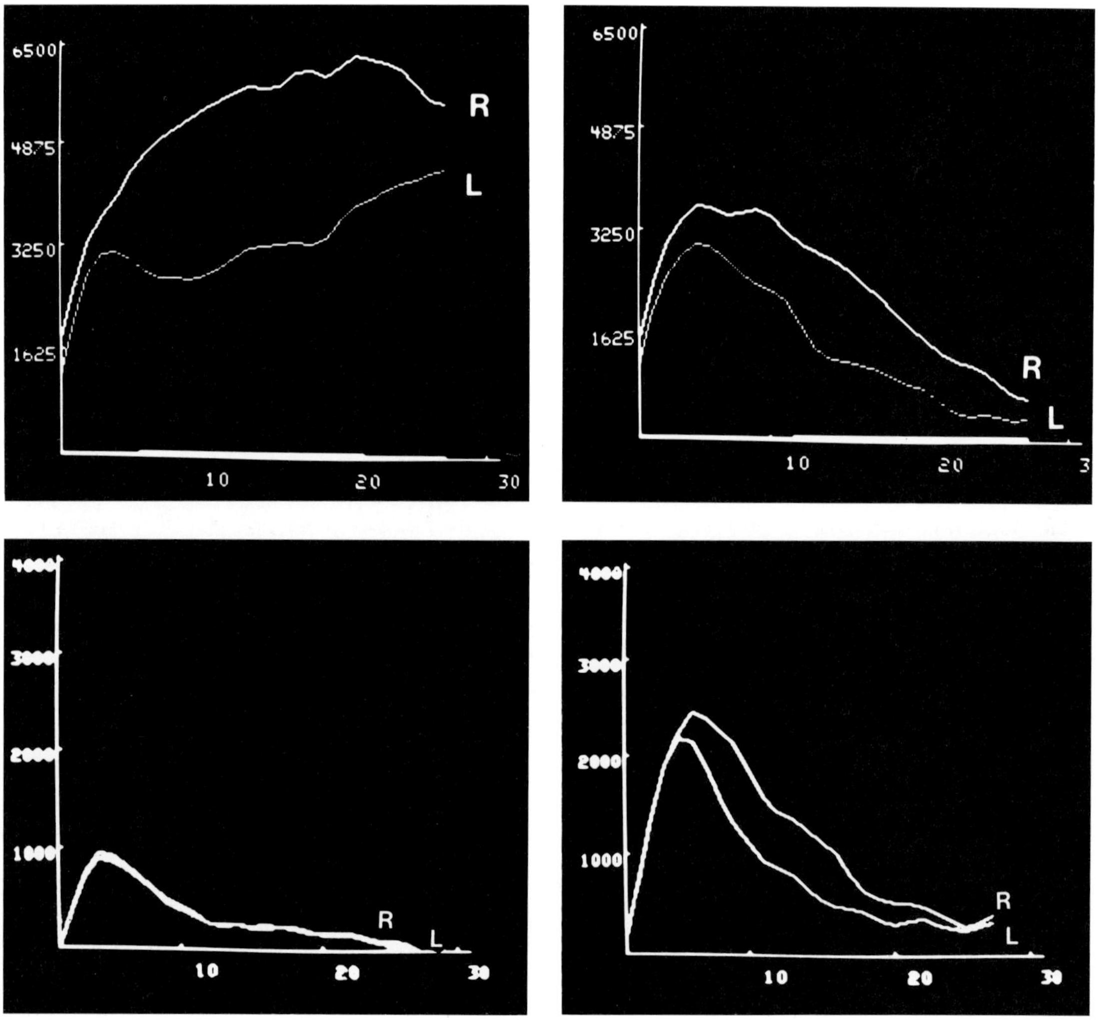

5–5 Effect of hydration state on renogram. Paraplegic patient studied 2 weeks apart in dehydrated (left panels) and normally hydrated (right panels) state. Effective renal plasma flow and differential function are not affected. Time-activity curve in dehydrated state mimics obstruction.

Conversely, creatinine clearance does not measure individual renal function unless ureteral catheterization is performed to collect urine from each kidney; urine leakage around the catheter and contamination of urine by the blood often invalidate the measurements.

Split (relative, differential) function studies have been used effectively in children with vesicoureteral reflux and in patients with obstructive uropathy before and after surgery, renovascular hypertension before and after angioplasty, or acute renal failure after medical treatment. The fact that urine collection is not required to obtain accurate measurement of individual renal function is particularly important in patients with spinal cord injury or ileal conduits, who are at high risk for renal disease and are unable to collect urine accurately.

Quantitation with DMSA

Uptake of DMSA correlates well with blood flow and glomerular filtration, and therefore can be used as an index of differential renal function. The best results have been obtained at 2 hr after DMSA administration. If renal function is asymmetric or low with a high background and substantial liver uptake, appropriate background subtraction is essential. A C-shaped region-of-interest laterally around each kidney gives the best results (Taylor 1982). An obstructed kidney should be evaluated carefully. Reduced or absent DMSA uptake does not necessarily imply irreversible damage, nor does it exclude possible recovery of function. Good uptake of DMSA in an obstructed or partially obstructed kidney indicates good function. DMSA is not recommended for measurement of the total renal function.

Quantitation with GH

Although GH is not removed from plasma by a single mechanism in the kidneys, the relative contribution of each kidney to total renal function can be measured by comparing background-corrected uptake in 1- to 3-min intervals after injection. Later frames should not be used for estimation, because accumulation of activity in the collecting system depends not only on the amount of radioactivity transported from the plasma into the urine but on such factors as renal pelvis anatomy, hydration status, and any pathology of the collecting system. GH uptake at intervals of 1–2 min or 2–3 min reveals good correlation with OIH uptake (Table 5–3).

Quantitation with OIH

Renal blood flow can be measured directly only by invasive methods. Noninvasive methods measure effective renal plasma flow. Smith introduced "effective" to emphasize the difference between true renal plasma flow and clearance of para-aminohippuric acid (PAH) (Goldring et al. 1936). The ideal material for estimation of ERPF should be completely extracted from the arterial blood and quantitatively excreted into the urine. PAH most closely meets these requirements, whereas OIH clearance is slightly lower, due to presence of free iodine in the preparation, plasma binding, and differences in tubular transport. The most accurate methods of global measurements of renal plasma flow utilize analysis of the OIH plasma disappearance curve constructed from multiple plasma samples. The single sample approach is widely used but is less accurate. Gamma-camera methods, which use uptake of OIH as a measure of renal plasma flow, although precise, are least accurate. Relative uptake by each kidney is measured between the first and second minute (Dubovsky, Russell 1982).

After injection of OIH, many parameters of renal and bladder function can be obtained. The 30-min imaging of the kidneys depicts uptake and kinetics of hippurate through the parenchyma and collecting system. Accumulated activity in the bladder at 30 min reflects the excretory function. A 44-min plasma sample is used to calculate global ERPF, which consequently aids in prediction of fractional excretion (Tauxe et al. 1971; Tauxe et al. 1982). Excreted activity is then compared to predicted excretion, and this ratio, termed the excretion index (EI), is calculated. On the scintigram, low EI is accompanied by retention of OIH either in the cortex or collecting system. Plasma flow in each kidney is estimated from the differential uptake in the 1- to 2-min frame. This study can be further modified by injecting furosemide (Lasix) to assess diuretic response of the kidneys and evaluate for an obstruction.

Quantitation with Glomerular Agents

Glomerular filtration rate (GFR), the volume of plasma ultrafiltrate produced in 1 min in renal glomeruli, cannot be measured directly. Conventional methods consist of clearance of inulin and creatinine. Initial radionuclide methods used ^{131}I-diatrizoate, a urographic contrast material, and achieved excellent correlation with inulin clearance (Bianchi et al. 1965). ^{125}I-iothalamate (Glofil) is approved for measurement of GFR in the United States. In Europe, the most commonly used agent is ^{51}Cr-EDTA (Brochner-Mortensen, 1985). Correlation of ^{99m}Tc-DTPA with inulin, ^{51}Cr-EDTA, and iothalamate is generally good, but accuracy depends on the degree of plasma protein binding, which varies among products. Global GFR with ^{99m}Tc-DTPA can be measured from a plasma disappearance curve constructed from multiple samples or a single sample drawn 3 hr after injection; differential GFR is determined from background and depth-corrected uptake between 1 and 3 min (Russell et al. 1985).

Currently, two camera methods of GFR estimation are widely used, and both require only a short imaging sequence. Uptake of DTPA by each kidney is measured as a fraction of the carefully calibrated standard dose (Gates 1982). A dose of 110 MBq of ^{99m}Tc-DTPA is counted in the syringe for 1 min at 30 cm from the center of the collimator. Data acquisition, initiated at time of injection, is performed in 15-sec frames and terminated after 6 min, and the syringe is again counted. Uptake is measured in the renal regions-of-interest after 50% background subtraction; the background is determined from semilunar regions-of-interest drawn under the kidneys. Renal depth is estimated from the patient's height and weight. Renal uptake in the 2- to 3-min interval is then calculated by adding right and left kidney counts corrected for background and depth, and expressed as a fraction of net standard counts. Glomerular filtration rate is estimated from a relationship between the uptake and creatinine clearance (Fig. 5–6).

The second camera method assumes that a negligible amount of ^{99m}Tc-DTPA leaves the kidneys during the first 3 min after injection and that the precordial curve is identical to the plasma curve. Calculated separate clearance values for each instance are derived by dividing the slope of background-corrected renal curves by plasma concentration obtained from the precordial curve and one plasma sample drawn at 20 min (Piepsz et al. 1977). Good correlation was obtained with the ^{51}Cr-EDTA method and creatinine clearance.

Summary

Estimation of ERPF with radioiodinated OIH and GFR with ^{99m}Tc-DTPA can be achieved in many ways. Each method yields clinically useful results. Since the method using blood samples is more accurate than camera methods alone, this author's preference is to use 1- to 2-min ^{131}I-OIH and 1- to 3-min ^{99m}Tc-DTPA uptakes to calculate differential (relative) ERPF or GFR; a single sample technique is used to calculate global ERPF (44 min) and global GFR (180 min). Renal scintigraphy is performed for at least 27 min, because additional information concerning radionuclide kinetics is often obtained. This is especially true in patients with obstructive uropathy, in whom di-

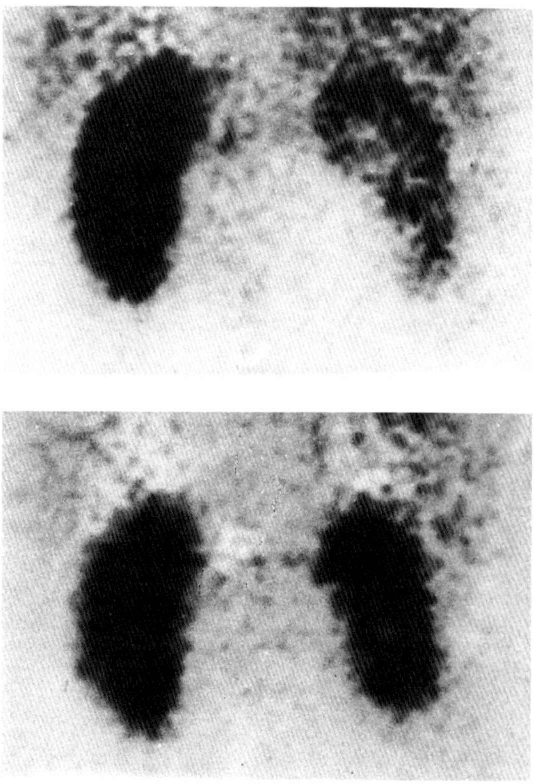

5–6 Glomerular filtration rate measured by method of Gates. Patient with obstruction in right collecting system caused by stone in distal ureter, studied before (upper panel) and after (lower panel) surgery, at which time right kidney glomerular filtration rate shows marked improvement. (Courtesy of G. F. Gates, Portland, OR.)

Table 5–4 Assessment of the Differential Function

$$\text{Function of the left kidney } \% = \frac{\text{Net counts in the left kidney}}{\text{Net counts in both kidneys}} \times 100$$

Radiopharmaceutical	Time	Comments
^{99m}Tc-DTPA	1–3 min	Measures relative glomerular filtration rate (GFR). Timing important.
^{99m}Tc-GH	1–3 min	Does not measure specific function. Timing important.
^{99m}Tc-DMSA	2–24 hr	Does not measure specific function. Any time after 90 min. In poorly functioning kidneys, best measured at 24 hr.
^{131}I-OIH	1–2 min	Measures relative effective renal plasma flow (ERPF). Timing important.

uretic response to furosemide may be tested concurrently (Table 5–4).

Diagnosis of Specific Problems

Acute Pyelonephritis

Acute bacterial pyelonephritis often presents with nonspecific symptoms and signs. Scintigrams performed with DMSA or GH using a high-resolution or pinhole collimator typically reveal multifocal areas of decreased uptake in enlarged kidneys, which return to homogeneous uptake after successful therapy (Fig. 5–7). Such an abnormal cortical scintigram, combined with increased uptake of ^{67}Ga-citrate or ^{111}Indium-labeled white blood cells in those areas, is diagnostic of kidney infection. Increase in ^{67}Ga uptake caused by extrarenal infection can be distinguished from acute pyelonephritis by ultrasonography or CT. Other causes such as vasculitis do not show cortical (flare pattern) defects seen on DMSA images. In addition, differential uptake can be evaluated on initial DMSA scintigrams and during treatment (Handmaker 1982).

Renal Trauma

For renal trauma, a ^{99m}Tc-GH scintiangiogram is followed by a few immediate static scintigrams (Berg 1982). Posterior, oblique, and anterior views are obtained 1 hr later. In renal contusion, there is compromised perfusion with decreased uptake in the involved kidney, which often appears smaller than the opposite one. In uncomplicated

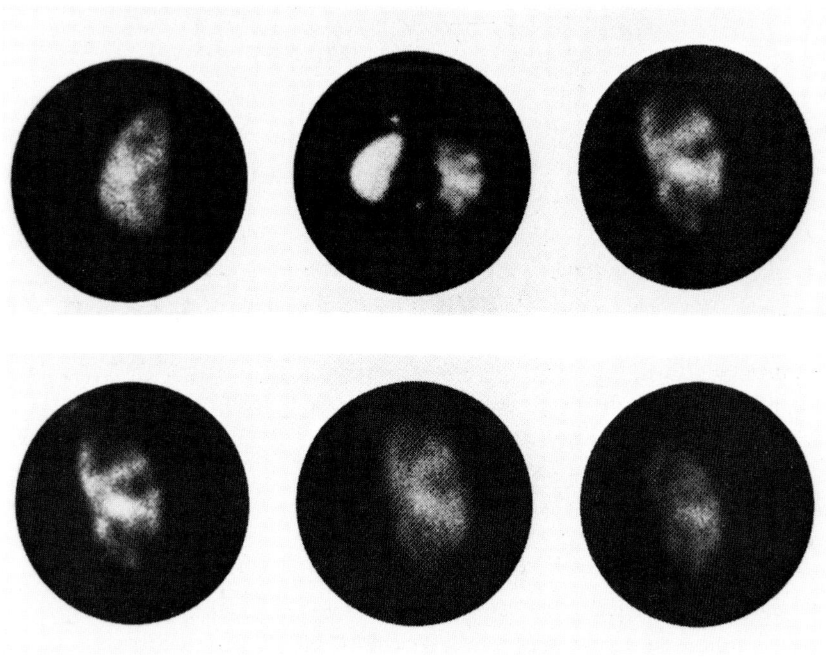

5–7 Eight-year-old male with severe right vesicoureteral reflux and recurrent infections. ^{99m}Tc-DMSA images reveal typical "flare" pattern of decreased activity on right side from hilum to periphery, multifocal in nature ("hot spots" in midline of posterior views are markers indicating 10-cm distance). (Reprinted, by permission, from Handmaker H: "Nuclear renal imaging in acute pyelonephritis." *Semin. Nucl. Med.* 12:246–253, 1982, Grune and Stratton, Orlando, FL.)

contusion, images return to normal within 48–72 hr. A contused kidney may bleed from a laceration, and the hemorrhage is usually seen on the perfusion study. Extrarenal hematoma will be seen as an area of reduced uptake best diagnosed on a combined liver-spleen-kidney scintigram as a photon-deficient area between the organs. Extravasation of urine from the injured kidney, ureter, or bladder causes an enlarging area of activity outside the collecting system. Urine leak and urinoma may also produce a pattern of ureteropelvic obstruction from external pressure on the ureter (Fig. 5–8).

The most severe renal trauma, avulsion of the renal pedicle, is seen as complete photopenia in the respective renal regions on the perfusion sequence and static scintigrams. Berg (1982) found that associated injuries of renal and hepatosplenic systems were common and, surprisingly, often clinically silent. An important advantage of radionuclide testing is the ability to evaluate the spleen and liver rapidly with ^{99m}Tc-sulfur colloid at the time of renal study.

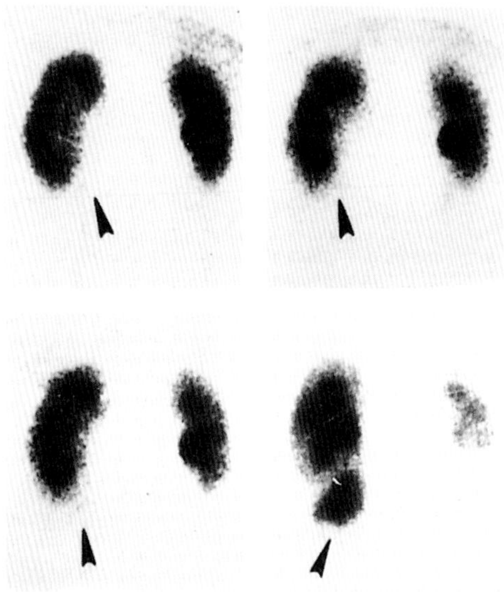

5–8 Examples of ^{99m}Tc-GH scintigrams (740 MBq) in evaluation of trauma. Urinary extravasation forming urinoma (arrow) and causing ureteropelvic junction obstruction. (Courtesy of B. C. Berg, Peoria, IL.)

Obstruction

Radionuclide renography plays an important role in the evaluation of patients with obstructive uropathy because location, degree of obstruction, and potential recoverability of renal function can be assessed (Scharf, Blaufox 1982). However, radionuclide scintigraphy provides only gross anatomic information as to the site of obstruction. This is more likely to be identified with OIH, which, although used in small quantities, is excreted almost quantitatively. Even in higher doses, DTPA and GH are excreted more slowly and do not provide expected diagnostic improvement over OIH. But the lower absorbed radiation dose of DTPA is advantageous for pediatric patients, in whom repeat studies are often required. In the future, MAG_3 may be the best alternative.

Dilatation of the collecting system, although well evaluated by radiologic techniques, does not always correlate with mechanical obstruction. Both congenital hydronephrosis with megaureters and postsurgical dilatation of the collecting system are sometimes difficult to differentiate from a true obstructive uropathy. The conventional Whitaker test directly measures the hydrostatic pressure through a needle or nephrostomy catheter inserted into the renal pelvis. Noninvasive radionuclide studies combined with renography can provide similar information.

Patients should be studied in a well-hydrated state. Besides the usual dynamic sequence, images of the kidneys should be obtained after voiding, since a distended bladder may prevent normal urine flow from the upper urinary tract. Consequently, children are often studied with an indwelling catheter in place. An additional view in the upright position can prove helpful, since stagnating urine in the dilated but nonobstructed pelvis will move into the bladder.

The diuretic renogram can help differentiate true mechanical obstruction from obstructive patterns caused by dilatation of the collecting system (Koff et al. 1979). It is performed with the usual dose of either OIH, MAG_3, or DTPA. Furosemide (0.5–1.0 mg/kg with maximum of 40 mg) is injected at 10 min when using OIH or MAG_3 and at 30 min with DTPA, and the patient is imaged for an additional 20 min. In mechanical obstruction, time-activity curves show a continuously rising curve. The washout pattern in hydronephrosis without a mechanical component is a sharp downturn of the renogram after furosemide (Fig. 5–9). The ambiguous response to furosemide results from incomplete, low-grade obstruction or inadequate diuretic response of the kidneys due to advanced parenchymal damage.

The most important application of the

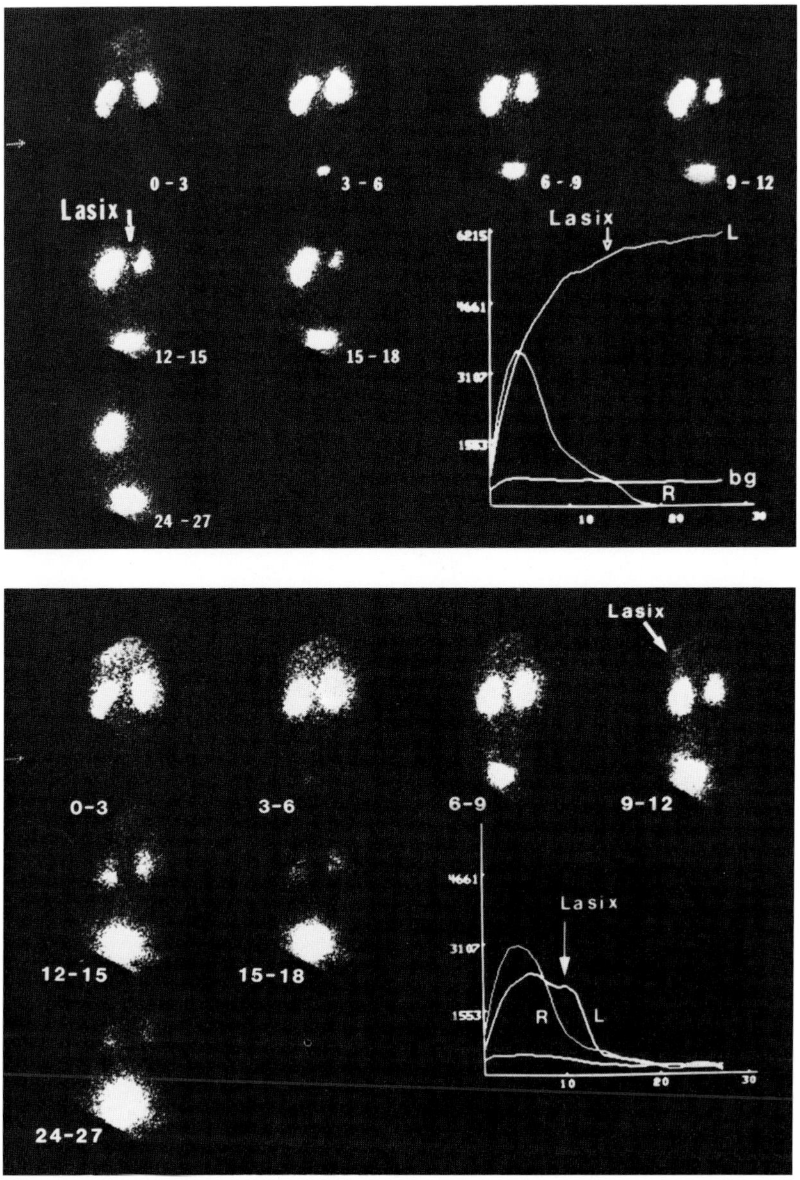

5–9 Diuretic renogram (3.7 MBq ^{131}I-OIH; 20 mg furosemide at 12 min) in 6-year-old girl with left flank pain (upper panel). Selected frames (0–3 min frame) present close-to-normal differential uptake with normal excretion from right kidney. Left kidney shows obstructive pattern without any washout after furosemide injection. Patient underwent pyeloplasty for ureteropelvic junction obstruction. Study performed 1 year later (lower panel) shows differential uptake unchanged, slight dilatation of left collecting system, but normal washout after furosemide.

radionuclide study in patients with obstruction is quantitative evaluation of renal function. Measurements of ERPF before and after surgery indicate that correction of ureteropelvic junction obstruction usually results in improved renal function, while improvement is less dramatic in longstanding distal ureteral obstruction (Belis et al. 1982).

Degree of obstruction and subsequent recovery of function were evaluated with encouraging results by deriving time-activity curves from region-of-interest over the renal cortex as well as from the whole renal region. When curves derived from the cortex had the same obstructive shape as the whole kidney curve, prognosis for functional improvement was less favorable. Cortical curves close to normal were associated with postoperative improvement. Clinical value of deconvolution analysis in obstruction was evaluated in a European cooperative study, in which mean transit time effectively discriminated between obstructive and nonobstructive renal disease.

In patients with acute and subacute obstruction, there is often poor correlation between degree of uptake and functional impairment. Recovery has been described in patients when no measurable ^{131}I-OIH uptake was seen in the kidney at 30 min (Fig. 5–10).

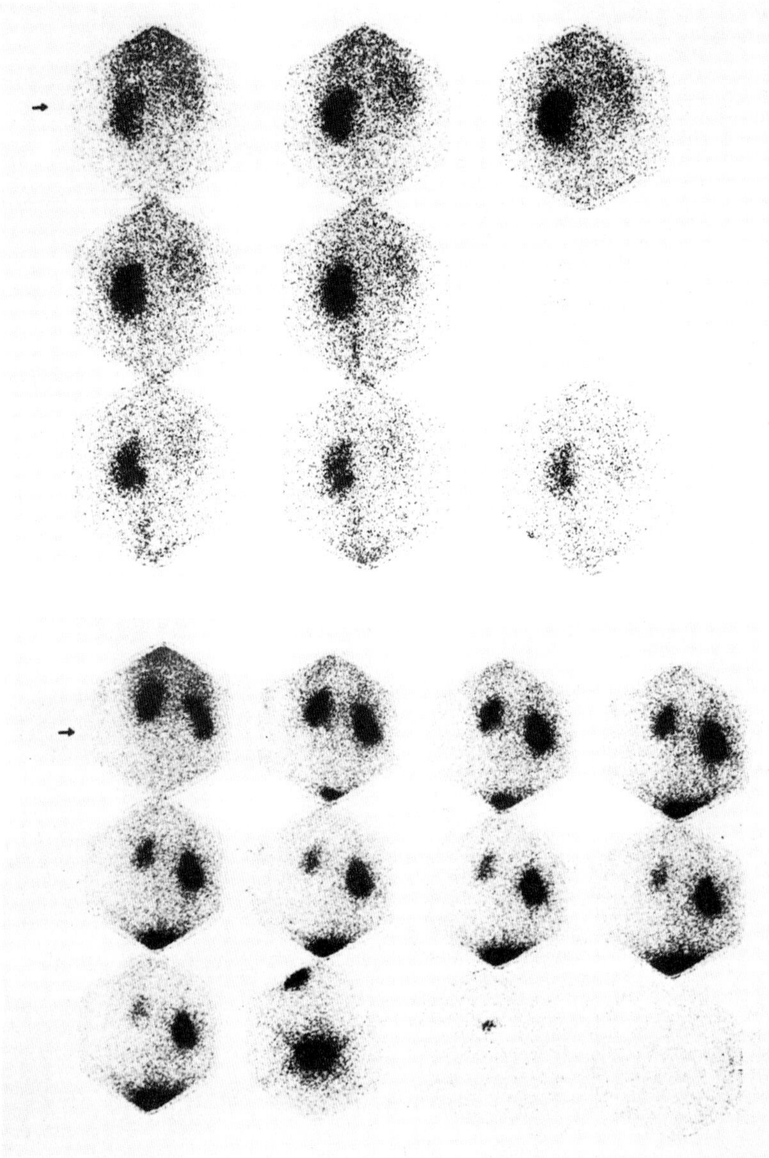

5–10 Thirty-eight-year-old female with congenital obstructive uropathy in right kidney, studied during acute episode of complete obstruction. Global effective renal plasma flow was 494 ml/min with no visible uptake in right kidney. Study was repeated after surgical correction (pyeloplasty). Results are presented in lower part of the illustration. Note lateral displacement of right kidney with prominent pelvic retention. Effective renal plasma flow in this kidney was 203 ml/min, 41% of global renal plasma flow.

Acute and Chronic Renal Failure

Acute renal failure may be caused by a variety of pathological processes, including cortical necrosis, acute tubular necrosis, hepatorenal syndrome, or acute interstitial nephritis. Bilateral acute pyelonephritis, bilateral renal artery obstruction, or renal vein thrombosis are less frequently observed. A typical scintigram of acute tubular necrosis, hepatorenal syndrome, and acute interstitial nephritis shows relatively good uptake, markedly prolonged transit, and very low urinary excretion of OIH. Differentiating acute noninfectious interstitial nephritis has been a diagnostic problem; however, an intense renal uptake of ^{67}Ga has been consistently noticed, a finding not present in patients with acute tubular necrosis. Scintiangiography and imaging with GH or DMSA are of diagnostic value in excluding or confirming the presence of renal infarction due to renal artery embolism.

Chronic renal failure is typically caused by chronic nonobstructive pyelonephritis, reflux nephropathy, renal vascular disease, or renal lymphoma. Other causes include longstanding, poorly controlled hypertension, diabetes mellitus, or lead poisoning. Radionuclide testing can effectively quantitate renal function and is more accurate in evaluation of degree of renal failure than plasma creatinine or creatinine clearance. Functional testing may be complemented by radionuclide cystography for reflux in children and by ^{67}Ga scintigraphy in patients with lymphoma.

Hypertension

Hypertensive patients were among the first studied with renograms, and early results were encouraging. Unfortunately, not all patients with anatomically present renal artery stenosis are hypertensive, and most hypertensions are not caused by the presence of a stenosis. Moreover, the same renographic patterns felt to be diagnostic of stenosis are described in other renal diseases, such as reflux and obstructive nephropathy or chronic pyelonephritis. Consequently, while renographic evaluation excluded the majority of patients without hemodynamically significant stenosis, positive predictive value was too low, and the radionuclide study was rejected as an unnecessary expense.

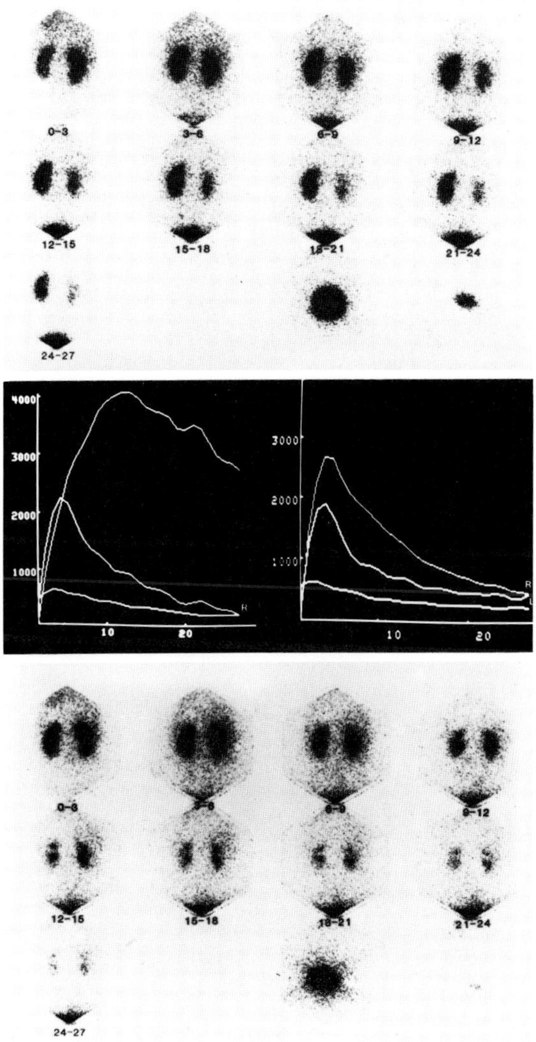

5–11 Scintigrams (posterior view) and renograms (11 MBq of ^{131}I-OIH) in hypertensive patient due to left renal artery stenosis (80%) before (upper and left middle panel) and after (right middle and lower panel) angioplasty. Note disappearance of cortical retention of OIH in left kidney (upper panel), which is the hallmark of an ischemic kidney.

This is not entirely justified, since there is a specific imaging pattern diagnostic of an ischemic kidney paralleling pathophysiologic findings of increased water reabsorption in the proximal tubules with generation of highly concentrated urine. The hallmark of this pattern is not the asymmetry in perfusion, in GFR, or in ERPF, which are nonspecific, but the prolongation of cortical transit of the radiopharmaceutical (Fig. 5–11). Captopril, an angiotensin-converting enzyme inhibitor, is now used to confirm suspicion of hemodynamically significant renal artery stenosis. Given 1 hr before the study, 25 mg of Captopril decreased GFR and therefore uptake of DTPA in the affected kidney. With OIH or MAG_3, the ERPF and uptake are not changed, while their cortical transit is markedly prolonged. This is seen on the images as cortical retention. Decrease in DTPA uptake or presence of cortical retention with OIH and MAG_3 after Captopril predicts curability of the lesion (Fig. 5–12) (Geyskes et al. 1987).

Renal Transplant Evaluation

In addition to HLA histocompatibility matching, living, related donors undergo examination of their renal anatomy and physiology. Many centers have recently added a radionuclide examination to their battery of tests as a noninvasive means of evaluating individual renal function. Quantitative data of individual renal function, such as ERPF or GFR, aid in predicting not only the function of the donor's remaining kidney but also the initial level of the recipient's function.

Certain complications occur at specific times following transplantation. Ischemic damage leading to acute tubular necrosis is commonly seen in cadaveric kidneys at the time of transplantation. The main cause is oxygenation and perfusion changes prior to the donor's demise. The degree of necrosis and recovery period are related to the

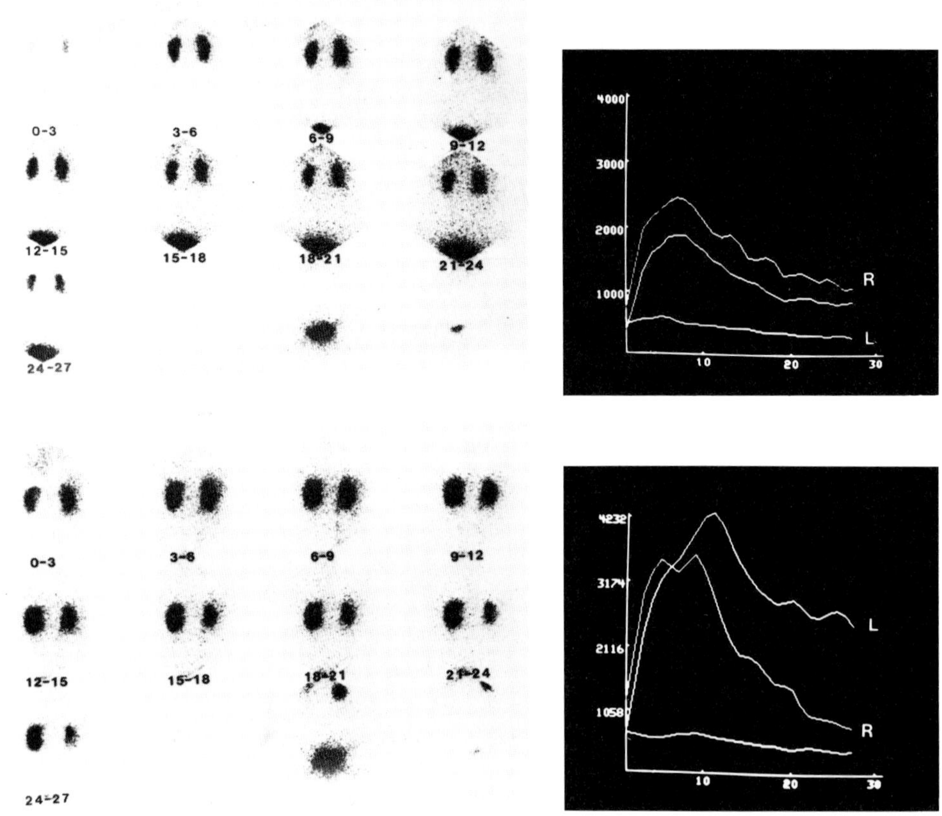

5–12 Scintigrams and renograms in hypertensive patient performed as baseline (upper panel) and repeated after 25 mg of Captopril (lower panel). Note enhancement of cortical retention in left kidney.

severity of ischemic insult. With the rare exception of irreversibly damaged kidneys, acute tubular necrosis resolves without treatment. Frequently, such kidneys subsequently develop immunologic complications, namely acute rejection.

Current classification of immunologic complications is based on histopathological features and on the time of their appearance.

Hyperacute rejection is a fulminating, irreversible process associated with the presence of preformed antibodies against the graft, which leads to intravascular thrombosis and cessation of function within minutes to hours after transplantation.

Accelerated rejection is a variant of acute rejection, occurring before the 5th postoperative day. It occurs in some patients who receive donor-specific transfusions before transplantation, a procedure found to modify immunologic tolerance, but which is not well understood.

Acute rejection is observed in the majority of recipients. It is a predominantly cell-mediated process occurring after the 5th day and during the first 3 months after transplantation. Clinical signs include fever, renal enlargement, and tenderness. Plasma creatinine levels are elevated. If acute rejection responds to therapy, function returns to normal.

Chronic rejection is a slow, insidious process suggestive of humoral mechanism, leading to injury of endothelial and interstitial cells. The narrowing vascular bed of the graft decreases renal blood volume and hence renal size. At the terminal stage, this leads to metabolic failure (acute tubular necrosis) and is often accompanied by hypertension.

Although monitoring with radionuclides is widely accepted as the best way to evaluate kidney graft performance, there is no universally accepted protocol. Most studies try to assess renal function and patency of the renal artery and collecting system. Although surgical complications, such as obstruction, urine leaks, and lymphocele, are relatively easily diagnosed from a single study, most immunologic or ischemic complications can be

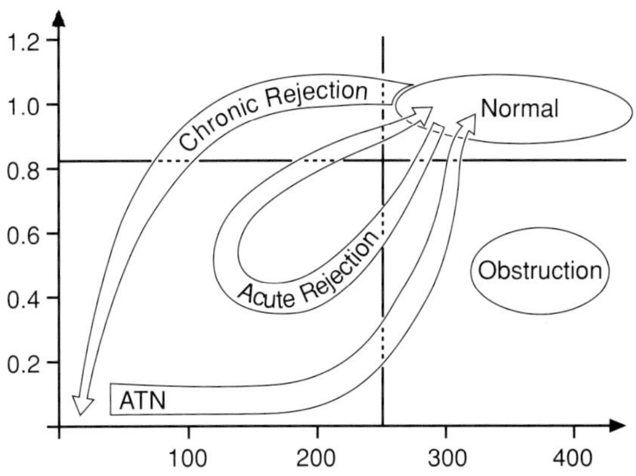

5–13 When ERPFs versus excretory indexes in renal transplants are plotted on horizontal and vertical axis, points fall into discrete areas relating to normal function, acute rejection, chronic rejection, acute tubular necrosis, and incomplete obstruction. Each complication has a typical temporal course, indicated by arrows. Combinations of complications or transitions between them in individual patients must be followed over time. In general, the ERPF provides an index of renal perfusion; the excretion index provides an index of renal transit time.

traced only with a sequence of tests (Fig. 5–13). Methods used most often employ ^{131}I-OIH and ^{99m}Tc-DTPA.

Monitoring with ^{131}I-OIH

OIH kinetics in a healthy graft and normal kidney are the same. Scintigrams and time-activity curves derived over the kidney, bladder, and background will therefore be indicative of renal function and patency of the collecting system.

Patients should be normally hydrated, because dehydration causes pooling of activity in the collecting system and simulates obstruction. Scintigrams are obtained in the anterior view for 30 min. Imaging again after voiding will reveal even mild cortical retention that might be obscured by bladder activity. Also, a small urinary leak, urinoma, or mild obstruction caused by lymphocele are better visualized after voiding. The usual dosage for OIH scintigraphy is 3.7–5.5 MBq per kidney (<1.5% of free iodide), with lower doses for children. Scintigraphic and renographic data may be complemented by measuring ERPF and excretory function using a single plasma sample at 44 min in adults and 53 min in children.

The uncomplicated course of normal graft function is documented by normal ERPF and excretory function.

Ischemic damage and acute renal failure are characterized by relatively good perfusion and uptake (ERPF low to normal) with disproportionately low excretory function (excretion index low to very low). Sometimes there is no urinary excretion. During this anuric phase, while plasma creatinine remains elevated, recovery of the graft function is most efficiently followed by ERPF, which should steadily increase. Markedly impaired excretory function, seen as prominent cortical retention and low activity output, rapidly improves when damaged tubular epithelium is replaced by normal cells. A smooth recovery is often complicated by superimposed rejection diagnosed by sudden decrease in ERPF and excretory function.

Acute rejection can develop rapidly. Scintigraphic evidence includes cortical retention and delayed appearance of the activity in the bladder. Severe rejection with markedly compromised renal plasma flow is often complicated by ischemic damage requiring dialysis. In the majority of patients, however, acute rejection is completely reversible with treatment.

In chronic or vascular rejection, ERPF steadily declines, while excretory function remains normal until metabolic requirements of the graft are compromised and cause ischemic damage. The first sign of vascular rejection is decreased graft size with declining radiohippurate uptake. This is often difficult to note on the scintigram, since excretory function remains normal until very late in its course (Fig. 5–13). A similar pattern of declining ERPF and normal EI is observed in transplant artery stenosis. These findings and hypertension are an indication for arteriography, which is best done with digital subtraction techniques to minimize contrast dosage (Curtis 1986).

Incomplete obstruction, easily detected as renal pelvic retention on scintigrams, exhibits normal ERPF and decreased EI. Complete obstruction remains a diagnostic problem that is best solved by sonography. Semiquantitative data derived from time-activity curves yield similar information as measurements of ERPF and excretory function. Investigators using ^{123}I-OIH can take advantage of the high count rate and better resolution and place two regions-of-interest (parenchyma and pelvis) or three regions-of-interest (cortex, medulla, pelvis) over the kidney. Curves derived from parenchymal samplings reflect prolongation of intrarenal transit time in acute tubular necrosis

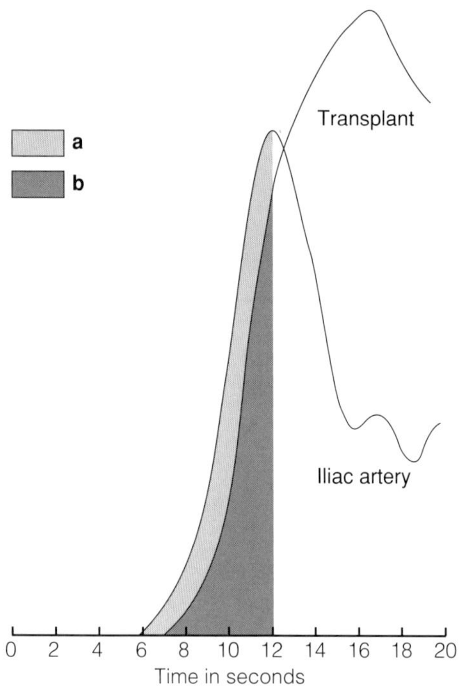

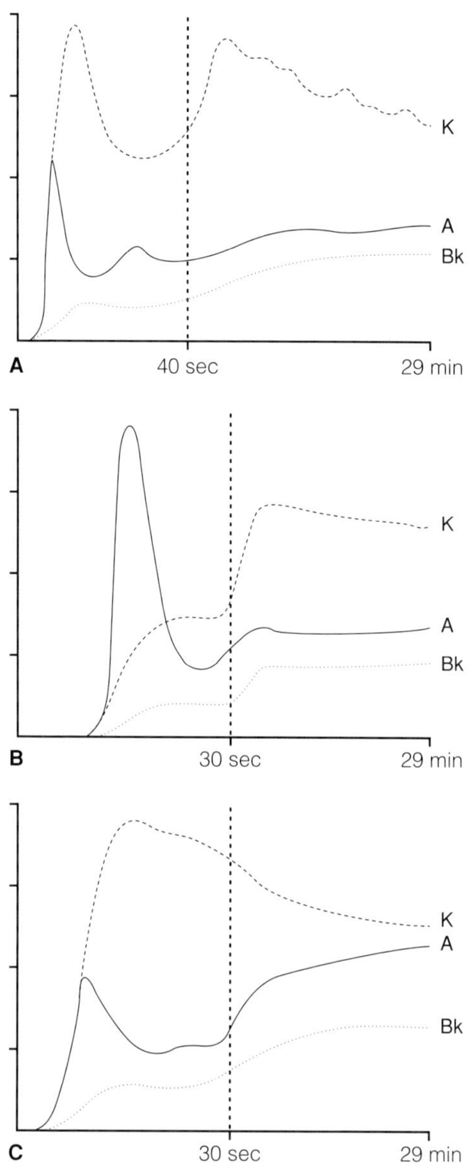

5–14 Perfusion index (area under arterial peak-a/area under renal peak-b × 100) is calculated from normalized curves obtained from region-of-interest over graft kidney (K) and iliac artery (A) distal to graft, as seen on left. Curves on right are generated from their respective region-of-interest in 1-sec frames for 40 sec, followed by 20-sec frames for 30 min and depicting: **(A)** normal function, **(B)** severe rejection, and **(C)** anuric acute tubular necrosis. Mean perfusion index in normals is 96, in acute tubular necrosis 153, and in acute rejection 256. There is, however, significant overlap in individual studies. (Bk = background.) (Reprinted, by permission, from Hilson AJW, Maisey MN, Brown CB, et al.: Dynamic renal transplant imaging with ^{99m}Tc-DTPA (Sn) supplemented by a transplant perfusion index in the management of renal transplants. *J. Nucl. Med.* 19:994–1000, 1978, The Society of Nuclear Medicine, New York, NY.)

and acute rejection, but are relatively normal in patients with incomplete obstruction.

Monitoring with ^{99m}Tc-DTPA

Scintiangiography with ^{99m}Tc-DTPA permits evaluation of perfusion. Semiquantitative monitoring by means of computer-generated time-activity curves requires only 60-sec data acquisition. Curves are derived from the regions-of-interest placed over the graft and over the aorta or iliac artery. Various flow patterns and indices calculated from the data are helpful in differential diagnosis of acute tubular necrosis and acute rejection (Fig. 5–14) (Hilson et al. 1978). Dynamic imaging follows the fast perfusion segment, and images assist in evaluating anatomy and detecting obstruction, urine leaks, or infarction. Similar quality images can be obtained with ^{99m}Tc-GH.

Rejection Testing

In addition to OIH and DTPA, which must be used in a temporal manner, the radiopharmaceuticals recommended in differentiating acute tubular necrosis from acute rejection include ^{99m}Tc-sulfur colloid, ^{125}I- and ^{131}I-fibrinogen, ^{67}Ga-citrate, and ^{111}Indium-labeled white cells or platelets. All of these, however, can give both false-positive and false-negative results.

Some newer drugs, such as cyclosporin, which suppresses the rejection process but is also nephrotoxic, make the differential diagnosis of impaired renal function even more difficult (Dubovsky, Russell 1988).

Radionuclide Cystography

The single most important indication for radionuclide cystography is the evaluation of vesicoureteral reflux, especially in children (Conway et al. 1975; Winter 1959). Reflux nephropathy, a major cause of chronic renal failure, may develop without clinically manifested infection; however, a coexisting infection often leads by a retrograde route to kidney disease, such as acute focal bacterial nephritis. The concept of reflux nephropathy includes entities such as chronic atrophic pyelonephritis, the Ask-Upmark kidney, renal segmental hypoplasia, and changes resembling those of obstructive nephropathy. Since reflux often remains undetected during childhood and early adulthood, the sequelae of renal failure may first become manifest later in life. Direct and indirect cystography are two methods of detecting vesicoureteral reflux.

Direct Cystography

Direct radionuclide cystography has become the test of choice in diagnosis and grading of ureteral reflux. When compared to conventional radiographic cystography, direct cystography demonstrates greater sensitivity for reflux detection, marked decrease in radiation exposure (μGy instead of mGy), and yields quantitative data of bladder function.

The patient's bladder is first catheterized and, after complete drainage of urine, the patient is placed on the imaging table and the catheter is connected to a bottle of saline. After free flow of saline (approximately 20 ml) is established into the bladder, 37 MBq of ^{99m}Tc-pertechnetate is injected into the injection section of the catheter. During the filling phase, the patient is supine with the detector underneath the table. The upper margin of the bladder is placed at the bottom of the imaging field, and the upper urinary tract is monitored closely on the persistence oscilloscope as the saline infusion continues. When reflux initially appears, the instilled volume of fluid is registered on a data sheet.

Sequential imaging begins after the bladder is sufficiently full. Scintigrams (300,000 counts) require approximately 5 min. Posterior and both posterior oblique views are also obtained. Signs of adequate filling of the bladder are leakage of urine

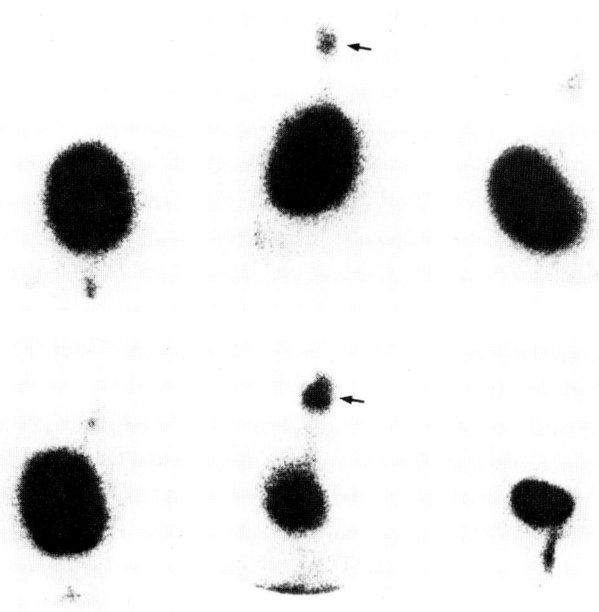

5–15 Cystogram (37 MBq ^{99m}Tc-pertechnetate) shows reflux in right pelvis (arrow) during filling phase (upper middle frame) and during voiding phase (lower middle frame).

around the catheter, cessation of flow from the saline bottle, excessive volume of instilled saline solution, and the patient's increasing discomfort. The usual bladder capacity in children is about 250 ml.

Before the patient voids, a 2-min posterior image of the bladder with low-intensity setting is obtained, and the total abdominal count is recorded. During the voiding phase after the catheter is removed, the patient's back is to the camera. Sequential images are obtained with high-intensity settings, and the volume of collected urine is measured and recorded. The 2-min postvoid image of the bladder (low-intensity settings) and counts are obtained for residual urine calculation. Other functional indices, such as actual volume refluxing into the pelvis, can be derived from the recorded data (Fig. 5–15).

Technical pitfalls include contamination by radioactive urine and, on occasion, ^{99m}Tc-pertechnetate is reabsorbed through the bladder mucosa and secreted by the gastric mucosa, thus simulating a reflux. In both cases, oblique and lateral projections are helpful.

Since reflux will stop spontaneously in at least 50% of children, temporal quantitative follow-up studies are indicated. The best indication of improvement is the increasing fluid volume at which the reflux occurs, since these patients have stable renal function and often the reflux disappears with age. In contrast, patients in whom the reflux occurs at decreasing bladder volumes often demonstrate progressive damage to renal parenchyma and usually require surgical treatment.

The direct radionuclide cystogram detects reflux better than contrast voiding cystography, but gives poorer anatomical definition of the genitourinary tract and will miss existing ureteroceles or lower ureteral reflux. Therefore, the standard contrast media cystogram is recommended as the initial test and the radionuclide test for follow-up.

Indirect Cystography

Indirect cystography was introduced to avoid bladder catheterization. Intravenous injection of ^{99m}Tc-DTPA or ^{99m}Tc-MAG$_3$ provides information not only on vesicorenal reflux but also on kidney function. The renal phase of the study is performed in the usual manner with data acquisition for 30 min.

After the renogram is completed, the patient is repositioned in front of the camera. Baseline data are acquired for 100 sec and the patient is asked to void, after which another 200-sec sequence follows. Girls should be sitting on a bedpan and boys holding a urine bottle. If there is significant residual activity in renal areas, the voiding study is delayed. However, renal regions do not have to be completely free of activity, since baseline data are available. Time-activity curves are generated from the renal, ureteral, bladder, and background regions. Normally, the bladder curve falls during the voiding phase, and no change is present in the renal curves. In patients with reflux, there is a drop in the bladder curve while kidney curves rise. Advantages of intravenous cystography lie in the physiologic nature of the test.

However, indirect cystography requires the patient to void on command, and transient reflux during the filling phase will be missed. Patients with markedly impaired renal function and hydronephrosis will retain large quantities of activity in the renal regions, and a small degree of reflux may be obscured.

Scrotal Scintigraphy

The main clinical indication for scrotal imaging is differentiation of spermatic cord torsion from other causes of painful hemiscrotum. The diagnosis must be established as soon as possible, since torsion of the spermatic cord with compromised perfusion of the testis leads to irreversible testicular necrosis after a few hours. Therapy is immediate surgical detorsion and orchiopexy.

Symptoms of acute onset and severe pain are not diagnostic of testicular torsion, because similar symptoms are present in patients with torsion of the testicular appendages, epididymitis, or traumatic orchitis. Scintigraphy of the scrotum reliably differentiates testicular torsion from other etiologies of acute scrotal pain. It is a simple and reliable method to evaluate the blood supply to the testes.

On the perfusion study, testicular torsion appears as lack of activity in the spermatic artery and a void in the scrotal blood pool on the static image. Epididymo-orchitis, on the other hand, depicts a normal blood supply and increased activi-

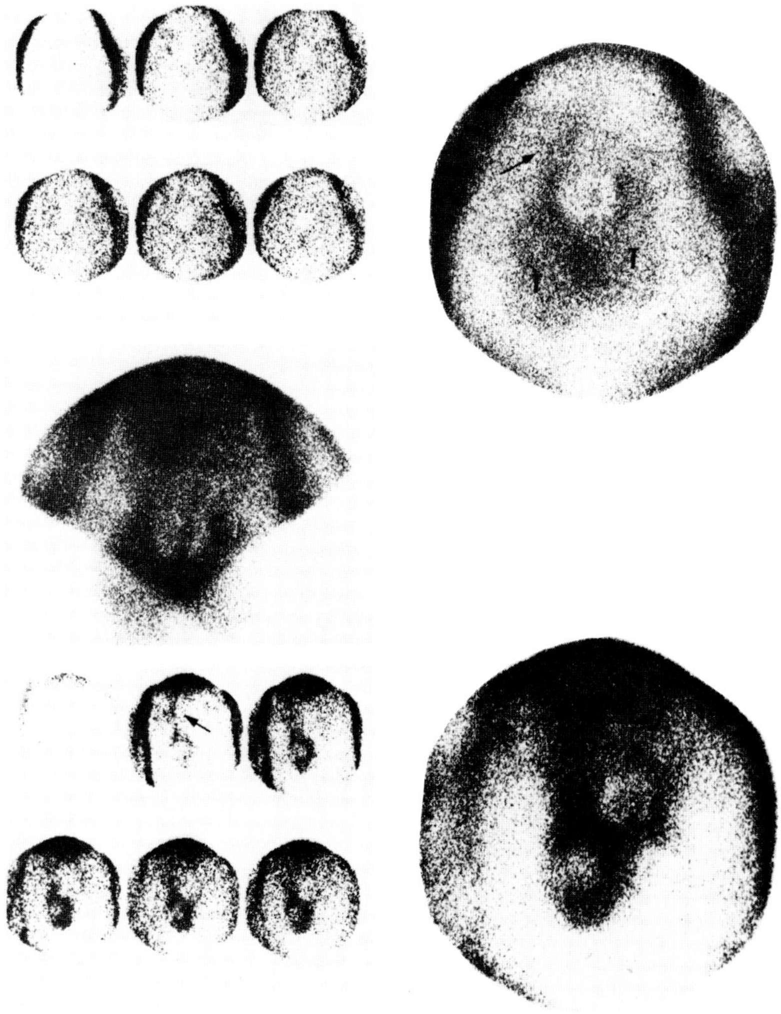

5–16 Panel 1 (upper): Testicular scan (550 MBq ^{99m}Tc-pertechnetate) in normal patient, showing normal, symmetrical perfusion (arrow) of both testes. Panel 2 (lower): Study in patient with right epididymitis showing increased vascularity during perfusion phase and tissue phase, consistent with inflammatory process. (Courtesy of L. E. Holder, Baltimore, MD.)

ty in the blood pool image because of hyperemic reaction (Holder et al. 1981).

The patient is injected while in a supine position with thighs slightly abducted. The scrotum is suspended on a tape cradle and the penis is taped over the symphysis pubis. In very young patients, a flexible lead shield may be used to decrease the body background. The gamma camera is positioned over the groin with the scrotum in the lower half of the field. In children, a converging collimator is essential in magnifying the image, but best results are obtained with a pinhole collimator. The adult dose of ^{99m}Tc-pertechnetate is 550–740 MBq; for children, the usual dose is 7.4 MBq/kg. After a rapid bolus injection, sequential 5-sec images are obtained for 1 min, followed immediately by static blood pool images (300,000 counts).

Normal scintigraphic findings are symmetric vascular supply and blood pool image with no difference between the two halves of the scrotum (Fig. 5–16). Normal testicular activity is of approximately the same intensity as the soft tissues of the thigh. Acute spermatic cord torsion shows decreased activity in both the perfusion and tissue phases in the affected side. If the condition is not diagnosed within 2 to 6 hr of onset of symptoms, the infarcted testis will become atrophic; a typical image of a "missed torsion" is characterized by a cold defect surrounded by a hot rim, caused by inflammatory changes in the surrounding scrotal tissue (Fig. 5–17). Testicular appendage torsion appears as slightly increased activity on static scintigrams. Rarely, a small cold defect is observed, and the diagnosis must be surgically established.

Scintigraphic findings in epididymo-orchitis are those of increased activity through both the dynamic and static phases (Fig. 5–16). If only the epididymis is involved, the increased uptake is

Table 5–5 Scintigraphic Findings in Scrotal Abnormalities

Condition	Dynamic Phase Blood Flow	Static Phase Cold Defect (testis)	Static Phase Scrotal Tissue (rim)
Normal	N[a]	–	N
Acute cord torsion	↓N	+	↓N
"Missed" torsion	↓N↑	+	N↑
Appendicular torsion	N↑	–	N↑
Epididymo-orchitis	N↑	–	↑
Abscess	↑	+	↑
Trauma	N↑	–	N↑
Hydrocele, spermatocele	N	+	N
Hematoma	N↑	+	N↑

[a] N, normal.

localized more in the lateral part of the scrotum, while involvement of the testis will show increased uptake in the entire hemiscrotum. Scrotal trauma usually increases blood flow and uptake, similar to those of epididymo-orchitis. Hematoma and hydrocele can cause a cold defect; since trauma sometimes precipitates testicular torsion, a scintigram may incorrectly diagnose a torsion (Table 5–5). Ultrasonography is then helpful.

Scrotal imaging is a sensitive test for diagnosing spermatic cord torsion. With knowledge of clinical history, correlation with physical findings and good technique, the true positive rate in testicular torsion approaches 100%.

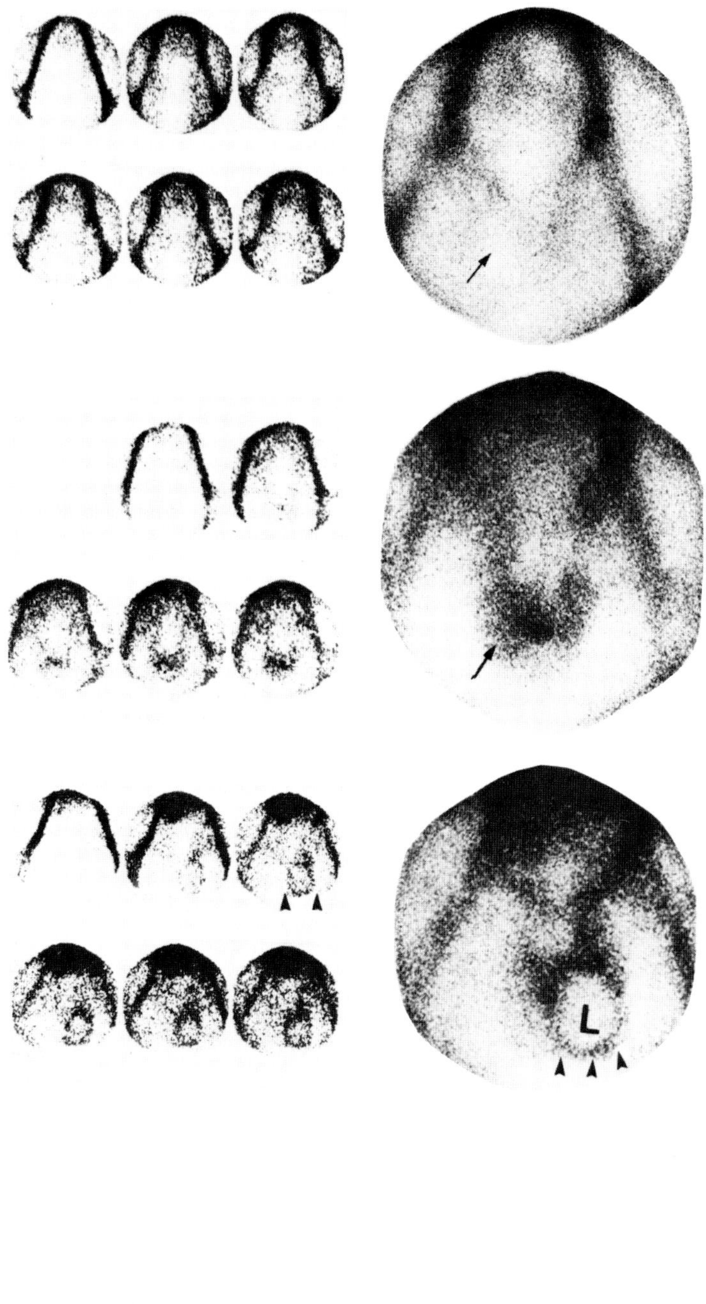

5–17 Panel 1 (upper): Testicular scan in patient with acute torsion of right testis (arrow). Panel 2 (middle): Same patient after manual detorsion, showing slightly increased uptake (arrow) characteristic of reperfusion. Panel 3 (lower): "Missed torsion" (in another patient) – cold lesion with hot rim – reflecting irreversible necrosis of testis (L) with inflammatory reaction in surrounding tissue (arrowheads). (Courtesy of L. E. Holder, Baltimore, MD.)

References

Arnold RW, Subramanian G, McAfee JG, et al.: Comparison of Tc99m complexes for renal imaging. *J. Nucl. Med.* 16:357–367, 1975.

Atkins HL, Thomas SR: Dosimetry of radiopharmaceuticals used in nephrologic investigation. *In* Tauxe WN, Dubovsky EV (eds.): *Nuclear Medicine in Clinical Urology and Nephrology.* Norwalk, CT, Appleton-Century-Crofts, 1985, pp. 31–37.

Belis JA, Belis TE, Lai JCW, et al.: Radionuclide determination of individual kidney function in the treatment of chronic renal obstruction. *J. Urol.* 127:636–641, 1982.

Berg BC: Nuclear medicine and complementary modalities in renal trauma. *Semin. Nucl. Med.* 12:280–300, 1982.

Bianchi C, Meozzi A, Zampieri A: Glomerular filtration rate measured by the urinary clearance of hyposulfite and radioiodine-labeled Hypaque in subjects with normal and impaired renal function. *Minerva Nucl.* 9:157–159, 1965.

Brochner-Mortensen J: Current status on assessment and measurement of glomerular filtration rate. *Clin. Physiol.* 5:1–17, 1985.

Chervu LR, Blaufox MD: Renal radiopharmaceuticals – an update. *Semin. Nucl. Med.* 12:224–245, 1982.

Conway JJ, Belman AB, Ring LR, et al.: Direct and indirect radionuclide cystography. *J. Urol.* 113:689–693, 1975.

Curtis JJ: Hypertension and kidney transplantation. *Am. J. Kidney Dis.* 7:181–196, 1986.

Dubovsky EV, Russell CD: Quantitation of renal function with glomerular and tubular agents. *Semin. Nucl. Med.* 12:308–329, 1982.

Dubovsky EV, Russel CD: Radionuclide evaluation of renal transplants. *Semin. Nucl. Med.* 18:181–198, 1988.

Gates GF: Glomerular filtration rate: Estimation from fractional renal accumulation of ^{99m}Tc-DTPA (Stannous). *Am. J. Roentgenol.* 138:565–570, 1982.

Geyskes GG, Oei HY, Puylaeret CBAJ, Dorhout-Mees EJ: Renovascular hypertension identified by Captopril-induced changes in the renogram. *Hypertension* 9:451–458, 1987.

Goldring W, Clarke W, Smith HW: The phenol red clearance in normal man. *J. Clin. Invest.* 15:221–228, 1936.

Handmaker H: Nuclear renal imaging in acute pyelonephritis. *Semin. Nucl. Med.* 13:146–153, 1982.

Hilson AJW, Maisey MN, Brown CB, et al.: Dynamic renal transplant imaging with ^{99m}Tc-DTPA(Sn) supplemented by a transplant perfusion index in the management of renal transplants. *J. Nucl. Med.* 19:994–1000, 1978.

Holder LE, Melloul M, Chen D: Current status of radionuclide scrotal imaging. *Semin. Nucl. Med.* 11:232–249, 1981.

Koff SA, Thrall JH, Keyes JW: Diuretic radionuclide urography: A noninvasive method for evaluating nephroureteral dilation. *J. Urol.* 122:451–454, 1979.

Older RA, Korobkin M, Workman J, et al.: Accuracy of radionuclide imaging in distinguishing renal masses from normal variants. *Radiology* 136:443–448, 1980.

Piepsz A, Dobbeleir A, Erbsmann F: Measurement of separate kidney clearance by means of ^{99m}Tc-DTPA complex and a scintillation camera. *Eur. J. Nucl. Med.* 2:173–177, 1977.

Russell CD, Bischoff PG, Kontzen F, et al.: Measurement of glomerular filtration rate: Single injection method plasma clearance without urine collection. *J. Nucl. Med.* 26:1243–1247, 1985.

Scharf SC, Blaufox MD: Radionuclides in the evaluation of urinary obstruction. *Semin. Nucl. Med.* 12:254–264, 1982.

Taplin GF, Dore EK, Johnson DE: The quantitative radiorenogram for total and differential renal blood flow measurement. *J. Nucl. Med.* 4:404–409, 1963.

Tauxe WN, Dubovsky EV, Kidd T, Jr., et al.: New formulae for calculation of effective renal plasma flow. *Eur. J. Nucl. Med.* 7:51–54, 1982.

Tauxe WN, Maher FT, Taylor WF: Effective renal plasma flow: Estimation from theoretical volumes of distribution in intravenously injected ^{131}I-orthoiodohippurate. *Mayo Clin. Proc.* 46:524–531, 1971.

Taylor A, Jr.: Quantitation of renal function with static imaging agents. *Semin. Nucl. Med.* 12:330–334, 1982.

Taylor A, Jr., Eshima D, Fritzberg AR, et al.: Comparison of iodine-131-OIH and technetium-99m-MAG$_3$ renal imaging in volunteers. *J. Nucl. Med.* 27:795–803, 1986.

Winter CC: A new test for vesicoureteral reflux: An external technique using radioisotopes. *J. Urol.* 81:105–111, 1959.

Suggested Reading

Bischof-Delaloye A (ed.): *Radionuclides in Nephrology.* Basel, Karger, 1987.

Dubovsky EV, Yester MV: Glomerular filtration rate, renal transit times, effective renal plasma flow, and differential renal function. *In* Gelfand MJ (ed.): *Effective Use of Computers in Nuclear Medicine.* New York, McGraw-Hill, 1987.

Fine EJ, Scharf SC, Blaufox MD: The role of nuclear medicine in evaluating the hypertensive patient. *In* Freeman LM, Weissman HS (eds.): *Nuclear Medicine Annual–1984.* New York, Raven Press, 1984.

Holder LE, Melloul M, Chen D: Current status of radionuclide scrotal imaging. *Semin. Nucl. Med.* 11:232–249, 1981.

Joekes AM, Constable AR, Brown NJG, et al. (eds.): *Radionuclides in Nephrology.* London, Academic Press, 1982.

Kirchner PT (ed.): *Nuclear Medicine Review Syllabus,* 3d ed. New York, Society of Nuclear Medicine, 1985.

O'Reilly PH, Shields RA, Testa HJ (eds.): *Nuclear Medicine in Urology and Nephrology,* 2d ed. London, Butterworth, 1986.

Renovascular hypertension. *Nephron.* 44(Suppl.), 1986.

Tauxe WN, Dubovsky EV (eds.): *Nuclear Medicine in Clinical Urology and Nephrology.* Norwalk, CT, Appleton-Century-Crofts, 1985.

Update on radionuclide assessment of the kidney-I. *Semin. Nucl. Med.* 12(3), July 1982.

Update on radionuclide assessment of the kidney-II. *Semin. Nucl. Med.* 12(4), Oct. 1982.

CHAPTER

6

Computed Tomography of Kidney, Adrenal, and Lower Urinary Tract

N. Reed Dunnick and Richard H. Cohan

Computed tomography (CT) combines computer technology with conventional radiography to reconstruct CT images. In conventional radiography, the intensity of a monochromatic X-ray beam is diminished in proportion to the thickness and density (attenuation coefficient) of the tissue through which it passes. CT uses these same monochromatic X rays, but measures intensity at many different projections and, using a complex series of calculations, generates an axial CT image.

The reconstructed CT image matrix is comprised of picture elements or pixels. Decreasing size of the X-ray beam and use of detectors with small apertures increases the spatial resolution. Early scanners produced a reconstructed matrix of 80×80 pixels with dimensions of 3 mm; current equipment uses matrices of 512×512 pixels with dimensions as small as 0.4 mm.

Spatial resolution or amount of blurring along the edge of a high-contrast object depends on detector geometry, reconstruction software, and the display pixel; it is independent of the intensity of the X-ray beam. The finer the X-ray beam collimation and the smaller the aperture of the detectors, the better the resolution. Software programs improve either high-contrast (bone) or low-contrast (soft tissue) resolution. The pixel size can be adjusted to fit the field of view and improve spatial resolution.

Contrast resolution, defined as the variability of the CT numbers of a uniform object, depends upon the X-ray intensity and dose. A CT number is used to define the attenuation coefficient of an object relative to air and water. Currently, CT numbers are called Hounsfield units (HU), named for Geoffrey Hounsfield, who developed the first clinically effective CT scanner. Air has a value of $^{-}1000$ HU and bone $^{+}1000$ HU, while soft tissue ranges from 40 HU to 70 HU.

The value of CT imaging over conventional radiography is due primarily to its axial projection of the image and its superior contrast resolution. The spatial resolution of current film screen combinations exceeds that of CT. Thus, conventional radiography may be more sensitive in detecting small lesions such as the mucosal irregularity of transitional cell carcinoma, while CT may be more useful in determining the precise radiodensity of an object, such as a radiographically lucent renal stone.

CT defines structures in the complex retroperitoneal region. The perinephric (Gerota's) fascia envelops the perinephric space, which includes kidney, adrenal, perirenal fat, vessels of the renal hilum, and proximal ureter. This space is further divided by bridging septae, which form a barrier to the dispersion of fluid collections. The anterior pararenal space contains the pancreas and portions of the duodenum and colon; the posterior pararenal space contains only fat.

Kidney

Computed tomography is the most sensitive method for detecting renal mass lesions. Precontrast scans detect calcification and renal stones, but contrast enhancement is essential for detecting parenchymal abnormalities. Unless a renal stone is suspected, the kidneys are routinely examined with contiguous 1-cm scans after intravenous contrast injection.

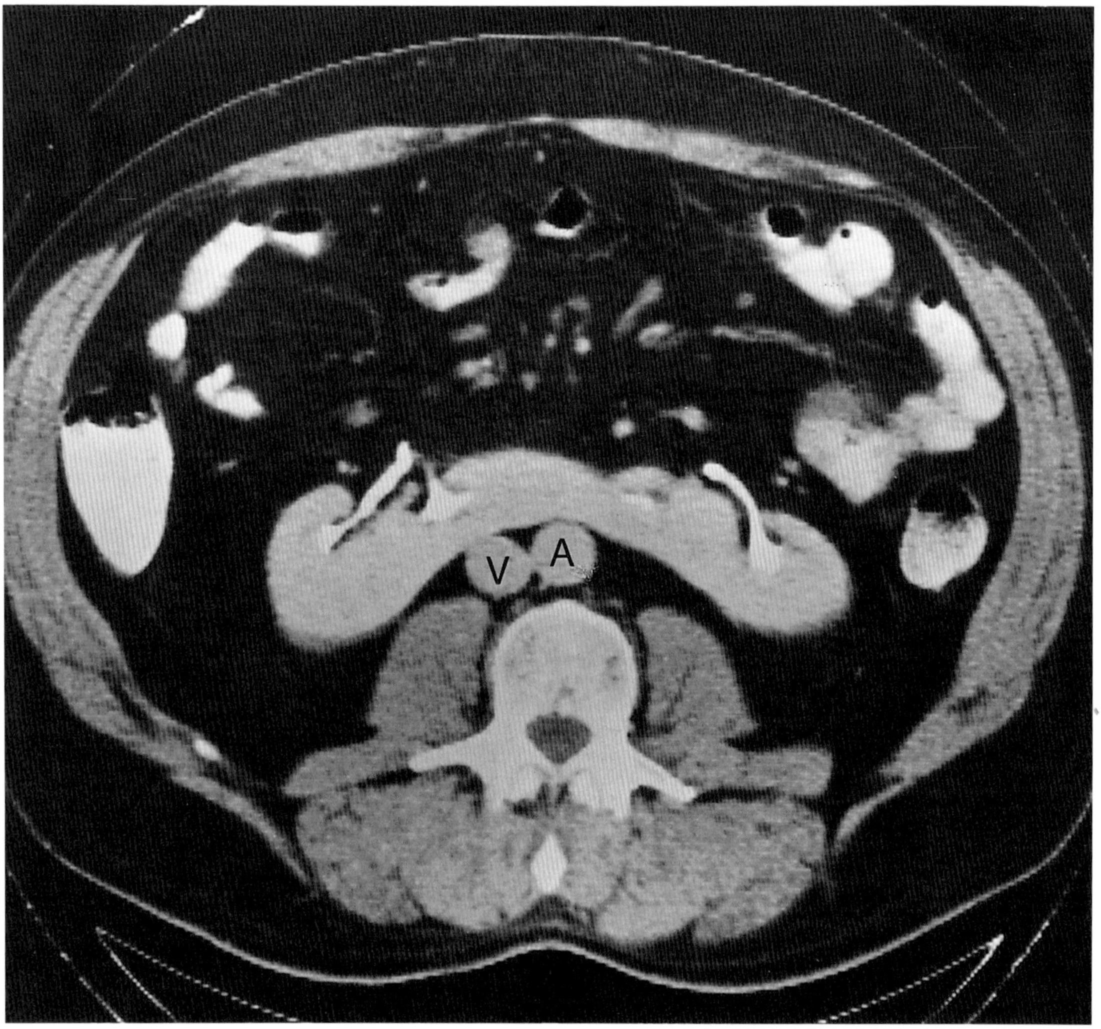

6–1 Horseshoe kidney. CT demonstrates isthmus of kidney anterior to aorta (A) and inferior vena cava (V).

Congenital Abnormalities

Congenital anomalies of the kidney such as a horseshoe kidney (Fig. 6–1), incomplete rotation, pelvic kidney, and crossed fused ectopia are usually identified with conventional urography. However, variations in the position of adjacent structures are much better delineated in the axial plane (Fig. 6–2), and CT may be needed to locate a safe path for percutaneous nephrostomy.

Abnormal renal morphology caused by splenic molding or renal duplication may be identified by CT, and unusual renal contours due to persistent fetal lobation or previous surgery can be clarified.

Renal Cysts

A benign cortical cyst is the most common renal mass. The periphery of the renal parenchyma is displaced as the cyst enlarges. CT shows a rounded homogeneous mass that has a clearly defined interface with normal renal parenchyma and an imperceptible thin wall (Fig. 6–3). In addition, the scan demonstrates a density near to that of water (0–15 HU) and no enhancement with intravenous contrast. These criteria must be fulfilled to diagnose a benign cyst. If one or more criteria is absent, further evaluation of the cystic mass is warranted.

High-density renal cysts, especially those in the 60–90 HU range, are most commonly due to hemorrhage, but can also be caused by high protein content of the cyst fluid or by diffuse calcifica-

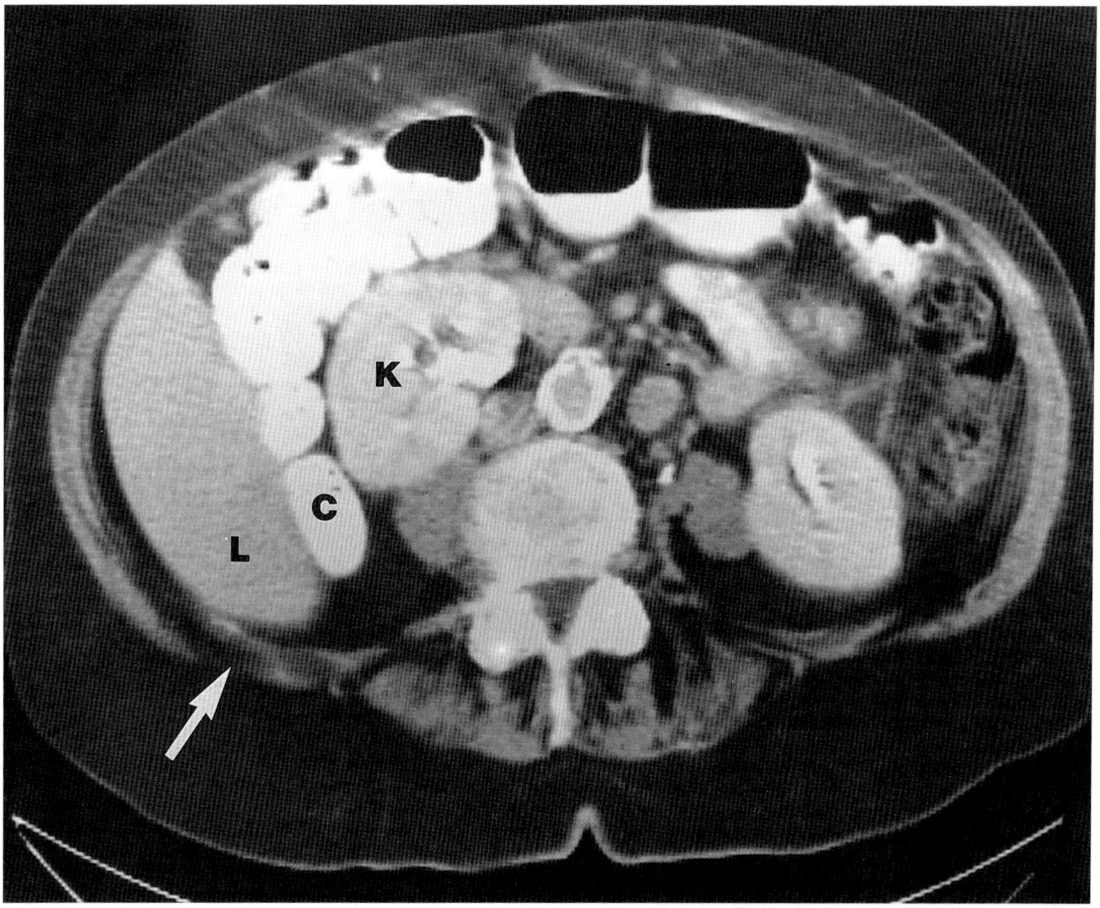

6–2 Abnormal renal position. Right kidney (K) lies anteromedial to its expected location. A percutaneous nephrostomy through the conventional route (arrow) would transverse both liver (L) and colon (C).

tion. If lesions conform to the criteria of a benign cyst with the single exception of the high density, they are usually benign. However, it is important to ensure that there is no contrast enhancement and that a soft-tissue mass or wall nodule is not associated with the cyst; either finding suggests malignancy (Dunnick et al. 1984). Ultrasonography confirms the cystic nature of these lesions (Foster et al. 1988).

Septations may occur in a simple renal cyst but are often too thin for CT imaging and may be detected only by sonography. These septated cysts are usually benign, but the presence of a soft-tissue mass adjacent to the cyst or thickening of the wall suggests a possible tumor (Rosenberg et al. 1985). Calcification in the wall of the cyst has little prognostic significance, unless it is associated with a tumor nodule.

If a cyst wall can be seen on a CT image, it is considered to be thickened. This may indicate reaction to previous infection, hemorrhage, or an abscess. Cysts with thick walls cannot be assumed to be benign; therefore, further evaluation such as ultrasound, cyst puncture, or surgery is suggested.

Parapelvic renal cysts usually cause stretching or compression of the collecting system (Fig. 6–4). They are commonly bilateral and frequently multiple. Parapelvic cysts are easily diagnosed on a contrast-enhanced scan, but they are not so obvious during sonography, when the multiple central cystic spaces may mimic hydronephrosis.

Adult-type polycystic renal disease is easily identified because both kidneys are riddled with innumerable, variable-size cysts (Fig. 6–5). One or more cysts may have a homogeneous high-density appearance indicating hemorrhage. Associated cysts in the liver are often present.

Patients undergoing long-term hemodialysis frequently develop benign cysts in their native kidneys. These kidneys have a higher incidence of

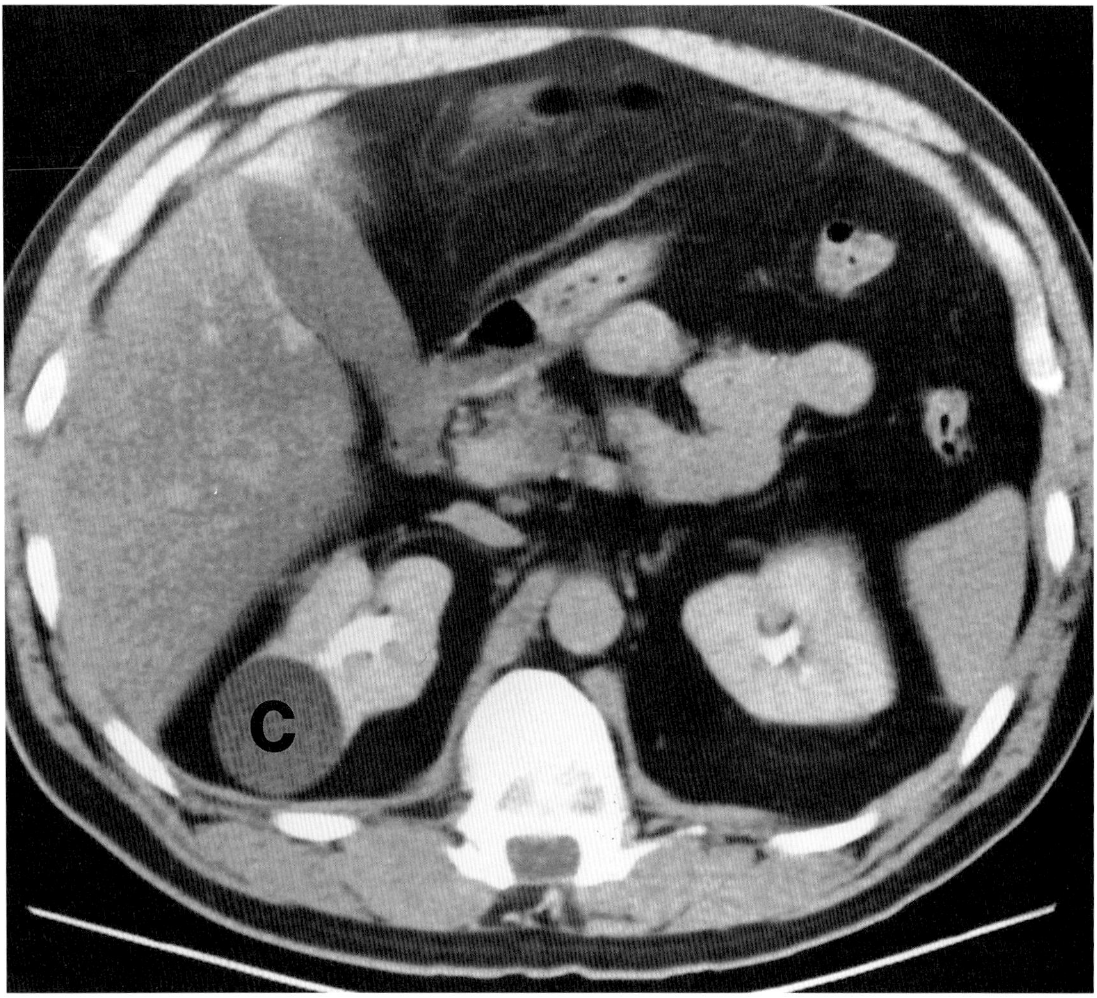

6–3 Benign cortical cyst. This well-defined water density mass (C) has an imperceptibly thin wall and does not enhance with intravenous contrast.

developing renal carcinomas (Petersen 1986). The kidneys in such patients are often small and contain multiple calcifications (Fig. 6–6), making these benign cysts difficult to distinguish from a solid tumor.

A multicystic dysplastic kidney is usually detected in childhood but may present incidentally in an adult, usually involving the whole kidney and consisting of a collection of cysts without functioning renal tissue. The ureter is atretic; the renal arteries and veins supplying the affected kidney are hypoplastic or absent.

Solid Renal Masses

Renal Adenocarcinoma

Any solid renal mass must be considered a renal adenocarcinoma until proven otherwise. Renal carcinoma appears as an irregular mass distorting the contour of the kidney (Figs. 6–7 and 6–8). Occasionally, smaller tumors produce no distortion and are difficult to detect without intravenous contrast revealing the lower-density tumor in the enhanced normal parenchyma. Even highly vascular renal carcinomas show less enhancement than the normal kidney (Johnson et al. 1987). However, without intravenous contrast, both may have similar density on CT; the tumor is "isodense" to the kidney. Calcification is more readily detected with

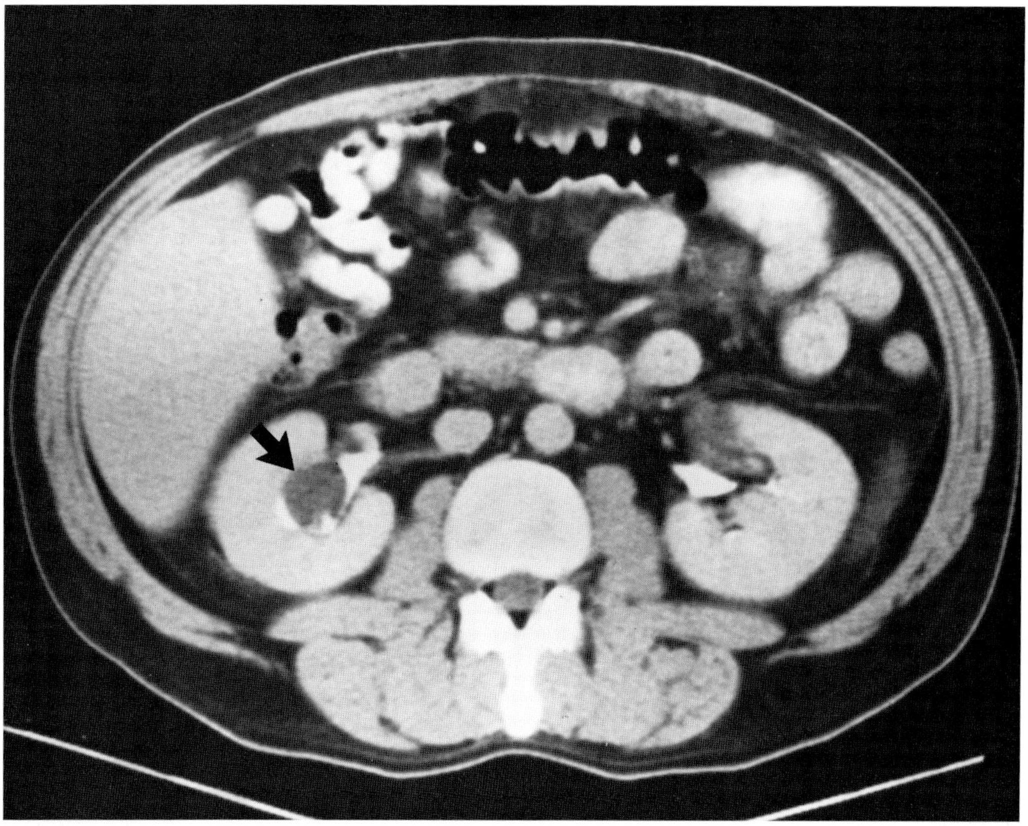

6–4 Parapelvic cyst. This cystic mass (arrow) does not opacify with excreted contrast material, but displaces renal collecting system.

CT than with urography. As many as 15% of renal adenocarcinomas are cystic (Fig. 6–7) and are distinguished from benign renal cysts by the irregular thick wall of the carcinoma and the poorly defined interface with the normal renal parenchyma.

Oncocytoma

Proximal renal tubular adenomas are benign solid neoplasms that do not metastasize or cause local invasion. They are usually asymptomatic and most commonly occur in older men. Most oncocytomas are single and 4 cm to 5 cm in diameter, but multiple and bilateral tumors have also been reported (Quinn et al. 1984). Larger oncocytomas may show a central stellate scar (Fig. 6–9) on CT, but this pattern may be closely mimicked by central necrosis of a renal carcinoma (Cohan et al. 1984). The findings by angiography of a spoke-wheel pattern are not pathognomonic, and surgery is needed. Since some renal adenocarcinomas may contain foci of oncocytes, needle biopsy is not sufficient. If the radiographic findings suggest oncocytoma, simple tumorectomy or excisional biopsy may be performed instead of radical nephrectomy.

Nephroblastoma

Nephroblastoma (Wilms's tumor), the most common abdominal malignancy in children, usually occurs before 5 years of age. It may be difficult to determine the tissue of origin in these frequently large tumors. Nephroblastoma is difficult to distinguish from a neuroblastoma, another common malignancy of infancy (Fig. 6–10).

Angiomyolipoma

Renal angiomyolipomas are benign hamartomatous lesions occurring in approximately 40% to 80% of patients with tuberous sclerosis. In these patients, the lesions are frequently multiple and

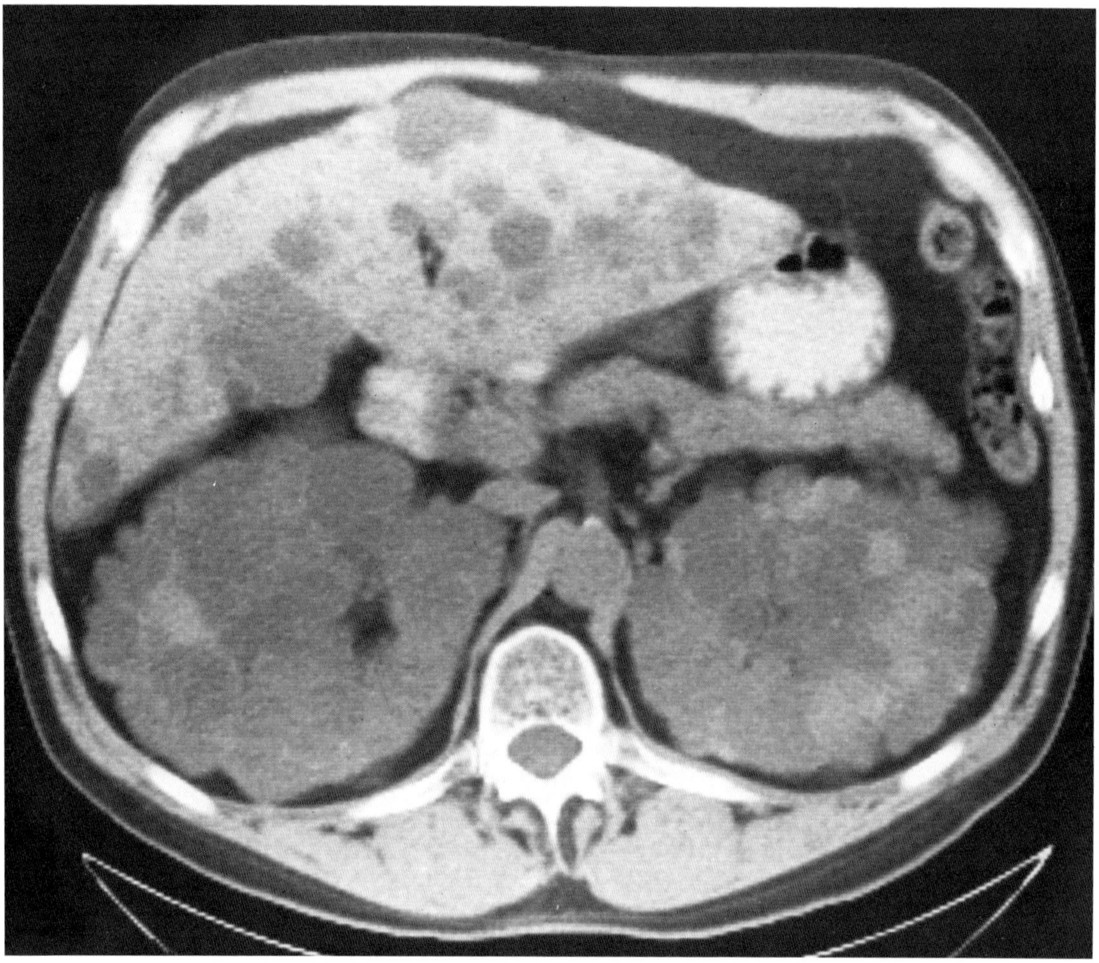

6–5 Polycystic kidneys. Innumerable cysts are present in both kidneys and the liver. High density of some of these renal cysts (arrows) indicates hemorrhage.

6–6 Hemodialysis-induced cysts. Small calcified kidneys ▶ with multiple small cysts are seen in this chronic hemodialysis patient.

6–7 Renal adenocarcinoma. Large irregular cystic mass ▶ distorts right kidney. Density of cyst content (17 HU) is greater than seen in simple cysts; thickened wall with nodular mass components indicates malignancy. Filling defect with inferior vena cava (arrow) could be followed as tumor thrombus extending from renal carcinoma.

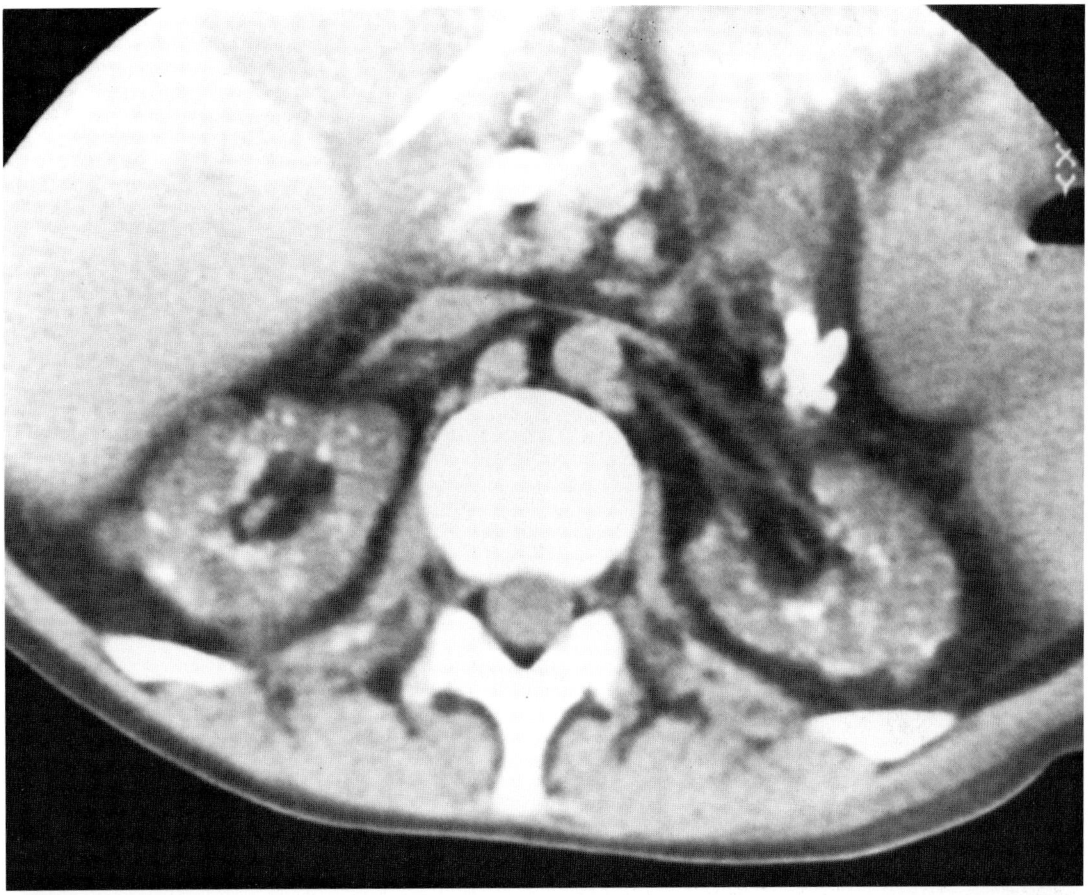

6–6

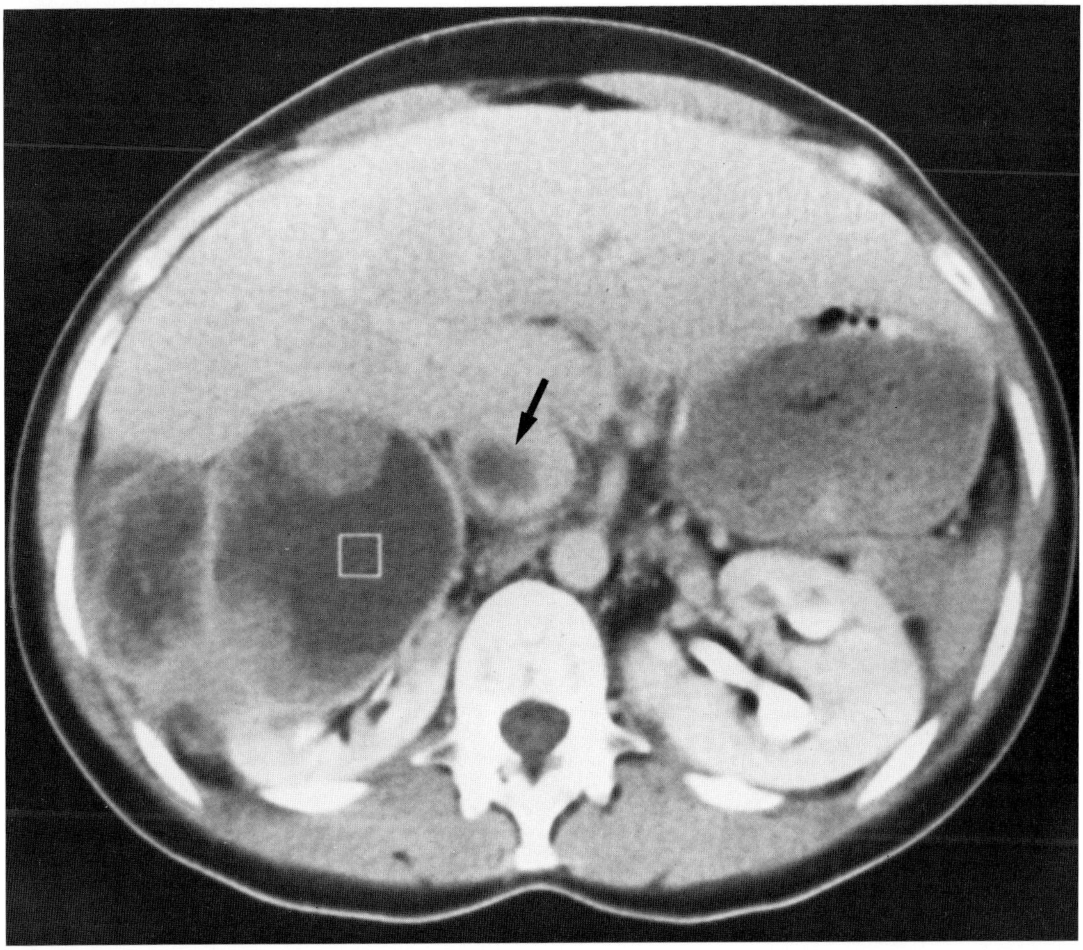

6–7

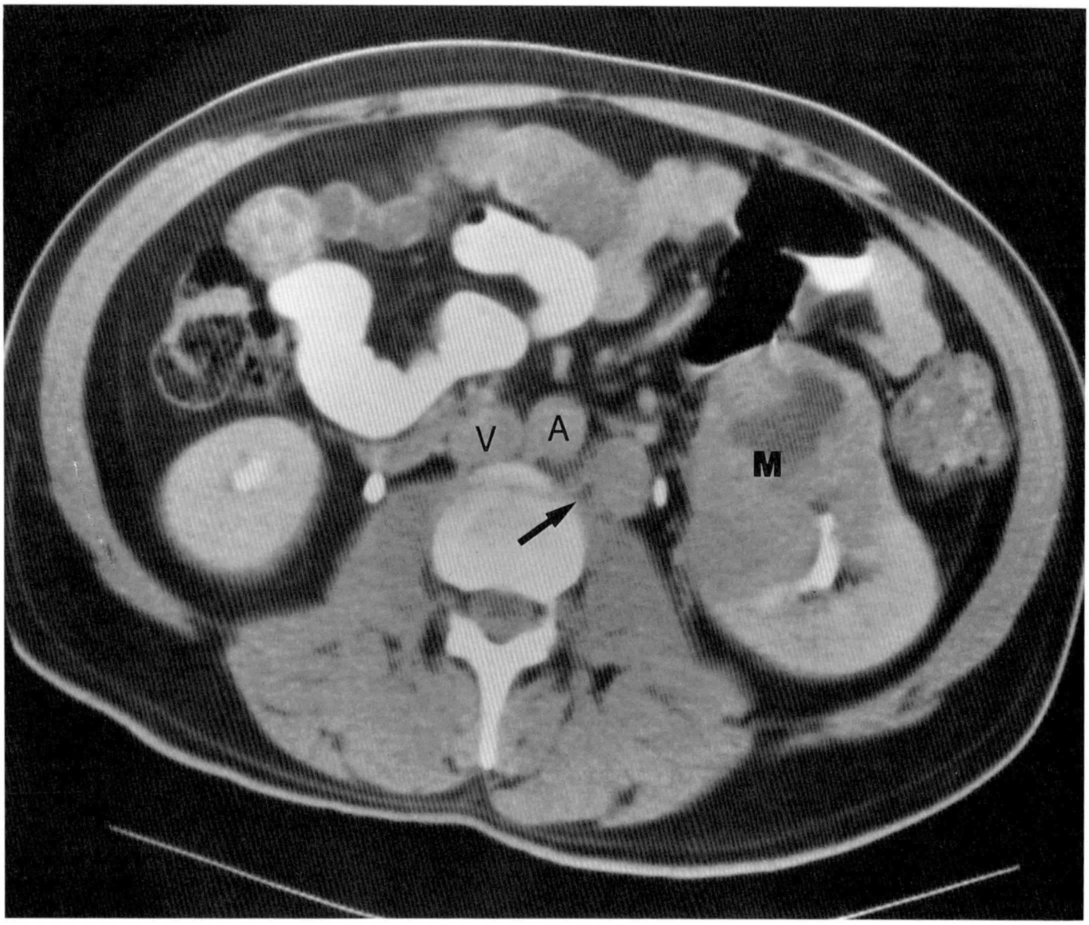

6–8 Renal adenocarcinoma. Mass (M) in left kidney is a primary renal adenocarcinoma. Enlarged left para-aortic mass (arrow) is a regional lymph node metastasis. A = aorta; C = cava.

6–9 Oncocytoma. Central stellate scar in this well-defined ▶ renal mass (arrows) suggests an oncocytoma. (Reprinted by permission, from Cohan RH, Dunnick NR, Degesys GE, Korobkin M: Computed tomography of renal oncocytoma. *J. Comput. Assist. Tomogr.* 8:284–287, 1984, Raven Press, New York, NY.)

6–10 Wilms's tumor. This large left renal mass (W) has ▶ distorted renal parenchyma (arrows). Low-density central portion indicates tumor necrosis. K = normal left kidney.

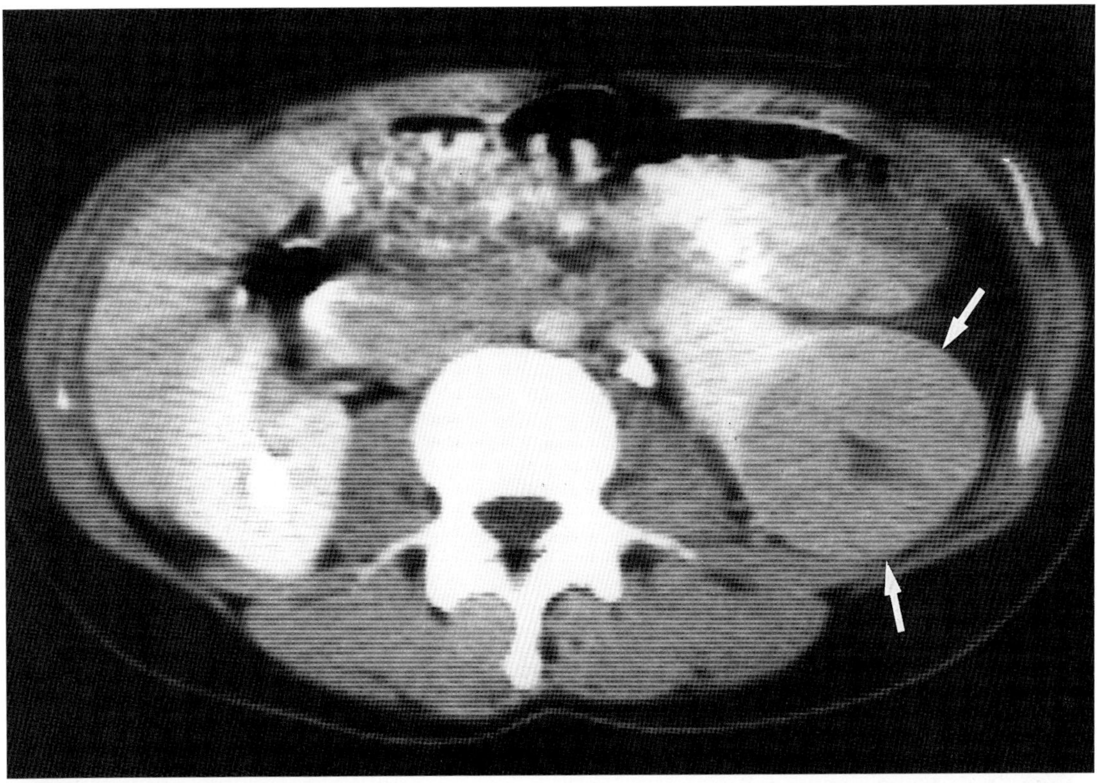

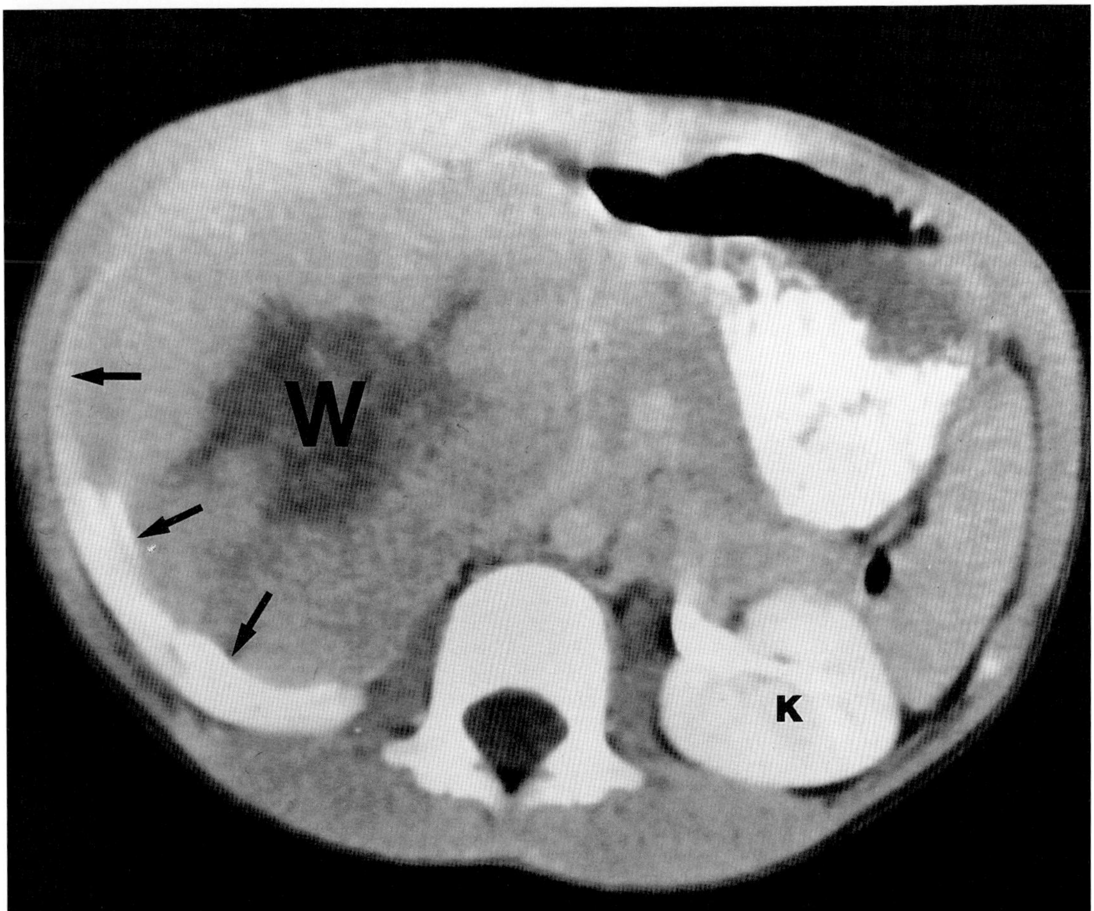
W
K

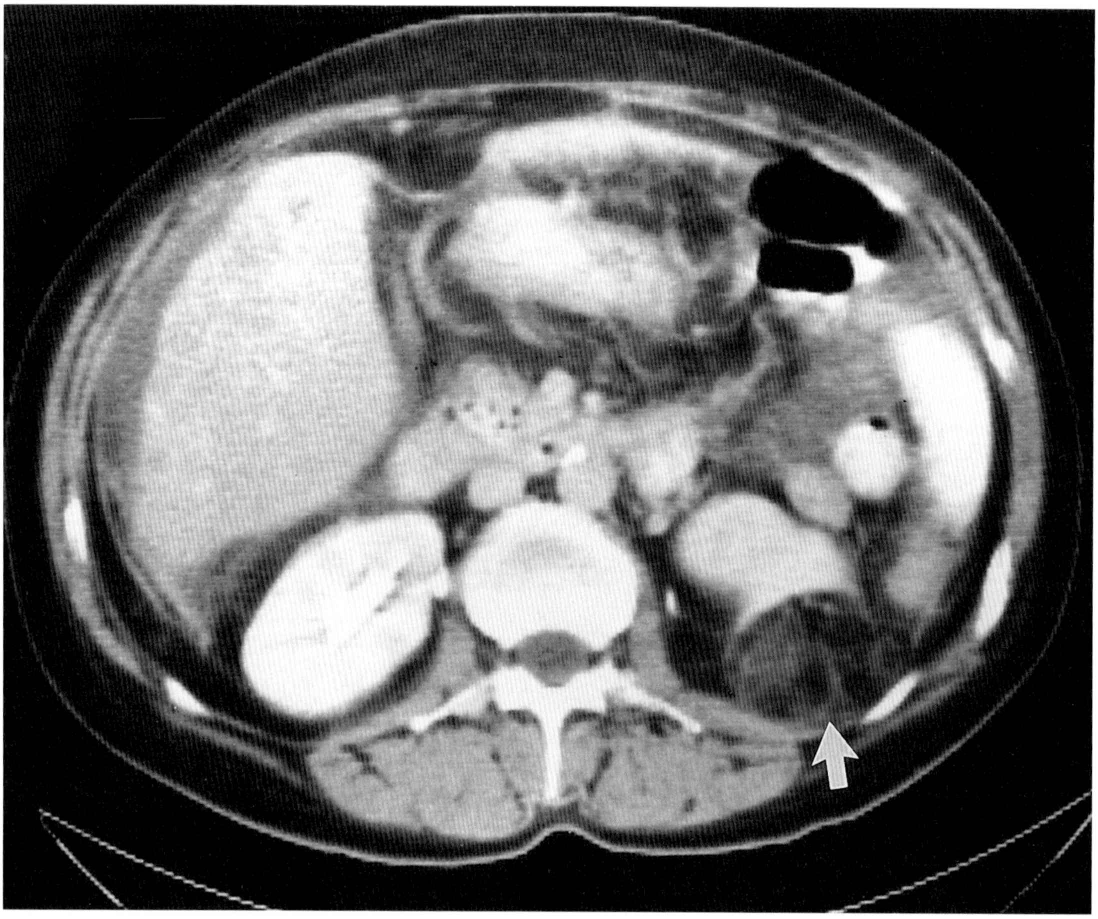

6–11 Angiomyolipoma. Fat density of left renal mass (arrow) characterizes an angiomyolipoma.

bilateral. With the more frequent use of CT and ultrasound, an increasing number of angiomyolipomas are detected as isolated lesions unassociated with tuberous sclerosis. These may be bilateral and are most commonly found in asymptomatic women.

Recognition depends on the low attenuation by CT or the high echogenicity by sonography of the fatty elements characteristic of this tumor (Fig. 6–11; Bosniak 1981; Bosniak et al. 1988). Angiomyolipomas that contain predominately vascular and muscle tissue and only a small amount of fat may not be distinguishable from other solid tumors of the kidney; however, these variations are rare.

Treatment has traditionally been surgical, but with increased confidence in the CT diagnosis of this benign tumor, most of these patients are being followed. Surgical or angiographic intervention and embolization is reserved for symptomatic or bleeding tumors.

Transitional Cell Carcinoma

Although transitional cell carcinoma is a common malignancy, only 2%–5% originate in the renal pelvis. Multiple tumors and recurrence are common. Bilateral synchronous tumors are rare, except in patients with analgesic or Balkan nephropathy. The radiographic appearance is a filling defect within the renal pelvis detected during excretory urography or retrograde pyelography (Fig. 6–12A). The filling defect arises from the wall and often has an irregular contour, allowing contrast material to penetrate the tumor.

CT excludes a renal stone as the etiology of the filling defect. The density of transitional cell carcinoma is greater than water but usually less than muscle or normal kidney. Since it is usually hypovascular, there is only slight contrast enhancement.

After intravenous contrast injection, the transitional cell tumor appears as a filling defect or

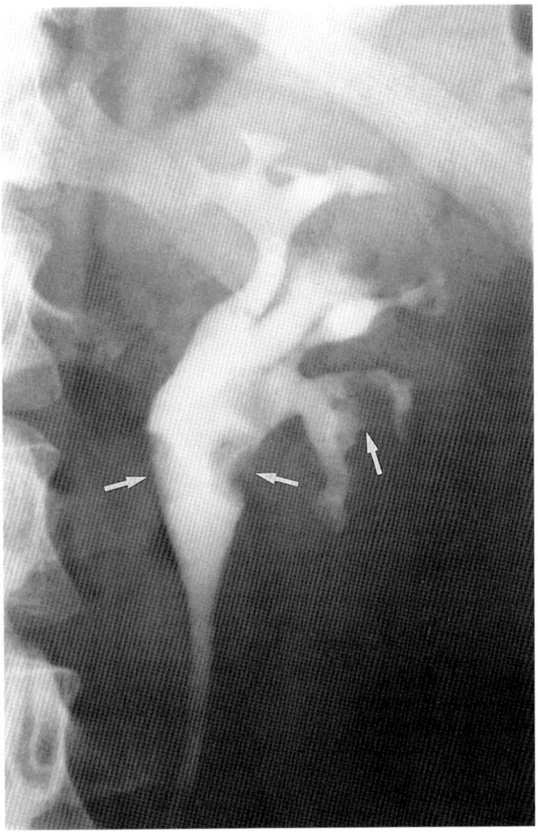

A

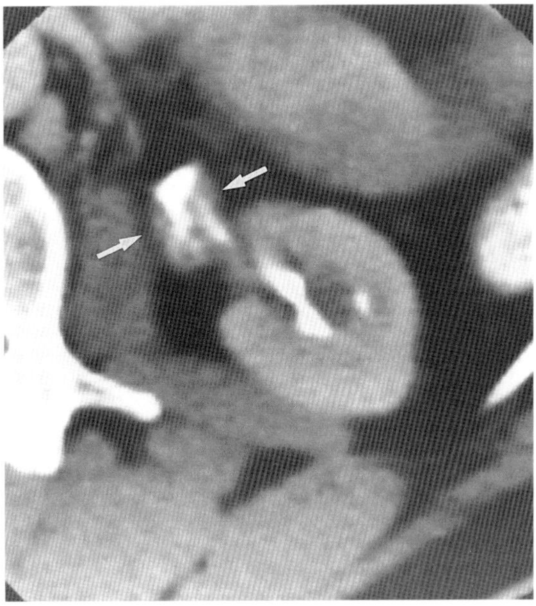

B

6–12 Transitional cell carcinoma. **(A)** Irregular filling defects (arrows) arising from wall of renal pelvis represent multifocal transitional cell carcinoma. **(B)** This correlates well with thickened renal pelvis (arrows) seen on CT.

thickening of the renal pelvic wall (Fig. 6–12B). Adjacent renal sinus fat may be compressed, and caliectasis indicates some degree of obstruction.

Metastases to the Kidney

Major advances in cancer therapy have resulted in prolonged survival for many patients. The natural history of many tumors is being altered, and metastases are being found in less common sites.

In autopsy series, renal metastases are usually from lung and breast carcinomas. They are more common than a second primary tumor (Pagani 1983). Since these metastases are usually small and clinically silent, occurring in patients with extensive metastatic disease, they may not be detected radiographically.

Precontrast scans may be normal unless the metastatic tumor causes some renal contour deformity. Metastases are usually hypovascular and are seen as low attenuation masses after intravenous contrast enhancement (Mitnick et al. 1985).

Lymphoma

Renal involvement by malignant lymphoma is found in about one-third of autopsy cases. Prior to CT and ultrasound, it was rarely detected except at autopsy. The kidney is involved more commonly with non-Hodgkin lymphoma than with Hodgkin's disease. Primary renal lymphoma is rare because lymphoid tissue is not normally found in the kidney.

Lymphoma of the kidney is due to either hematogenous dissemination or to direct extension from the retroperitoneum (Hartman et al. 1982). Hematogenous dissemination most commonly results in variable-size lymphomatous nodules or masses in the renal cortex. Diffuse infiltration of the kidney, a less common form, is found in about 10% of cases. Direct extension from para-aortic lymph nodes may also occur.

On unenhanced scans, lymphoma may present as a mass distorting the renal contour; however, lymphoma confined entirely within the kidney may not be recognized, since the density is similar to normal renal parenchyma.

After contrast injection, the lymphomatous

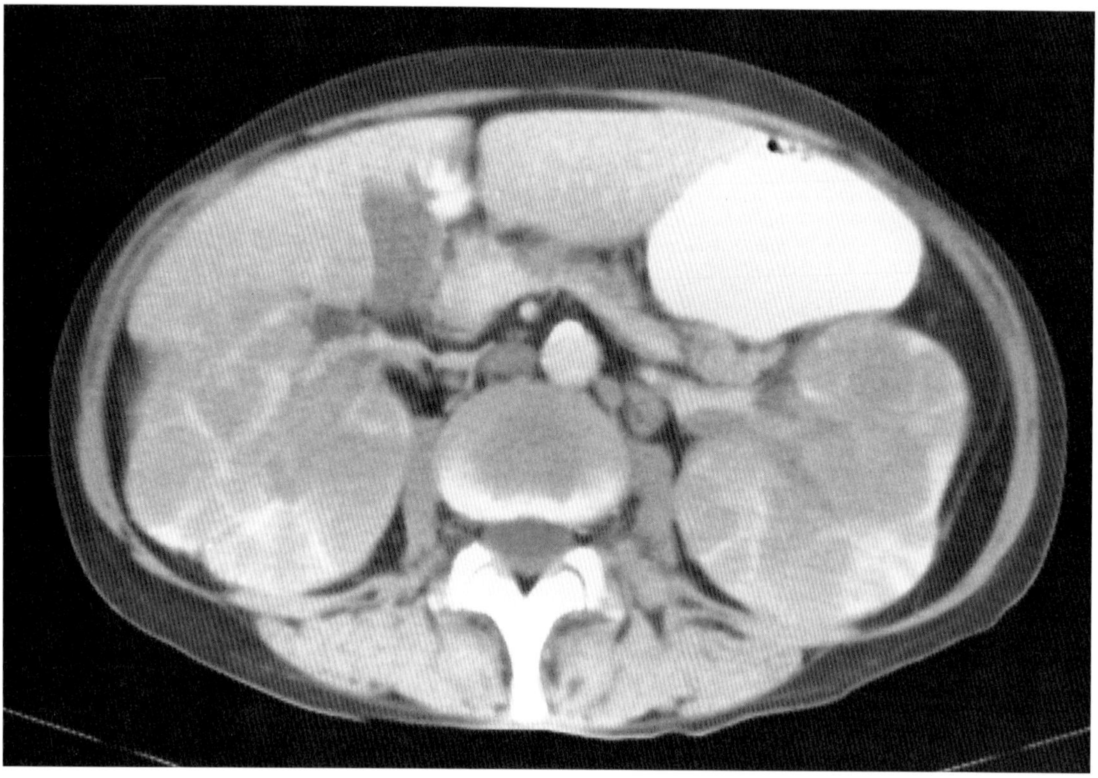

6–13 Renal lymphoma. Multiple low-density masses interspersed between functioning renal parenchyma represent lymphomatous nodules.

tissue is easily recognized because it does not show as much contrast enhancement as the normal kidney (Jafri et al. 1982). The tumor mass is homogeneous and is typically well defined (Fig. 6–13); calcification and central necrosis are rare. Many patients with renal lymphoma also show involvement of retroperitoneal lymph nodes, which reinforces the CT diagnosis.

Calculi

Excretory urography remains the primary imaging modality for urinary tract stone disease. However, 10%–20% of renal stones are poorly calcified and may not be seen well on an abdominal radiograph. During urography, nonopaque calculi are seen as a filling defect within the collecting system and must be differentiated from transitional cell carcinoma, blood clot, sloughed papilla, or fungus ball (Parienty et al. 1982).

CT can distinguish differences in density as small as 0.5%, whereas plain film radiography requires a difference of at least 5% (Federle et al. 1981). Thus, even lucent stones not seen on an abdominal radiograph are readily detected by CT (Fig. 6–14).

The intrarenal collecting system should be studied with contiguous 1-cm sections without intravenous contrast injection. Overlapping sections will decrease the chance of missing a calculus, owing to change in position of the kidney from breathing. In addition, section thickness should approximate stone diameter when imaging for small calculi, to minimize the problem of partial volume averaging. The partial volume effect of density, or volume averaging, occurs when an object such as a cyst, mass, or stone does not fully occupy the thickness of the CT section. When small stones are suspected, thin sections of 1.5 mm, 3 mm, or 5 mm should be used.

Once intravenous contrast has been administered, the entire collecting system becomes dense and the stone is obscured. If the filling defect is not a renal stone, contrast material may be useful because it can be seen around the tissue density of the tumor or blood clot.

Treatment of urinary tract calculi depends partly on the type of stone (Hillman et al. 1984). CT can measure the density to help determine the type of stone. Uric acid stones are the least dense, measuring 200–600 HU. Calcium oxalate stones are the densest, usually ranging from 800–1,000 HU and over. Struvite stones have an intermediate density and show some overlap with the other calculi. Many renal stones have more than one component.

Inflammatory Lesions

Pyelonephritis

Urinary tract infections that respond to antibiotic therapy do not require radiologic imaging. Imaging is needed, however, to identify complications such as abscess formation. In patients with repeated urinary tract infection, imaging helps detect a possible morphologic or physiologic abnormality.

Acute bacterial pyelonephritis produces edema and swelling of the kidney. The intrarenal vessels are narrowed, and the nephrogram shows delayed

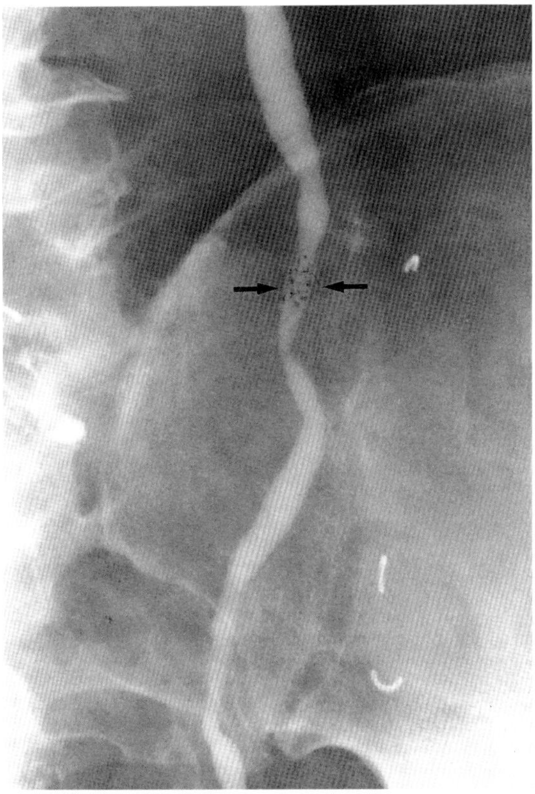

A

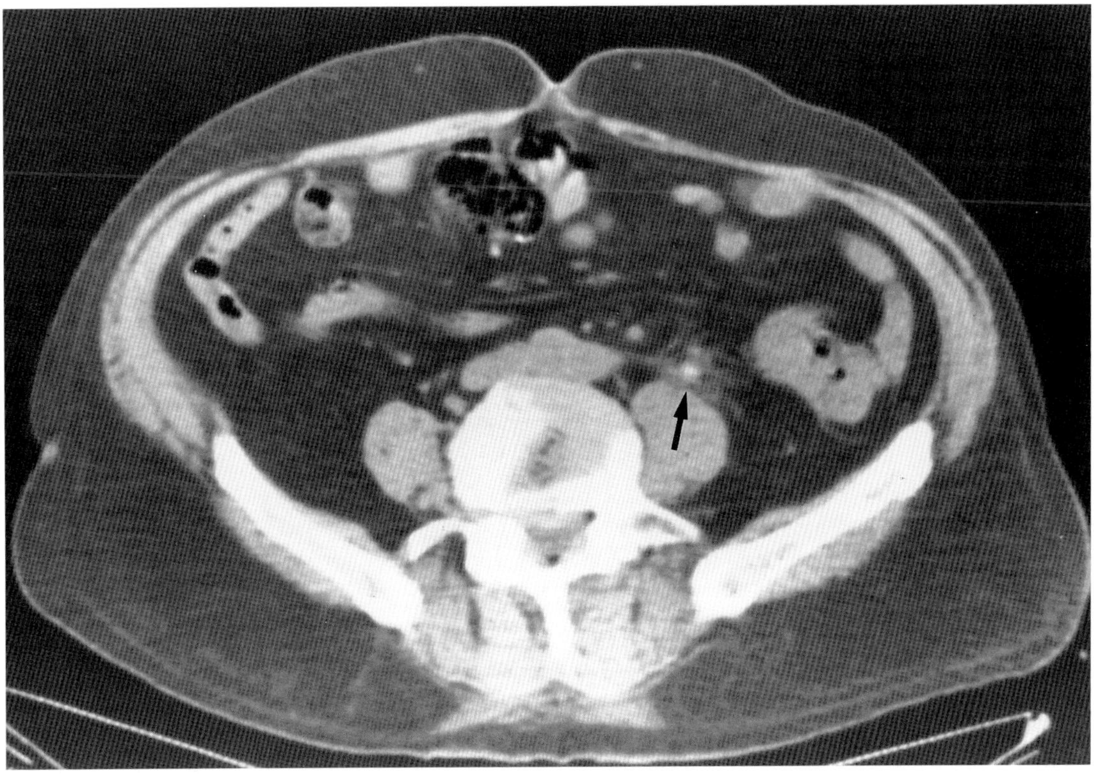

6–14 Ureteral stone. **(A)** Filling defect (arrow) is seen in left ureter on a retrograde pyelogram. **(B)** High-density (arrow) on CT done without contrast indicates that this is a nonopaque ureteral stone.

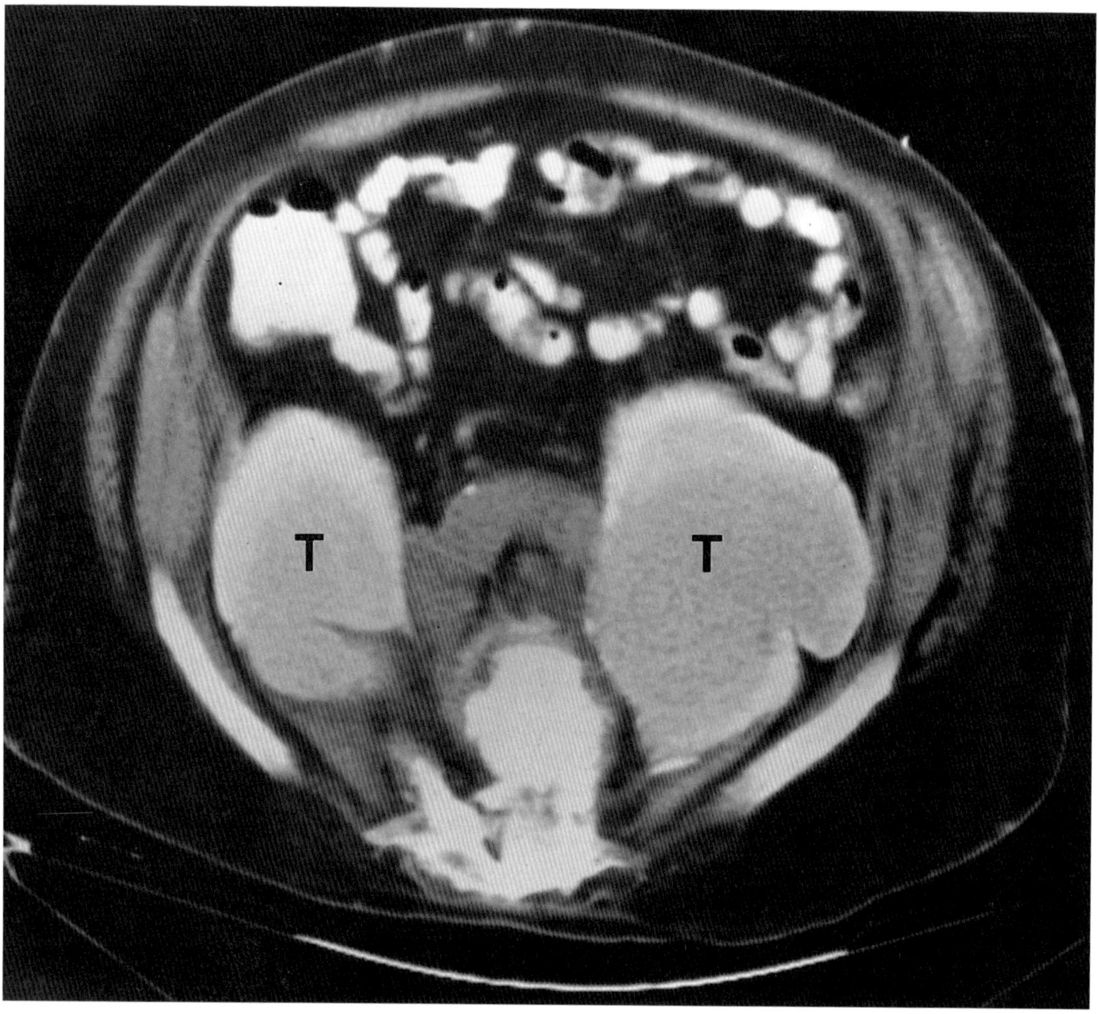

6–15 Tuberculosis. Large calcified paraspinal masses (T) are sterile abscesses in this patient with Pott's disease.

contrast appearance and less intensity than that of a normal kidney. Renal function is impaired, and the collecting system is attenuated. These changes can be seen on both excretory urography and CT. CT may also demonstrate the characteristic striated pattern of renal parenchyma opacification due to local edema compressing the vessels and tubules, which prevents normal contrast excretion (Gold et al. 1983).

If only a portion of the kidney is affected, it is termed acute lobar nephronia and is seen as a focal mass with CT or ultrasound (Rosenfield et al. 1979). Percutaneous needle aspiration may be needed to distinguish this mass from renal carcinoma.

Chronic pyelonephritis is usually an incidental finding on CT. The kidney is small with an irregular contour; caliceal detail cannot be evaluated, but areas of marked parenchymal loss can be seen.

Tuberculosis

Infection of the urinary tract from pulmonary tuberculosis can occur years after the primary lung infection. Typically, the kidneys are infected by blood-born bacilli; the lower urinary tract is involved only after direct extension down the ureter.

The earliest radiographic finding of caliceal blunting or obliteration is best detected by excretory urography. Subsequently, parenchymal loss with irregular cortical scarring is similar to that seen with chronic pyelonephritis. CT can be useful in evaluating genitourinary tuberculosis, because the lumbar spine or psoas muscles can be evaluated for involvement (Fig. 6–15; Goldman et al. 1985).

Xanthogranulomatous Pyelonephritis

Xanthogranulomatous pyelonephritis is a rare inflammation typically seen in middle-aged women and associated with chronic urinary tract infections and renal calculi. It is characterized by the formation of xanthomatous tissue comprised of lipid laden macrophages and usually involves the entire kidney, but segmental xanthogranulomatous pyelonephritis can occur. *Proteus* or *E. coli* are the most common infecting organisms.

The kidney is enlarged, but the reniform shape is preserved. Parenchyma is usually thinned, and the calices are markedly dilated (Goldman et al. 1984). Contrast enhancement differentiates the thin parenchymal rim from the dilated calices. Contrast enhancement of the renal parenchyma reflects only the vascularity of the inflammatory tissue, since there is usually no renal function. The renal pelvis is often contracted and may contain an obstructing stone or staghorn calculus; smaller calculi may be seen. Inflammation extending into the perinephric space is common.

Abscess

An intrarenal abscess may arise from either a preexisting renal infection or from another primary site of infection. The most common hematogenously spread infectious agent is *Staphylococcus aureus*, while those arising from the kidney are *E. coli*, *Proteus*, and *Pseudomonas*.

A renal abscess is seen on CT as an ovoid mass within the parenchyma. Density of the central portion is near or slightly greater than water. The abscess wall is thick and enhances with intravenous contrast; the margin between the abscess and normal parenchyma is indistinct (Morgan, Nyberg 1985). Occasionally, an intrarenal abscess will contain gas. There may also be thickening of the renal capsule and of Gerota's fascia.

Trauma

Computed tomography is more sensitive than excretory urography in detecting injuries resulting from trauma. Renal, splenic, or hepatic injury suspected with abdominal trauma may all be examined at the same time by CT. In the pelvis, CT can demonstrate bladder injury or contrast extravasation, and may also provide valuable information about the extent and location of any pelvic fractures. Excretory urography will correctly stage 60%–85% of trauma patients. CT may still be appropriate if the urogram is nonspecific, or if there is clinical suspicion of renal injury (Bretan et al. 1986).

Renal contusion occurs when urine and blood extravasate into the renal parenchyma but remain contained within the kidney. This presents as an area of poor renal function due to the interstitial edema. It does not require surgical intervention.

Laceration is a parenchymal injury that extends to the periphery of the kidney. If the renal capsule remains intact, a subcapsular hematoma or urinoma results. If the renal capsule is disrupted, urine and blood will spill into the perinephric space. Renal fracture is a disruption that separates the major fragments (Fig. 6–16). Opacification and function of these parts depend upon the integrity of the vascular supply.

Although most cases of trauma are treated conservatively, suspected renal artery injury is an indication for arteriography (Lang et al. 1985). Arterial injury can be diagnosed with CT, especially dynamic CT, by the absence of opacification of the ipsilateral kidney.

The most common kidney injury detected by CT is a perinephric hematoma confined by Gerota's fascia and by the many septae found in the perinephric space. An acute hematoma can be diagnosed by its high density of 60–90 HU.

With a subcapsular hematoma the strong renal capsule confines the blood; the parenchyma contour is often flattened and deformed. These patients should be observed for the development of hypertension or Page kidney during the subsequent year.

Adrenal

Current-generation CT scanners identify the adrenal glands in nearly all patients. Abnormalities are usually detected in symptomatic patients with functional neoplasms of the adrenal cortex or medulla; the rest are found incidentally.

Functional Lesions

Cushing's Syndrome

Cushing's syndrome results from increased glucocorticoid secretion and is characterized by truncal obesity, hypertension, glucose intolerance,

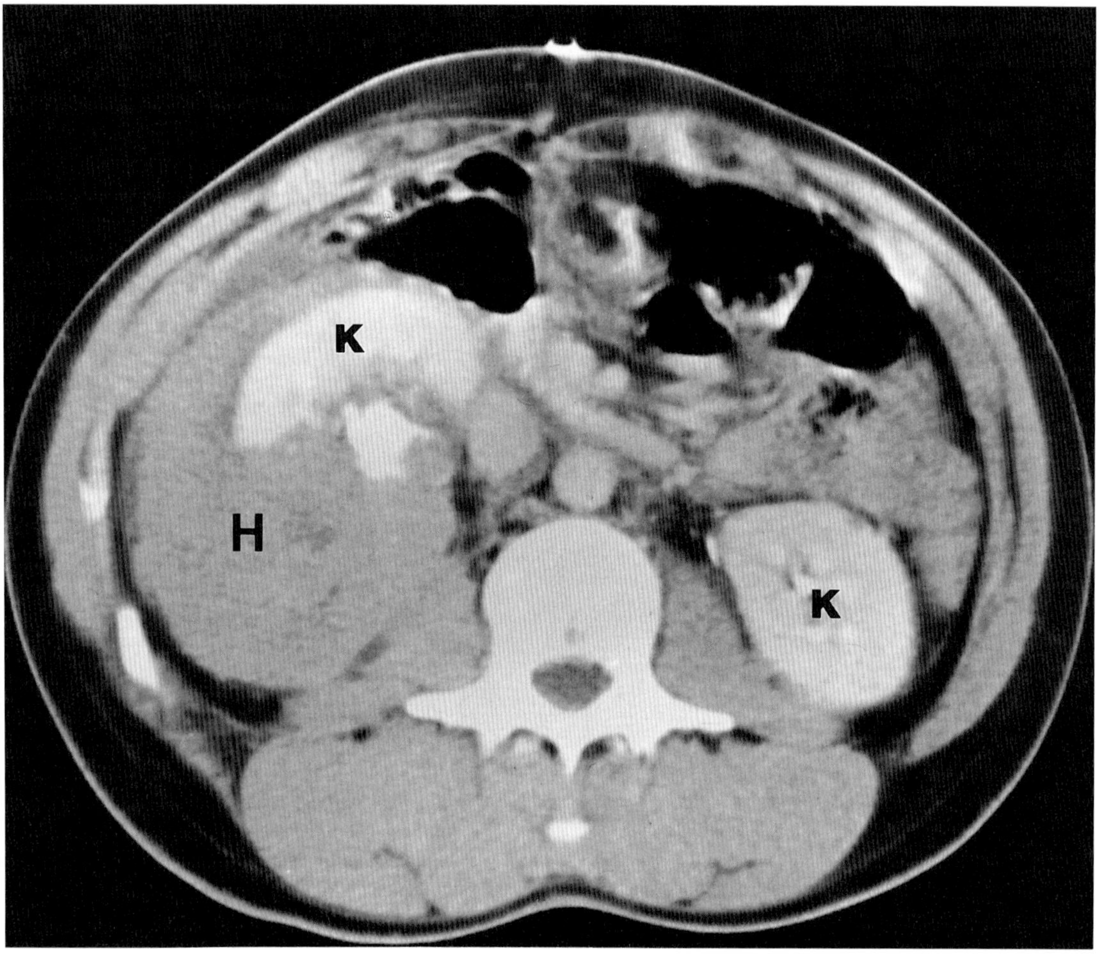

6–16 Renal fracture. A large perinephric hematoma (H) and one portion of fractured right kidney are seen on this CT image. K = kidney.

6–17 Adrenal hyperplasia. Both adrenal glands (arrows) ▶ are enlarged, but they maintain a normal configuration and have no focal masses.

osteoporosis, hirsutism, muscular atrophy, and abdominal striae. The most common cause is adrenal hyperplasia resulting from excess adrenocorticotropic hormone (ACTH). This is usually secondary to a pituitary adenoma, but is occasionally due to ACTH production by other neoplasms, such as oat-cell carcinoma or bronchial adenoma. On CT, generalized enlargement of the adrenals is noted (Fig. 6–17). The adrenal glands maintain their normal configuration, although the individual limbs may appear elongated.

An apparently normal adrenal CT does not exclude the diagnosis of hyperplasia. In some cases, particularly in children, hyperplasia may appear nodular and difficult to distinguish from multiple adrenal adenomas.

The most common adrenal neoplasms causing Cushing's syndrome are adenomas. These tumors average 4 cm in size. Adrenal adenomas are homogeneous, round adrenal masses of soft tissue or water density surrounded by abundant retroperitoneal fat (Dunnick, Doppman et al. 1982). The apparent water density results from volume averaging of soft tissue and fat and not from fluid; calcification is rare.

Occasionally, Cushing's syndrome can be secondary to primary adrenal carcinoma, as over 50% of these neoplasms will produce recognizable hormones, most commonly cortisol. Primary adrenal cancers grow rapidly and present clinically usually at 6 cm or greater (Fig. 6–18). Central necrosis and dystrophic calcification are often seen (Dunnick, Heaston et al. 1982).

CT scans of adrenal carcinomas must include evaluation of the left renal vein and inferior vena cava, because tumor thrombus commonly spreads from the adrenal veins into these vessels. Invasion can often be detected by enlargement of the left

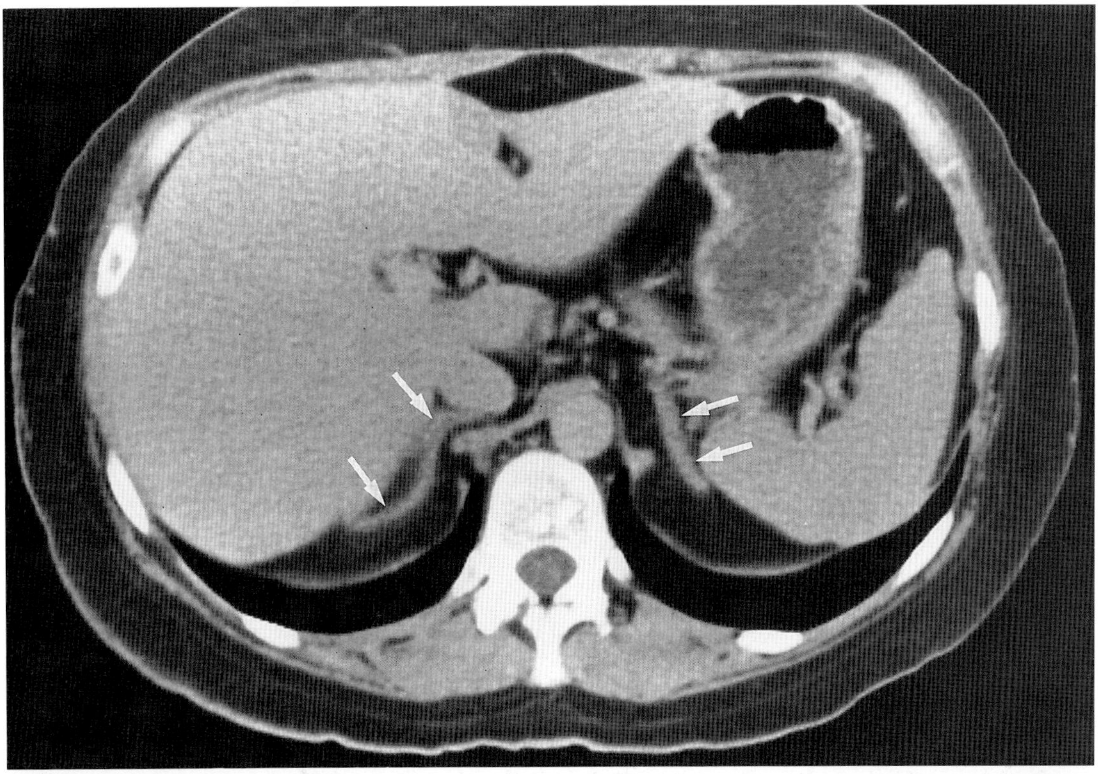

6–17

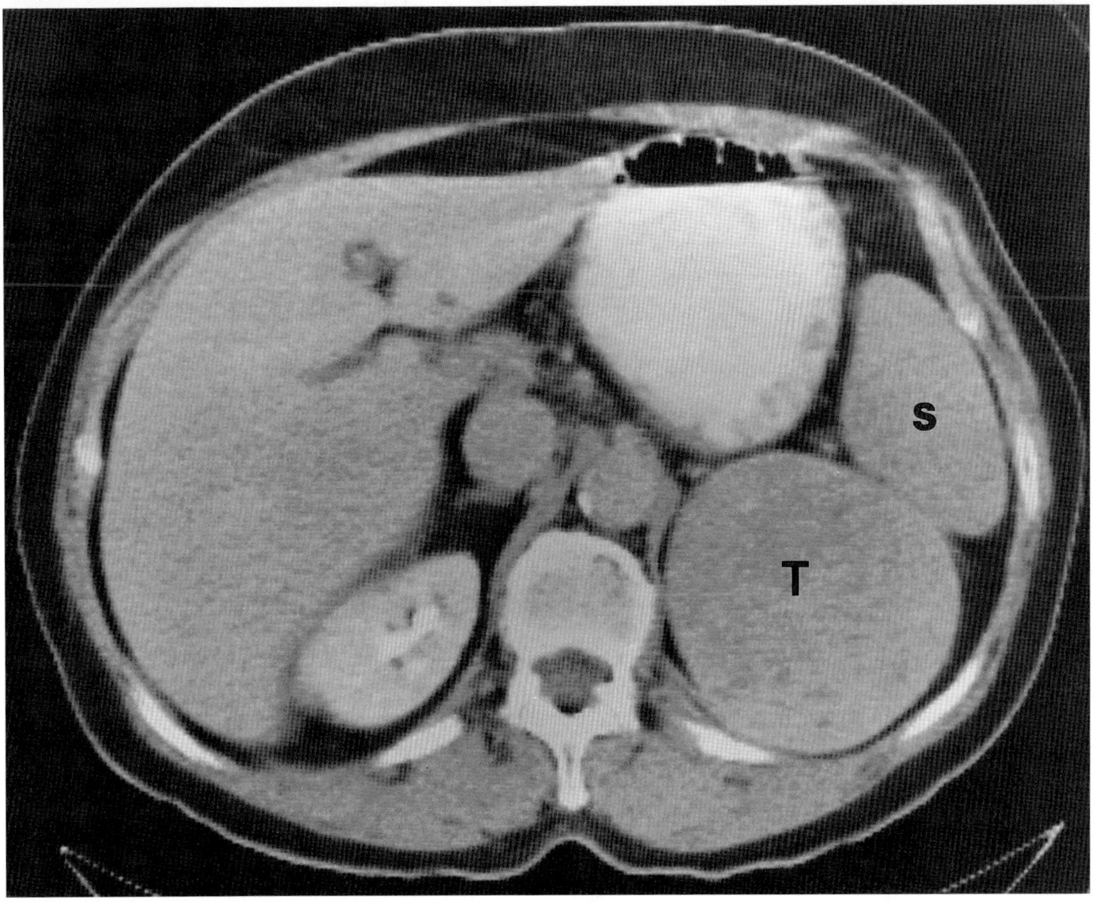

6–18 Adrenal carcinoma. This large left adrenal tumor (T) displaces adjacent organs. S = spleen.

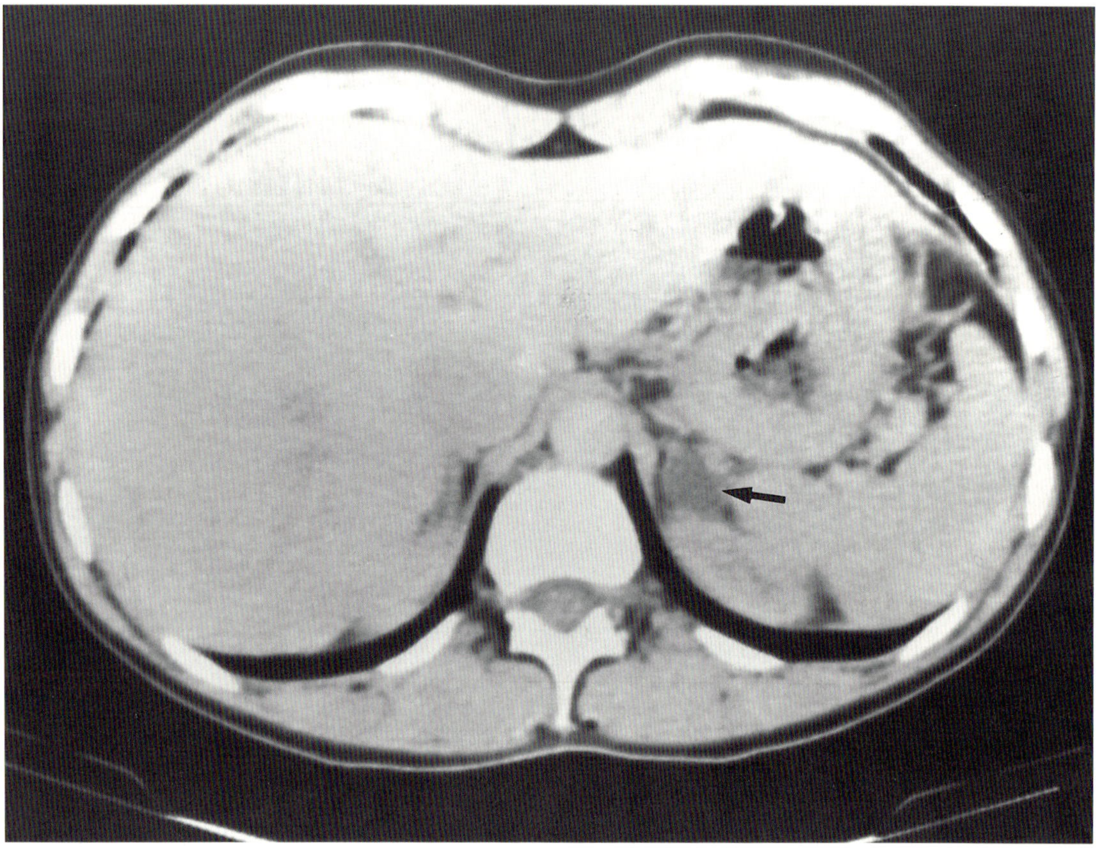

6–19 Aldosteronoma. Small mass in left adrenal gland (arrow) is an aldosterone-secreting adenoma in this patient with Conn's syndrome.

renal vein or inferior vena cava with or without identifiable intraluminal lucency. Venography may be required to exclude the presence of clot in patients with normal CT scans, although magnetic resonance imaging will likely supplant venography for evaluation of the vessels. Invasion of adjacent organs such as the liver, spleen, or kidneys can preclude surgery. A fat plane between the neoplasm and the adjacent organ means there is no invasion; however, absence of a fat plane is inconclusive.

Conn's Syndrome

Patients with primary aldosteronism present with hypertension and hypokalemia. Elevated aldosterone levels also result in low serum renin levels. Most commonly, Conn's syndrome is caused by a functioning adrenal adenoma rather than hyperplasia; etiology is important, since adenomas require surgery and adrenal hyperplasia is treated medically.

Aldosteronomas tend to be the smallest of the functioning adrenal adenomas, averaging under 2 cm in diameter (Fig. 6–19). In these cases CT must be performed using contiguous scans of 5-mm thickness at 5-mm intervals. Intravenous contrast is usually not needed. Even using this technique, only about 70% of adenomas will be identified; consequently, patients with biochemical evidence of an aldosteronoma require adrenal venous sampling for optimal localization. (Dunnick et al. 1982.)

Pheochromocytoma

Patients with pheochromocytoma typically present with recurrent attacks of palpitations, sweating, and pounding headaches. Hypertension is usually persistent but fluctuating. Measurement of urinary catecholamines, metanephrines, and vanillylmandelic acid provide a sensitive screening examination for pheochromocytoma. However, the rare nonfunctioning pheochromocytoma does not release excess catecholamines unless provoked, and will escape detection by these screening assays. The diagnosis is by measurement of 24-hr urinary concentrations of metanephrine or vanillylmandelic acid.

In 90% of cases, these tumors originate in the adrenal medulla. Pheochromocytomas are nearly always larger than 2 cm when they become clinically apparent; thus, a CT scan of the adrenal area can be obtained at 1-cm intervals. Since the tumors are moderate to large and elevation of catecholamines can occur with intravenous contrast, the scan should be done without intravenous contrast. Oral contrast is still used to opacify the bowel.

A pheochromocytoma appears as a round or oval mass of soft-tissue density. Central regions of low attenuation representing necrosis or cystic degeneration have been reported in up to 23% of patients. Calcification has been described in only 7%.

Ten percent of pheochromocytomas are extra-adrenal. Ectopic pheochromocytomas can be located anywhere from the base of the brain to the epididymis, although most occur along the sympathetic chain, usually at the organ of Zuckerkandl, in the retroperitoneal para-aortic region. Thus, scans should be continued inferiorly at least to the level of the aortic bifurcation in an attempt to identify an extra-adrenal pheochromocytoma. If no abnormal mass is identified after performing these additional scans, further evaluation with ^{131}I-metaiodobenzylguanidine (MIBG) is recommended. This radiopharmaceutical helps localize extra-adrenal pheochromocytomas.

Ten percent of adrenal pheochromocytomas are multicentric, with 5% being bilateral adrenal tumors; thus, once an abnormal mass is identified, others should be sought. Particular attention should be given to the contralateral adrenal gland and to the previously described common extra-adrenal sites.

Neuroblastoma

Neuroblastoma, the most common solid tumor in children, is derived from neural crest cells and can occur in any location where these cells are present. It most commonly originates in the adrenal gland or abdomen (70%). Children with neuroblastomas frequently present with a palpable abdominal mass, weight loss, and abdominal pain.

CT is the most sensitive imaging test for detection and staging of neuroblastoma. The lesions appear as soft-tissue retroperitoneal masses often with central cystic and necrotic areas. Calcification is present in most patients either as rings, multiple stippled flecks, or dense clumpy aggregates. These tumors can frequently infiltrate the adjacent mesenteric vessels so that no fat plane is detected between the aorta, inferior vena cava, celiac, or superior mesenteric artery and the mass.

Nonfunctional Mass Lesions

Nonfunctioning Adenomas

Nonfunctioning adrenal adenomas have been detected in 1.4%–33% of autopsies. Most of these adenomas are microscopic and are not usually identified on a CT scan. Glazer and colleagues (1982) found unsuspected adrenal masses in 0.6% of abdominal CT scans.

As with functioning adenomas, nonfunctioning adenomas are usually less than 3 cm and homogeneous. They may have water or soft-tissue attenuation. Calcification is rare. Occasionally, the lesions may be large and contain areas of necrosis.

If an adrenal mass is incidentally noted in a patient without biochemical abnormalities or a primary malignancy elsewhere, and if the lesion is under 3 cm in size, it can be followed by CT at 3-, 6-, and 12-month intervals and considered a nonfunctioning adenoma. If the adrenal mass exceeds 3 cm, further evaluation is warranted.

Adrenal Metastases

Almost any malignant neoplasm can metastasize to the adrenal gland, but lung, breast, renal carcinoma, and melanoma are the most common. Adrenal metastases have been found at autopsy in as many as 26% of cases of malignancies; however, half of these are microscopic and would not be detectable by CT.

Adrenal metastases may be small, homogeneous, and indistinguishable from nonfunctioning adenomas. They normally show soft-tissue attenuation. Larger metastatic masses more frequently contain low-attenuation areas of necrosis or hemorrhage than do their adenomatous counterparts.

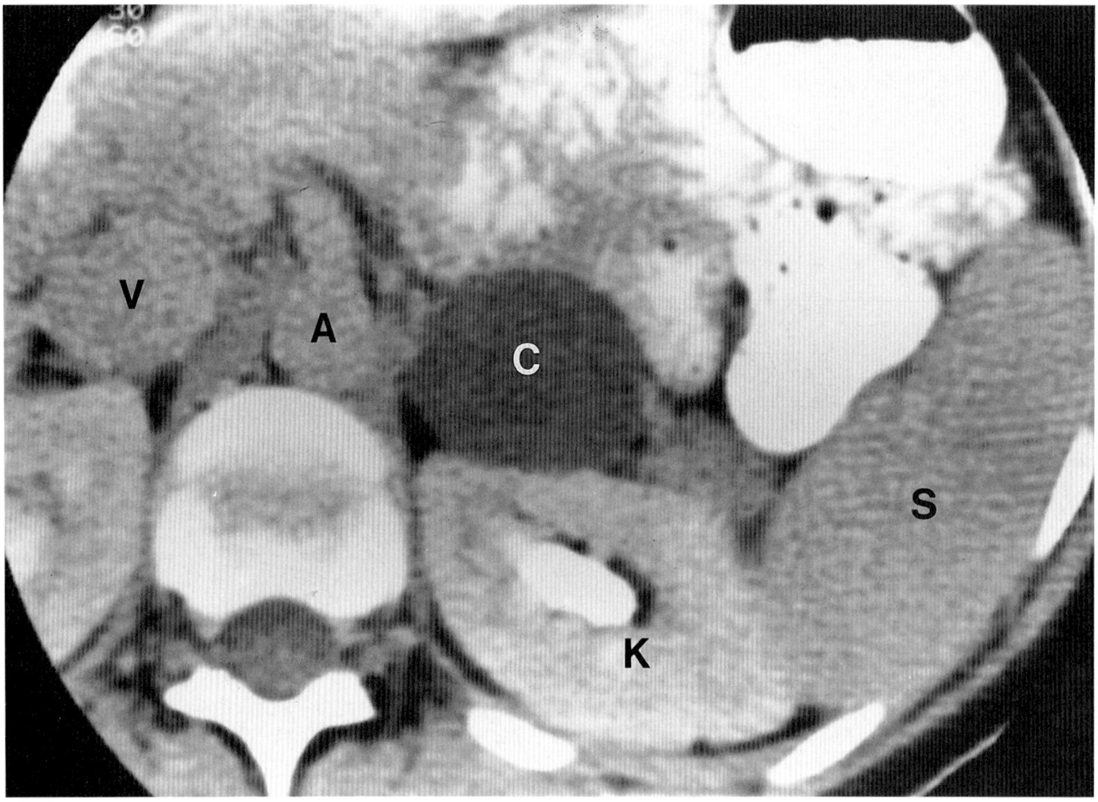

6–20 Adrenal cyst. This homogenous water density mass (C) in left adrenal gland has characteristics of a benign adrenal cyst. V = inferior vena cava; A = aorta; K = kidney; S = spleen.

Because of the difficulty in differentiating a metastasis from an adenoma by CT appearance alone, any adrenal mass in an oncology patient requires evaluation by CT-guided percutaneous biopsy. Aspiration of malignant cells can establish the correct diagnosis. If no malignant cells are isolated, results are inconclusive.

Recently, several articles have compared the appearance of adrenal metastases, adenomas, and pheochromocytomas using magnetic resonance imaging. Malignant adrenal masses and pheochromocytomas have significantly higher signal intensity on T2 weighted images than benign adenomas. This distinction may offer another characterization of the adrenal mass discovered in an oncology patient.

Adrenal Cysts

Adrenal cysts are rare, occurring in less than 1 in 1,600 patients at autopsy, with most cysts too small to be detected by CT. These benign lesions are commonly endothelial lined, suggesting lymphangitic or angiomatous origin. Other etiologies include pseudocyst formation secondary to necrosis or liquifaction of a hematoma after hemorrhage into a normal gland or an adrenal adenoma; epithelial (glandular or retention) cysts; or parasitic cysts (usually echinococcal) (Johnson et al. 1985).

Adrenal cysts occur most frequently in middle-aged women. On CT, the cysts are usually homogeneous water attenuation masses (Fig. 6–20). Peripheral calcification has been noted in approximately 15% of these cysts. A noncalcified cyst cannot be differentiated from a water density adenoma by CT, but can be distinguished by ultrasound. Treatment is only required if the cyst is large enough to cause symptoms.

Adrenal Hemorrhage

Adrenal hemorrhage in adults is associated with the stress of surgery, trauma, burn injury, or septic shock. Occasionally, it is found in patients with disseminated intravascular coagulation, thrombocytopenia, or those on anticoagulant therapy.

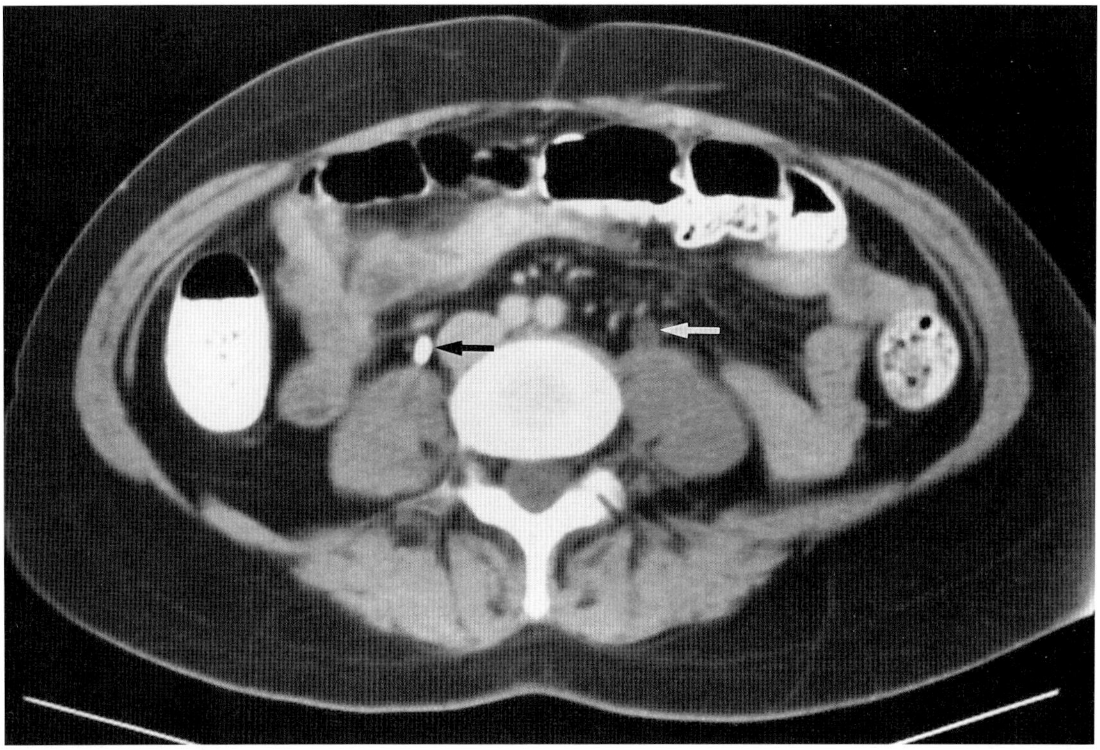

6–21 Ureteral obstruction. Right ureter (black arrow) is opacified by excreted contrast material. Obstructed left ureter (white arrow) is dilated and filled with nonopacified urine.

CT examinations of patients with adrenal hemorrhage demonstrate either unilateral (usually right) or bilateral adrenal masses of soft-tissue attenuation. These may contain small areas of decreased and increased attenuation, indicating liquifaction of portions of the hematoma and fresh bleeding, respectively. The appearance of an adrenal hematoma is often nonspecific.

If there is high density, or if follow-up scans reveal a decrease or disappearance of the mass along with decreasing attenuation values, the diagnosis of adrenal hemorrhage is established. Ultimately, calcifications may form.

Myelolipoma

The adrenal myelolipoma is a rare benign neoplasm containing fat and bone marrow cells. These tumors have no malignant potential and are nonfunctioning. They are readily recognized by their predominantly fatty density and soft tissue strands. Areas of calcification and hemorrhage may also be present. They are similar in CT appearance to the angiomyolipoma of the kidney.

Lower Urinary Tract

Ureter

Prior to CT, the retroperitoneum was evaluated by opacification of the ureter. Deviation or extrinsic compression of the ureter by retroperitoneal masses such as lymph node metastases can now be directly assessed. Bulky metastases commonly cause lateral deviation of the proximal ureters but do not usually obstruct the ureter unless there is extensive tumor encasing it. At the sacrum, the ureter passes medial to the iliac vessels and lymph nodes; thus, lymphadenopathy will push the distal ureter medially.

Ureteral obstruction can be recognized on CT by dilation of the ureter and a delay in opacification by excreted contrast material (Fig. 6–21). With high-grade obstruction, the affected ureter will not usually opacify but can still be identified as a tubular structure just lateral to the aorta or inferior vena cava and anterior to the psoas muscle. CT can delineate a mass causing ureteral obstruction (Megibow et al. 1982).

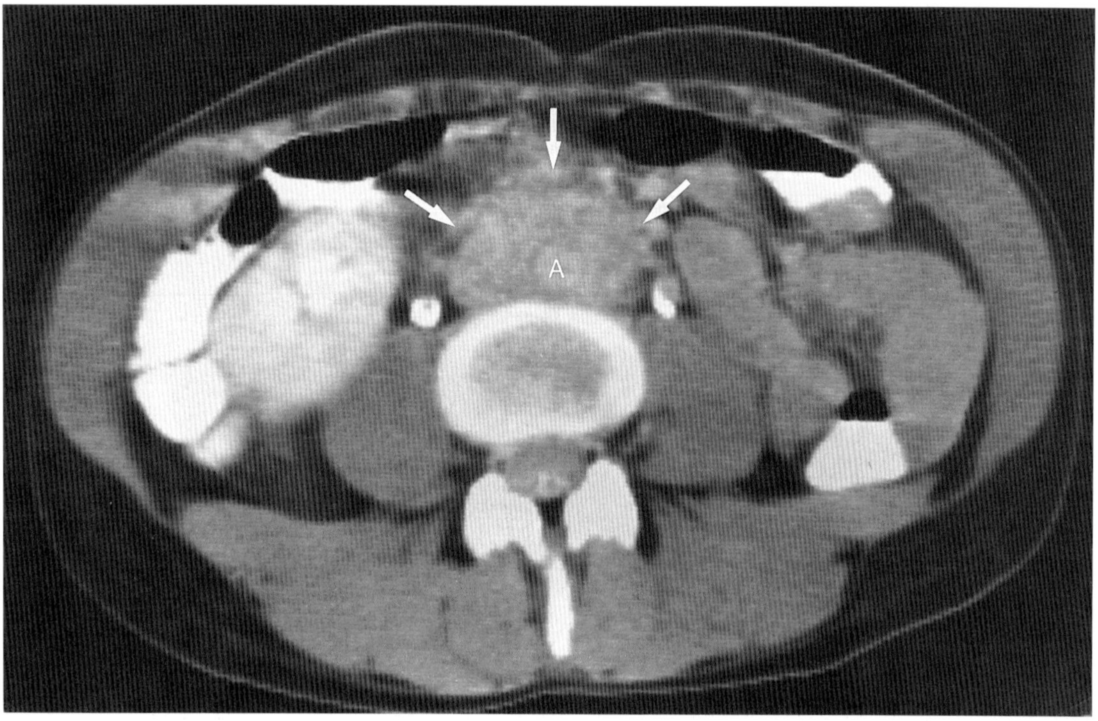

6–22 Retroperitoneal fibrosis. Para-aortic soft-tissue mass (arrows) envelopes aorta (A) and inferior vena cava. (Reprinted by permission, from Degesys GE, Dunnick NR, Silverman PM, Cohan RH, Illescas FF, Castagno A: Retroperitoneal fibrosis: Use of CT in distinguishing among possible causes. *Am. J. Roentgenol.* 146:57–60, 1986, American Roentgen Ray Society.)

Since spatial resolution on CT is less than that of film screen combination, it has not been used often for evaluation of intrinsic ureteral lesions. However, CT can help identify ureteral stones, since even a calculus nonopaque by radiograph is clearly visible by its high density on CT (Fig. 6–14).

Retroperitoneal Fibrosis

Retroperitoneal fibrosis usually occurs in middle-aged men. Etiology is usually unknown, but it is sometimes related to methysergide (Sansert) ingestion or caused by retroperitoneal tumor or perianeurysmal fibrosis. CT appearance is of a soft-tissue mass enveloping the ureters and great vessels (Fig. 6–22). It is most common at the L4–5 level, but may extend from the renal hilum to the true pelvis. It has also been associated with mediastinal fibrosis.

Idiopathic retroperitoneal fibrosis cannot be distinguished radiographically from retroperitoneal lymphoma, lymph node metastases, or diffusely infiltrating tumor; biopsy is required. However, marked anterior displacement of the great vessels may be seen with a tumor but not with retroperitoneal fibrosis (Degesys et al. 1986). Furthermore, the lateral contour of fibrosis often has a sharp linear border with the adjacent fat rather than the lobulated margins of retroperitoneal metastases.

Bladder

Intrinsic diseases of the bladder are amenable to direct cystoscopic examination. CT delineates masses causing extrinsic compression on the bladder. It is used to stage bladder carcinoma.

Carcinoma

Carcinoma of the bladder, the most common malignancy of the urinary tract, usually occurs in men over 50 years of age. Transitional cell cancers account for over 90% of cases. CT significantly improves preoperative staging by identifying extension to the pelvic sidewall and distant metastases (stages C and D) (Amendola et al. 1986). Spread to retroperitoneal lymph nodes can be detected by CT only if the nodes are enlarged.

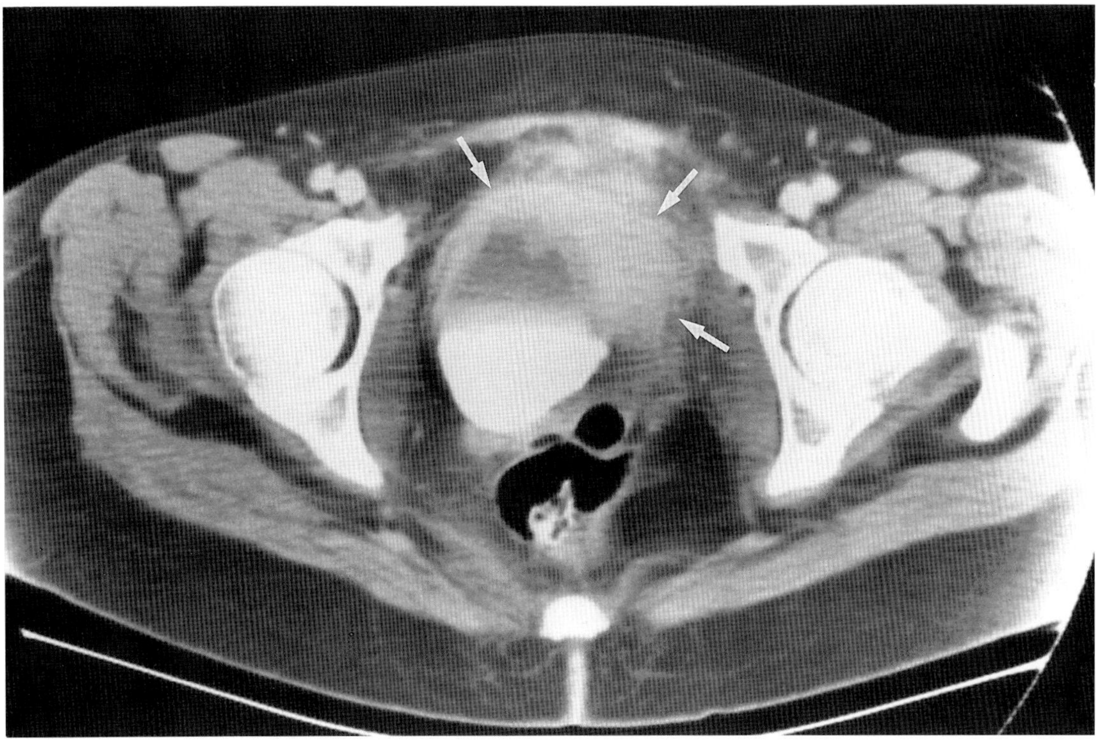

6–23 Bladder carcinoma. Thickened wall and soft-tissue mass (arrows) in anterolateral portion of bladder indicate carcinoma, which was responsible for left ureteral obstruction in Fig. 6–21.

Hematogenous metastases occur most frequently in the liver and lung.

Bladder tumors can be recognized on CT if they have sufficient mass to thicken or deform the bladder wall (Fig. 6–23). This appearance may be mimicked by changes due to previous surgery and biopsy, inflammation, or radiation therapy (Weinerman et al. 1983). Loss of tissue planes or a soft-tissue mass extending into the perivesical fat indicate local tumor extension. Since bladder tumors often begin in the trigone region, obstruction of one or both ureters is common. They may also extend directly posterior into the seminal vesicles.

Although CT improves the ability to stage bladder carcinoma, it has a low accuracy rate compared to surgery. CT cannot differentiate nonspecific inflammatory changes in the perivesical fat from tumor infiltration. Enlarged retroperitoneal lymph nodes may be due to benign reactive changes, and small tumor deposits may be present in normal size lymph nodes. Percutaneous fine-needle aspiration confirms tumor involvement in indeterminate cases.

Extrinsic Masses

Pelvic lipomatosis causes compression and elevation of the bladder into a vertical, almost pear-shaped configuration. On CT, excessive fat is seen in the pelvis, which confirms the diagnosis. A similar urographic appearance is seen with pelvic fractures where a large hematoma is responsible for the bladder compression. Bilateral processes such as lymphoceles or bulky adenopathy from malignant lymphoma may also appear similar. Each of these causes can be discerned by the combination of a plain pelvic radiograph and a CT scan.

Prostate

In situ carcinomas have been incidentally found in 80% of men over 80 years of age. Since malignant and benign prostatic enlargement both have the same density, it is impossible to predict prostate carcinoma by CT. A lobulated contour may be more common in patients with prostate cancer (Fig. 6–24 A), but this has little clinical value, as the diagnosis is best made by physical examination

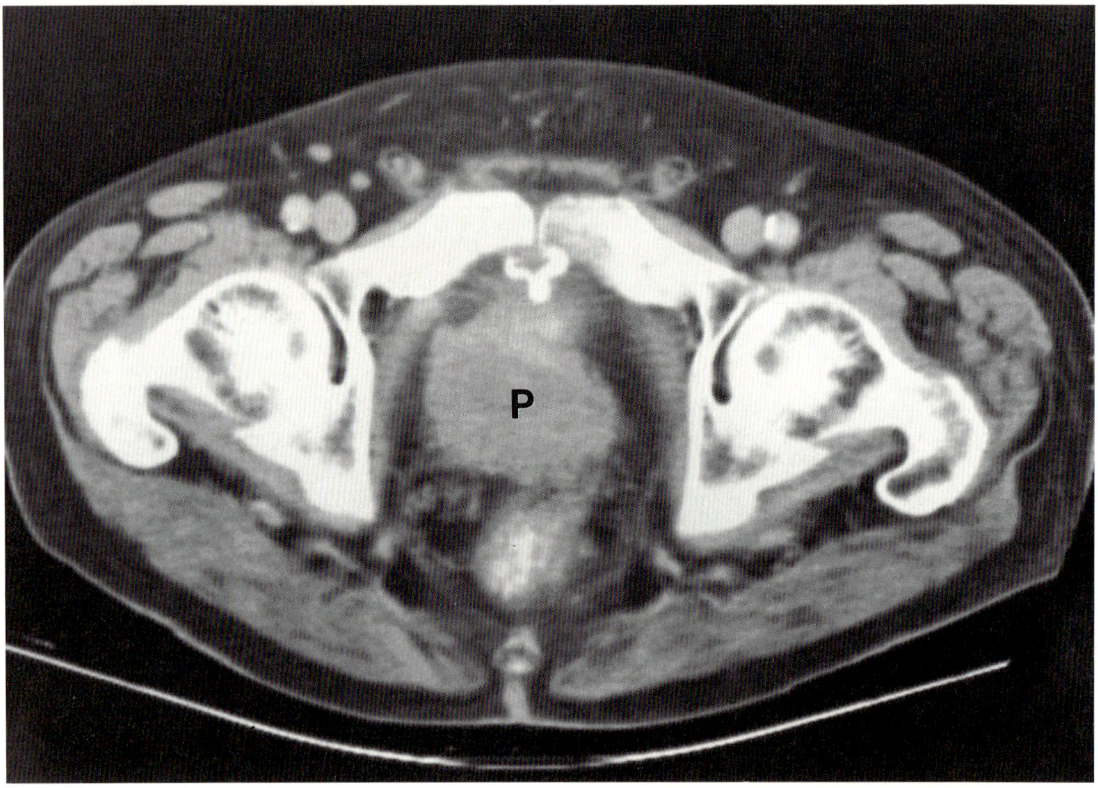

A

6–24 Prostate cancer. **(A)** Irregular contour of this enlarged prostate (P) suggests carcinoma. However, biopsy is needed for confirmation. **(B)** Metastases cause enlargement of iliac lymph nodes (arrows). **(C)** Para-aortic lymph nodes (arrows) are enlarged by metastatic disease. A = aorta; V = inferior vena cava.

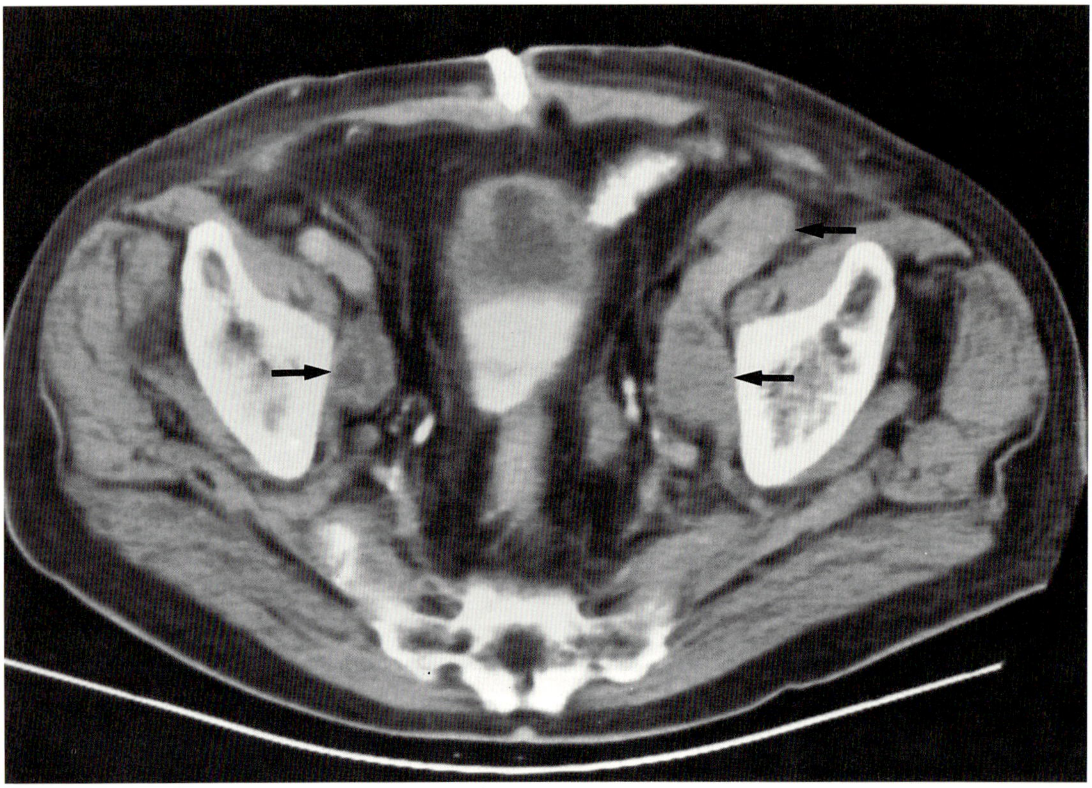

B

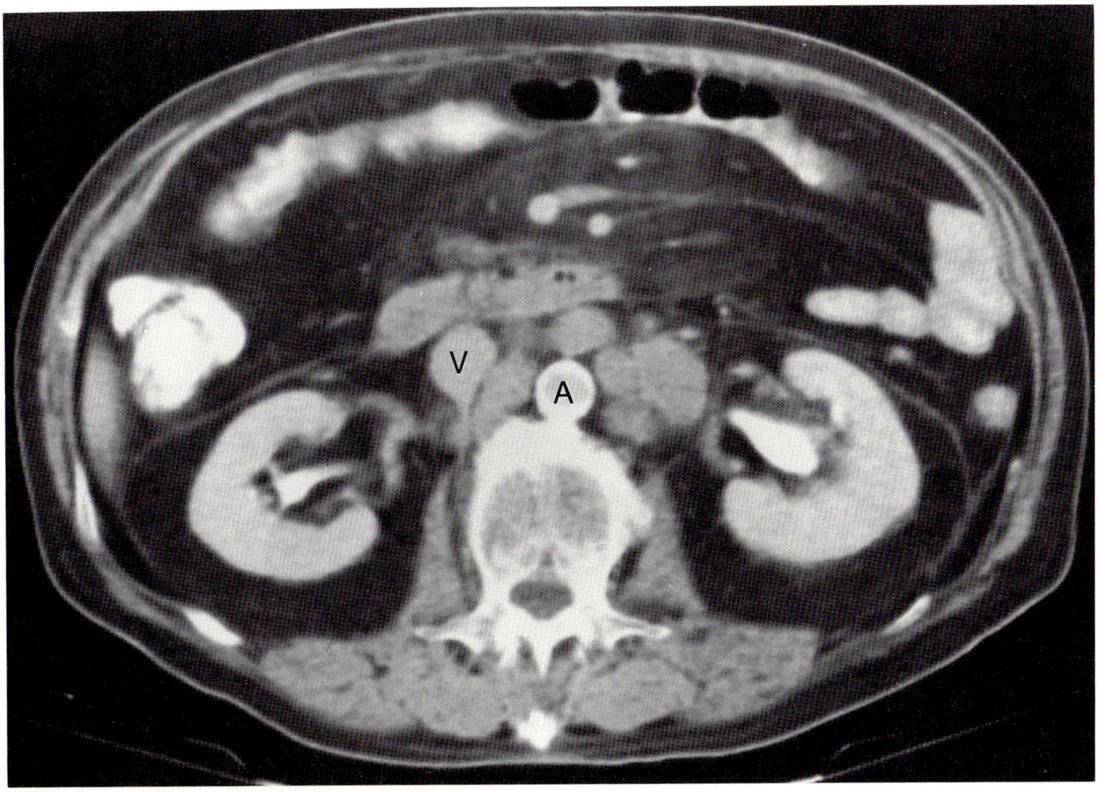

C

or transrectal ultrasound (Rifkin 1987) and needle biopsy. CT primarily assists in disease staging; however, as with bladder carcinoma, CT is limited to defining extension of tumor beyond the gland (stages C and D).

Prostate carcinoma may extend directly through the capsule to involve adjacent structures such as the seminal vesicles, bladder, or rectum. Involvement can be suggested by CT when there is loss of the normal fat plane. Tumor spread to the pelvic sidewall and enlargement of local lymph nodes may also be defined (Fig. 6–24B).

Stage D disease includes hematogenous metastases or involvement of retroperitoneal lymph nodes (Fig. 6–24C). The sensitivity of CT in detecting lymph node involvement is limited unless the nodes are enlarged; it will miss small metastatic deposits (Weinerman et al. 1983). Bone involvement can be more efficiently determined by radionuclide scintigraphy.

Testes

CT is used primarily to look for intra-abdominal extension of testicular neoplasms and to determine the location of an undescended testis.

Carcinoma

Testicular tumors are the most common cause of cancer death in males between 25 and 35 years of age. Tissue subtypes include teratoma, embryonal cell carcinoma, seminoma, and, rarely, choriocarcinoma. Patients present with pain, a palpable testicular mass, or symptoms of tumor dissemination.

Testicular tumors commonly spread along the lymphatic pathways, which parallel the gonadal veins. On the left side, the lymph channels course to the level of the renal vein before entering the para-aortic chains; on the right side, the lymphatics drain directly to the paracaval chains at approximately the L–2 or L–3 level. If there has been no prior scrotal surgery, the first site of metastases from a left testicle tumor is in the region of the left renal hilum and para-aortic lymph nodes at the L–1/L–2 level. For right-sided tumors, it is to the paracaval lymph nodes just above the aortic bifurcation. Extensive retroperitoneal tumor or prior surgery may result in pelvic or inguinal metastases.

Lymphography is occasionally used with CT to stage testicular neoplasms. Lymphography can detect tumor within normal-sized lymph nodes based on changes in the internal architecture. CT

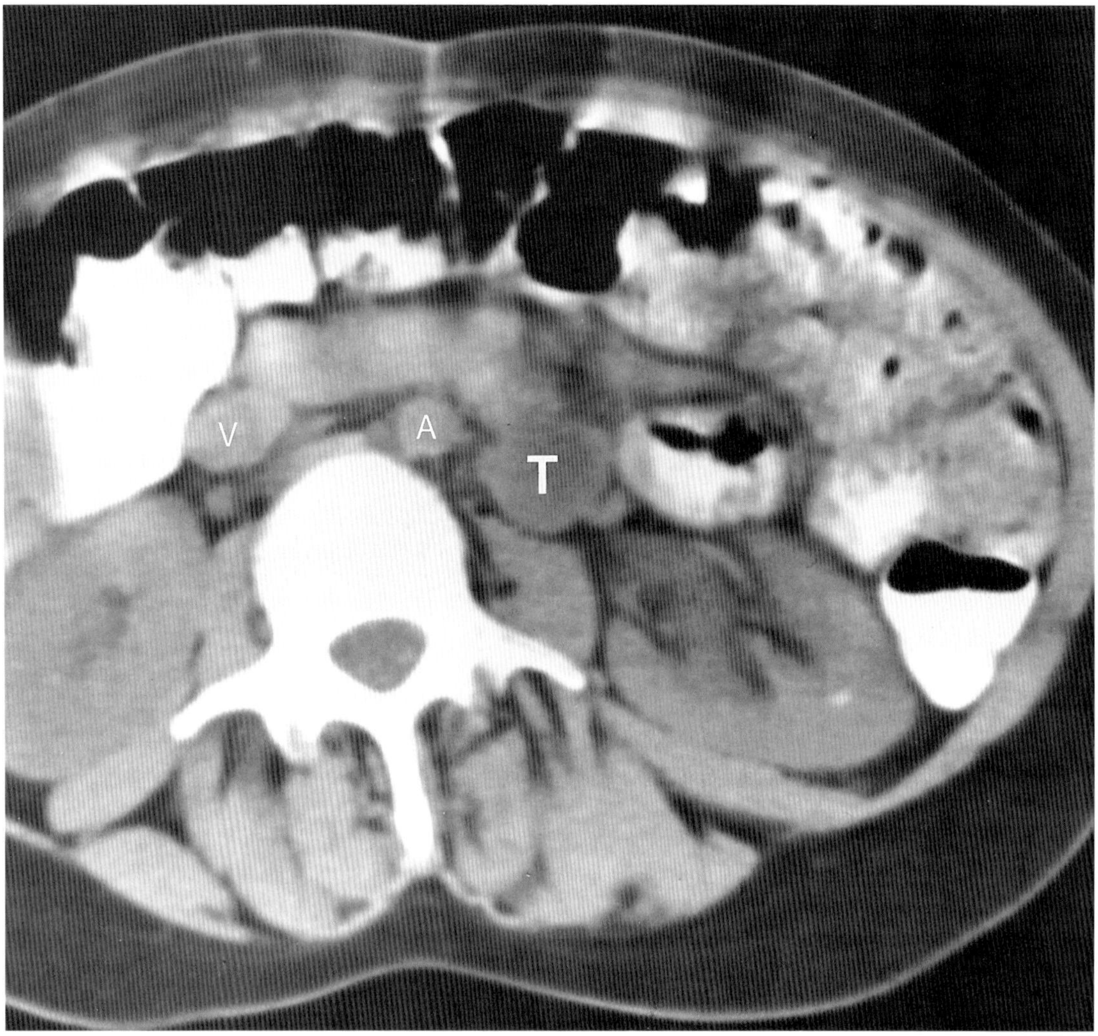

6–25 Testicular carcinoma. Metastatic tumor (T) from left testis ascends along lymphatic chain to para-aortic chain at level of left renal vein. A = aorta; V = inferior vena cava.

delineates the extent of tumor better and can identify disease in lymph nodes not opacified by lymphography. With the increasing resolution and availability of equipment, CT is becoming the primary staging method.

Involved lymph nodes are detected by their increased size (Fig. 6–25). Nodes larger than 1 cm in diameter in the retroperitoneum are considered metastases if their location is consistent with the expected drainage route. Large nodal metastases may undergo central necrosis and even calcification. This is, however, different from benign teratomatous degeneration, which may occur with effective therapy. These benign cystic masses may increase in size, while solid tumor deposits decrease in size with treatment. Biopsy may be needed to make this distinction.

Undescended Testes

Cryptorchoid testes may be detected radiographically by ultrasound, CT, testicular venography, or magnetic resonance imaging. Sonography is useful primarily when the testis lies in the inguinal canal. CT can localize intra-abdominal testes as well, but uses ionizing radiation. Testicular venography is the most accurate method of identifying gonadal tissue but requires considerable technical expertise. Magnetic resonance imaging holds promise as the most effective and least invasive diagnostic method.

Undescended testes lie along the path of testicular migration and may be located anywhere from the lower pole of the kidney to the scrotum. The majority, however, lie in or near the inguinal canal; thus, careful examination of this region by contiguous sections is essential. An undescended testis can be recognized as an ovoid soft-tissue mass along the course of testicular descent. Oral contrast for opacification of adjacent loops of bowel and intravenous contrast for identification of pelvic vessels are helpful.

References

Kidney

Bosniak MA: Angiomyolipoma (hamartoma) of the kidney: A preoperative diagnosis is possible in virtually every case. *Urol. Radiol.* 3:135–142, 1981.

Bosniak MA, Megibow AJ, Hulnick DH, Horii S, Raghavendra BN: CT diagnosis of renal angiomyolipoma: The importance of detecting small amounts of fat. *Am. J. Roentgenol.* 151:497–501, 1988.

Bretan PN, Jr., McAninch JW, Federle MP, Jeffrey RB, Jr.: Computerized tomographic staging of renal trauma: 85 consecutive patients. *J. Urol.* 136:561–565, 1986.

Cohan RH, Dunnick NR, Degesys GE, Korobkin M: Computed tomography of renal oncocytoma. *J. Comput. Assist. Tomogr.* 8:284–287, 1984.

Dunnick NR, Korobkin M, Silverman PM, Foster WL, Jr.: Computed tomography of high density renal cysts. *J. Comput. Assist. Tomogr.* 8:458–461, 1984.

Federle MP, McAninch JW, Kaiser JA, Goodman PC, Roberts J, Mall JC: Computed tomography of urinary calculi. *Am. J. Roentgenol.* 136:255–258, 1981.

Foster WL, Jr., Roberts L, Halvorsen RA, Dunnick NR: Sonography of small renal masses with indeterminant density characteristics on computed tomography. *Urol. Radiol.* 10:59–67, 1988.

Gold RP, McClennan BL, Rottenberg RR: CT appearance of acute inflammatory disease of the renal interstitium. *Am. J. Roentgenol.* 141:343–349, 1983.

Goldman SM, Fishman EK, Hartman DS, Kim YC, Siegelman SS: Computed tomography of renal tuberculosis and its pathological correlates. *J. Comput. Assist. Tomogr.* 9:771–776, 1985.

Goldman SM, Hartman DS, Fishman EK, Finizio JP, Gatewood OMB, Siegelman SS: CT of xanthogranulomatous pyelonephritis: Radiologic-pathologic correlation. *Am. J. Roentgenol.* 141:963–969, 1984.

Hartman DS, Davis JC, Jr., Goldman SM, Friedman AC, Fritzsche P: Renal lymphoma: Radiologic-pathologic correlation of 21 cases. *Radiology* 144:759–766, 1982.

Hillman BJ, Drach GW, Tracey P, Gaines JA: Computed tomographic analysis of renal calculi. *Am. J. Roentgenol.* 142:549–552, 1984.

Jafri SZH, Bree RL, Amendola MA, Glazer GM, Schwab RE, Francis IR, Borlaza G: CT of renal and perirenal non-Hodgkin lymphoma. *Am. J. Roentgenol.* 138:1101–1105, 1982.

Johnson CD, Dunnick NR, Cohan RH, Illescas FF: Renal adenocarcinoma: CT staging of 100 tumors. *Am. J. Roentgenol.* 148:59–63, 1987.

Lang EK, Sullivan J, Frentz G: Renal trauma: Radiological studies (comparison of urography, computed tomography, angiography, and radionuclide studies). *Radiology* 154:1–6, 1985.

Mitnick JS, Bosniak MA, Rothberg M, Megibow AJ, Raghavendra BN, Subramanyam BR: Metastatic neoplasm to the kidney studied by computed tomography and sonography. *J. Comput. Assist. Tomogr.* 9:43–49, 1985.

Morgan WR, Nyberg LM: Perinephric and intrarenal abscesses. *Urology* 26:529–536, 1985.

Pagani JJ: Solid renal mass in the cancer patient: Second primary renal cell carcinoma versus renal metastasis. *J. Comput. Assist. Tomogr.* 7:444–448, 1983.

Parienty RA, Ducellier R, Pradel J, Lubrano JM, Coquille F, Francois R: Diagnostic value of CT numbers in pelvicaliceal filling defects. *Radiology* 145:743–747, 1982.

Petersen RO: *Urologic Pathology*, 1st ed. Philadelphia, J. P. Lippincott, 1986, p. 35.

Quinn MJ, Hartman DS, Friedman AC, Sherman JL, Lautin EM, Pyatt RS, Ho CK, Csere R, Fromowitz FB: Renal oncocytoma: New observations. *Radiology* 153:49–53, 1984.

Rosenberg ER, Korobkin M, Foster W, Silverman PM, Bowie JD, Dunnick NR: The significance of septations in a renal cyst. *Am. J. Roentgenol.* 144:593–595, 1985.

Rosenfield AT, Glickman MG, Taylor KJW, Crade M, Hodson J: Acute focal bacterial nephritis (acute lobar nephronia). *Radiology* 132:553–561, 1979.

Adrenal

Dunnick NR, Doppman JL, Gill JR, Jr., Strott CA, Keizer HR, Brennan MF: Localization of functional adrenal tumors by computed tomography and venous sampling. *Radiology* 142:429–433, 1982.

Dunnick NR, Heaston D, Halvorsen R, Moore AV, Korobkin M: CT appearance of adrenal cortical carcinoma. *J. Comput. Assist. Tomogr.* 6:978–982, 1982.

Glazer HS, Weyman PJ, Sagel SS, Levitt RG, McClennan BL: Non-functioning adrenal masses: Incidental discovery on computed tomography. *Am. J. Roentgenol.* 143:121–128, 1982.

Johnson CD, Baker ME, Dunnick NR: CT demonstration of an adrenal pseudocyst. *J. Comput. Assist. Tomogr.* 9:817–819, 1985.

Lower Urinary Tract

Amendola MA, Glazer GM, Grossman HB, Aisen AM, Francis IR: Staging of bladder carcinoma: MRI-CT-surgical correlation. *Am. J. Roentgenol.* 146:1179–1183, 1986.

Degesys GE, Dunnick NR, Silverman PM, Cohan RH, Illescas FF, Castagno A: Retroperitoneal fibrosis: Use of CT in distinguishing among possible causes. *Am. J. Roentgenol.* 146:57–60, 1986.

Megibow AJ, Mitnick JS, Bosniak MA: The contribution of computed tomography to the evaluation of the obstructed ureter. *Urol. Radiol.* 4:95–104, 1982.

Rifkin MD: Endorectal sonography of the prostate: Clinical implications. *Am. J. Roentgenol.* 148:1137–1142, 1987.

Weinerman PM, Arger PH, Coleman BG, Pollack HM, Banner MP, Wein AJ: Pelvic adenopathy from bladder and prostate carcinoma: Detection by rapid-sequence computed tomography. *Am. J. Roentgenol.* 140:95–99, 1983.

CHAPTER

7

Magnetic Resonance Imaging of the Genitourinary Tract

Joseph P. LiPuma, Patrick J. Bryan, and Harold E. Butler

Magnetic resonance (MR) imaging is a relatively new method of imaging the central nervous system and the body. Lauterbur first recognized MR's potential as an imaging modality in 1973. Diagnostic scans have recently become possible, making MR an exciting method of clinical imaging and research in radiology. The National Institutes of Health (NIH) MR Consensus Panel recommends several areas in the genitourinary tract that are amenable to MR evaluation, including staging of pelvic and renal malignancies.

Magnetic resonance images represent proton distribution in the body. They are based on rates of dissipated energy following external stimulation by a radio frequency of known intensity. A basic MR system consists of a powerful magnet (cryogenic, electromagnetic, or permanent magnet), a radiofrequency coil (transmit, receive, or transmit and receive), gradient coils, data acquisition/processing computers, and the power supply.

The magnet generates a homogeneous static magnetic field that aligns protons (hydrogen nuclei) (Fig. 7–1A and 7–1B). The most powerful magnetic fields are created by cryogenic magnets supercooled with liquid nitrogen or helium. The strength of the magnetic field is measured in kiloGauss (kG) and tesla, which are units of magnetic field strength. By definition, 1 tesla (T) equals 10 kG. As a frame of reference, the earth's magnetic field is 0.6 Gauss. Therefore, a system operating at 10 kG or 1 T has a magnetic field strength approximately 20,000 times stronger than the earth's magnetic field. Currently available imaging systems using cryogenic magnets can develop field strengths up to 2 T. The resistive electromagnets can generate field strengths up to 1.5 kG (0.15 T). Permanent systems can generate field strengths up to 0.4 T. The issue of optimal field strengths for body imaging is a subject of ongoing research; regardless of the type and strength of the magnet, the resultant magnetic field must be uniform.

The radiofrequency (RF) coil generates a pulse that perturbs the equilibrium of proton nuclei already aligned in the magnetic field by adding energy to the system and raising the energy level of the protons to a higher state (Fig. 7–1C). When the RF transmission stops, the energized protons return to their aligned position in the magnetic field (equilibrium state), and the previously absorbed energy is emitted as a radio frequency (Fig. 7–1D).

Depending upon the design of the system, an RF receiver coil is used to receive the reradiated RF signal and localize the protons in a given area within the specimen. The receiver coils can either be body coils, which receive signal from the entire excited volume (body), specially designed head coils, or surface coils, the latter of which read signals from a smaller volume defined by the diameter of the coil. Surface coils provide improved spatial resolution and signal-to-noise ratio in the smaller volume that is evaluated.

A gradient coil is used to electronically select the imaging plane that can be either transverse, sagittal, or coronal, or in any other desired oblique plane. The system computer then processes the acquired information and generates the diagnostic image. Unlike computed tomography (CT), this system allows for examination of an area in multiple planes without requiring a special computer for image reconstruction.

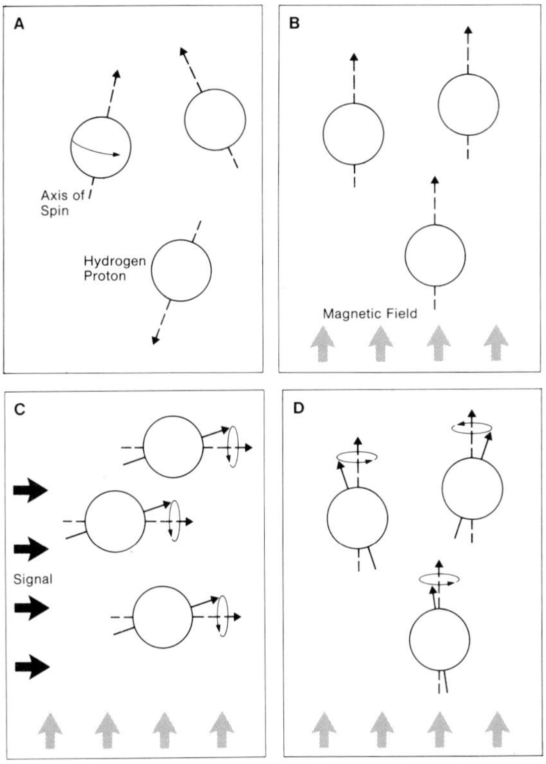

7–1 Concept of magnetic resonance. **(A)** Typical random orientation of spinning hydrogen protons. **(B)** Magnetic field applied. Axis of spin aligned with magnetic field. **(C)** Radio frequency signal applied at 90° to magnetic field. Force tips protons from alignment with magnetic field to alignment with radiosignal and causes wobble motion called precession. Protons precess in synchronized rotation initially. **(D)** Radio signal turned off. Protons realigned with magnetic field, giving off energy until precessional rotation becomes random. T1 is measure in milliseconds of time taken by protons to realign with magnetic field once radio signal is turned off (i.e., the time they are giving off their absorbed energy). T2 is time taken by protons to go from synchronized rotation under effect of radio frequency signal to random rotation when it is turned off. (Reprinted, by permission, from Hashimoto B et al.: Magnetic resonance imaging. *Virginia Mason Clinic Bulletin* 40 [4] [Winter 1986–1987], 139–148.)

Physical Principles of MR

MR images are derived from a series of complex physical phenomena, including the following:

1. An atomic nucleus with an odd number of protons or neutrons, or an unpaired electron, has an intrinsic spin. The intrinsic spin of each nucleus with its associated electrical charge generates a small magnetic field, so that each nucleus behaves like a small bar magnet. This is called paramagnetic behavior. The orientation of these miniature nuclear magnets is random (Fig. 7–1A).

2. If nuclei that demonstrate paramagnetic behavior are exposed to a strong magnetic field, such as in an MR system, they align themselves so that their individual magnetic fields parallel the lines of force of the magnetic field to which they are exposed (Fig. 7–1B). As a result of nuclear alignment, the intrinsic nuclear spins are directed around the axis of the applied magnetic field. This spinning is referred to as precession of the nucleus. The rate or frequency of precession is determined by the Larmor equation $W_0 = \gamma H_0$, where W_0 = angular frequency of precession, γ= gyromagnetic ratio (nuclear constant), and H_0 = strength of the magnetic field. So long as the magnetic field remains on, the nuclei in the strong magnetic field achieve a new equilibrium state different from the random equilibrium state when the magnetic field is not present.

3. If the nuclei, which are at equilibrium within the magnetic field of an MR imaging system, are exposed to an RF pulse, energy is added to the system and nuclei are raised to a higher energy state. In this state, the nuclear bar magnets are no longer aligned with the magnetic field of the instrument (Fig. 7–1C). This high-energy state results in an unstable equilibrium that can only be maintained if the RF pulse continues to be applied. When the RF pulse is turned off, the nuclei return to the original equilibrium state within the static magnetic field (Fig. 7–1D). The release of energy during the return to the equilibrium state results in the reradiation of the previously absorbed RF energy as a characteristic radio frequency. T1 (longitudinal or spin-lattice relaxation time) and T2 (transverse or spin-spin relaxation time) are used as parameters to describe the return of the excited nucleus to the resting state.

4. Resonance or maximum nuclear excitation is the basis of the MR imaging technique. When the radio frequency of the RF pulse used equals the precession frequency of the excited nucleus, resonance occurs.

5. The behavior of the protons in a system is described as the sum of the individual behaviors. In an MR system, the net magnetization vector refers to the sum of all the individual nuclear magnetic fields of the nuclei being observed at the time of the examination.

Although MR imaging derives all of its signal from body protons that are found in fat and water, current technology does allow for imaging other nuclei such as carbon, phosphorus, and sodium on a limited basis. In anatomic areas where there is little or no influence of motion, such as the head, spine, and extremities, MR has been rapidly incorporated into daily practice. On the other hand, MR images of the body have been hampered by lower spatial resolution, lower signal-to-noise ratios, and motion-related artifacts.

T1 and T2 Parameters

T1 and T2 characterize the loss of energy by the excited protons. T1 measures the time needed to dissipate energy to the surrounding medium (lattice) and return to the equilibrium state. T2 measures the time for nuclei to begin precessing out of phase because of the influence of the protons on each other due to their inherent magnetic fields. In solids, T1 is long because little molecular motion can occur in a solid lattice to dissipate energy to the medium; T2 is short because nuclei in close proximity have a greater influence on each other and facilitate dephasing of the nuclear precession. Conversely, in liquids, T1 is short because the nuclei are mobile, which allows for the absorbed energy following an RF pulse to dissipate rapidly to medium (lattice); T2 is long because the nuclei in motion tend to be farther apart, exert less influence on each other, and take longer to dephase each other's spins. T1 and T2 are complex exponential functions.

Although T1 and T2 are significant influences in the generation of the MR signal, other factors are important. The number of protons in the imaged area, the rate of flow of protons through the imaged area, and the RF pulse sequence influence signal intensity. Consequently, MR images are complex views of the body that contain a great deal of physiological information.

The RF pulse sequence used to perturb protons is not constant. The sequence used determines whether T1, T2, or proton density is emphasized in a particular image. For instance, in T2-weighted images, a pulse sequence is chosen that emphasizes the T2 properties of the samples more than other factors. The pulse sequence selected dramatically changes the appearance and information of the resulting images. In the abdomen and pelvis, pulse sequences that are T1 weighted and proton density weighted are useful for screening purposes because fat is bright under these conditions and organs can be outlined readily. In the central nervous system, T2-weighted images are favored because pathology in the central nervous system changes tissue T2 more (prolongs it), so that changes are best differentiated using T2-weighted images.

Interpreting MR Scans

The rules regarding "black and white" areas on CT images have no application when reviewing MR images. Black and white areas on CT images are related to attenuation of the X-ray beam by the tissue, as with conventional radiographic techniques. Areas that attenuate the beam least appear black, while those that attenuate the beam the most appear white. On the other hand, the MR image results from complex interrelationships between T1, T2, number of protons in the imaged area, rate of flow of protons through the imaged area, and RF pulse sequence used. Furthermore, the significance of black and white areas in T1 and T2 images is not constant because of the different pulse sequences used.

In T1-weighted spin echo images, the white or bright areas (high MR signal intensity) correspond to areas of high proton density or short T1 of the specific tissue. Dark areas correspond to areas of low proton density, long T1 values, or areas where protons have a high rate of flow or velocity through the area imaged (for example, flowing blood). Gray areas, therefore, represent intermediate values of proton density and relaxation times. Fat in the perinephric space, the retroperitoneum, renal sinus, bone marrow, and pathological areas such as an angiomyolipoma appear white because of the high proton density and short T1 time of fat. Conversely, cortical bone (few protons), circulating blood (motion), urine-containing structures (long T1 of urine), and air in the lungs and bowel (few protons) appear black. Organs and muscles appear as varying shades of gray, depending on interaction of the various factors responsible for the MR signal.

Renal Imaging

The kidney is evident in the retroperitoneum, surrounded by high signal intensity retroperitoneal fat. Regardless of the pulse sequence or coil used to image the kidney, the renal capsule is not visualized. Visualization of a low signal intensity renal margin on T1-weighted scans is due to chemical shift artifact and should not be mistaken for thickened renal capsule. This artifact is determined by the direction of the "read" gradient. It appears as an area of decreased signal on one side and increased signal on the opposite side (Fig. 7–2 A). The cortex and medulla can be readily differentiated in normal kidneys on T1-weighted scans without contrast (Fig. 7–2 A, B).

MR provides a clear delineation of the internal structure of the kidney using a T1-weighted image (spin echo TR 500 msec/TE 30 msec). If the images are performed in the body coil, both kidneys can be included on a single transverse or coronal scan. If a surface coil is used, high-resolution, high signal-to-noise, small field-of-view scans of a single kidney can be obtained (Fig. 7–2 B). The cortex has a higher signal than the adjacent renal medulla because the renal medulla has longer relaxation times, in particular a longer T1. As the TR and TE of a particular sequence are prolonged and the scans become more heavily T2-weighed, the ability to discriminate the cortex and the medulla decreases significantly, because the medulla has a long T2 and becomes isointense with the cortex on T2-weighted images.

The renal sinus is usually identified by sinus fat, which appears as a bright area centrally in the kidney on both T1- and T2-weighted sequences because of the short T1 and long T2 associated with fat. The pelvocaliceal system and proximal ureters are not visualized consistently in the absence of a dilated collecting system. These structures have a low signal intensity on T1-weighted images because of the long T1 of urine, but if a T2-weighted sequence is used, there is a relative increase in signal intensity due to the long T2 of urine. The renal vascular pedicle is identified as low signal intensity tubular structures (Fig. 7–2 A, B). The arteries and veins can be differentiated by following the structures back to their respective communications with the aorta and inferior vena cava. The lack of signal from flowing blood occurs because the protons do not remain within a selected slice long enough to generate a signal. Gerota's fascia may be seen as a zone of low intensity dividing the perirenal and pararenal spaces, if thickening is present due to underlying disease. As in CT examination, normal thin fascial planes are not consistently visualized.

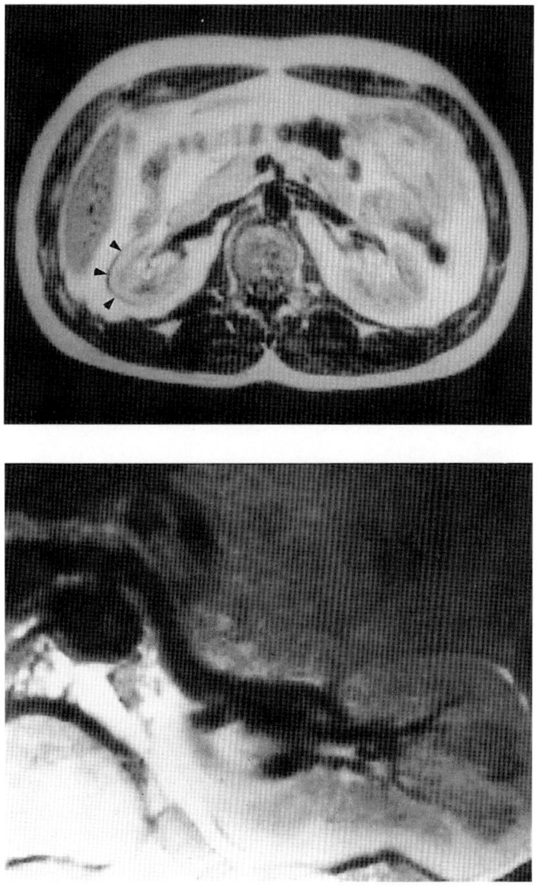

7–2 Normal renal anatomy. **(A)** Body coil image including both kidneys. Chemical shift artifact (arrow heads) alternating bands of decreased and increased signal, not to be confused with renal capsule. Corticomedullary differentiation is readily apparent; white cortex (short T1) and dark medulla (longer T1). **(B)** Surface coil image of left kidney: increased SNR and improved resolution are evident. Anatomy described in 7–2 A is better visualized.

The radiographic evaluation of renal masses fits into a well-defined algorithm, which includes urography, ultrasonography, computed tomography, and angiography. Given the current state of technical development of MR imaging and recent NIH recommendations, MR has no place as a primary screening modality for renal masses, but has value for staging renal malignancies.

Simple Renal Cysts

Simple renal cysts are easily detected and defined by MR. As in other modalities, strict criteria must be fulfilled to accurately differentiate a simple cyst from a solid lesion or complex cystic lesion (Fig. 7–3). The fluid in a simple cyst is similar to urine, having a long T1 and T2. On T1-weighted

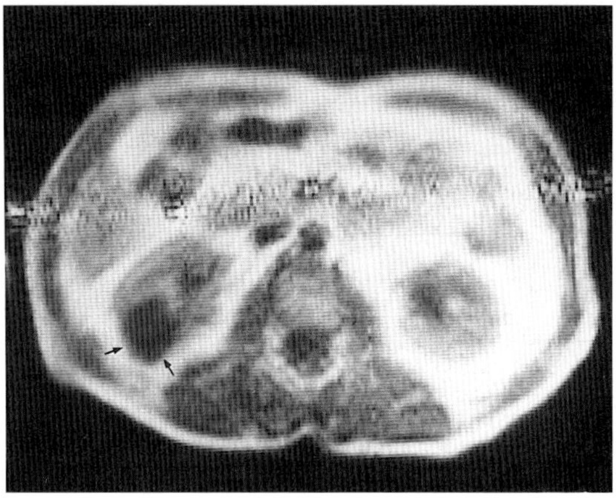

7–3 Simple renal cyst, right kidney. Low signal mass in right kidney (arrow); no perceptible wall; homogenous internal architecture without nodules or internal septa; smooth interface with adjacent normal renal parenchyma.

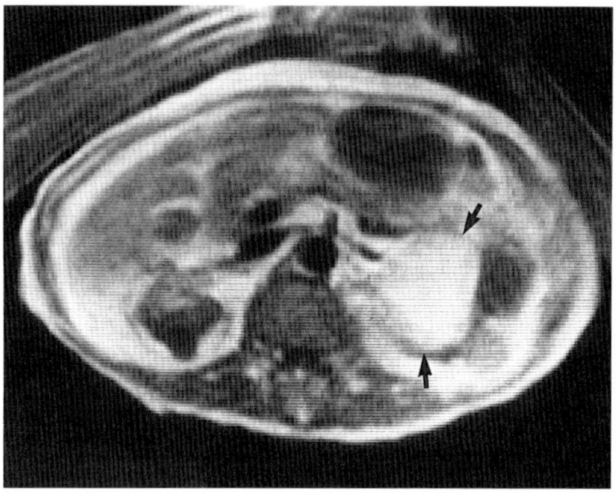

7–4 Hemorrhagic renal cysts, left kidney. Dialysis patients with chronic renal failure. These patients have a higher incidence of cysts and tumors. Small simple cyst posterior aspect of right kidney. Large hemorrhage cyst (arrows) (T1 scan) medial aspect of left kidney, with marked increase in signal; two adjacent small older hemorrhagic cysts of increased signal but less than new hemorrhage. Chronic renal disease evidenced by decreased renal parenchyma and loss of corticomedullary junction. Note thickened Gerota's fascia on the right. It is important to realize that a high signal is now known not to be specific for hemorrhage and can be seen related to infection and high protein content. (Reprinted, by permission, from LiPuma JP: Magnetic resonance image of the kidney. *Radiol. Clin. North Am.* 22:925–941, 1984, W. B. Saunders Co., Philadelphia.)

sequences urine is dark and on T2-weighted sequences urine is bright; it may become brighter than fat on heavily T2-weighted sequences. Morphologic characteristics are important and similar to those noted on a CT scan (i.e., no perceptible wall where the cyst projects into the perinephric fat, homogeneous internal architecture without nodules or internal septa, and a smooth interface with the adjacent normal renal parenchyma). In the authors' and others' experience, no simple cysts have been confused for complex cysts or solid lesions if these criteria are satisfied (Hricak et al. 1983; LiPuma et al. 1983).

Complex Renal Cysts

These cysts have atypical findings such as inhomogeneous contents, irregular walls, and septations or calcifications. Experience with these types of lesions is limited and mostly involves hemorrhagic cysts (Fig. 7–4). Cysts containing nonclotted hemorrhagic fluid demonstrate a characteristically high signal intensity on T1-weighted sequences, due to the short T1 of subacute nonclotted blood (extracellular methemoglobin). The signal brightens as T2-weighting is increased to a point where the signal is greater than fat, due to the long T2 of nonclotted blood. Compared with simple renal cysts, the signal from hemorrhagic cysts is greater on T1- and T2-weighted scans, regardless of pulse sequence used. As these cysts age, the corresponding image intensity of the blood diminishes on both T1- and T2-weighted images but never approaches the low signal of simple cyst fluid on T1 scans. Some authors have noted fluid/fluid levels in hemorrhagic cysts and suggested that this finding correlated with benign hemorrhage (Hilpert et al. 1986; Marotti et al. 1986). Since this is related to gravitational layering of cyst contents, there is no basis in relating this finding to the benign nature of a hemorrhagic cyst.

The problem in evaluating complex cysts stems from encountering one of these lesions during a time when the image intensity overlaps that from other lesions such as a neoplasm. Given current MR technology, no reliable method exists to differentiate hemorrhagic cysts, infected cysts, and cysts associated with malignancy. All these lesions may show similar imaging characteristics at different times in their evolution. Another shortcoming of MR evaluation of complex masses is the inability to define calcification in masses, since calcification is such an important finding in complex masses.

Solid Renal Masses

MR imaging has proved disappointing for evaluating solid masses. Hricak reported 100% detection rate and 96% staging accuracy of renal masses for MR. Conversely, some investigators, including the current authors, have not had a similar experience (Quint et al. 1987; Schmidt et al. 1985). Solid renal masses, including renal cell carcinomas, have variable signal intensities, from hyperintense to hypointense (Fig. 7–5). The extremes are readily identified, but when the mass is isointense to normal parenchyma, it may go undetected if MR is used as a primary screening exam. Studies by Quint et al. (1987), Schmidt et al. (1985), and Fein et al. (1987) demonstrate clearly that a significant number of solid renal masses in each of their series were isointense to normal renal parenchyma when using spin-echo techniques. Advent of different pulse sequences or a suitable intravenous contrast agent for MR imaging may improve MR status for primary detection of solid masses in the kidney.

The authors believe MR to be most useful in the staging of previously identified renal masses. The advantages of MR imaging include better evaluation of tumor thrombus in renal veins and inferior vena cava; ability to optimally differentiate invasion of adjacent tissues; ability to image and differentiate enlarged nodes from adjacent vascular structures; and ability to image in multiple planes.

In routine spin-echo images, vessels are devoid of signal under normal circumstances. Appearance of increased signal in a vessel can be due to tumor thrombus, presence of clot, or change in flow due to compression by extrinsic tumor (Fig. 7–6). Manipulation of flow-related characteristics, such as even-echo rephasing and flow-related enhancement, can be used to differentiate tumor thrombus from blood clot and flow-related changes. Furthermore, vessels enlarged by high flow can be differentiated from those veins enlarged by tumor invasion without the use of contrast. Unlike CT, MR's multiplaner imaging allows for direct visualization of the entire length of a vessel. Coronal and sagittal sections, in particular, allow for evaluation of tumor extent and definition of the interfaces with adjacent organs.

Pulse sequence manipulation allows for optimizing contrast between soft tissues and im-

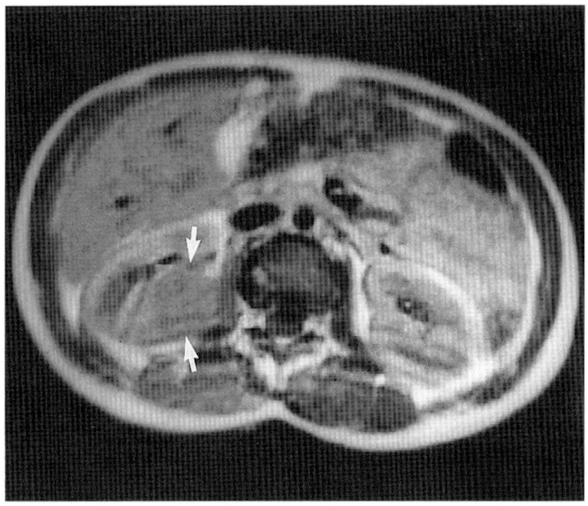

7–5 Solid renal mass, right kidney. Solid mass (arrows) arising centrally in right kidney. Signal intensity is intermediate between normal cortex and medulla. To date, no characteristics to distinguish different types of solid mass have been elucidated.

provement of differentiation between displacement and invasion of an adjacent organ (Figs. 7–6 and 7–7). Early invasion of adjacent perinephric fat is detectable by the superior contrast resolution of MR imaging. This is seen as disruption of the smooth renal margin and as a decreased signal in the fat adjacent to the mass (Hricak et al. 1985). However, there are problems with the evaluation of early fat infiltration; motion artifacts currently associated with abdominal MR imaging can cause irregular margins at the fat/mass interface. MR evaluation of lymph nodes is not improved over CT, since both modalities depend on contour change and increase in size to detect metastases; neither modality is capable of detecting tumor deposits in normal-sized lymph nodes.

Preoperative evaluation can help the urologist determine the type and extent of surgery needed. MR, like CT, is capable of staging renal cell carcinoma using Robeson's criteria. The reported accuracy for contrast-enhanced CT staging of renal malignancy is 91%, with a comparable accuracy for MR in one study of 27 patients (Marotti et al. 1986). Despite seeming advantages for MR over CT, larger series are required to make results statistically significant. For the time being, the authors agree with Glazer (1988), who recommends that MR imaging of the kidney be limited to "a) use as replacement for CT in evaluation of known or suspect renal masses in patients with contraindication to urographic contrast material

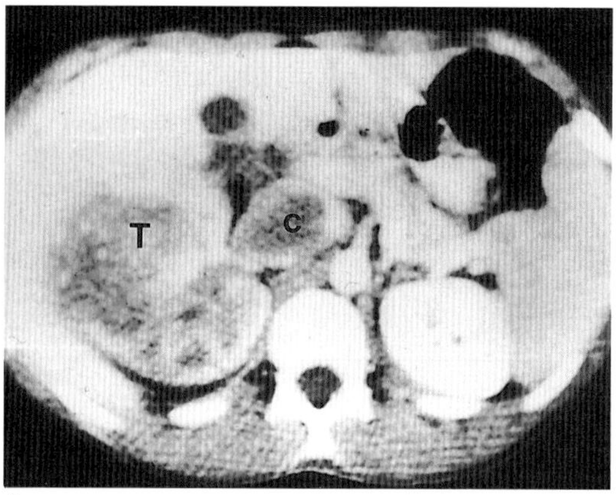

A

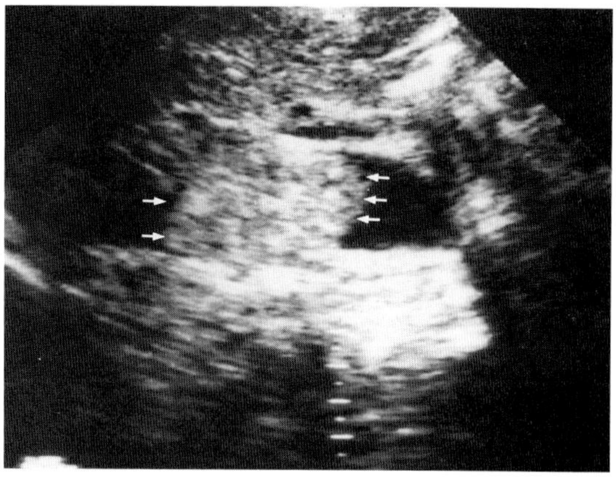

B

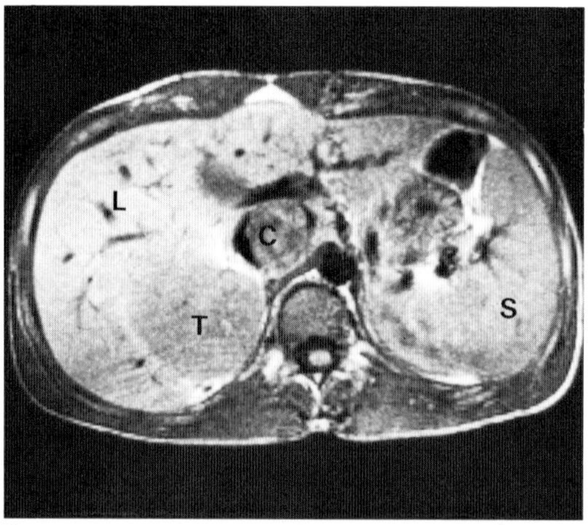

C

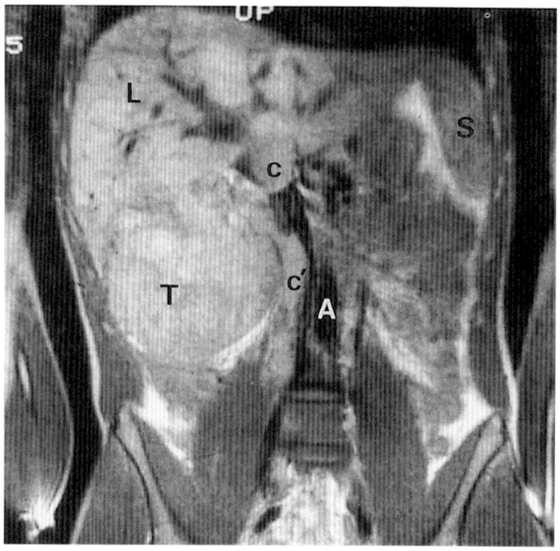

D

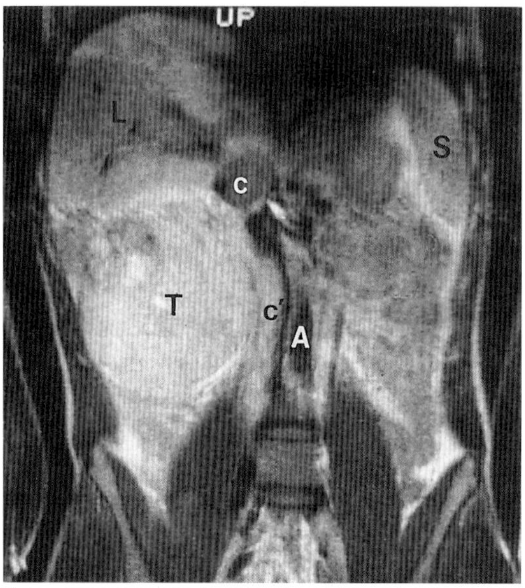

E

7–6 Vascular staging of renal carcinoma. **(A)** Bolus CT: right renal tumor mass (T) involving anterolateral aspect of upper pole. Invasion of inferior vena cava (C) with question of hepatic invasion because clear plane between the mass and liver could not be established. **(B)** Ultrasonography: longitudinal image demonstrating localized tumor (arrows) in inferior vena cava. **(C)** MR: axial T1 scan corresponding to level of CT exam shown in (A). (L = liver, S = spleen, C = tumor thrombus in inferior vena cava, T = tumor mass.) Question of hepatic invasion remains unanswered; there is no evidence of metastasis. **(D)** MR: coronal T1 scan demonstrating tumor thrombus in upper inferior vena cava (C) and signal in lower cava (C'). It could not be determined on T1 scans whether this lower area in the cava represented flow abnormality, thrombus, or tumor thrombus. (T = tumor mass, L = liver, S = spleen, A = aorta.) **(E)** MR: coronal T2 scan cleared up several unanswered questions; a cleavage plane appears to be evident between renal mass and hepatic parenchyma, and the signal in the lower cava did not increase, suggesting that this signal was not due to slow turbulent flow. At surgery the tumor had not invaded the liver, and there was tumor thrombus in cava. (T = tumor mass, L = liver, A = aorta.)

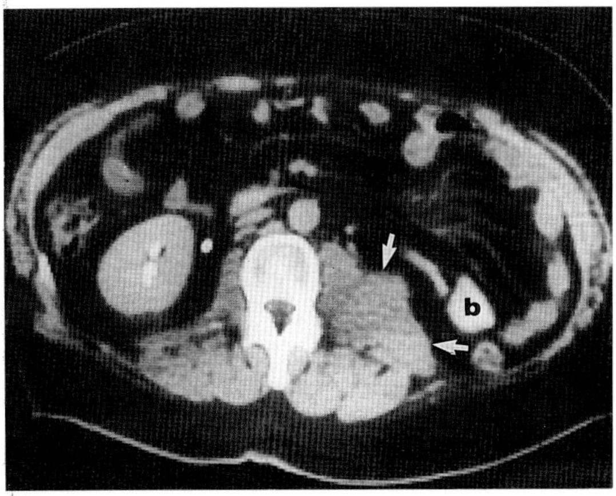

A

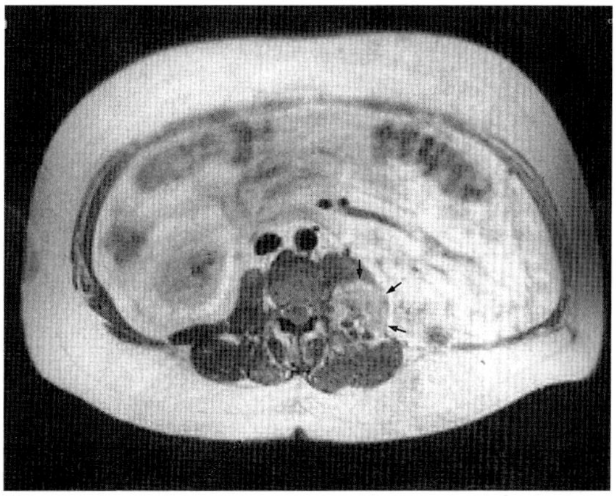

B

7–7 Left renal fossa post nephrectomy. **(A)** Axial CT image demonstrating shift of bowel (b) into left renal fossa and diffuse enlargement of left psoas muscle (arrows). **(B)** Axial T2 MR scan demonstrates psoas invasion in discrete fashion, as high signal mass (arrows) within psoas. Superior contrast resolution facilitates better definition of extent of disease.

and b) use as an alternative to CT in staging of renal cell carcinomas."

Other Diseases

Initially, many investigators hoped that visualization of the corticomedullary junction without contrast would allow evaluation of medical renal parenchymal diseases. Unfortunately, current MR imaging shows gross anatomic change, such as loss of corticomedullary differentiation; this is a nonspecific indicator seen in multiple renal medical diseases including renal transplant rejection (Fig. 7–8), glomerulonephritis, hydronephrosis, renal vascular obstruction, and acute and chronic renal failure, and can also be seen in simple dehydration. Changes on renal MR imaging have also been noted in paroxysmal nocturnal hemoglobinuria and in 11 children with sickle cell disease where the signal from the cortex is decreased on T2-weighted scans (Laude et al. 1986; Mulopulos et al. 1986). This phenomenon has been related to iron deposits (hemosiderin) in the cortex, which decrease T2.

The inability to identify calcifications (Fig. 7–9), including renal calculi, occurs because there are not enough protons to generate a signal. This significantly hinders renal imaging, since calcifications in renal carcinoma and complex cysts cannot be detected primarily, and renal calculi can go undetected. Manipulations exist that help practitioners identify calcifications if it is known they are present, but this does not help in cases of primary detection. Thus, renal imaging has substantial limitations.

Imaging the Normal Pelvis

Pelvic anatomy can be well displayed in multiple planes. Unlike the upper abdomen, motion is not a major problem in the pelvis. Transverse sections are comparable to CT, but the direct visualization of the pelvic anatomy in coronal and sagittal planes is far superior (Fig. 7–10) (Bryan et al. 1984). Pelvic imaging is performed with a spin-echo technique using a double echo and providing proton density and T2-weighted scans of the same area simultaneously. High signal intensity fat surrounds much of the pelvic viscera. Musculature and pelvic viscera are visualized as anatomical structures of varying shades of gray. On T1-weighted scans, striated muscle, with its moderately long T1 and short T2, has a low signal intensity compared with adjacent viscera and fat. On T2-weighted scans, the short T2 of striated muscle decreases the signal intensity compared to viscera and fat.

Urine in the bladder has a long T1 and T2 (Fig. 7–10). On T1-weighted scans, urine has a low signal intensity, even lower than striated muscle. On a T2-weighted scan, the signal from urine decays less than the signal of tissue with shorter T2s, so that urine can have a higher signal intensity than fat as the TE is prolonged. When the urine is high in signal intensity, the bladder wall can be seen in relief between high intensity urine and fat.

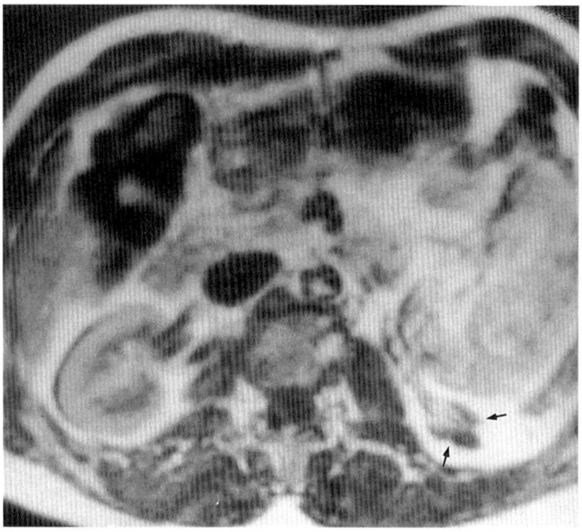

A

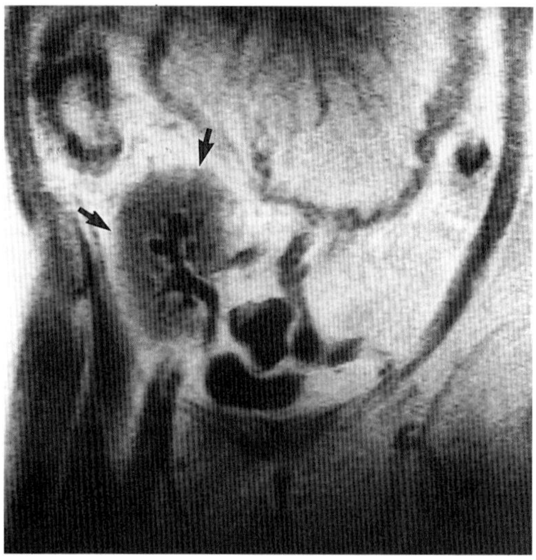

B

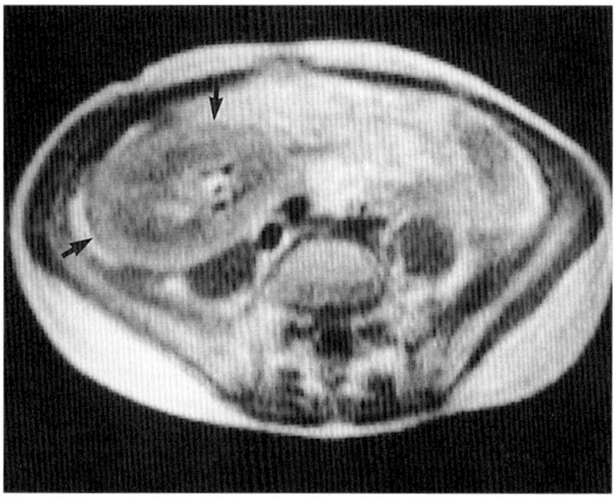

C

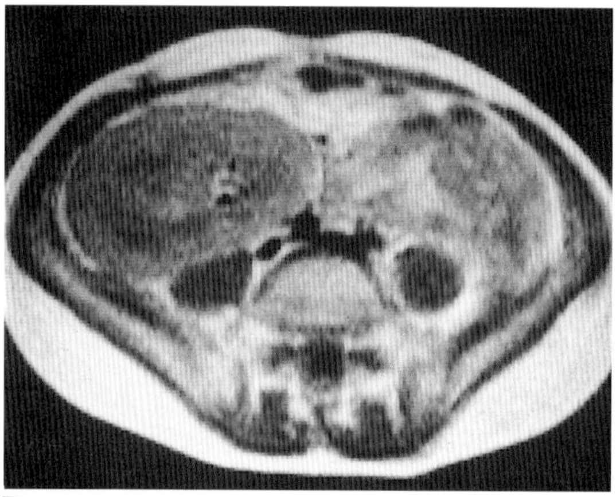

D

7–8 Loss of corticomedullary junction. Although this is a nonspecific finding in medical renal disease and dehydration, if noted it should raise clinical suspicion of problems. **(A)** Atrophied left kidney (arrow) secondary to infections in childhood. Normal right kidney and corticomedullary junction. **(B)** Coronal T1-weighted image of transplant kidney in right iliac fossa (arrows) shows dilated collecting system secondary to chronic ureterovesical junction obstruction; corticomedullary junction is absent. **(C)** Normal renal transplant (arrows) demonstrating distinct corticomedullary junction (T1-weighted image). **(D)** Same patient as **(C)**, 4 weeks later, demonstrating loss of corticomedullary junction (T1-weighted image; biopsy proven). Note increase in renal size secondary to edema.

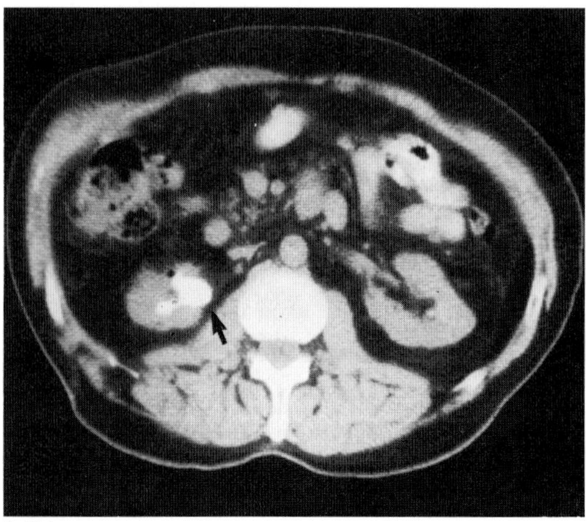

7–9 A

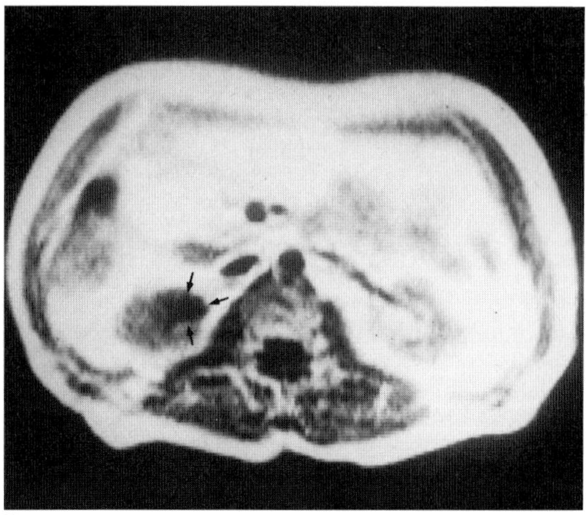

B

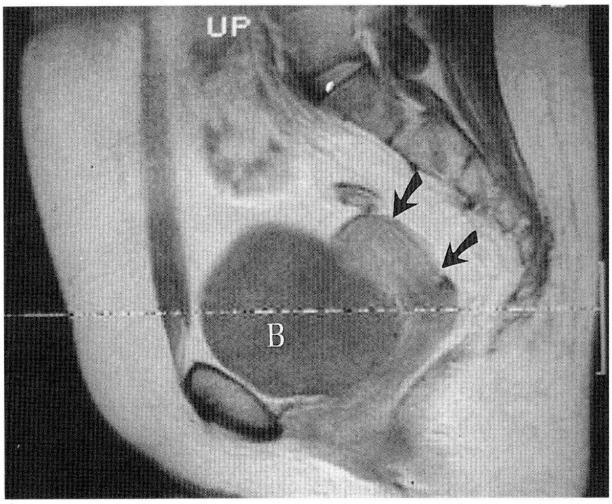

A

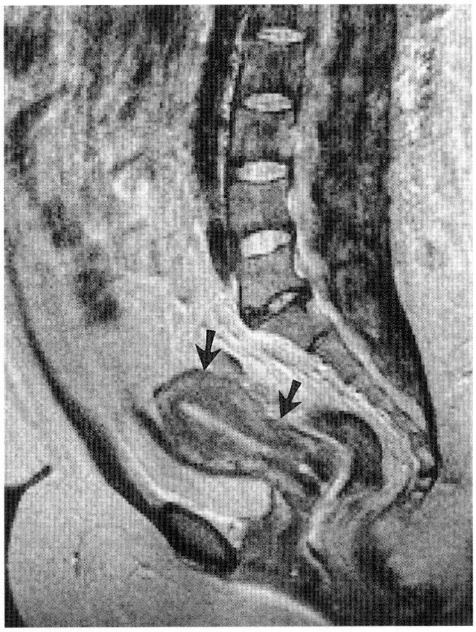

B

7–10 Normal pelvic anatomy: female. **(A)** Sagittal MRI (proton density) of bladder (B) and uterus (arrows). Intermediate signal from bladder contents and nonvisualization of the wall is characteristic. Uterus demonstrates slight increase in endometrial signal but no evidence of differentiation between junctional zone and myometrium. **(B)** Sagittal MRI (T2): Uterus (arrows) demonstrates high signal endometrial area, intermediate signal peripheral myometrium, and very low signal area between endometrium and myometrium, known as the junctional zone. **(C)** Coronal MRI (proton density): Intermediate signal from ovaries (arrows), superior to bladder. **(D)** Coronal MRI (T2): Signal from ovaries has increased, as has signal from urine. Note that relative signal from striated muscle decreases as compared to **(C)** because of a short T2, and urine increases because of a long T2.

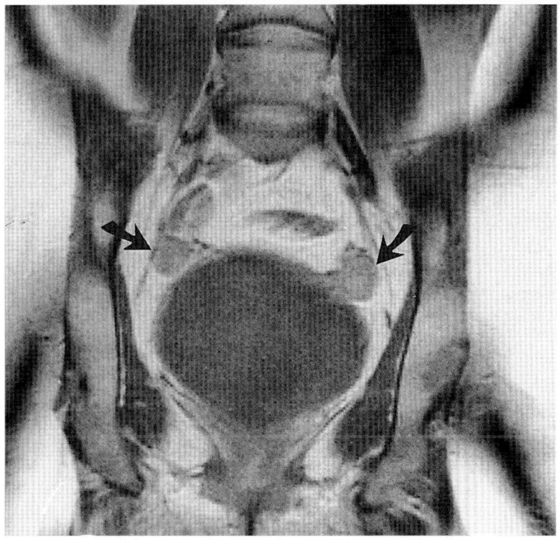

C

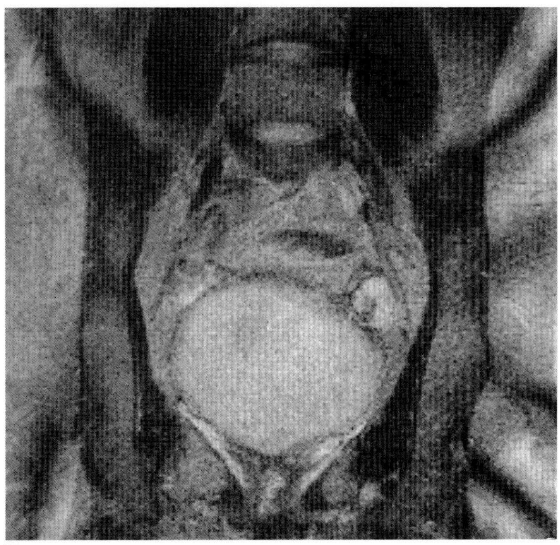

D

The rectum is most easily identified when it contains gas (low signal intensity) (Fig. 7–11); lack of gas can make differentiation from adjacent structures difficult. The levator ani muscle, which forms the floor of the pelvis and acts as a demarcating point between the pelvis and perineum, is readily identified on coronal scans.

Normal lymph nodes and metastatic lymph nodes less than 1 cm may not be distinguished. Nodes larger than 1 cm can easily be visualized, although benign (reactive or inflammatory) nodes cannot be differentiated from malignant replace-

◀ **7–9** Calcifications. Inability to visualize calcifications is a major shortcoming in renal evaluation. This will severely limit its use in patients with hematuria for stone disease or malignancy and evaluation of complex cysts found by other modalities. **(A)** Axial CT image demonstrating large staghorn calculus (arrow) in right kidney. **(B)** Axial MRI (T1) demonstrating no signal in right collecting system (arrows); without prior history, differentiation from hydronephrosis would be impossible, since corticomedullary junction is not appreciated (chronic renal disease?).

ment in the authors' experience. Early reports that there are T2 differences between acute inflammatory nodes and all other causes of nodal enlargement have not been substantiated.

In general, three basic MR sequences are used in the evaluation of the pelvis of both males and females. T1-weighted scans are used to maximize contrast between muscle and fat; these scans help identify early extension of tumors beyond the margins of the organ of origin (Fig. 7–12 A, C). Proton density scans, on the other hand, are very high signal-to-noise scans, which provide excellent anatomic images (Fig. 11 A–C). Finally the T2-weighted scans provide high contrast and are useful in evaluating the internal architecture of structures (Fig. 11 D, E). Proton density and T2-weighted scans can be obtained simultaneously with a double echo spin-echo technique. Selection of imaging plane is based on the structure to be examined and its relationship to adjacent structures.

Female Pelvis

In the female pelvis, the uterus is best demonstrated with a sagittal scan (Fig. 10). On T1-weighted images it is a homogenous structure of intermediate intensity located between the rectum and bladder. On T2-weighted scans, a distinction between myometrium and endometrium can be made (Fig. 7–10 B). Furthermore, in response to hormonal stimulation, the cyclical variation in endometrial thickness can be observed.

In women taking oral contraceptives or gonadotropin-releasing hormones and analogs, the endometrium appears atrophic, as one would expect physiologically. A middle zone, the junctional zone, surrounds the endometrium and is continuous with the fibrous stroma of the cervix; on T2-weighted scans this zone is low in signal intensity (Fig. 7–10 B). The significance of this zone is uncertain and there is no histological correlate for the junctional zone known at this time. Lee et al. (1985) report that this is due to flow phenomenon, but confirmatory evidence is lacking.

Three distinct zones are also seen in the cervical area, as well as a transition zone from the corpus of the uterus to the cervix. The high signal intensity located centrally in the cervix is believed to represent cervical mucous, both intra- and extracellular, separated from the outer muscularis by a band of low image intensity that is assumed to be stromal tissue of the endocervix. The fibrous stroma of the cervix is low in signal intensity, due to the short T2 of fibrous tissue.

The ovaries can be identified with MR scanning. Consistency of identification depends upon the technique used and the age of the patient. Thin contiguous slices are most reliable in identification of the ovaries, but this, of course, increases scan time. The ovaries are most easily identified in women of reproductive age and are more difficult to identify in the atrophic state in postmenopausal women. On T1-weighted scans, the ovaries are seen as areas of intermediate signal intensity, similar to striated muscle. This intermediate signal facilitates separation from surrounding fat in T1-weighted images. On proton density scans, imaging can be more difficult because there is a slight increase in the signal of the ovaries; they are slightly greater than striated muscle (Fig. 7–10 C). Ovaries containing follicles have high signal (greater than fat) on T2-weighted scans.

The vagina is best demonstrated on sagittal scans. The vaginal walls are low in signal intensity on T2-weighted images, due to the short T2 of smooth muscle.

Male Pelvis

MR scans of the male pelvis can duplicate the anatomic relationship between the prostate, bladder, and seminal vesicles described in axial CT scans (Fig. 7–11). The ability of MR to do direct coronal and sagittal scans enhances the evaluation of these relationships. On T1-weighted scans, the normal fat space separating the seminal vesicles from the posterior wall of the bladder (except in the midline) can readily be identified in axial, sagittal, and coronal scans. The seminal vesicles and prostate have similar signal intensities on T1-weighted scans, less than those of the surrounding fat. As the T2-weighting increases, the signal intensity of both the prostate and seminal vesicles increases. In heavily T2-weighted scans the fluid-containing seminal vesicles are brighter than the surrounding fat (Fig. 7–11 E). If surface coils are used with T2-weighting, internal anatomy of the prostate can also be identified.

The peripheral zone of the prostate composes 70%–75% of the glandular tissue, and makes up the posterior, lateral, and caudal aspects of the

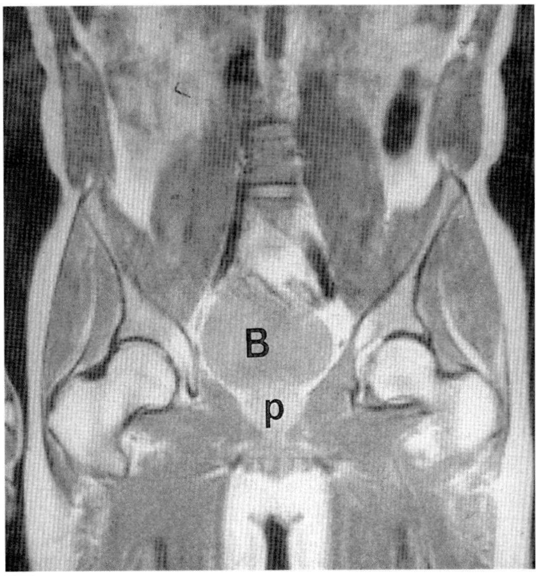

A

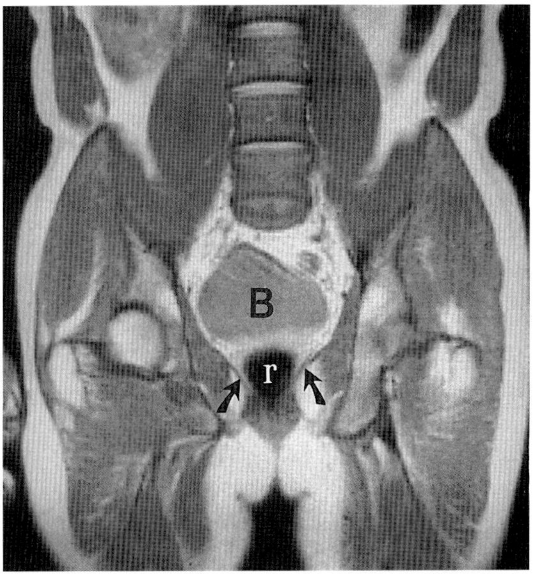

B

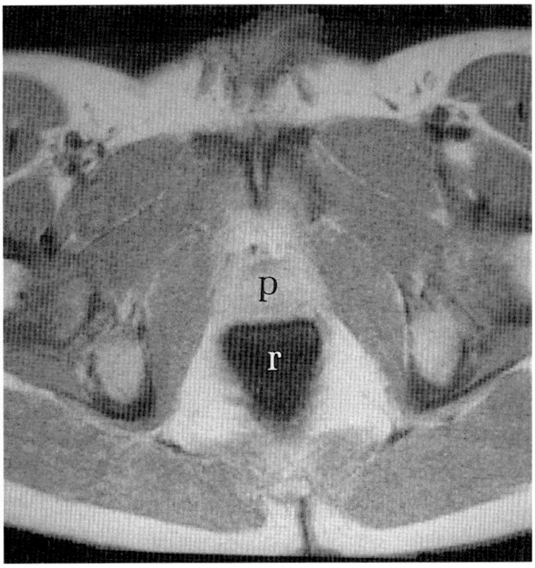

C

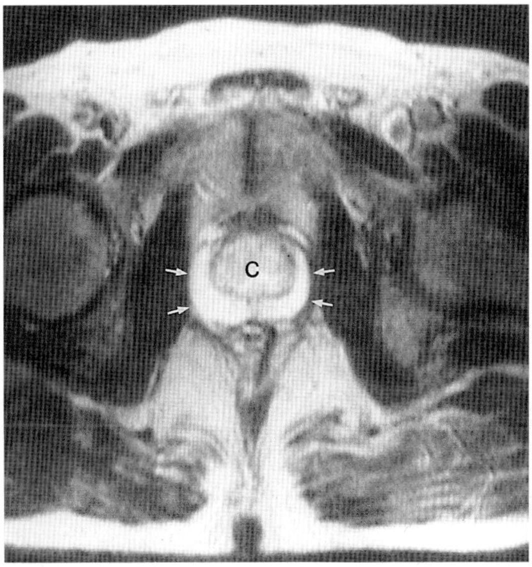

D

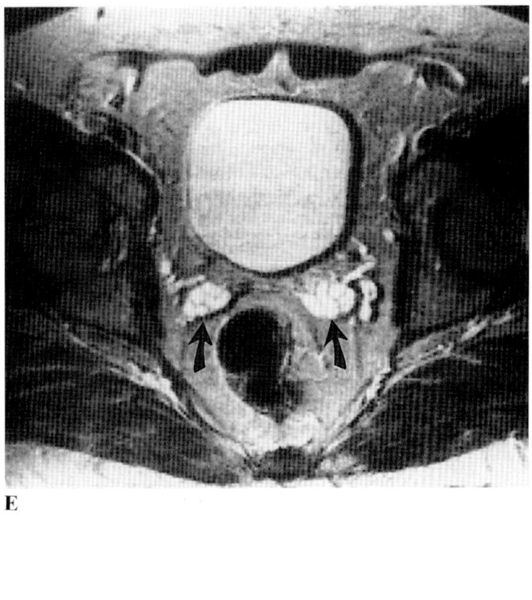

E

7–11 Normal male pelvic anatomy: Coronal and axial images through male pelvis. **(A)** Coronal, proton density: bladder (B) and prostate (p). **(B)** Coronal, proton density: Bladder (B), seminal vesicles (s), rectum (r), levator muscles (arrows). **(C)** Axial, proton density: Prostate (p) and rectum (r). **(D)** Axial, T2: Prostate. Note differentiation between central (c) and peripheral zones (arrows). **(E)** Axial, T2: Convoluted seminal vesicles (arrows). Note chemical shift artifact, causing apparent thickening of left wall of bladder.

gland. This portion of the gland has the highest incidence of carcinoma. The central zone represents a cone of tissue with its base postero-inferior to the bladder neck and its apex at the verumontanum. This portion of the gland surrounds the ejaculatory ducts. The smallest portion of the gland, accounting for a maximum of 5% of the gland, is the transitional zone. Anatomically it blends with the periurethral glands and periprostatic sphincter and is an anatomically distinct area, but its MR signal is similar to the central zone, so that this area cannot be directly visualized. This area is thought to be responsible for benign prostatic hypertrophy.

As noted earlier, differentiation of the central and peripheral zones is best on T2-weighted images (Fig. 7–11 D); the peripheral zone is high in signal intensity, whereas the transitional and central zones tend to have an intermediate signal. Differentiation of these two zones is optimal in younger subjects. In older patients, the central zone is not reliably seen. When it was first noted that internal prostatic anatomy was discernible on MR imaging, it was hoped that the definition between the zones would facilitate differentiation of benign from malignant disease. This has not so far proven to be the case.

The seminal vesicles vary in intensity from low signal on T1-weighted images to a high signal on T2-weighted images (Fig. 7–11). Disruption of the high signal on T2 images identified tumor invasion into the seminal vesicles.

The periprostatic venous plexus is visualized on T2-weighted scans as a high signal at the base of the bladder surrounding the upper portion of the prostate gland. The high signal is attributed to even-echo rephasing and slow-flowing blood in the veins. Once again disruption of the high signal is used as an indicator of invasion by carcinomas either from the base of the bladder or the prostate.

The penis is best identified on sagittal scans. Again T2-weighted scans are best for delineating internal anatomy. On these scans the corpora cavernosum and spongiosum are high in signal intensity. Midline sagittal slices readily identify the course of the urethra. Results of scrotal imaging using surface coils and high field strength magnets have recently been published (Baker et al. 1987; Rholl et al. 1987). The signal from the testes is low to intermediate on T1-weighted and proton density scans and relatively high on T2-weighted sequences. In contrast, the tunica albuginea, epididymis, and mediastinum testis are lower in signal and can be readily differentiated.

Bladder Pathology

Bladder studies normally employ two sequences, one to provide a T1-weighted image and a second double echo sequence to provide both proton density weighted images and T2-weighted images. Although it would be ideal to examine all bladders in the axial, coronal, and sagittal planes, this is not usually done because of increased scan time. Axial scans plus a sagittal scan, which is optimal for evaluation of the base, dome, and bladder neck, should provide a complete study of the bladder.

Imaging the bladder is useful for the evaluation of primary tumors or tumors invading from adjacent organs such as the prostate, rectum, or uterus. The TNM system of staging bladder carcinoma is given in Table 7–1.

Table 7–1 TNM Method of Bladder Tumor Staging

TNM Stage	Description
Stage T1S	In situ lesion
Stage T1	Lesion confined to mucosa
Stage T2	Lesion involving mucosa and superficial muscle
Stage T3A	Involvement of mucosa, superficial muscle, and deep muscle
Stage T3B	Local extension beyond adventitia
Stage T4A	Extension to bowel and seminal vesicles
Stage T4B	Extension to pelvic sidewalls

MR clearly demonstrates the extent of papillary growth into the bladder and differentiates stages T3B and T4 from those confined to the bladder wall (Fig. 7–12). In the authors' experience, degrees of bladder wall involvement defining stages T1, T2, and stage T3A cannot be discriminated because the different layers of the bladder wall cannot be distinguished. It is possible grossly to identify intraluminal lesions using a T1-weighted image or proton density weighted image to allow determination of the intraluminal extent of a papillary tumor. Invasion of the wall is seen as thickening of the wall on the proton density images and as increase in signal of the bladder wall on T2-weighted images. Invasion of perivesical fat causes an irregular decrease in the signal of the fat, best seen on T1-weighted images.

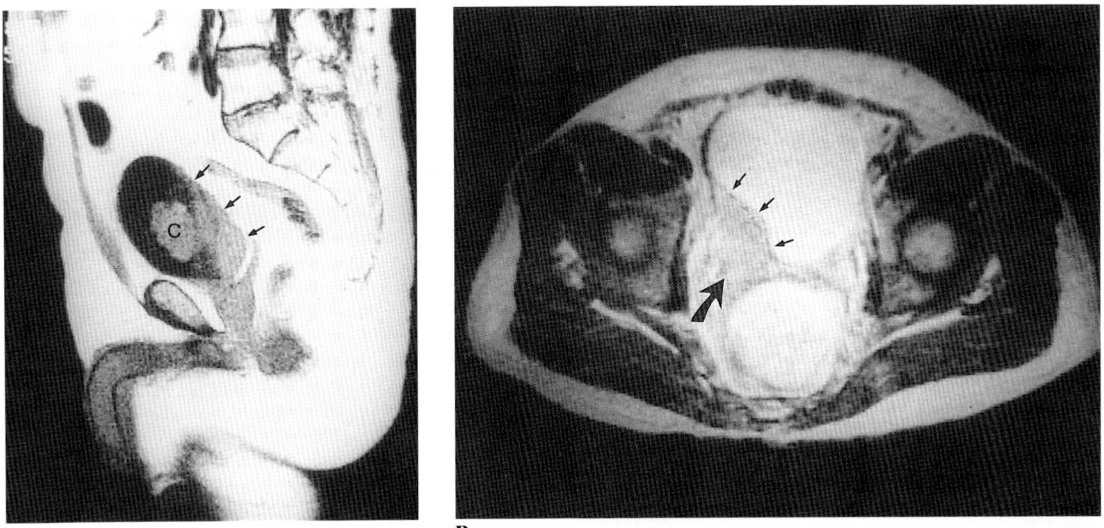

A B

7–12 Bladder carcinoma. **(A)** Sagittal MRI (T1) demonstrating low signal urine and large papillary carcinoma (c) in bladder. There is extensive tumor along posterior bladder wall (arrows) but no extension to perivesical fat. **(B)** Axial T2 scan demonstrating case of T4A bladder carcinoma (small arrows) invading right seminal vesicle (large arrow). **(C)** Axial T1 scan demonstrating case of T4B bladder carcinoma infiltrating perivesical fat anteriorly (arrows), enlarged left pelvic node (arrowhead), and large bladder mass (m).

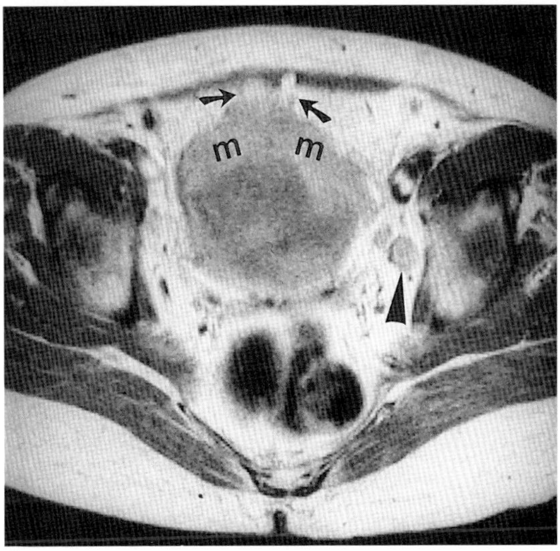

C

Invasion of the seminal vesicles (stage T4A) is best seen by using both T1- and T2-weighted sequences (Fig. 7–12B). Involvement of the pelvic sidewalls is facilitated by using coronal or axial scans to check for nodal enlargement and change in contour and size of the adjacent musculature. The main advantage of MR is differentiation of stages T3B and stage 4 from lower stages. These changes are sometimes subtle and can be difficult to detect on CT examinations. In the authors' experience, MR has a slight but definite advantage over CT in detecting extravesical spread.

Pathology in the Male Pelvis

Evaluation of Prostatic Disease

Carcinoma of the prostate is listed as the second or third most common cause of cancer deaths in males. Autopsies performed on males over 50 years of age reveal that 14%–46% have evidence of carcinoma of the prostate. In staging prostatic disease, stage A disease *(in situ)* and stage B (intracapsular) are readily amenable to surgery, and most patients are effectively cured. Therapy of stages B2 and early stage C is controversial. Stage B2 represents intracapsular disease that involves the prostatic capsule. Early stage C represents early extension of carcinoma beyond the capsule without evidence of direct involvement of either the seminal vesicles or periprostatic veins. In these cases, there is a question whether the patient should be treated surgically or with radiation therapy, the latter of which is usually reserved for cases of stage C and D disease.

Current methods for evaluating prostatic disease are suboptimal because they underestimate the extent of the disease. It was hoped that CT would improve staging, but CT has not proven to be completely satisfactory. In particular, prostatic disease tends to replace rather than enlarge nodal tissue, and without an increase in size, involvement of these nodes could not be detected. Lymph-

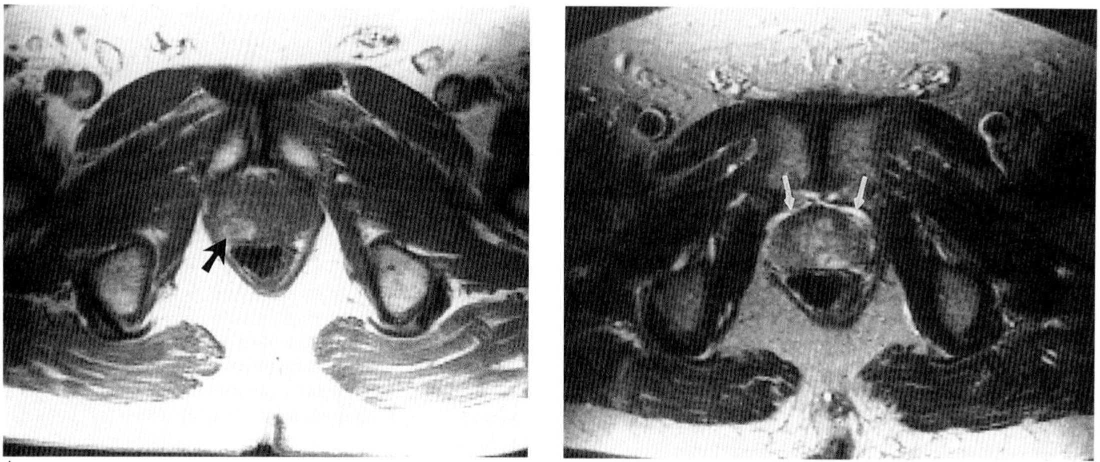

A B

7–13 Prostatic carcinoma. **(A)** T1-weighted scan showing area of increased signal posterolaterally on right side arrow). **(B)** Tumor is less obvious on this T2-weighted image, but there is slightly diminished signal in corresponding area of prostate compared to the remainder of the gland. Note the brighter signal of periprostatic venous plexus.

angiography can detect lymph node involvement but is limited by its inability to detect local extension and distal metastases. It does not always opacify affected pelvic nodes.

The promise of MR is based on its potential to differentiate degrees of local invasion. MR can clearly demonstrate the periprostatic fat, periprostatic venous plexus, seminal vesicles, and levator ani muscle, which are critical in differentiating stage B and C disease at a local level.

Despite early research suggesting that the appearance of the prostate gland on MR could be used to differentiate between benign prostatic hypertrophy and carcinoma of the prostate, this has not proved possible. Signals from malignant prostatic nodules can be either increased or decreased relative to the surrounding prostate on both T1- and T2-weighted images (Bryan et al. 1986) (Fig. 7–13).

Penile and Scrotal Disease

MR readily demonstrates local and adjacent global anatomy of the penis and scrotum. However, the role of MR in the evaluation of penile pathology is unsubstantiated. On T2-weighted scans testicular pathology has been identified as low signal intensity relative to the high signal of normal testes. There have been isolated reports of MR's value in diagnosing hydroceles, ependymal cysts, and epididymitis, but the number of cases is too small to be meaningful. Since ultrasound is readily suited to evaluation of the scrotum and is less expensive, there appears to be no justification for primary MR scanning of the scrotum.

Pathology in the Female Pelvis

Uterus

A solid mass in the uterus requires differentiation between a leiomyoma and uterine carcinoma. Although other potential lesions exist, they are uncommon. The leiomyoma is the most common uterine tumor. Uncomplicated fibroids are characteristically hypointense relative to normal myometrium on all pulse sequences, due to their low mobile proton content (Fig. 7–14 A, B). Degenerated fibroids have a long T2 value and a relatively intense signal on T2-weighted images.

T2-weighted sequences are best suited for the differentiation of fibroids from normal myometrium, whereas proton density and T1 sequences are least reliable. T2 scans clearly demonstrate number of lesions, size, precise location, and presence and extent of degeneration. Hricak et al. (1986) have suggested that MR provides useful therapeutic information regarding the location of a leiomyoma. They observed that leiomyomas associated with hypermenorrhea produce anatomic disruption of the junctional zone, and that since small lesions can be removed by hysteroscopic surgery, MR identification can be valu-

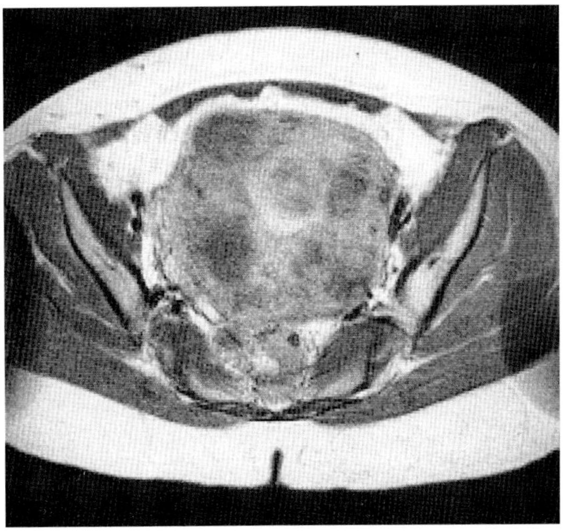

A

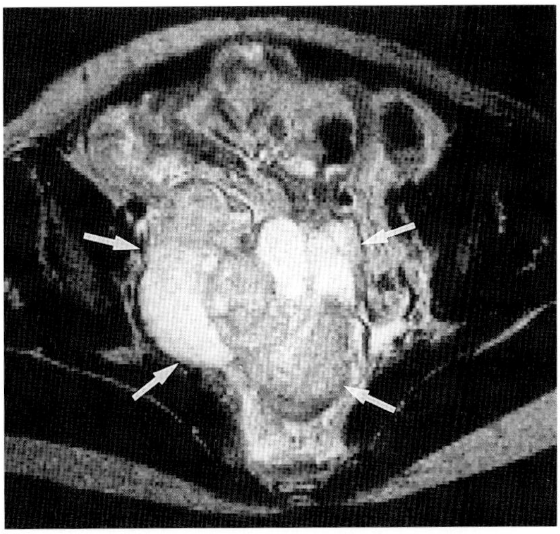

B

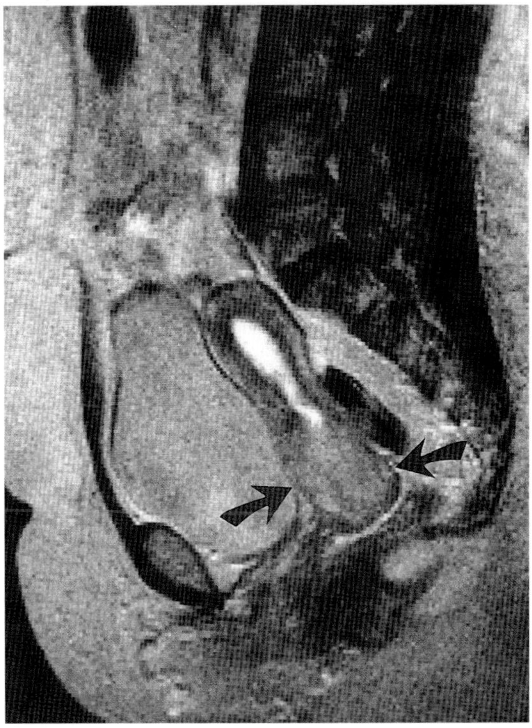

C

7–14 MR imaging of uterine tumors. **(A)** Proton density scan through massively enlarged uterus with multiple fibroids. Signal from fibroids tends to be lower than normal myometrium. Within individual fibroids, high signal areas are attributed to hemorrhage, myxomatous, or fatty degeneration, and low signal is attributed to calcification and hyalinization. **(B)** Endometrial carcinoma. Transverse T2-weighted scan. There is a large irregular tumor with inhomogenous strong signal on the T2-weighted image (arrows). Myometrium is extensively invaded by tumor. **(C)** Carcinoma of cervix. T2-weighted image in sagittal plane shows irregular enlargement of cervix (arrows), with extension into body of uterus. Note high signal in endometrial canal, due to obstruction by cervical carcinoma.

able. Furthermore, lesions can be treated hormonally and followed for size reduction and removed. Except for identification of disruption of the junctional zone, ultrasound can accomplish the same goals at less cost. Like ultrasound, MR is unable to determine if malignant degeneration is present from tissue characteristics. It depends on gross morphological changes with regard to size and disruption of anatomical planes and associated clinical findings.

Adenomyosis

The authors have had no direct experience with adenomyosis. Marks et al. (1987) have reported a characteristic picture as a poorly marginated low signal area contiguous and isointense with the junctional zone containing a central high signal area attributed to ectopic endometrium. If the high signal area is not present, the lesion appears undistinguishable from leiomyoma with diminished signal.

Endometrial Carcinoma

The most obvious manifestation of endometrial carcinoma on MR is complete derangement of the normal layered uterine architecture, with associated uterine enlargement. If the size of the uterus is normal, the disappearance of the junctional zone between the endometrium and myometrium can be the sole indicator of myometrial spread. This finding has limitations, since the junctional zone is absent in postmenopausal women. The authors have observed that although the junctional zone is absent as a distinct layer, if postmenopausal women are not on steroids, the interface between the endometrium and myometrium is smooth; therefore, irregularity suggests tumor invasion (Butler et al. 1984).

As in CT evaluation, distention of the endometrial canal should raise the possibility of endometrial or cervical carcinoma in postmenopausal women. The authors are in agreement with Hricak et al. (1987) that MR is an excellent modality for staging endometrial carcinoma. Hricak et al. report a staging accuracy of 92%. The improvement over CT staging is based on MR's ability to visualize internal uterine architecture. Unlike CT, MR is not limited to evaluating only for extra-uterine disease such as distant metastasis, lymphodenopathy, and invasion of pelvic sidewalls.

Gestational Trephoblastic Disease (Molar Pregnancy)

The authors have used MR on two patients with this tumor. Uterine enlargement was seen in both cases, with associated disruption of zonal anatomy by high signal tumor on both T1- and T2-weighted scans. High signal on T1-weighted scans is attributed to hemorrhage. Hricak et al. (1986) reported the same finding but also noted abundant feeding vessels in the adnexa and a thecalutein cyst. They found MR useful in follow-up, since seeing a return of three-layered internal uterine architecture can be used in conjunction with observation of decreasing B-HCG levels.

Cervical Carcinoma

In the authors' experience, cervical carcinoma presents either as a small mass within the cervix that disrupts the relationship between the high signal endocervical area and lower signal peripheral zone, or as a large expanding mass replacing the cervix (Fig. 14C) (Butler et al. 1984). The tumor has a higher signal intensity than the normally low signal fibrous stroma of cervix on the T2-weighted scan and can be identified disturbing the zonal architecture of the cervix even if size is not increased. Togashi et al. (1986) agree with the current authors' findings and further state that in stage 0 or 1A (microscopic) disease, the cervix appears normal on MR.

Ovaries

Simple Ovarian Cysts

This lesion is the most common pathological finding in the female adnexa on ultrasound examination. The most common MR description is that of a rounded well-defined, low signal area with imperceptible walls, in addition to nonvisualized septa on T1 examination and relatively high signal on T2 examination (Fig. 7–15A). Signal intensity of cyst contents on T1-weighted images can vary widely. The authors have found signal intensity of cyst fluid to correlate with triglyceride and cholesterol content.

Hemorrhagic Cysts

There is no characteristic picture of a hemorrhagic cyst. The signal from a particular hemorrhagic cyst is a function of age of the hemorrhage. Fresh blood, clotted blood, and old hemorrhagic blood that is breaking down each generate different signals. Fresh blood has a high signal on both T1- and T2-weighted images, due to short T1 and long T2s. As blood clots and breaks down, signal in the clot decreases. Hemorrhagic changes seen on body MR have not been as well substantiated pathologically as they have been in the central nervous system.

Teratomas

Teratomas consist of fat and various amounts of fibrous tissue, hair, and calcification. The signal from the contained fat parallels the signal from subcutaneous fat but decreases as the amount of other contained elements increases. The authors have evaluated 11 pathologically proven teratomas, 9 of which contained fat, making the diagnosis simple (Fig. 7–15B). In 2 lesions the fat content was markedly diminished, making diagnosis difficult. The appearance of nonfatty components varied from wall nodules to contained, rounded nodules of decreased signal, and more unusually to free-form configurations. Togashi et al. (1987) found that dermoid fat demonstrated a pathognomonic chemical shift artifact pattern that differentiated this high signal lesion from a high signal endometrial cyst. They also described gravity-dependent layering, fat-fluid levels, floating debris, globular calcifications, and palm-treelike

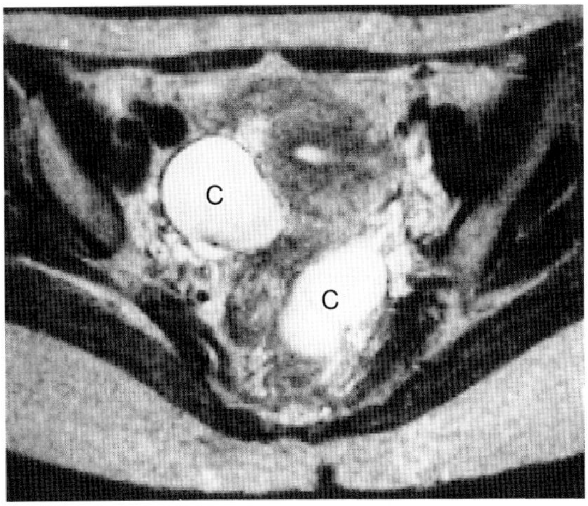

A

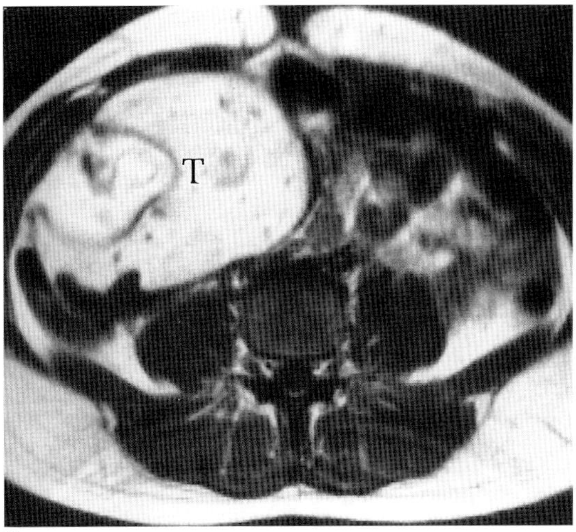

B

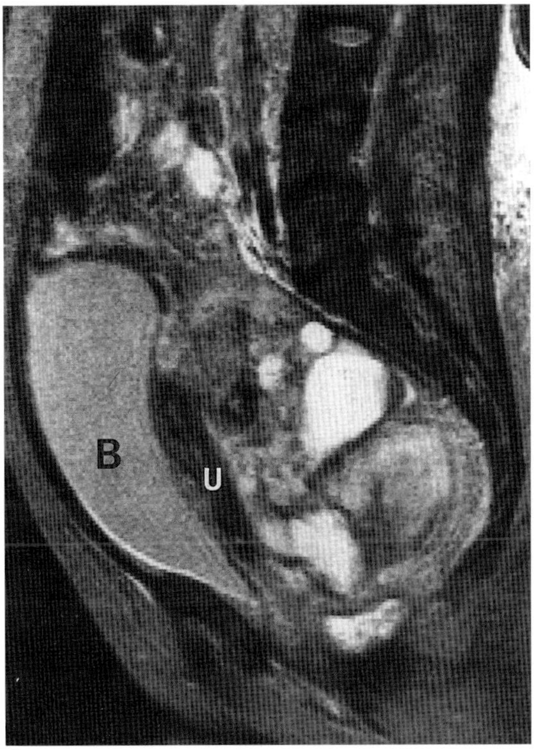

C

7–15 **(A)** Bilateral ovarian cysts. Due to long T2 of the cyst (c) contents, they have high signal on T2-weighted images. The signal intensity of T1-weighted images varies greatly, depending on exact composition of the fluid. **(B)** Ovarian teratoma. Teratoma (T) has mixed signal intensity, due to its varying components, on the T1-weighted image. Note the bright signal from the fatty components. **(C)** Cystadenocarcinoma of ovary. T2-weighted image in sagittal plane. A large tumor of mixed signal occupies most of pelvis, displacing uterus and bladder anteriorly. Uterus (u) is identified as relatively low signal structure between ovarian tumor and bladder (B).

protrusions within the lesion, which they claim increase the certainty of the diagnosis. As in other pathological processes, it is unlikely that MR can permit a tissue-specific diagnosis and definitively rule out malignant degeneration.

Ovarian Tumors

Experience with cystadenomas (serous and mucinous), cystadenofibromas, and cystadenocarcinomas remains small, but these tumors have signal characteristics that would be expected in mixed cystic and solid tumors (Fig. 15C). Given current experience, MR does not appear as useful as CT or ultrasonography. Ultrasonography is better suited to evaluate and delineate the characteristic of the lesion itself, while CT is better suited for metastatic evaluation – in particular, delineation of peritoneal implants.

Endometrioma

In our experience, an endometrioma has the appearance of a loculated pelvic mass. The septa and locules are thicker than those associated with simple cysts (Fig. 7–16). The individual locules are generally not rounded, as in a simple cyst, but have sharp angles. The angular character of these locules is attributed to adhesions secondary to extensive hemorrhage. MR signal is usually high because of contained, clotted blood. Nishimura et al. (1987) agree, but add that adhesions to surrounding organs, seen as a loss of clear margins and tethering, should be looked for. Exceptions to these findings, particularly a diminished T1 signal, have been noted by the current authors and others

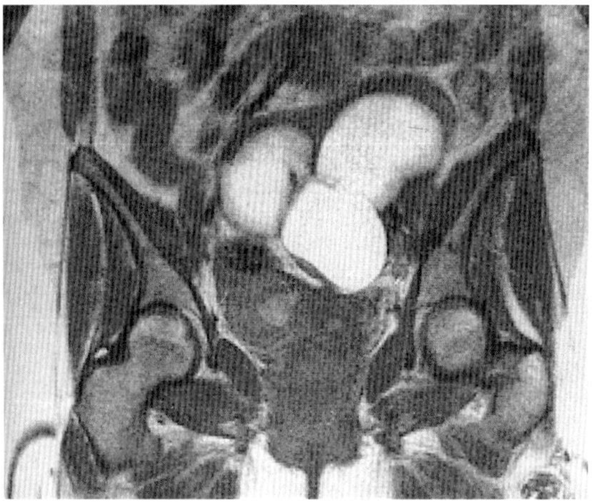

7–16 Endometrioma. Spin density weighted image in coronal plane shows lobulated masses of high signal intensity. Endometriomas usually have high signal intensity on all pulse sequences, due to contained blood.

and has been attributed to the presence of blood breakdown products, deoxyhemoglobin, or hemosiderin. Overall the role of MR in the evaluation of endometriosis remains unclear (Butler et al. 1984). MR's global view of the pelvis improves on ultrasonography, but decreased resolution limits MR's use for small lesions, and MR completely misses tiny implants visible to the laparoscopist. Overall, this evaluation appears to remain the domain of the laparoscopist.

Conclusion

MR evaluation of the genitourinary tract is in its infancy. To date, there are no primary indications for MR that cannot be performed by other modalities at far lower costs.

The NIH consensus panel recommendations are as follows:

1. MR equals CT in renal mass evaluation. Limitations were noted for small renal masses, isointense renal masses, and calcified masses. MR is recommended when CT is equivocal or when contrast is contraindicated.

2. MR applications in gynecological disease remain undetermined. MR is not a screening modality in the female pelvis. MR shows excellent potential in staging endometrial carcinoma and cervical carcinoma. MR provides a global view of the pelvis and is able to depict concomitant pelvic lesions.

3. MR is at least equal to CT in the male pelvis. MR is a promising method of staging prostatic cancer outside of the capsule.

4. MR is probably superior to CT in staging of bladder carcinoma.

At University Hospitals of Cleveland the authors continue to explore staging potentials of MR for malignancies involving the kidney, uterus, cervix, bladder, and prostate. Preliminary data suggest MR is better than CT in staging many of these areas. The authors continue to conduct both tests in hopes of confirming MR's superiority in these areas.

References

Baker LL, Hajek PC, Burkhard TK, et al.: MR imaging of the scrotum: Pathologic conditions. *Radiology* 163:93–98, 1987.

Bryan PJ, Butler HE, LiPuma JP: Magnetic resonance imaging of the pelvis. *Radiol. Clin. North Am.* 22:897–906, 1984.

Bryan PJ, Butler HE, Nelson AD, LiPuma JP, et al.: Magnetic resonance imaging of the prostate. *Am. J. Roentgenol.* 146:543–548, 1986.

Butler HE, Bryan PJ, LiPuma JP, et al.: Magnetic resonance imaging of the female pelvis. *Am. J. Roentgenol.* 143:1259–1266, 1984.

Fein AB, Lee JKT, Batte DM, et al.: Diagnosis and staging of renal cell carcinoma. A comparison of MR imaging and CT. *Am. J. Roentgenol.* 148:749–753, 1987.

Glazer GM: MR imaging of the liver, kidneys, and adrenal glands. *Radiology* 166:303–312, 1988.

Hilpert PL, Friedman AC, Radecki PD, et al.: MRI of hemorrhagic renal cysts in polycystic kidney disease. *Am. J. Roentgenol.* 146:1167–1172, 1986.

Hricak H, Crooks LE, Shelden PE, et al.: Nuclear magnetic resonance imaging of the kidney. *Radiology* 146:425–432, 1983.

Hricak H, Demas BE, Braga CH, et al.: Gestational trephoblastic neoplasm of the uterus: MR assessment. *Radiology* 161:11–16, 1986.

Hricak H, Demas BE, Williams RD, et al.: Magnetic resonance imaging in the diagnosis and staging of renal and perirenal neoplasms. *Radiology* 154:709–715, 1985.

Hricak H, Stem JL, Fischer MR, et al.: Endometrial carcinoma staging by MR imaging. *Radiology* 162:297–305, 1987.

Hricak H, Tscholakott D, Heinrichs L, et al.: Uterine leiomyomas: Correlation of MR, histopathological findings, and symptoms. *Radiology* 158:385–391, 1986.

Hricak H, Williams RD, Spring DB, et al.: Anatomy and pathology of the male pelvis by magnetic resonance imaging. *Am. J. Roentgenol.* 146:1101–1110, 1983.

Laude IM, Glazer GM, Sarnaik S, et al.: Sickle cell nephropathy: MR imaging. *Radiology* 158:385–391, 1986.

Lee JKT, Gersell DJ, Balfe DM, et al.: The uterus: In vitro MR-anatomic correlations of normal and abnormal specimens. *Radiology* 157:175–179, 1985.

LiPuma JP, ElYousef SJ, Bryan PJ, et al.: Renal NMR. Paper presented at the 69th Annual Meeting of RSNA, Chicago, November 1983.

Marks AS, Hricak H, Heinrichs LW, et al.: Adenomyosis and leiomyoma: Differential diagnosis with MR imaging. *Radiology* 163:527–529, 1987.

Marotti M, Hricak H, Fritzsche P, et al.: Complex and simple renal cysts: Comparative evaluation with MR imaging. *Radiology* 162:679–684, 1986.

Mulopulos GP, Tumer DA, Schwartz MM, et al.: MRI of the kidney in paroxysmal nocturnal hemoglobinuria. *Am. J. Roentgenol.* 146:51–52, 1986.

Nishimura K, Togashi K, Itoh K, et al.: Endometrial cysts of the ovary: MR imaging. *Radiology* 162:315–318, 1987.

Quint LE, Glazer GM, Chenevert TL, et al.: MRI of renal tumors: Histopathological correlation with in vivo and in vitro imaging (abstr.) *In Book of Abstracts, Society of Magnetic Resonance in Medicine,* p. 219. Berkeley CA: Society of Magnetic Resonance Imaging in Medicine, 1987.

Rholl KS, Lee JKT, Ling D, et al.: MR imaging of the scrotum with a high-resolution surface coil. *Radiology* 163:99–103, 1987.

Schmidt HC, Tscholakoff D, Hricak H, et al.: MR image contrast and relaxation times of solid tumors in the chest, abdomen, and pelvis. *J. Comput. Assist. Tomogr.* 9:738–748, 1985.

Togashi K, Nishimura K, Hon K, et al.: Uterine cervical cancer: Assessment with high field imaging. *Radiology* 160:431–435, 1986.

Togashi K, Nishimura K, Itoh K, et al.: Ovarian cystic teratomas: MR imaging. *Radiology* 162:669–673, 1987.

CHAPTER
8
Lymphography and Fine-Needle Aspiration Biopsy in Staging of Urologic Tumors

Reiley Kidd

Evaluation of lymph nodes is important in the staging and follow-up of patients with urologic malignancies, since these tumors generally metastasize by the lymphatic system. Tests available for this purpose are computed tomography (CT), ultrasound, magnetic resonance (MR) imaging, or lymphography with or without fine-needle aspiration biopsy.

Pedal lymphography is an examination where pelvic and para-aortic lymphatic channels and nodes are filled with Ethiodol, an oil-based radiopaque contrast material. Lymphography combined with fine-needle aspiration biopsy is useful for evaluating patients with advanced local carcinoma of the prostate (stage C) and bladder (stages B2 or C). For lower stages of these tumors with an aggressive histology, it may also be helpful. Lymphography, even with fine-needle biopsy, is not useful in staging tumors of lesser histologic grade or clinical stage.

Pathophysiology

Each organ has its own lymphatic drainage pattern, and lymphogenous spread of a tumor usually occurs along known lymphatic drainage routes. These normal patterns may, however, be altered by disease, previous surgery, or radiation therapy.

Normal lymphatic drainage of the prostate and bladder are similar, with first echelon visceral nodes lying deep in the pelvis adjacent to these organs. Lymphatic metastases will spread to these nodes first. Subsequently, the tumor will spread to the medial chain of nodes in the external iliac group or to internal iliac (hypogastric) or presacral nodes. Once these nodes are involved, cephalad spread may occur, first to the common iliac and then to the para-aortic nodes. Bladder or prostate cancer rarely spread to para-aortic nodes directly.

Lymphatic drainage of the testicle differs from that of the bladder and prostate in that the primary echelon nodes of the testes are in the para-aortic or paracaval area, rather than in the pelvis. Testicular lymphatics accompany venous drainage. The first echelon node of the right testis usually lies at the entrance of the right testicular vein into the inferior vena cava, typically at about the level of the 3rd lumbar vertebra. However, it may be found anywhere from the 4th lumbar vertebra caudally to as high as the 11th thoracic vertebra. The first echelon node on the left is usually found at the junction of the left testicular vein with the left renal vein. From there, lymphatic flow is to nearby para-aortic nodes and then cephalad to retrocrural nodes. Usually there is no lymphatic spread to pelvic nodes, unless a transscrotal biopsy has been performed or lymphatic obstruction by initial metastases to higher nodes has allowed retrograde spread through the lymphatics.

Lymphography only opacifies pelvic and para-aortic (paracaval) nodes in the pathway of lymphatic flow from the feet. Unfortunately, visceral, internal iliac, and presacral nodes rarely fill. The first echelon nodes of the testes, particularly the left, may also not fill. This is one of the main reasons for the relatively high false-negative rate of this test.

Controversy exists about whether the obturator node, a common site of early metastases in bladder and prostate tumors, is opacified by lymphography. Studies (Zoretic et al. 1983) indicate that the surgical obturator node is routinely opacified by lymphography.

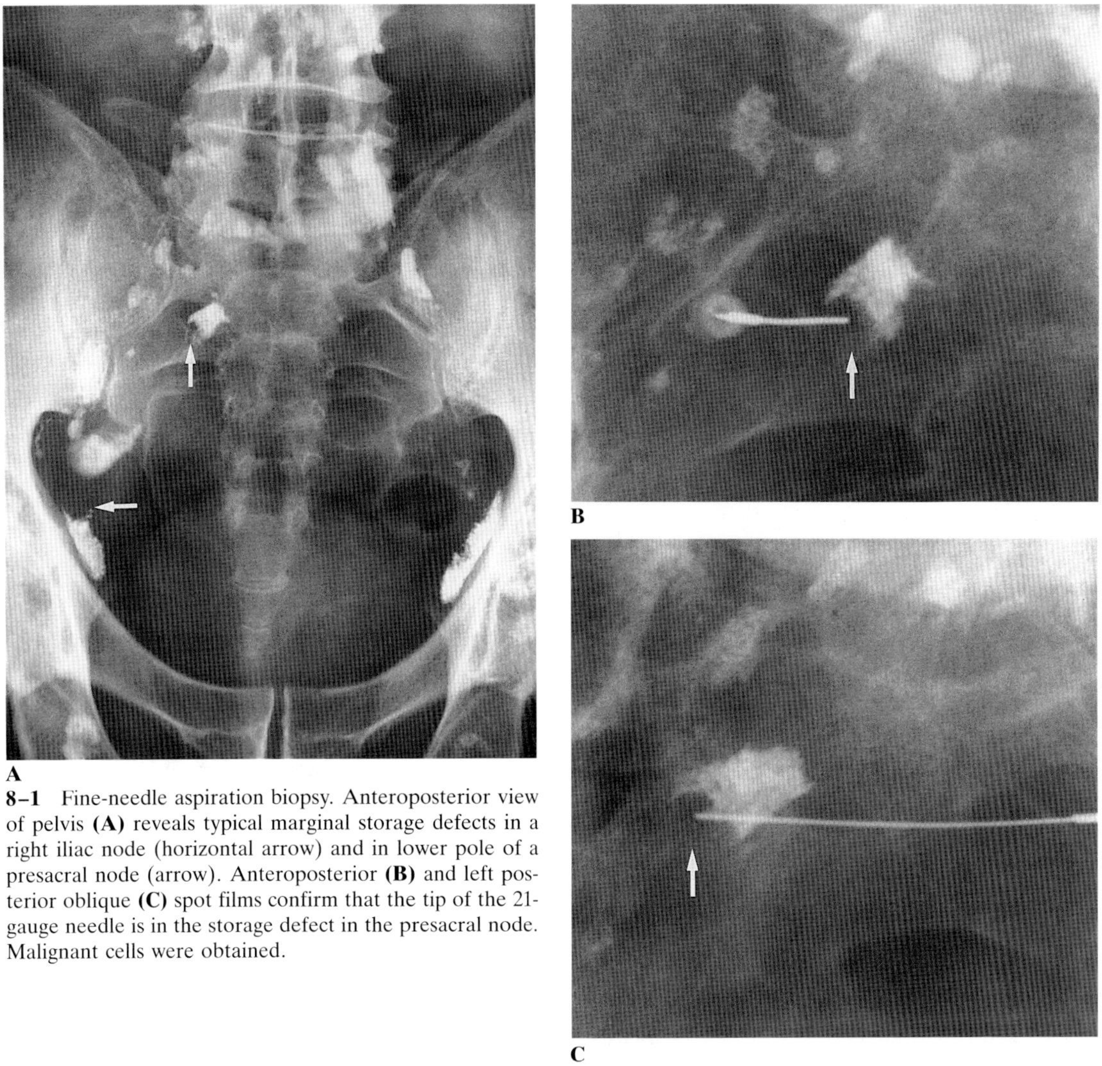

8–1 Fine-needle aspiration biopsy. Anteroposterior view of pelvis **(A)** reveals typical marginal storage defects in a right iliac node (horizontal arrow) and in lower pole of a presacral node (arrow). Anteroposterior **(B)** and left posterior oblique **(C)** spot films confirm that the tip of the 21-gauge needle is in the storage defect in the presacral node. Malignant cells were obtained.

Technique

Examination of lymph nodes is done on 2 successive days without hospitalization. To initially locate the lymphatics, blue dye is injected intradermally. Patients should be forewarned that the dye may temporarily color their urine. A lymphatic channel on the dorsum of each foot is cannulated with a 27-gauge needle, and contrast material is infused, filling lymphatic channels to the midlumbar region. This usually requires 5–6 ml of Ethiodol; no more than 7 ml per side should be injected to minimize oil embolization to the lungs (see paragraph on "Complications"). The first set of radiographs is obtained after 1–2 hr to demonstrate lymphatic flow. This is termed the vascular phase.

Contrast gradually enters the lymph nodes, and radiographs are obtained on the second day (18–24 hr after contrast infusion) to demonstrate the nodal architecture.

Fine-needle aspiration biopsy is an essential adjunct to lymphography. Introduced by Gothlin in 1976, the procedure consists of passing a 21- to 23-gauge needle percutaneously into an abnormal-appearing lymph node or a suspected tumor using fluoroscopy, computed tomography, or ultrasound for guidance. Fluoroscopy, especially multidirectional fluoroscopy, is best for aspiration of small nodal defects found at lymphography. Cells are aspirated, stained, and examined by a cytologist. Fine-needle biopsy is a safe procedure, which is routinely performed on an outpatient basis.

Fine-needle aspiration biopsy can confirm a positive diagnosis by lymphography (Fig. 8–1). It can also eliminate the false-positive and equivocal lymphographic diagnosis; if lymphography is posi-

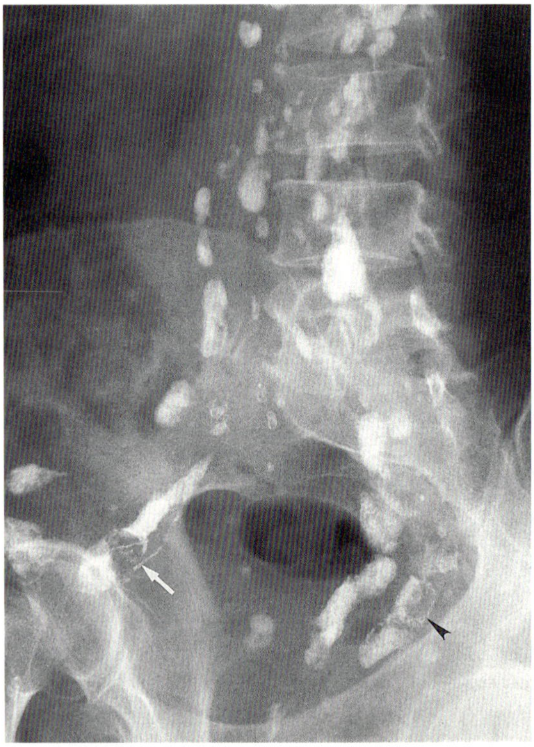

A

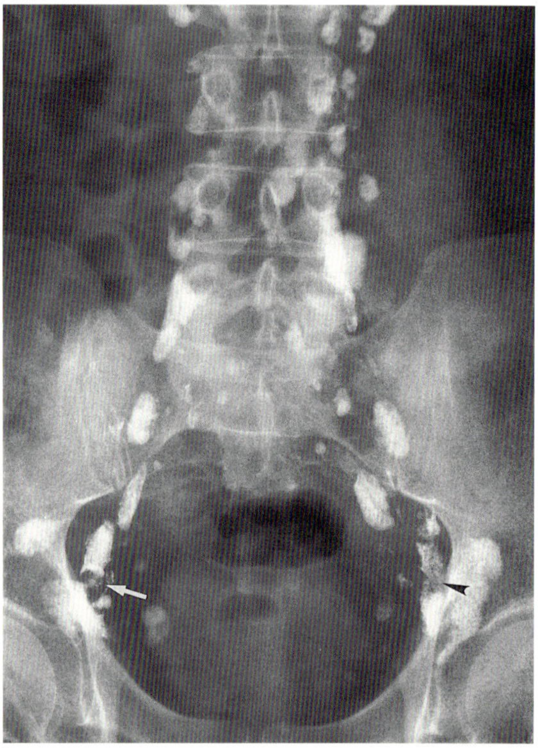

B

8–2 False-positive lymphography. Right posterior oblique (**A**) and anteroposterior (**B**) views of pelvis demonstrate a 14-mm crescentic defect at caudal end of right surgical obturator node (white arrows) not traversed by lymphatics. Node appears focally enlarged, with splaying of the opacified node at its junction with the defect. Left surgical obturator node (black arrows) shows incomplete opacification with frayed posterior margin. Right node was considered positive for metastasis; the left was equivocal. Fine-needle aspiration biopsy of both nodes was negative, and a subsequent lymph node dissection revealed no metastases. There was radiographic confirmation that both nodes had been excised. (Reprinted, by permission, from Kidd R, Crane RD, Dail DH: Lymphangiography and fine-needle aspiration biopsy: Ineffective for staging early prostate cancer. *Am. J. Roentgenol.* 141:1007–1012, ©1984, American Roentgen Ray Society.)

tive, but needle biopsy of the abnormal nodes is cytologically benign, the lymphographic diagnosis is revised to negative (Fig. 8–2).

We therefore believe that fine-needle aspiration biopsy should be performed for all positive or equivocal lymphograms.

Appearance of Metastases

Most metastases appear as crescent-shaped filling defects, 8 mm or more in diameter, in the margin of an opacified node (Fig. 8–3). Defects smaller than 8 mm are usually due to a benign cause, such as previous inflammation or normal nodal involution. Differentiation between benign nodal defects or metastases can be made by fine-needle aspiration biopsy, as already discussed. Large metastases may completely replace the node, leaving only a thin rim of contrast-filled sinusoid peripherally, creating the so-called ghost node (Fig. 8–4). Further tumor growth will result in complete obstruction, with nonfilling of nodes in the involved chain and persistent filling of the lymphatics. Lymphatic rupture with extravasation of Ethiodol and collateral flow are other manifestations of lymphatic obstruction.

Occasionally, a metastasis will infiltrate the node diffusely, resulting in generalized nodal enlargement and a foamy appearance (Fig. 8–5),

8–4 Ghost node. Oblique radiograph of pelvis following ▶ lymphangiogram reveals a thin rim of Ethiodol outlining an enlarged external iliac node (arrow) in a man with cancer of the prostate. Fine-needle aspiration biopsy of this node confirmed metastasis.

8–5 Foamy appearance of metastases on lymphography. ▶▶ A left posterior oblique radiograph of pelvis in man with carcinoma of the prostate shows several enlarged, foamy-appearing nodes in left common and external iliac groups, the largest measuring 13 mm × 19 mm (arrow). Fine-needle aspiration biopsy of this node was positive.

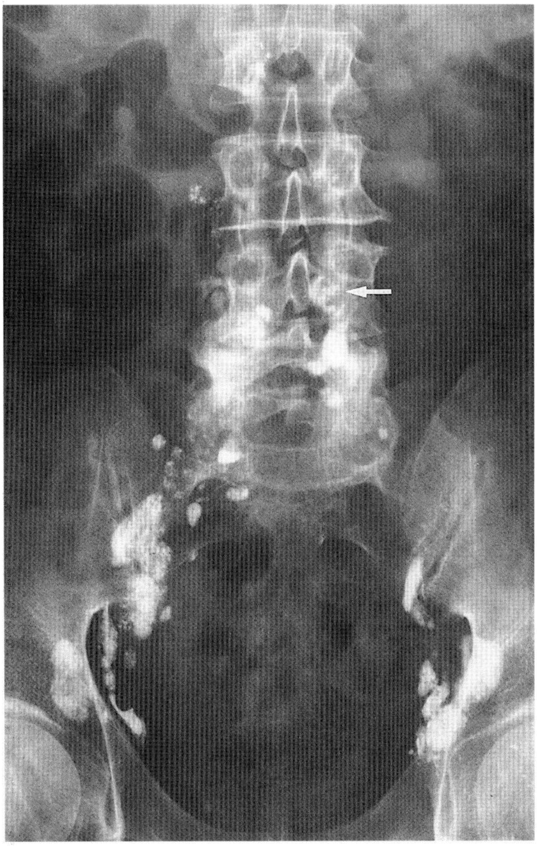

A

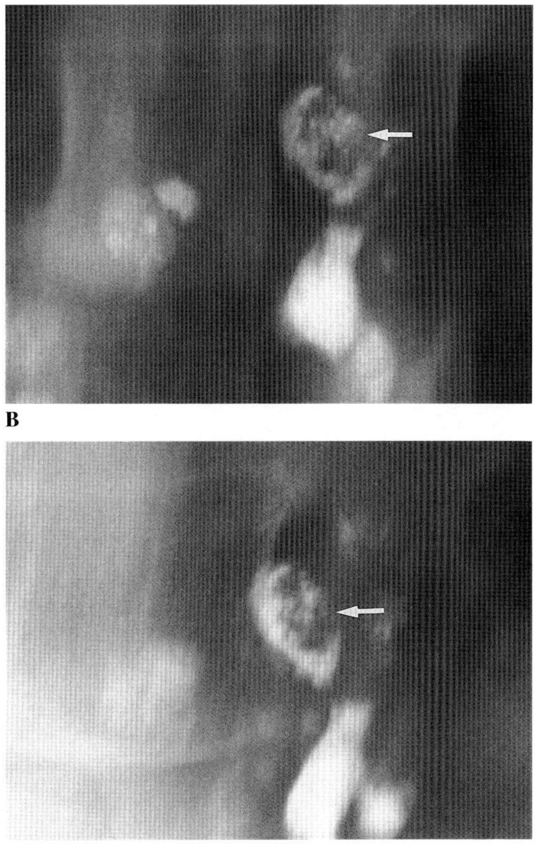

B

C

8–3 Typical appearance of metastasis. Anteroposterior film of abdomen **(A)** demonstrates crescentic filling defect in a lower para-aortic node (arrow). Anteroposterior **(B)** and left posterior oblique **(C)** tomography confirm typical crescentic peripheral filling defect produced by metastasis. Aspiration biopsy was positive.

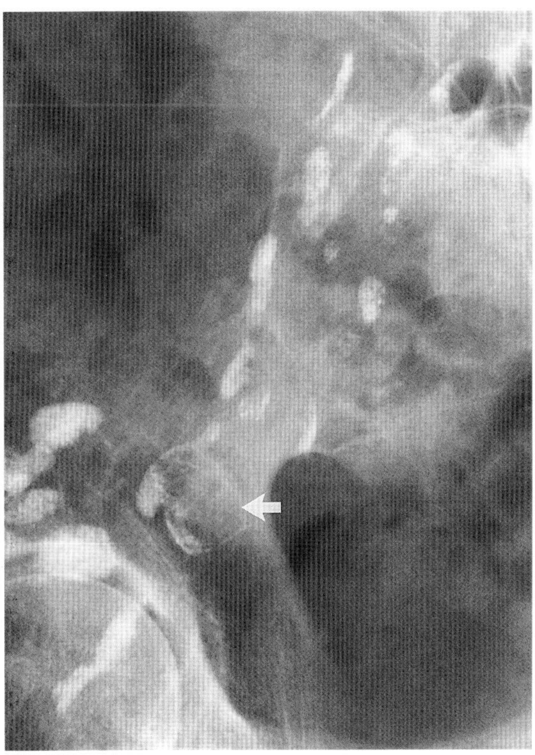

8–4

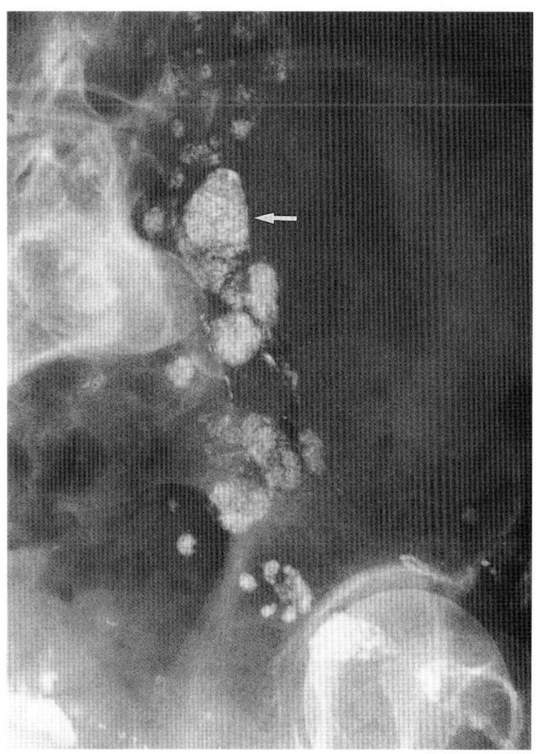

8–5

a pattern usually associated with lymphoma. This pattern is usually seen in metastases from seminomas and rarely in other tumors.

Accuracy

The ability of a test to detect disease is termed the sensitivity of the test. The sensitivity of any test depends upon the study population. Studies containing a predominance of patients with advanced tumor stages inevitably demonstrate a much higher sensitivity for a given test than studies with patients in earlier stages of disease. Comparison of the reported accuracy of lymphography with that of any other imaging technique is hampered by the variable and usually unspecified distribution of early versus advanced disease patients in these studies.

In general, lymphography is specific but insensitive. Its true positive rate is generally 90%–95%; it approaches 100% with the addition of fine-needle aspiration biopsy. However, the false-negative rate can be as high as 30%–50%, resulting in as many as half of the patients with nodal metastases having negative lymphography. This is primarily because lymphography is a macroscopic test, incapable of detecting microscopic deposits of tumor in nodes. Lymphography also does not fill many nodes that may be involved with metastases.

Needle aspiration does not impact the high false-negative rate. Aspiration of nodes appearing normal on lymphangiography helped in one series (Gothlin, Hoiem 1981), but not in this author's experience (Kidd, Correa 1984). In addition, fluoroscopically guided needle aspiration cannot be done on nodes that do not opacify.

Complications

About a third of patients undergoing lymphography will experience fever or chills the night after contrast infusion. This is a self-limited response to the contrast, which may be treated symptomatically. It is not serious unless accompanied by signs of respiratory distress.

Local complications related to the incision site are uncommon and are minimized by good technique and thorough irrigation of the incisions with saline prior to suturing.

Several studies have shown a transient decrease in pulmonary diffusion capacity in most patients undergoing lymphography, presumably due to Ethiodol reaching the pulmonary capillary bed via the thoracic duct. However, this is rarely symptomatic. Respiratory impairment due to pulmonary embolization of contrast is minimized by avoiding lymphography in patients with symptomatic lung disease, and by monitoring the cephalad flow of contrast with intermittent radiographs, terminating the infusion before contrast reaches the thoracic duct. As stated earlier, no more than 7 ml per side should be infused.

Allergic reactions, such as skin rash, itching, and wheezing, occur less frequently than with other iodinated contrast materials, and are usually mild. More severe reactions, such as cardiorespiratory arrest and death, have occurred, but are extremely rare.

Another rare complication, chemical pneumonitis, can occur as the embolized oil is hydrolized in the lungs into fatty acids that irritate the alveolar lining. This reaction develops in the first 24–48 hr after contrast infusion. The first signs are fever, cough, sputum that may be bloody, and respiratory distress. Reducing the volume of Ethiodol has greatly decreased this complication.

Contraindications

Contraindications to lymphography are respiratory impairment and lower extremity vascular insufficiency. Virtually 100% of patients undergoing the test embolize the oily contrast medium in the pulmonary arterial bed, since the thoracic duct empties directly into the central venous system. Although only a small fraction of the pulmonary arterial bed is affected, patients without pulmonary reserve can go into respiratory failure. Patients at increased risk include those with chronic lung diseases, previous lung irradiation, and extensive lung metastases.

Lower extremity vascular insufficiency, especially in insulin-dependent diabetic patients, may impair the healing of the incisions on the feet, and may result in infection or ulceration.

A relative contraindication is a previous anaphylactoid reaction to iodinated contrast agents. Where clinically indicated, the test can usually be accomplished following pretreatment with steroids and antihistamines.

Role of Lymphography

Prostatic Carcinoma

The likelihood of prostate cancer spreading to lymph nodes correlates with the clinical stage and histologic grade of the tumor. Urologists performing lymph node dissections in patients with newly diagnosed prostate cancer have reported nodal metastases in 14%–21% of patients with clinical stage B1 disease, in 23%–28% with A2 disease, in 30%–50% with B2 disease, and in 39%–63% with stage-C disease.

The efficacy of lymphography is also related to clinical stage and histologic grade. In studies that include information on clinical stage of disease, positive lymphograms are extremely rare in stages A1 and B1, and unusual in stages A2 and B2. The largest study that considered histologic grade and clinical stage of prostate cancer (Kidd et al. 1984) combined lymphography and fine-needle aspiration biopsy and confirmed metastases in none of 116 patients with B1 disease, 1 of 40 (3%) with A2 disease, and 1 of 73 (1%) with stage B2 disease; results were positive in 33 of 203 (17%) patients with clinical stage-C disease. Thus, lymphography found substantially fewer metastases than expected in each stage, and results were poorest in early stage disease. In this study, all of the patients whose nodal metastases were detected by the combined tests had a histologic Gleason score of 6 or greater. Based on this information, this author and colleagues believe that lymphography, even combined with needle aspiration, is ineffective in staging A or B prostate cancer.

In patients with clinical stage-C disease, lymphography combined with fine-needle aspiration biopsy identifies only one-third to one-half of those with nodal metastases. However, a positive needle aspiration biopsy in these patients spares them the morbidity and expense of a staging lymph node dissection, and allows for a more confident selection of appropriate therapy. Patients whose combined procedure is negative are not excluded from subsequent staging surgery. Therefore, lymphography and fine-needle aspiration biopsy are most useful in patients with clinical stage-C disease or with high-grade histologic (Gleason score 8 or higher) stage-A2 and stage-B2 tumors, so long as a positive result will alter the treatment plan or obviate staging lymphadenectomy.

A negative lymphogram should not be equated with the absence of nodal metastases, since the false-negative rate of lymphography is 30%–50% or greater, especially in earlier stages of disease.

Bladder Carcinoma

Because carcinoma of the bladder is less prevalent than prostatic carcinoma, and because it metastasizes later, there are fewer reports on the efficacy of lymphography in patients with bladder cancer. As with prostate cancer, lymphography and needle aspiration biopsy appear to be most useful in the higher clinical stages and histologic grades, and of little or no value in early disease. The false-positive rate of lymphography alone, without fine-needle aspiration, is higher in patients with bladder cancer compared to those with prostate cancer, because nodal enlargement and filling defects are common in the absence of nodal metastases. Fine-needle aspiration biopsy is essential to avoid a false-positive diagnosis.

Tumors of the Testis

Since the first echelon node of the testis, especially the left, may not opacify by lymphography, most radiologists currently prefer computed tomography. CT defines the volume and extent of bulky metastases more completely than lymphography and is a less invasive test. CT-guided fine-needle aspiration biopsy can confirm a positive scan.

Theoretically, lymphography can detect metastases in normal-sized nodes, whereas computed tomographic diagnosis of nodal metastasis depends solely on nodal enlargement. Some radiologists advocate lymphography for patients with testicular carcinoma if the initial staging CT scan is negative. This policy will yield a minimal increase in confirmed nodal metastases.

Other Urologic Malignancies

Patients with carcinoma of the kidney or ureter are usually staged with computed tomography or magnetic resonance imaging. Carcinoma of the seminal vesicle is rare; however, lymphography may benefit patients with this disease, since lymphatic drainage of the seminal vesicles resembles that of the prostate and bladder.

Conclusions

In patients with prostate or bladder carcinoma, lymphography combined with fine-needle aspiration biopsy is useful primarily for advanced local disease: stage C in carcinoma of the prostate and stage B2 or C in carcinoma of the bladder. In patients with histologically aggressive tumors, the procedures may be helpful in earlier stages. While fine-needle aspiration biopsy and lymphography will miss as many as half of those patients with lymph node metastases, a positive result can obviate lymphadenectomy for staging and allow for confident selection of therapy. This should not be done if the results will not alter the treatment plan.

In patients with testicular carcinoma, computed tomography is preferable as the initial staging test. If CT is negative and treatment would be altered by the presence of macroscopic nodal metastases, lymphography can be performed and will occasionally detect a metastasis to a nonenlarged node.

Fine-needle aspiration biopsy should be performed routinely in all cases of positive or equivocal lymphography to confirm the lymphography diagnosis and to eliminate false-positive diagnoses.

Lymphography is helpful when positive and confirmed by needle aspiration. It is meaningless when negative, due to a false-negative rate of 30%–50% or more, especially in lower tumor stages. This limitation cannot be overcome by needle aspiration of lymphangiographically normal nodes.

References

Gothlin JH, Hoiem L: Percutaneous fine-needle biopsy of radiographically normal lymph nodes in the staging of prostatic carcinoma. *Radiology* 141:351–354, 1981.

Kidd R, Correa RJ, Jr.: Fine-needle aspiration biopsy of lymphangiographically normal lymph nodes: A negative view. *Am. J. Roentgenol.* 132:1005–1007, 1984.

Kidd R, Crane RD, Dail DH: Lymphangiography and fine-needle aspiration biopsy: Ineffective for staging early prostate cancer. *Am. J. Roentgenol.* 141:1007–1012, 1984.

Zoretic SN, Wajsman Z, Beckley SA, Pontes JE: Filling of the obturator nodes in pedal lymphangiography: Fact or fiction? *J. Urol.* 129:533–535, 1983.

Suggested Reading

Clouse ME (ed.): *Clinical Lymphography,* 2d ed. Baltimore, Williams & Wilkins, 1985.

Marincek B, Brutschin P, Triller J, Fuchs WA: Lymphography and computed tomography in staging non-seminomatous testicular cancer: Limited detection of early stage metastatic disease. *Urol. Radiol.* 5:243–246, 1983.

Spellman MC, Castellino RA, Ray GR, Pistenma DA, Bagshaw MA: An evaluation of lymphography in localized carcinoma of the prostate. *Radiology* 125:637–644, 1977.

Strijk SP, Debruyne FMJ, Herman CJ: Lymphography in the management of urologic tumors: Radiologic-pathologic correlation. *Radiology* 146:39–45, 1983.

Thomas JL, Bernardino ME, Bracken RB: Staging of testicular carcinoma: Comparison of CT and lymphography. *Am. J. Roentgenol.* 137:991–996, 1981.

CHAPTER

9

Arteriography and Venography of the Urinary Tract

William H. Bush

In the 1960s and 1970s, vascular studies were the primary method for diagnosing disorders of the richly perfused urinary system. During the past decade, however, with the development of ultrasonography, dynamic computed tomographic scanning, and magnetic resonance imaging, profound changes have occurred in imaging the retroperitoneum and pelvis. Angiography is no longer a primary diagnostic tool for the urinary tract.

Nevertheless, arteriographic and venographic techniques remain the foundation for many interventional and other diagnostic procedures, including: venous sampling of the adrenal gland for aldosteronoma; embolization of traumatic injuries to the kidney; and vascular embolization to control bleeding from pelvic organs or after pelvic fracture. Moreover, arteriography is the most accurate method of diagnosing renal vascular hypertension and provides the route by which renal artery stenosis can often be corrected.

Vascular Anatomy

Renal Arteries and Veins

Renal vascular variation is affected principally by the origin of the kidney from the metanephrogenic mass and its initial origin in the pelvis, at the caudal end of the mesonephric mass. Likely based on differential growth, under stimulation of the ureteric bud, the renal mass "migrates" cephalad to the L2 level. It assumes parts of the freely anastomosing series of arteries arising from the aorta called the "rete arteriosum urogenitale" (Hollinshead 1966). Variations in ascent, rotation, and position influence the vascular supply of the organ.

The renal arteries commonly originate at the first or second lumbar level from the lateral or anterolateral aspect of the aorta, just below the origin of the superior mesenteric artery (Oedman, Ranniger 1968). The right renal artery courses beneath the inferior vena cava, while the left renal artery lies behind the main left renal vein, crossing to join the inferior vena cava (Fig. 9–1). Although both major renal arteries lie posterior to or behind their respective veins, some of the segmental branches of the right renal artery commonly course anterior to the vein near the renal hilum.

Supernumerary accessory renal arteries are found in over 37% of patients. These may originate anywhere from the T4 to L4 level (Hollinshead 1966; Merklin, Michels 1958). An accessory artery more often originates from the ventrolateral or ventral aspect of the aorta. Of the one-third of kidneys that deviate from the single artery pattern, 12% have two or more arteries of aortic origin that enter the hilus; 12% have two arteries of aortic origin, one entering the hilus and the other a renal pole; and 13% have polar arteries (usually upper) derived from a source other than the aorta (e.g., phrenic artery) (Merklin, Michels 1958). A frequent accessory artery is to the lower pole of the kidney; this may arise from above or below the origin of the main renal artery.

The kidney is perfused from anterior and posterior divisions, the latter supplying the posterior aspect of the kidney, except for the lower pole. The anterior division supplies about two-thirds of the kidney, including the lower pole (Fig. 9–2). The medial apex supply may involve both divisions. There are no anastomoses between the

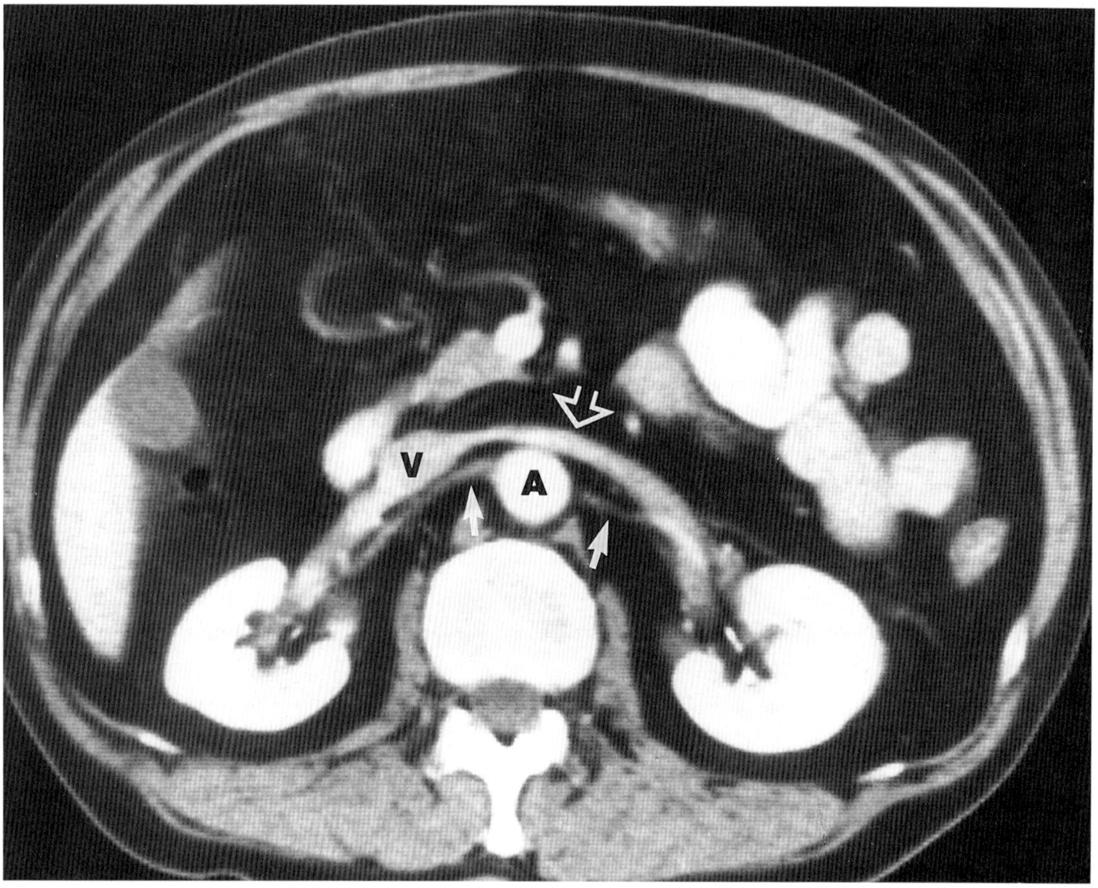

9–1 Relationships of renal arteries and veins. Axial CT scan at renal level shows both arteries and veins. Arteries (arrows) arise anterolaterally from aorta (A) and lie posterior to veins. Left renal vein (open arrow) courses over aorta to reach IVC (V).

branches of the renal artery, so that each branch is an end artery. The major intrarenal vessels are the interlobar arteries, which course peripherally from the segmental vessels to form the arcuate arteries at the corticomedullary junction; small interlobular vessels arising from the arcuates are best seen on magnification angiography (Fig. 9–3).

Other branches of the main renal artery, or one of the segmental arteries, are those to the adrenals, renal capsule, and ureter. The right inferior adrenal artery usually arises from the main renal artery and tends to be prominent and variable. It may be multiple, also giving rise to capsular vessels or arteries to the renal parenchyma of the upper pole.

A varying number of capsular vessels arises from the main renal artery or its major segmental branches. These capsular arteries course over the kidney through the fat in Gerota's space; in addition, capsular arteries communicate with the interlobular and interlobar arteries of the kidney through direct perforating branches (Luzsa 1974). A fairly constant branch from a major segmental renal artery is the ureteric artery; from this, the inferior capsular branch to the kidney often arises (Fig. 9–4). The gonadal arteries typically originate from the anterior aspect of the abdominal aorta below the renals, although occasionally from a renal artery.

The venous anatomy is less variable. The right cardinal vein persists as the inferior vena cava and the adrenal, renal, and gonadal veins develop from segments of the extensive cardinal vein anastomotic venous complex of the mesonephric period. As is true in the arterial system, more than one of the veins draining the nephrogenic ridge may persist, giving rise to multiple renal veins (Hollinshead 1966). A retroaortic left renal vein (Fig. 9–5) is due to persistence of the dorsal part of the supracardinal-subcardinal anastomosis. Similarly, if a renal vein arises low enough, it will cross anterior

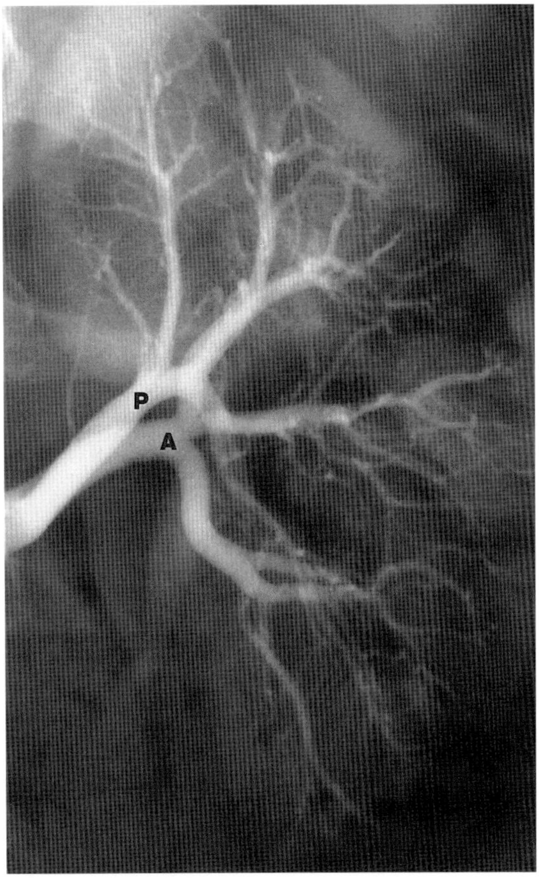

9–2 Normal left renal arteriogram illustrating posterior and anterior divisions. Posterior division (P) typically supplies posterior aspect of kidney, but not lower pole. Anterior divisions (A) supply about two-thirds of the kidney, including lower pole.

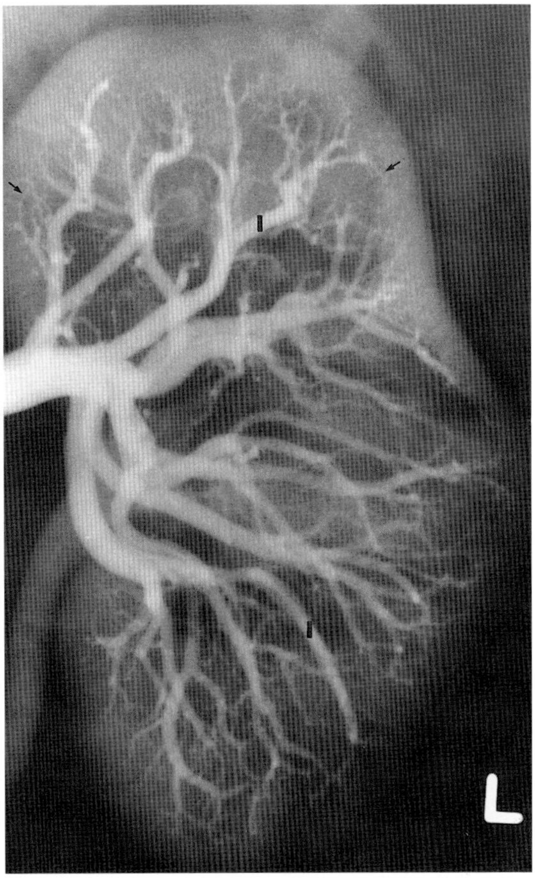

9–3 Selective renal arteriogram. Interlobar vessels (I) course peripherally to form arcuate vessels (arrows) at corticomedullary junction. The most peripheral interlobular vessels can be seen in the cortex of this modified (1.5×) magnification view.

to part of the inferior vena cava, which at that level is derived from the dorsally situated supracardinal vein (Hollinshead 1966).

Unlike the arteries, the intrarenal veins have numerous anastomoses (Fig. 9–6). Two or three major renal vein trunks emerge from the renal hilum to form the renal vein. The right renal vein or veins are usually short, and multiple veins are common (20%–25%); multiple veins are much less frequent on the left (1%–4%) (Hollinshead 1966). The renal veins are located anterior to the artery, although on the right, one or more arterial branches frequently lie in front of the vein trunk.

Arteries and Veins of the True Pelvis

The arterial supply to the organs of the true pelvis (bladder, uterus, prostate) was detailed exquisitely by Nilsson (1967). The main arterial supply to the bladder, uterus, and prostate are the inferior gluteal, internal pudendal, obturator, and visceral arteries. They arise from the anterior division of the internal iliac (hypogastric) artery (Fig. 9–7).

The inferior gluteal and internal pudendal arteries most commonly arise as a common trunk. The small sciatic branch of the inferior gluteal artery accompanies the sciatic nerve. From the internal pudendal artery originate the middle hemorrhoidal artery, small branches to the bladder, and branches to the perineum, urethra, and external genitalia. The obturator artery courses along the pelvic wall with branches to the viscera; just before it enters the obturator canal it gives off a pubic branch. These visceral arteries from the internal iliac (hypogastric) artery vary widely in pattern.

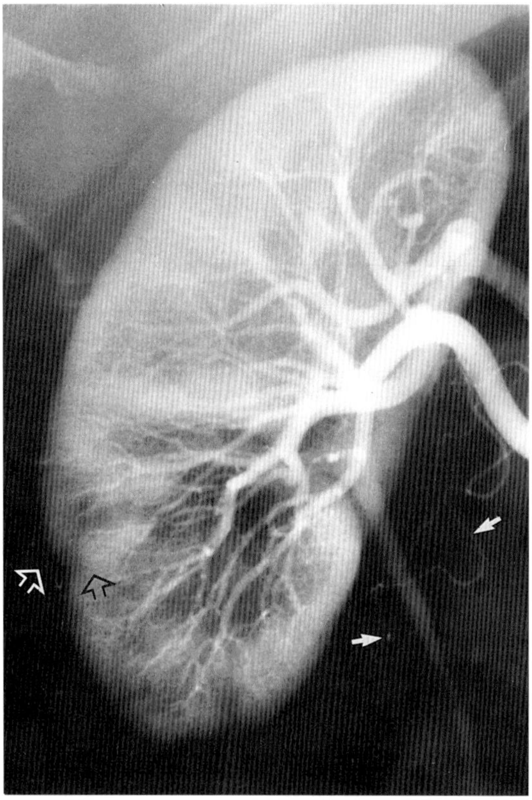

9–4 Ureteric and capsular branches. Ureteric artery (arrows) will usually arise from caudal branch of multiple renal arteries. It may arise from an accessory vessel, making it vulnerable during surgery to harvest a donor kidney for renal transplant. Capsular branches arise at hilum but also as perforating branches from interlobar vessels (open arrows).

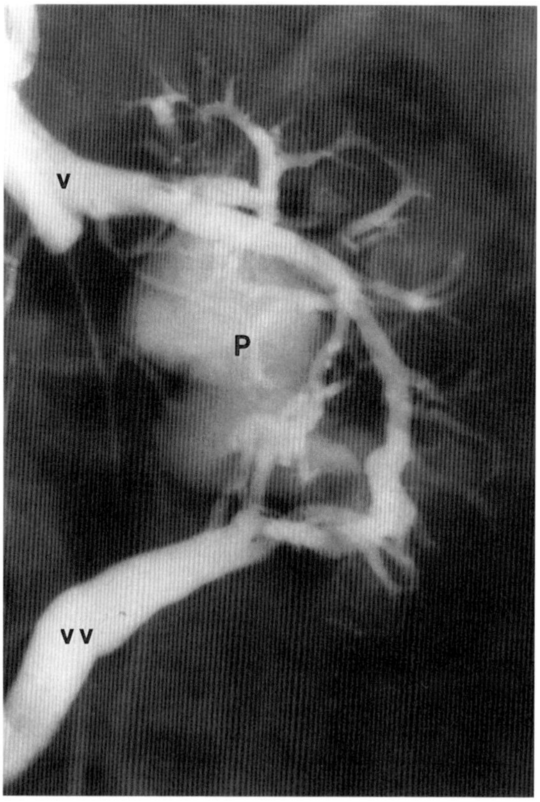

9–5 Renal vein variation. Two major veins on left side: Upper vein (V) is near usual position, and a large second vein (VV) courses in a lower retroaortic position to join cava. P = renal pelvis, also showing congenital variation.

The entire upper part of the bladder is supplied by the unobliterated part of the umbilical artery, called the superior vesical artery; it usually arises from the pudendogluteal trunk (75%) or the internal pudendal artery (20%). The floor of the bladder as well as the prostate and vagina are supplied by the inferior vesical artery, which arises from the internal iliac artery or one of its branches. The various arteries of the bladder arborize in the wall of the bladder and anastomose with each other and those of the other side.

Vessels of the Adrenal Gland

The adrenal arteries are derived from three divisions on each side (Fig. 9–8). The superior adrenal artery originates from the inferior phrenic artery, which in turn has its origin as a branch off

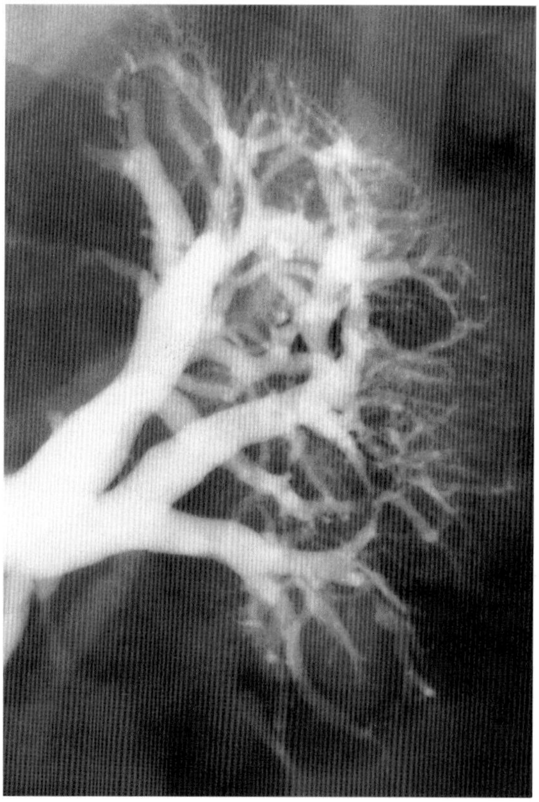

9–6 Normal left renal venogram showing usual freely anastomosing branches.

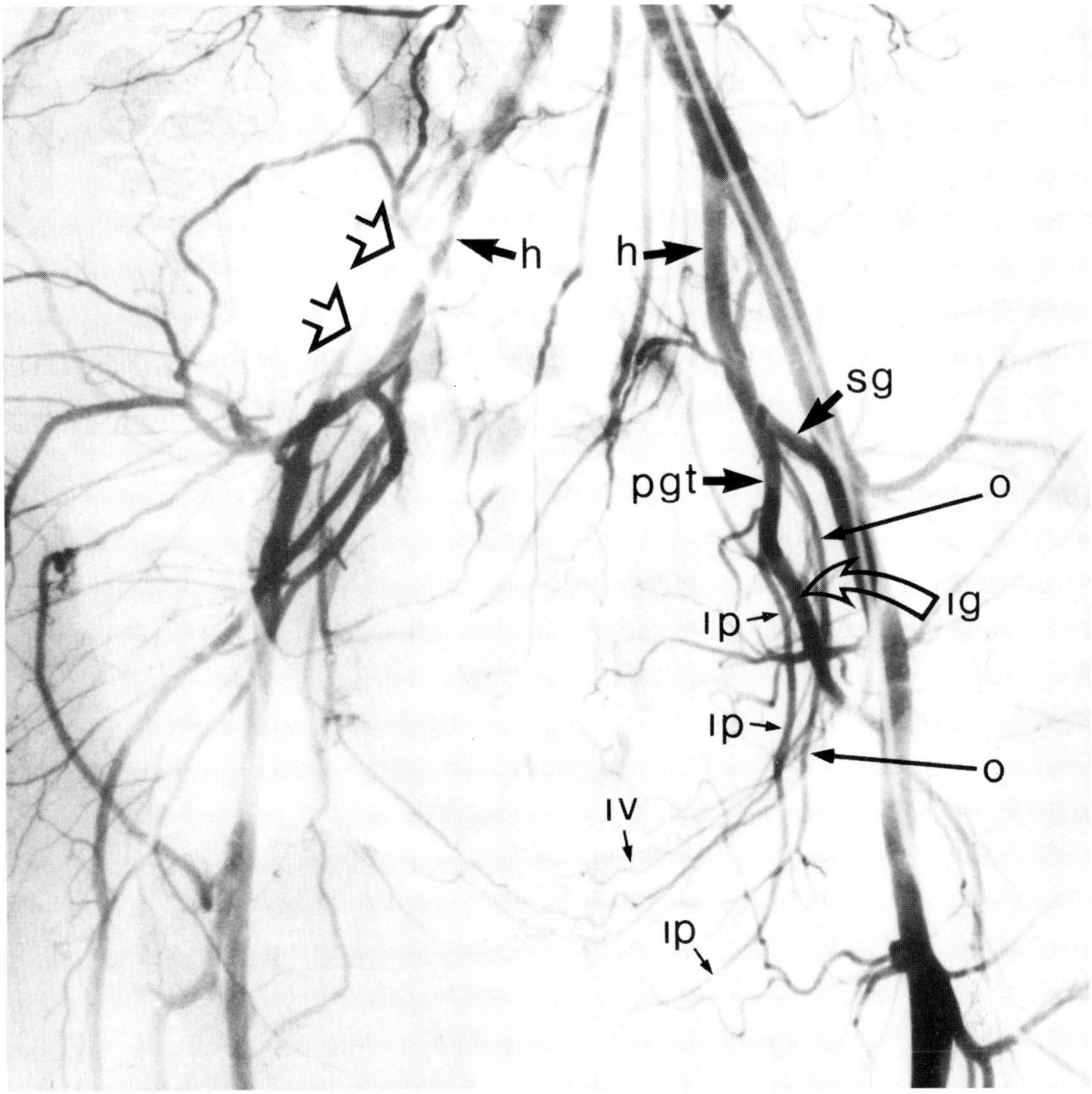

9–7 Pelvic arteriogram done to evaluate arterial supply in patient with recurrent right ureteral carcinoma causing claudication. Right external iliac artery (two open arrows) is encased and markedly narrowed; there is also narrowing of the adjacent internal iliac (hypogastric) artery (h). Branches of left hypogastric artery (h) are: sg = superior gluteal artery; pgt = pudendo-gluteal trunk; ig = inferior gluteal artery (open curved arrow); ip = internal pudendal artery; o = obturator artery; iv = inferior vesical artery.

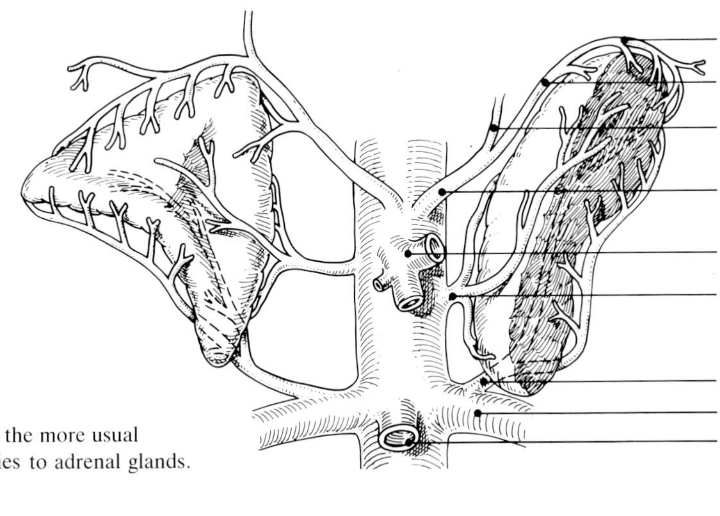

9–8 Illustration of the more usual distribution of arteries to adrenal glands.

the aorta just cephalad and lateral to the celiac artery or directly from the proximal celiac trunk (Kahn 1967). In addition, major supply comes from the inferior adrenal artery, which on the right side is often a major branch of the main renal artery or an upper segmental renal artery. Vascular supply to renal parenchyma in the upper pole of the kidney may also arise from the inferior adrenal artery. The left adrenal artery is less dominant, arising usually from the aorta, and is frequently difficult to selectively define angiographically. The middle adrenal arteries bilaterally are small, often multiple, and difficult to selectively demonstrate.

Technique for Arteriography

Informed consent should be obtained before angiography or interventional procedures. If the patient has a history of an anaphylactoid reaction to contrast or of severe asthma or allergy, nonionic contrast combined with premedication is recommended.

Patients should maintain a light food but large liquid intake before angiography to minimize nephrotoxicity from the contrast media. If oral fluid intake is low, intravenous fluids should be given before and during angiography. A full meal just before angiography should be avoided because of potential nausea, emesis, and aspiration. Moreover, in the setting of interventional angiography, emergency surgery may be necessary.

Creatinine level should be measured, especially if the patient is an insulin-dependent diabetic or has small-vessel renal disease. Hematologic studies are obtained routinely in patients with bleeding disorders, severe liver disease, or those taking anticoagulants or large doses of aspirin; preferably, aspirin should be discontinued 1 week before the examination. Mild sedation such as 10 mg of diazepam (Valium) is given by mouth; analgesics are usually not necessary. The groin or axilla is liberally infiltrated with 0.25% bupivacaine hydrochloride (Marcaine) using a 1½-inch 25-gauge needle.

Arteriography is usually done by a transfemoral route using the Seldinger method of insertion. An 18-gauge needle with hollow stylet and blunt needle shaft is suggested (Pott's needle). A straight or movable J-tipped wire is commonly used. The transfemoral route has advantages over

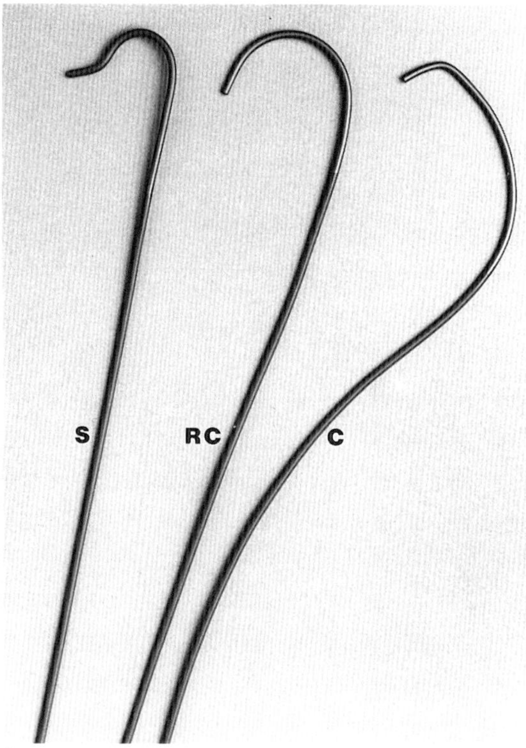

A

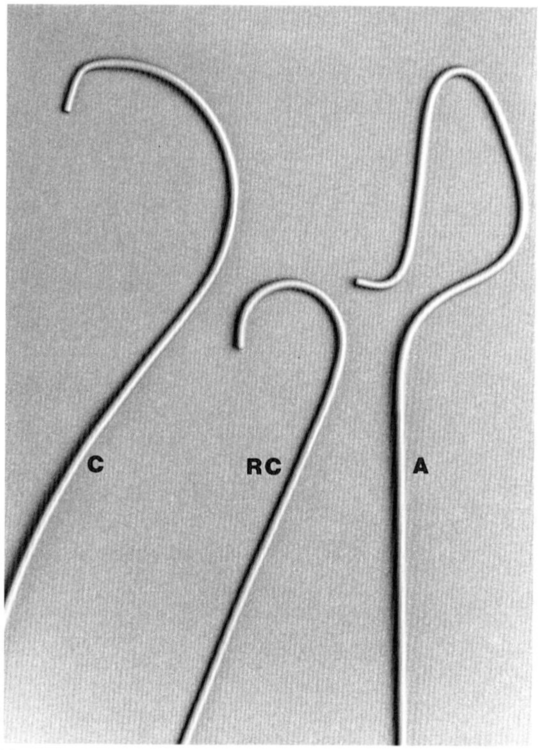

B

9–9 A, B Photographs of various catheter shapes available for urologic angiography. RC = simple curve (Rösch Celiac); S = shepherd's hook; C = cobra-shaped; A = adrenal venous catheter.

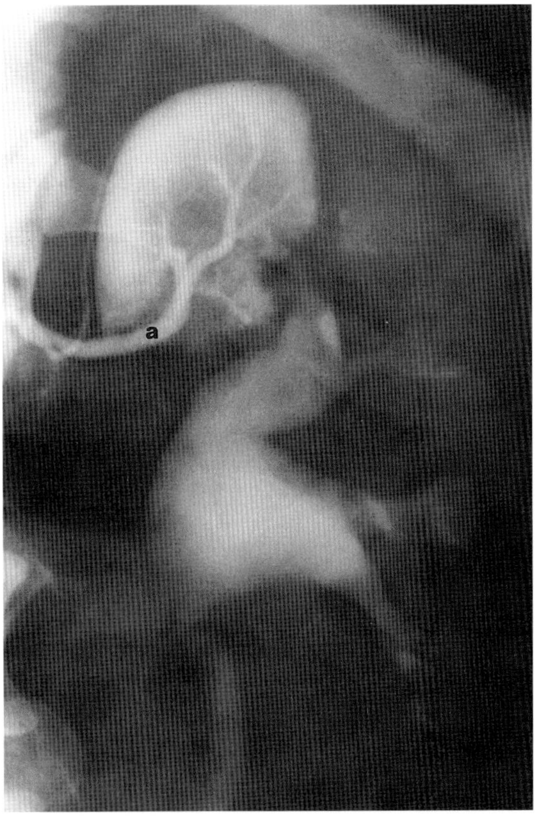
A

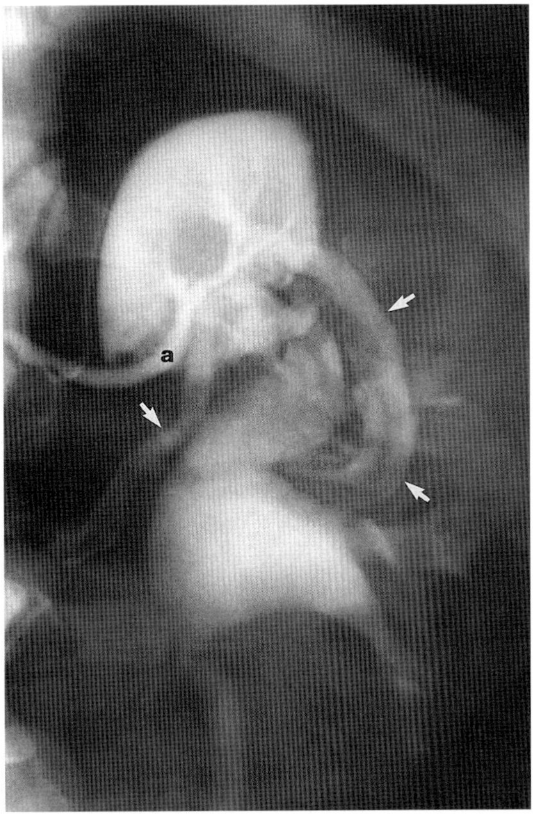

B

9–10 "Pseudo" arteriovenous fistula. **(A)** Selective injection into accessory artery (a) to upper left kidney. **(B)** Continued injection causes forceful shunting into venous system (arrows), mimicking an arteriovenous fistula. This phenomenon occurs when a small vessel is occluded by the injecting catheter and an excessive forceful injection of contrast media is made. a = accessory artery.

an axillary artery approach for most renal and adrenal studies; the risk of vertebral artery embolization is avoided, as is a hematoma in the axillary sheath, which can cause a serious neurologic deficit. Sometimes an insertion of catheters via the left axillary artery is necessary to accomplish selective renal studies or angioplasty of a downward coursing renal artery; if approached from the transfemoral route, an acute angle may preclude insertion of balloon dilating catheters.

Catheters

For aortography a recommended catheter is a 5F, 65-cm high-pressure catheter with a pigtail tip. A 4F pigtailed catheter with high flow rates is also available. Selective renal arteriography is most readily accomplished with either a shepherd's hook or a cobra-shaped catheter (Fig. 9–9). Occasionally a C-curve will be helpful, or even the small C-curve (inferior mesenteric, RIM). For selective studies, a 5F torque control catheter is suggested. For steeply oblique renal arteries, a Simmons or Mikelson-shaped catheter is helpful. The angiographer should become familiar with four or five basic catheter shapes and use those for most procedures. A selection of intricate shapes can be reserved for special problems.

Arteriography of the pelvic organs is best accomplished by inserting the catheter via the contralateral femoral artery to the side being examined. A C-curve or Simmons curve catheter or a deflector wire is used for passage over the iliac artery bifurcation. A cobra-shaped catheter, exchanged over a wire, provides the optimal shape and control for selectively catheterizing the individual vessels of the internal iliac (hypogastric) artery.

Contrast Material and Filming Sequence

For aortography, contrast with a higher concentration of iodine is used. Warming the contrast will reduce substantially its viscosity. Conventional ionic contrast media with a high concentration of iodine causes an intense heat sensation and pain because of its high osmolality (e.g., 2,500 mOsm). Therefore, low osmolar contrast is now recommended for aortography and large-volume visceral studies. Conventional ionic contrast, if used at all, is limited to "test" injections during catheter manipulations and for small-volume visceral injections. For aortography, 50 ml is injected at a rate of 20 ml/sec, and filming is done using the sequence of 2 films/sec for 3 sec, 1 film/sec for 3 sec, and 1 film every 3rd sec for 9 sec. The filming sequence for evaluating patients for renal vascular hypertension is changed so that the initial series is done at 3 films/sec for 3 sec to specifically image the proximal renal arteries in a high-pressure, high-flow system.

For selective renal arteriography, 10–12 ml is injected at a rate of 5 ml/sec. Filming is done at a rate of 2 films/sec for 3 sec, 1 film/sec for 3 sec, and 1 film every 3rd sec for 9 sec. This provides an arterial phase, a parenchymal phase, and the venous phase.

Changes can occur during arteriographic injection that can mimic vascular disease. Mild contraction waves can occur in the renal arteries (Meaney, Buonocore 1966). If a small vessel is forcefully injected, rapid opacification of the vein will occur (Fig. 9–10). This artificial "shunting" must not be mistaken for an arteriovenous malformation (Meng et al. 1974). Intrarenal vascular spasm can occur due to catheter or guide-wire manipulations; this can result in intense spasm of an isolated vessel or more generalized spasm that will mimic vasculitis and parenchymal disease (Fig. 9–11) (Elkin 1975). Guide-wire and catheter manipulations in the renal artery should be avoided for 5–10 min. Flushing the vessel with saline and using an antispastic agent such as the calcium-channel blockers verapamil or nifedipine can help reverse this. Verapamil, 2.5 mg, can be given intra-arterially through the catheter into the specific vessel. Nifedipine, 10 mg, is given as a sublingual gelatin capsule. Both must be used very cautiously in patients with cardiac disease. Repeat injection with a low-osmolar contrast agent will also help.

Need for Aortogram

Opinion differs as to the need for an aortogram prior to selective renal arteriography. If the question involves the site or number of renal arteries or integrity of the renal artery ostium, then aortography is essential. If the procedure is to define an intrarenal process previously diagnosed by ultrasound or CT, then the examination can begin with a selective renal study, concluding with the aortogram if necessary. Often, however, an initial aortogram can facilitate the examination and minimize selective catheter manipulations, since the vessel locations and variations have been defined. The aortogram should be deferred in the patient with renal failure, to minimize use of contrast; arteriography with digital subtraction technique in this setting is the optimal technique because contrast volume can be minimized.

Magnification

Magnification techniques, whereby the patient is moved away from the film and closer to the X-ray tube to magnify the image, were developed when angiography was a primary diagnostic method. These techniques are no longer justified for routine use because of increased radiation to the patient. They should be reserved for special situations when demonstration of detailed intrarenal anatomy is essential.

Digital Subtraction Angiography

Digital subtraction angiography (DSA) makes it possible to obtain images of the arterial system by a venous injection or to greatly reduce the amount of contrast necessary to obtain images during an arterial injection. The arterial injection with digital subtraction is of particular importance for patients with worsening renal failure due to renal artery stenosis and for patients with diabetic nephropathy.

9–11 Vascular spasm during renal arteriography, causing ▶ patchy parenchymal changes mimicking disease. Spasm was induced by catheter and guide wire and resolved spontaneously over 15 min. **(A)** Right renal arteriogram showing decreased perfusion of lower two-thirds of kidney (arrows). Compare with Fig. 9–11 C. **(B)** Same injection, parenchymal phase. Thinned, patchy appearance to cortex (arrows) is caused by vascular spasm rather than true renal or vascular pathology. (Compare with Fig. 9–11 D.) **(C)** Repeat injection 15 min later, showing normal vessels and cortex, after spontaneous resolution of vascular spasm. **(D)** Parenchymal phase of second injection is now normal.

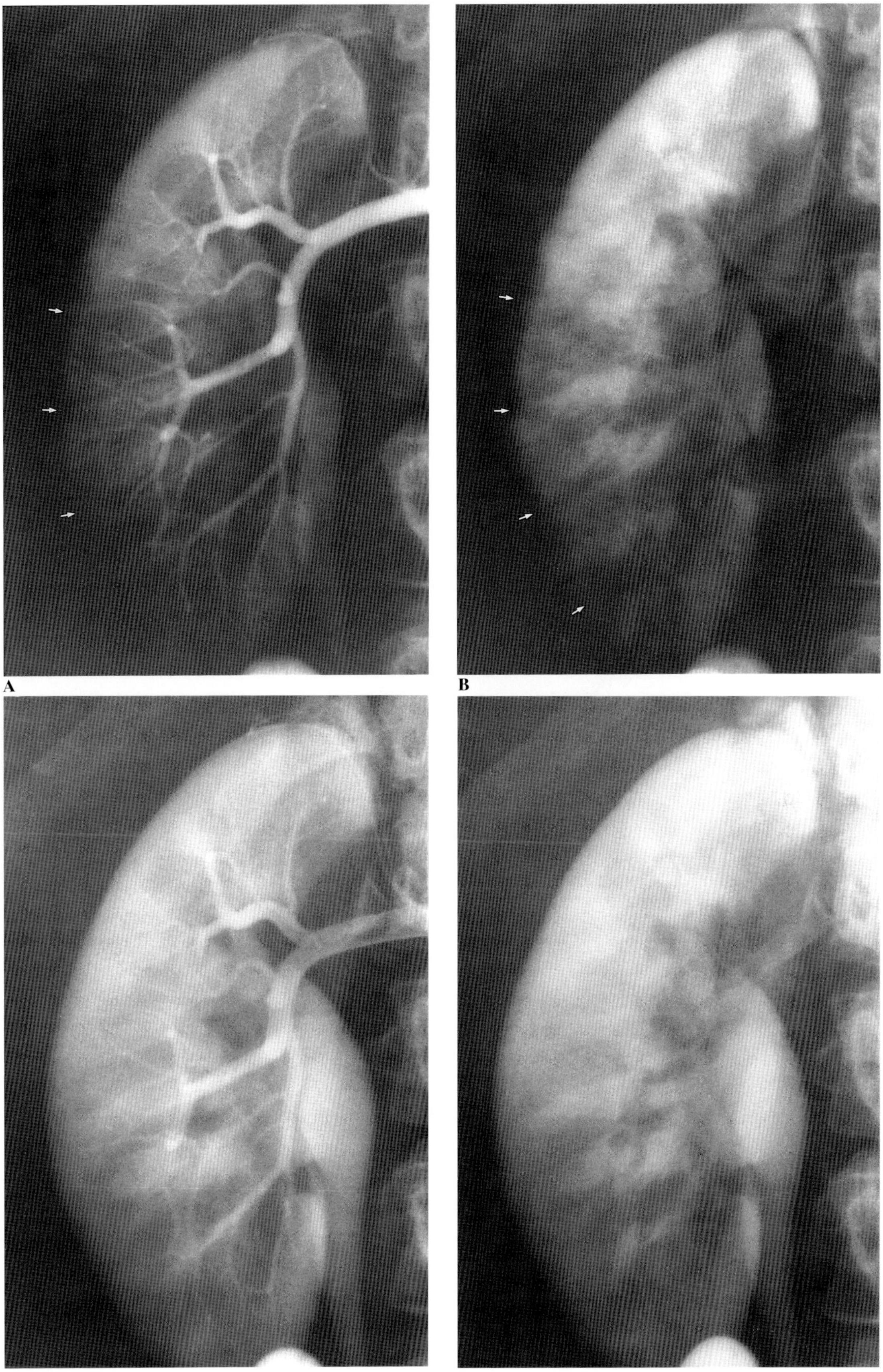

A B C D

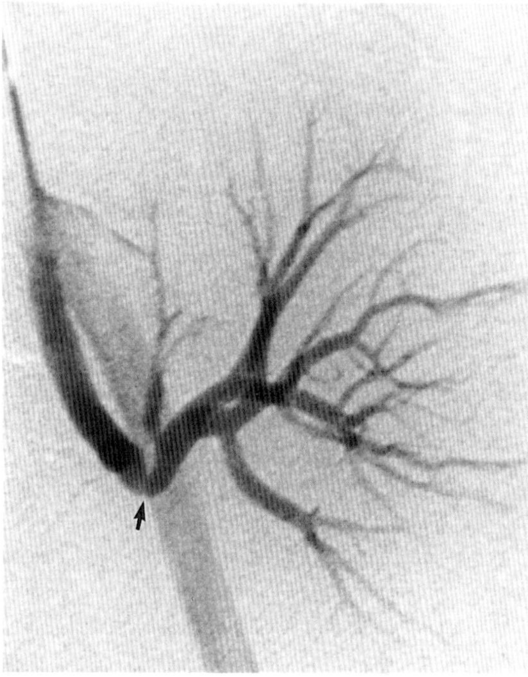

9–12 Digital subtraction studies permit use of minimal amounts of contrast in studying abnormally functioning renal transplant kidneys. Arterial DSA study of left transplant kidney showing 70% stenosis (arrow) of artery near anastomosis with hypogastric artery. Only 3 ml of contrast, diluted to 10 ml with saline, was necessary to obtain this image. Stenosis was then dilated successfully.

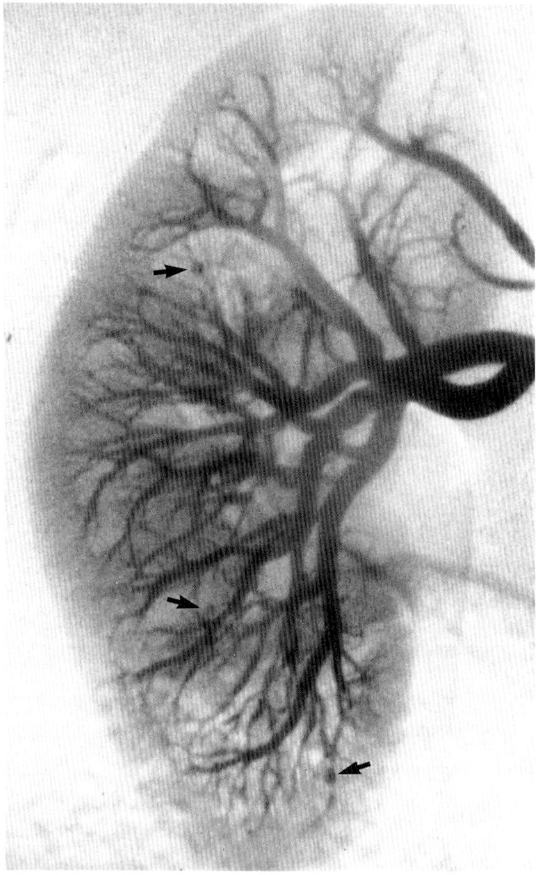

9–13 Renal arteriogram of 29-year-old woman, with arthritis and hypertension, confirming vasculitis presumably caused by collagen vascular disease. Note small subtle aneurysms (arrows). (Arteriogram courtesy of Harvey M. Goldstein, San Antonio, TX.)

DSA uses computer processing to enhance further the image obtained from the image intensifier of the fluoroscope. An image intensifier is coupled to a video camera with an excellent signal-to-noise ratio. The analog video image is electronically amplified and then converted to digital form for storage. The digitized images are viewed on a monitor where they can be further enhanced by subtracting various initial background images (mask) from an image obtained during contrast injection, leaving only the image of the contrast-filled vessel. Because of the electronically enhanced image, much less contrast density is needed to visualize a vessel.

Arterial DSA

Arterial DSA provides excellent definition of small vessels using diluted contrast (1:2, 1:3). Motion and cardiac factors are nearly eliminated during direct arterial injection. Thus, a limited arterial contrast study is possible for patients at high risk for contrast-induced renal failure, such as those with diabetic nephropathy or other causes of small vessel renal disease. In evaluating renal transplants for presence of stenosis, images can be obtained in multiple planes with minimal contrast (Fig. 9–12). Likewise, arterial DSA is of great value during transluminal renal artery angioplasty or embolization procedures, again because it requires much less contrast media.

Intravenous DSA

Intravenous DSA can be done as an outpatient procedure and eliminates the small risk associated with arterial catheter manipulation. A 5F pigtail high-pressure catheter is inserted percutaneously with the Seldinger technique via an antecubital vein or, if necessary, a femoral vein. The catheter is advanced to the superior vena cava at the right atrium. A 50-ml injection of high-strength contrast (e.g., 350 mg I/ml or 370 mg I/ml) is given at a rate of 20 ml/sec, and images are obtained of the area

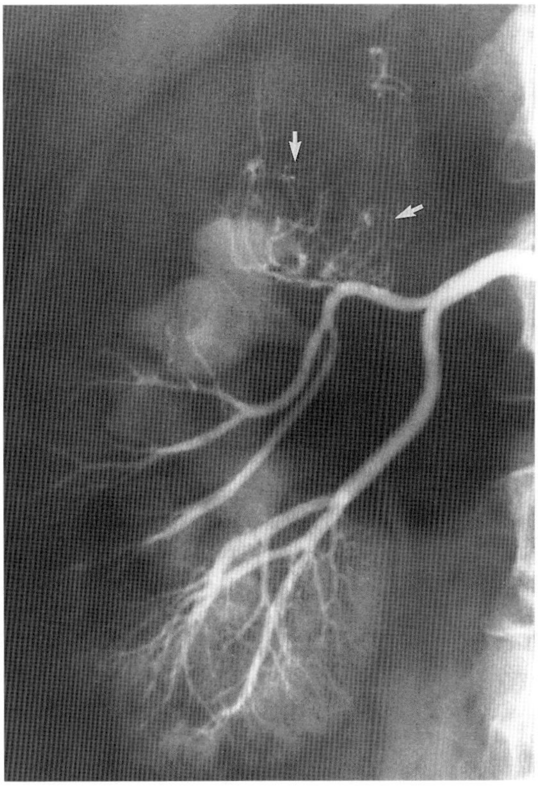

9–14 Renal arteriogram (selective injection of one of two vessels) confirming tumor vascularity (arrows) of small mass in upper central right kidney.

of interest beginning just before the contrast "arrives" in the arterial system, to provide at least one image without contrast, which gives the background "mask" for obtaining the "subtraction" image. With newer high-pressure, high-flow 4F catheters, many centers are now using outpatient arteriography (film and/or DSA) instead of outpatient venous DSA. The motion and cardiac problems that can severely compromise venous DSA are thereby eliminated.

Film versus DSA

The resolution of a video image, although good, does not equal that of film. Breathing motion and bowel peristalsis between the time of the mask image and the desired image with contrast are the primary causes of image degradation. Bowel peristalsis can be reduced or eliminated by giving 1 mg (1 ml) of glucagon intravenously.

Poor cardiac function causes the other major problem with intravenous digital subtraction angiography. Slow, ineffective cardiac output has the effect of diluting the contrast and prolonging arrival time, thereby increasing the chance for misregistration or motion artifact. Artifacts along the edges of pulsatile vessels can also cause errors in interpretation even on arterial DSA studies. DSA, however, has proven to be a great asset in permitting multiple injections to be obtained in various projections, in providing detailed images of small vessels filled with dilute contrast, and in permitting full examinations to be completed with only a small amount of contrast media.

Indications for Arteriography

Vascular Anatomy for Surgery

Aortography can be extremely helpful to the urologic surgeon in deciding whether an organ or parts of an organ can be resected and how many arteries may be encountered. Vessels to a horseshoe kidney or pelvic kidney can be evaluated preoperatively. The combination of a cut-film series plus digital subtraction arteriography is suggested.

Selective renal arteriography on cut-film, augmented by regular film subtraction techniques, is unsurpassed in providing renal and adrenal vascular detail. This may confirm vasculitis (Fig. 9–13) of a kidney, such as polyarteritis nodosa with its small vessel aneurysms. Confirmation of renal tumor neovascularity can, at times, assist the surgeon in making preoperative decisions (Fig. 9–14). A need for this type of detail is, in the author's opinion, the main justification for using magnification techniques in cut-film angiography.

Arteriographic patterns of the adrenal gland are nonspecific, and preoperative arteriography of the adrenal to diagnose a pheochromocytoma should be avoided. Whenever contrast studies of patients with a possible pheochromocytoma are done, adequate beta-adrenergic blockade with Dibenzyline is advocated, and intravenous Regitine or nitroprusside should be available. Regitine is given intravenously in 5-mg increments.

Since crossover perfusion between the right kidney and adrenal is common, arteriography is no longer recommended for differentiating renal and adrenal masses. Magnetic resonance imaging is the best means of differentiating masses of adrenal or renal origin, in that it can provide images in the sagittal or coronal planes.

Renal Transplant

Screening of kidney donors using digital subtraction angiography has not proved sufficiently effective, because its accuracy in determining the number of renal arteries is at best 91%, and in a recent series was only 82% even using arterial DSA (Cho et al. 1987; Hillman 1985). This percentage is not felt to be adequate by most transplant surgeons, as an unexpected vessel may jeopardize an already risky procedure. Regular or cut-film arteriography provides the most accurate assessment of renal artery anatomy.

Angiography of a transplanted kidney poses special problems. It is imperative that the angiographer talk with both the urologic surgeon and the nephrologist to ascertain the type of vascular anastomosis (end-to-end, end-to-side) and the site of anastomosis (hypogastric, external iliac artery). The angiographer also needs to know whether stenosis, acute tubular necrosis, or rejection reaction is suspected.

An end-to-end arterial anastomosis to the hypogastric artery is best approached by a femoral puncture of the contralateral side. For the usual contralateral approach to a hypogastric anastomosis, a cobra-shaped catheter is suggested. An axillary artery approach may be necessary, particularly if balloon catheter angioplasty is to be done. An end-to-side external iliac artery anastomosis is best approached from the ipsilateral side.

The venous anastomosis is usually an end-to-side connection to the external iliac vein, so that an ipsilateral approach with a partial C-curved catheter is used. A 5F polyurethane catheter heated to give a 45-degree angle works quite well, especially when combined with a C-curved wire.

The multidirectional fluoroscopic unit used for digital subtraction angiography is invaluable for assessing stenosis at the anastomotic site postoperatively (Fig. 9–10A). Evaluation of intrarenal vasculature to differentiate acute tubular necrosis from rejection reaction is best done with regular X-ray film techniques. It is often not definitive but can be suggestive (Castaneda-Zuniga 1986; Foley et al. 1985).

Renovascular Hypertension

Digital subtraction angiography is used in the outpatient evaluation of patients with possible renovascular hypertension. A definitive diagnosis was achieved in 94% of cases by Hillman (1985). Dunnick et al. (1987) found intravenous DSA to have a sensitivity of 96% and a negative predictive value of 98% in screening patients for suspected renovascular hypertension. Digital subtraction angiography is more accurate than either urography or radionuclide renography in detecting a renal artery cause of hypertension, and is simpler than sampling for renal vein renins. Outpatient intravenous digital subtraction angiography is recommended as the screening test for renal artery stenosis in patients with newly discovered hypertension (Dunnick et al. 1987; Hillman 1985).

Since renovascular hypertension has only a 5% incidence and medical therapy effectively controls blood pressure in most patients, procedures such as digital subtraction angiography could be limited to patients unresponsive or intolerant to medical therapy, or to those with unusual clinical manifestations. Hillman, on the other hand, argues convincingly that if interventional therapy would be used to reduce or eliminate medical therapy of the hypertension, a digital subtraction study is economically justified as a screening test (Hillman 1985).

Patients with newly diagnosed hypertension, or whose hypertension has become difficult to control medically, undergo a vascular study for diagnosis at this author's medical center, the Virginia Mason Clinic in Seattle. If the patient is young, or has a good cardiac output, then outpatient venous DSA is selected. Otherwise, aortography is done as an outpatient procedure, using standard film techniques. If an angioplasty is likely, the author and colleagues at the clinic do a standard arteriogram and proceed immediately with angioplasty if the stenosis is greater than 50%. Determination of renal vein renin before treatment is reserved for diagnostic problem cases.

Trauma

Angiography is reserved for cases of renal trauma that are unclarified by CT or magnetic resonance imaging, or for patients who are unresponsive to medical therapy. Dynamic CT scanning has proved most effective in evaluating renal trauma (Lang et al. 1985). However, for pelvic trauma with continued hemorrhage, arteriography can identify the source of bleeding and at the same time provide a route for embolization of the vessel.

Other Applications

Arteriography can help to define the bleeding site in tumors of the bladder, uterus, cervix, or prostate, and can provide a route for embolization.

Arteriography of the hypogastric arteries to evaluate for stenosis and possible dilation as a cause of impotence seems indicated, but its use in evaluating small vessel disease awaits further study (Bookstein 1987).

Technique for Venography

Venography is best accomplished via the transfemoral route. The adrenal, renal, gonadal, and pelvic veins are all readily accessible. The right femoral vein provides easier access to the inferior vena cava and its branches because of its straight course. Initial puncture using the Seldinger technique, preferably using a Potts needle, is facilitated by having the patient perform the Valsalva maneuver during needle placement, as this distends the femoral vein. This author prefers this method over aspirating the needle with a syringe. The force of venous flow during the Valsalva maneuver is surprising. If the Valsalva maneuver is used, there is no chance of plugging the needle with tissue or vein wall, as can occur with aspiration.

After the vein has been correctly entered and the guide wire inserted, the vein wall should be dilated before inserting a curved-tipped catheter. Although the jugular approach has been advocated for gonadal vein catheterization and embolization, this author has rarely found this necessary. Newer catheter equipment allows nearly all studies to be done via the simpler femoral approach.

Indications for Venography

Adrenal Vein Sampling

Diagnostic venography of the adrenals is seldom indicated, as it is not specific and there is risk of adrenal hemorrhage or infarction. Diagnosis of an adrenal mass is best made by CT or magnetic resonance imaging. However, adrenal vein catheterization for venous sampling is still the most specific test for establishing the site of an aldosterone-secreting adenoma.

Since the left adrenal vein consistently arises from the upper aspect of the main left renal vein, the specially designed adrenal catheter is optimal (Fig. 9–9). The adrenal veins on the right are small and enter the inferior vena cava posterolaterally rather than anterolaterally, like the renal veins or accessory hepatic veins. This can be confusing if orientation and appearance during a modest contrast injection are not observed closely. In the author's experience, successful sampling from the right veins has been achieved in 80%–85% of the cases; a C-curve or cobra-shaped catheter has proved to be more effective than the dedicated adrenal catheter for the right adrenal vein.

Renal Tumor

Some tumors (transitional cell carcinoma, lymphoma) diffusely infiltrate the kidney and yet are hypovascular by arteriography, causing only minimal arterial abnormalities. Because venous walls are thin, encasement and deformity of the intrarenal veins occur much earlier than arterial changes, and epinephrine-enhanced venography can confirm gross tumor disease when arteriographic changes are minimal (Smith et al. 1975). These encasement changes on venography, however, are nonspecific and can be caused by an inflammatory process.

To opacify the intrarenal veins, renal artery flow is slowed by the injection of 8–10 μg of epinephrine through a renal artery catheter. Approximately 15 sec later, the venous catheter is injected with 20–30 ml contrast at a rate of 10–12 ml/sec. The volume and flow rate depend on catheter position and size of the vein. If the venous catheter tip is in a main renal vein, up to 45 ml of contrast media injected at a rate of 15 ml/sec may be necessary. For an intrarenal injection, 20–25 ml at 8–10 ml/sec is suggested. One or two side holes near the catheter tip help prevent recoil of the catheter with these larger-volume injections. Filming is done at the rate of two films/sec for 5 sec. Excellent intrarenal venograms can be obtained by this method (Goldman et al. 1978; Kahn 1969).

Renal Vein Thrombus

Definition of thrombus in the renal veins of a patient with membraneous glomerulonephritis can

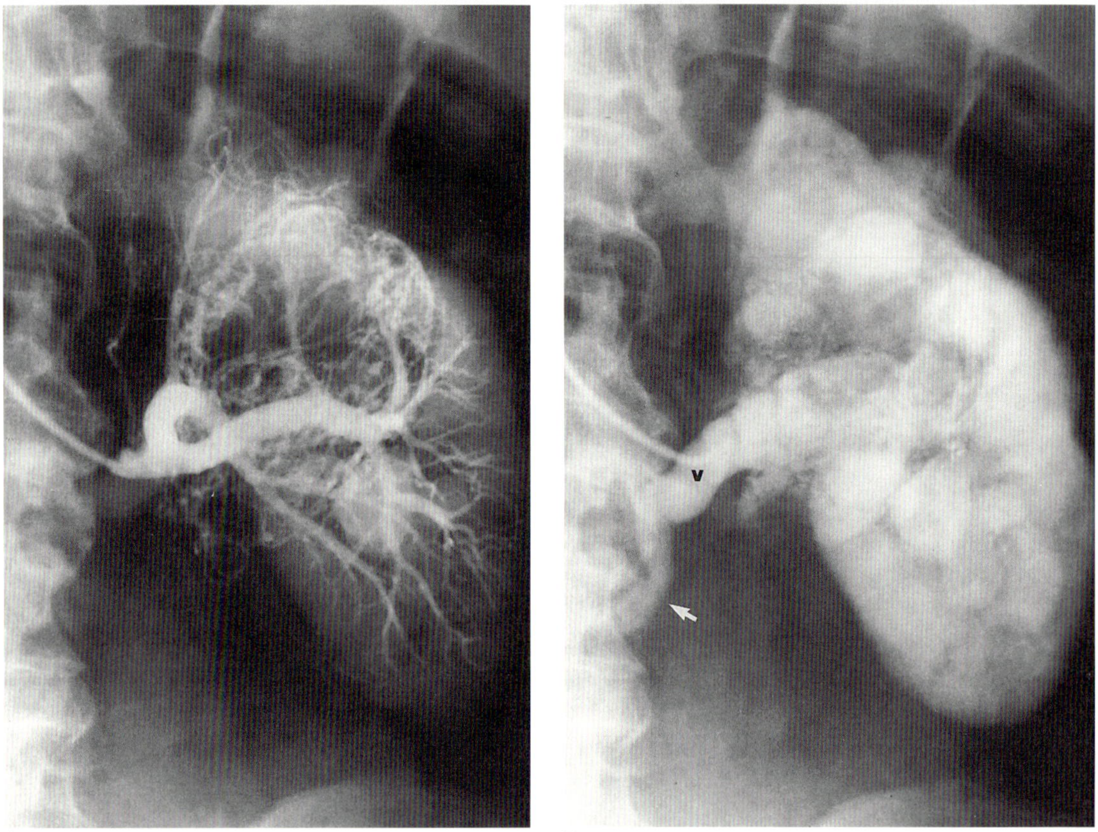

A

B

9–15 Use of arterial injection to opacify renal vein. **(A)** Large left renal tumor with prominent neovascularity. **(B)** Renal vein (V) was opacified, confirming freedom from tumor, by injecting 40 ml of contrast intraarterially at 5 ml/min and filming a long sequence (1 film/sec × 12). Large volume injected is acceptable because kidney is to be resected. Note retroaortic vein position (arrow).

assist the clinician in decisions regarding anticoagulant therapy (Clark et al. 1979; Llach et al. 1975). Intrarenal detail requires injection of epinephrine in the renal artery via an arterial catheter to slow blood flow, but gross evaluation of the main renal vein for clot or to confirm a large tumor thrombus can be done with only a venous catheter in the main renal vein using digital subtraction techniques.

However, magnetic resonance imaging now offers excellent definition of major vessels and will supplant venography for evaluating the major renal veins or inferior vena cava in most cases of renal tumor. As an additional technique, excellent opacification of the renal veins at the time of selective renal arteriography can be achieved by injecting 40 ml of contrast into the tumor-containing kidney and filming during the venous phase (Fig. 9–15). This large-volume renal injection is only done when the kidney is to be resected, but can provide clear detail as to patency or tumor thrombus in the renal vein.

Other Applications

Renal venography is helpful to identify a venous varix as a cause of unexplained hematuria. This is done after renal arteriogram is found to be normal; 8–10 μg of epinephrine is then injected through the arterial catheter, so that detailed renal venous anatomy can be obtained during the venous injection. Venous sampling for renin determination is used to confirm renal artery stenosis as a cause for hypertension. Sampling on the left side should be done proximal to the left gonadal vein. Selective intrarenal vein sampling is done for cases with segmental artery stenoses.

Varicocele

Embolization of the gonadal vein with detachable balloon or stainless steel coils is becoming the accepted method to treat varicoceles contributing to infertility or causing pain (White et al. 1981). Gonadal vein catheterization for venography is done as an outpatient procedure and provides both the diagnosis and an immediate route for treatment. About 90% of the time, the left gonadal vein is the cause of the varicocele and requires occlusion.

The left gonadal vein normally arises from the left renal vein, though it can arise from an accessory renal vein or retroaortic left renal vein. The right gonadal vein usually originates from the inferior vena cava at about the L3 level; however, in 20% of patients, it can arise from the right renal vein. There are often small, retroperitoneal communications to the gonadal vein that are not important because of the presence of valves and direction of flow. However, careful venography is required to detect paralleling collateral gonadal veins that may subsequently enlarge and reform a varicocele after embologic occlusion of only a main vein (Kaufman et al. 1983) (Fig. 9–16).

The catheter for the initial diagnostic venogram should have a side hole near the tip to allow aspiration and clearing of the catheter after cannulization of the renal vein. Venous injection, while the patient does a Valsalva maneuver, is done with a contrast dose of 15–25 ml at 5–10 ml/min, again depending on the size of the vein. There is no need to slow renal artery flow with epinephrine.

CT eliminated the need for most diagnostic venography in detecting undescended testicle, and magnetic resonance imaging now provides such detail that it is the recommended test for undescended testicle not found clinically or by ultrasonography.

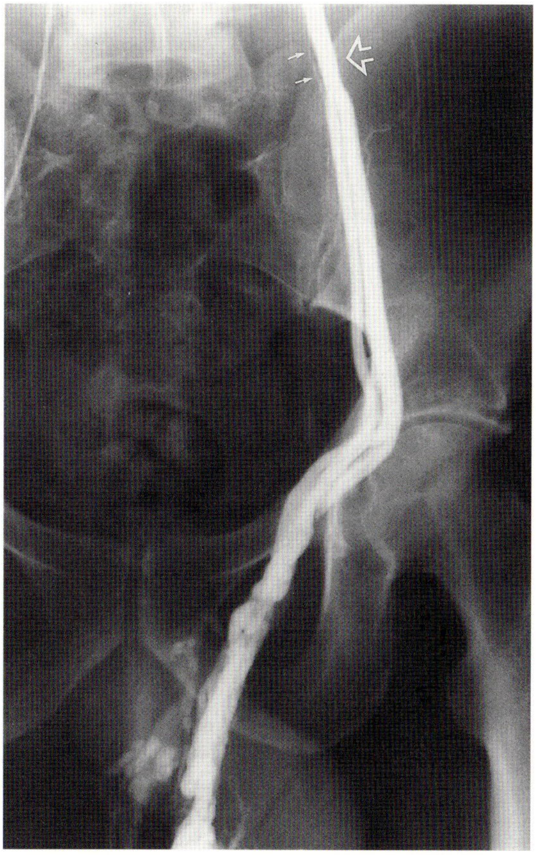

9–16 Left gonadal venogram. Catheter inserted in right femoral vein and tip placed in upper left internal spermatic vein via left renal vein. Contrast injection shows two large veins above internal inguinal ring and in inguinal canal, forming large varicocele in scrotum. A very small vein is visible along main spermatic vein (arrow). Balloon placement for occlusion will need to be above major division (open arrow). A second balloon may be necessary above small collateral if it persists on injection of upper internal spermatic vein after initial balloon placement.

Impotence

Corpora cavernosography, including drug injection for the manipulation of venous flow patterns, is currently being investigated as a means of diagnosing and possibly treating impotence.

Corpora cavernosography is easily accomplished as an outpatient procedure. A 19-gauge butterfly needle is inserted into one of the corpora cavernosa on the distal shaft of the penis just proximal to the corona. The area of needle insertion is anesthetized locally with a small amount of 0.25% bupivacaine using a 25-gauge needle. The entire venous system of the penis fills with only one injection, as there is free cross-communication between the corpora cavernosum. Detailed venous anatomy and pathologic changes are discussed in the article by Bookstein (1987).

References

Bookstein JJ: Cavernosal venoocclusive insufficiency in male impotence: Evaluation of degree and location. *Radiology* 164:175–178, 1987.

Castaneda-Zuniga WR (ed.): *Radiologic Diagnosis of Renal Transplant Complications*. Minneapolis, University of Minnesota Press, 1986.

Cho WH, Jacobs SC, Lawson RK: Digital substraction angiography for renal donor evaluation. *Urology* 30:289–292, 1987.

Clark RA, Wyatt GM, Colley DP: Renal vein thrombosis: An underdiagnosed complication of multiple renal abnormalities. *Radiology* 132:43–50, 1979.

Dunnick NR, Svetkey L, Braun SD, Cohan RH, Newman GE, Himmelstein SI, Klotman PE: Intravenous digital subtraction angiography for the detection of renovascular hypertension. Paper presented at Society of Uroradiology meeting, Orlando, FL, Jan. 31, 1987.

Elkin M: Radiology of the urinary tract: Some physiologic considerations. *Radiology* 116:259–270, 1975.

Foley WD, Bookstein JJ, Tweist M, Gikas RW, Mayor GH, Turcotte JG: Arteriography of renal transplants. *Radiology* 116:271–277, 1975.

Goldman ML, Gorelkin L, Rude JC, Sybers RG, O'Brien DP: Epinephrine renal venography in severe inflammatory disease of the kidney. *Radiology* 127:93–101, 1978.

Hillman BJ: Renal digital subtraction angiography. *Urol. Clin. North Am.* 12(4):699–713, 1985.

Hollinshead WH: Embryologic and anatomic considerations. *In* Kincaid OW (ed.): *Renal Angiography*, Chicago, Yearbook Medical Publishers, 1966.

Kahn PC: Selective angiography of the inferior phrenic arteries. *Radiology* 88:1–8, 1967.

Kahn PC: Selective venography in renal parenchymal disease. *Radiology* 92:345–349, 1969.

Kaufman SL, Kadir S, Barth KH, Smyth JW, Walsh PC, White RI: Mechanism of recurrent varicocele after balloon occlusion or surgical ligation of the internal spermatic vein. *Radiology* 147:435–440, 1983.

Lang EK, Sullivan J, Frentz G: Renal trauma: Radiological studies. Comparison of urography, computed tomography, angiography, and radionuclide studies. *Radiology* 154:1–6, 1985.

Llach F, Arieff AI, Massry SG: Renal vein thrombosis and nephrotic syndrome. *Ann. Intern. Med.* 83:8–14, 1975.

Luzsa G: The renal arteries, their branches, and their collateral circulation. *In* Luzsa G (ed.): *X-Ray Anatomy of the Vascular System*. Philadelphia, J. P. Lippincott, 1974, p. 243.

Meaney CH, Buonocore E: Contractions of the renal arteries during arteriography. *Am. J. Roentgenol.* 86:41–48, 1966.

Meng CH, Adler J, Elkin M: Early renal vein opacification during selective renal angiography: Trueta phenomenon or technical artifact. *Radiology* 112:61–67, 1974.

Merklin RJ, Michels NA: The variant renal and suprarenal blood supply with data on the inferior phrenic, ureteral, and gonadal arterico. *J. Int. Coll. Surgeons* 29:41–76, 1958.

Nilsson J: Angiography in tumors of the urinary bladder. *Acta Radiol.* 263(suppl):1–130, 1967.

Oedman P, Ranniger K: The location of the renal arteries. An angiographic and postmortem study. *Am. J. Roentgenol.* 104:283–288, 1968.

Smith JC, Roseck J, Athanasoulis CA, Baum S, Waltman AC, Goldman M: Renal venography in the evaluation of poorly vascularized neoplasms of the kidney. *Am. J. Roentgenol.* 123:552–556, 1975.

White RI, Kaufman SL, Barth KH, Kadir S, Smyth JW, Walsh PC: Occlusion of varicoceles with detachable balloons. *Radiology* 139:327–334, 1981.

Suggested Reading

Boatman DL, Cornell SH, Koelln CP: The arterial supply of horseshoe kidneys. *Am. J. Roentgenol.* 113:447–451, 1971.

Chait A: Current status of renal angiography. *Urol. Clin. North Am.* 12(4):687–697, 1985.

Chait A, Molta A, Nelson JH: The collateral arterial circulation of the pelvis. *Am. J. Roentgenol.* 102:392–399, 1968.

Fankuchen E: Techniques of renal angiography. *In* Taveras JM, Ferrucci JT (eds.): *Radiology: Diagnosis-Imaging-Intervention*. Philadelphia, J. P. Lippincott, 1986, chap. 10, pp. 1–5.

Gill WM, Pudran WR: The arteriographic diagnosis of renal parenchymal diseases. *Radiology* 96:81–84, 1970.

Graves FT: The anatomy of the intrarenal arteries in health and disease. *Br. J. Surg.* 43:605–616, 1956.

Kincaid OW: *Renal Angiography*. Chicago: Yearbook Medical Publishers, 1966.

Mitty HA, Goldman H: Angiography in unilateral renal bleeding with a negative urogram. *Am. J. Roentgenol.* 121:508–517, 1974.

Pingoud EG, Glickman JG: Angiography. *In* Rosenfield AJ, Glickman MG, Hudson J (eds.): *Diagnostic Imaging in Renal Disease*. New York, Appleton-Century-Crofts, 1979, pp. 51–62.

CHAPTER

10

Radiation Dose to Patient and Personnel during Uroradiologic Procedures

William H. Bush and Douglas Jones

The use of X rays has increased to the extent that half of the U.S. population receives some medical radiation each year. The risk versus the benefit of medical radiation must always be considered. More than 125 million people benefit from X-ray diagnosis per year. However, this same radiation is projected to cause 350–600 leukemias, 1,000–2,000 solid tumors, and 130–2,400 genetic anomalies (Hall 1984).

The total bone marrow or whole body radiation dose from all sources including medical radiation prorated over the entire U.S. population averages 203 mrem/yr; exposure from background (nonmedical) radiation averages 110 mrem/yr (Hall 1984; National Academy of Sciences 1980). There are large variations in exposure from terrestrial sources; for example, average exposure on the Colorado Plateau is 90 mrem, compared to a yearly average of 23 mrem on the Gulf Coastal Plain. If the contribution from cosmic radiation is added, the difference is more exaggerated, so that the naturally occurring exposure to individuals in Denver is almost three times that of people living in Houston. Furthermore, there are much larger variations throughout the world, mainly as a result of pockets of naturally occurring radionuclides.

Effects of Radiation

The effects of low doses of radiation include: 1) genetic effects, 2) leukemogenesis and carcinogenesis, and 3) somatic effects on the embryo and fetus.

Genetic Effects

The popular concept is that radiation produces bizarre mutants that are easily recognized; this is not the case. Radiation increases slightly the incidence of the same mutations that occur spontaneously; consequently, radiation effects must be assessed against the relatively high (10%) natural background of mutations (Hall 1984). From 1% to 6% of spontaneous mutations may be attributed to nonmedical background radiation. The absence of observable genetic effects in the survivors of Hiroshima and Nagasaki has led to the current thinking that genetic hazards of radiations at low doses are probably less important than the carcinogenic effect of radiation.

Carcinogenic Effects

Data used to assess radiation-induced malignancies in humans consist of relatively few cases of cancer in a few thousand individuals exposed to large doses of radiation, in excess of 1 Gy (100 rad). The data are too limited to define a dose-response relationship. To obtain risk estimates at low doses, an extrapolation of high-dose data is necessary; a linear extrapolation assumes that the effect per rad is the same at all doses; a linear-quadratic relationship is the model that finds wide acceptance today. The concept of a threshold dose is no longer accepted.

Effects on Embryo and Fetus

The principle effect of radiation throughout organogenesis and into the fetal period is microcephaly and mental retardation. The so-called 10-day rule, applied to elective procedures, is that women of childbearing age should be exposed to radiologic procedures involving the pelvis or lower abdomen only during the first 10 days after the onset of a menstrual period of normal intensity and duration. If a procedure is deferred because of a possible pregnancy, and the patient proves to be pregnant on the return visit a few weeks later, the embryo is likely to be in organogenesis. Enforcement of the 10-day rule may require a 9-month delay in completion of the diagnostic examination.

Terminology

The term *radiation* commonly refers to ionizing radiation, that is, radiation that is sufficiently energetic to disrupt the chemical bonds of the body's molecules directly. X rays are electromagnetic waves with high energy and a short wave length. At the other end of the electromagnetic spectrum are nonionizing radiations such as microwaves and radiowaves.

Radiation exposure or ionization in air is measured in roentgens (R); 1 R = 1,000 milliroentgens. The radiation dose is measured in terms of absorbed energy (100 erg/g), which is termed a *rad* (acronym for radiation absorbed dose); 1 rad = 1,000 mrad. The international unit (SI) for absorbed dose is the gray (Gy), named after the British physicist and radiobiologist. One gray equals 100 rad, or 1 rad equals 1 centigray. Some radiations (for example, alpha-radiation) have a more potent biological effect than X rays; this effect in humans is equated and referred to as rem (radiation equivalent man). For X rays in humans the biological quality factor is 1; therefore the quantities are numerically equal. The international unit for this equivalent radiation effect is the sievert (Sv), named after the Swedish physicist; 1 Sv = 100 rem (Wyckoff 1978). The radiation dose associated with radiologic examinations in urology is usually expressed as mrem or microsievert (1 mrem = 10 μSv). Previously, the curie was the unit used to describe the activity of radioactive materials, named in honor of Pierre and Marie Curie. The new SI unit for describing activity of a radioactive substance is the becquerel (Bq), named after the discoverer of radioactivity; 1 Bq = 1 disintegration per second.

Although 1.15 R = 1 rad = 1 rem, and R is exposure in air rather than absorbed dose, for ease of clinical application, R, rad, and rem are often used interchangeably.

Direct and Scattered Radiation

Radiation dose to the patient or personnel is a summation of direct beam and scattered radiation. Direct radiation exposure is that diverging beam or pyramidal-shaped cone of X rays generated by the small focal spot in the X-ray tube. This primary beam traverses the patient and is attenuated in passage through the patient to create the image on the X-ray film or on the fluoroscope, image intensifier, and ultimately the television monitor. This high-intensity beam of radiation shows rapid drop-off at its margins and can be defined by collimation or coning of the field with the X-ray apparatus.

Scattered radiation results from interactions of the primary radiation with the patient; scattered radiation is also an important part of the X-ray dose to personnel. Whereas primary beam radiation can be avoided readily, scattered radiation is more difficult to avoid and requires more conscientious shielding.

There is a rapid decrease in radiation dose with increasing distance from the X-ray source. This concept, termed the *inverse square law*, applies to a small X-ray source (the primary beam); for example, a 100 mR exposure at 1 ft from the source drops to 6 mR at 4 ft. Because the patient behaves as a large source of scattered radiation, the dose due to scatter does not drop off as rapidly, but does decrease substantially with the distance.

Radiation Dose Limits for Personnel

Recommended annual dose limits vary slightly according to whether one uses the figures given by the International Commission on Radiation Protection (ICRP) or those of the U.S. Nuclear Regulatory Commission (NRC). For persons exposed occupationally to external radiation, the ICRP recommends an annual dose limit to the whole body, lens, and marrow, of 50 mSv (5 rem); to hands of 750 mSv (75 rem); and to skin of 300 mSv (30 rem). The NRC recommends an annual dose limit to occupationally exposed personnel as fol-

Table 10–1 Radiation Dose to Patient during Standard Radiologic Imaging Examinations

	Female Gonad (mrem)	Male Gonad (mrem)	Skin Surface (mrem)
PA and lateral chest	0.1	0.05	45
Lumbar spine (2-view)	204	30	400–1,800
KUB	50	20	160–300
IVP (8-view)	450–800	100	2,100–4,000
Upper GI	10–125	10	2,800–7,000
Barium enema	1,000–2,000	200–300	4,000–11,000
CT scan (abdomen and pelvis)	1,400	100–1,000	4,400

Source: Data compiled and calculated from: Antoku, Russell 1971; Finston 1983; Gray et al. 1981; Judy, Zimmerman 1986; Whalen, Balter 1984.

lows: to the whole body or trunk, 50 mSv (5 rem); to the lens of the eye, 150 mSv (15 rem); to the hands and forearms, 500 mSv (50 rem); and to skin, 500 mSv (50 rem).

The concept of allowable limit is now superseded by the rationale, "as low as reasonably achievable" (ALARA). In this scheme, the user of ionizing radiation is obliged to consider alternatives to current practice that will result in lower radiation exposure even though the current practice does not result in exposure levels that exceed the maximum permitted.

Anyone working with radiographic equipment should wear a radiation-monitoring badge, which is checked monthly. The badge is worn outside the lead apron at the collar level.

Radiation Doses during Urologic Procedures

X-ray dose to the skin does not maintain a direct relationship to the risk of leukemia or cancer. Arithmetic conversions of skin surface dose to specific target organ dose must be made for each radiation energy and field size. Similarly, in relating bone marrow dose to risk of leukemia, the amount of active marrow irradiated must be calculated and the relative risk of leukemia known for a total body (total bone marrow) dose must be reduced accordingly.

Radiation dose to a small field (6-in fluoroscope, field size <13 cm diameter) does not equate to total body dose in calculating limitations recommended by the NRC or the ICRP. Skin dose values for a small field of X-ray exposure are to be compared to similar skin doses from other procedures and not to organ or total body values.

Radiation doses to patients during standard radiologic examination are listed in Table 10–1. Gonad doses vary considerably, depending on whether the gonads are in or near the field of exposure; note the difference in dose between an upper gastrointestinal study and a barium enema. Organ or gonad dose during CT (computed tomography) scanning is greater, relative to surface or skin dose, because the X-ray tube rotates about the body, causing summation of internal doses. Radiation doses to the patient during other uroradiologic examinations are shown in Table 10–2 (Judy, Zimmerman 1986).

Table 10–2 Radiation Dose to Patient during Uroradiologic Examinations

Test	Ovary (mrem)	Testis (mrem)	Skin Surface (mrem)
Cystography	300	700	1,500
Retrograde pyelography	400	50	2,000
Lymphangiography	450	60	2,400

Source: Judy, Zimmerman 1986.

Radiation doses to the urologist during cystoscopy, retrograde studies, and ureteroscopy depend on many variables such as amount of fluoroscopy or filming, distance from the X-ray tube, and whether the X-ray tube for fluoroscopy is under or over the table (the under-table tube reduces scatter radiation from the patient). Distance is also the

Table 10–3 Radiation Dose to Patient during Percutaneous Stone Removal

Area	Average Dose (Range)
Anterior skin surface at kidney (small vol.; patient prone)	25 (10–129) rem
Female gonad region (surface dose)	580 (110–2,050) mrem
Male gonad region (surface dose)	180 (10–770) mrem

Source: Bush et al. 1984.
Note: Average fluoroscopy time was 24 min (range, 9–75).

Table 10–4 Radiation Dose to Personnel during Percutaneous Stone Removal

Personnel	Mean Dose (mrem)	Range (mrem)
Radiologist		
Neck	10	2–32
Hand	27	10–200
Urologist	10	1–38
Assisting nurse	4	1–11
Anesthesiologist	3	1–10
Radiologic technologist	4	1–10

Source: Bush et al. 1985.
Note: Radiation dose to personnel was calculated from measurements during single-stage percutaneous nephrostolithotomy in which 135 calculi were removed from 102 patients. Not all personnel were involved in all procedures. Average fluoroscopy time was 24 min (range 9–75 min).

urologist's ally (inverse square law); one should always step back during filming. Freeze-frame imaging during fluoroscopy will also help decrease radiation to both patient and physician.

Radiation doses to the patient and attending personnel during percutaneous stone removal are detailed in Tables 10–3 and 10–4, respectively; comparative doses from other radiologic procedures are listed in Tables 10–5 and 10–6. Radiation to the radiologist during a percutaneous nephrostomy should be less than that incurred during access and dilation for percutaneous stone removal; for the more complex nephrostolithotomy, dose to the radiologist's neck averaged 10 mrem and to the hands, 27 mrem (see Table 10–4).

Radiation doses to the patient and other personnel incurred during extracorporeal shock wave lithotripsy (ESWL) are listed in Tables 10–7 and 10–8. During ESWL, radiation dose to the patient can be minimized with the following strategies: use of a retrograde catheter or stent to localize small or faintly opacified calculi, especially in large patients; appropriate fluoroscopic collimation; minimizing fluoroscopy during patient positioning; and minimizing the number of video spot images and their attendant high radiation exposure.

Table 10–5 Dose to Patient during Percutaneous Stone Removal Compared to Other Interventional Procedures

Procedure	Female Gonad	Male Gonad	Skin Surface
Abdominal angiography	–	31 mrem[a]	–
Cardiac catheterization	–	–	<33 rem
Carotid angiography	–	–	23 rem[b]
Percutaneous stone removal	580 mrem	180 mrem	25 rem[b]

Source: Data compiled and calculated from Antoku, Russell 1971; Bush et al. 1984; Kaude, Svahn 1974; Pavlicek et al. 1982; Stacey et al. 1974.
[a] Range, 2–110 mrem.
[b] Average.

Table 10–6 Dose to Personnel during Percutaneous Stone Removal Compared to Other Interventional Procedures

Procedure	Fluoroscopy Time (min) Mean (Range)	Dose (mrem) to Radiologist: Mean (Range)		Dose (mrem) to Assisting Nurse: Mean (Range)
		Forehead/Neck	Hand/Finger	
Percutaneous transhepatic cholangiography	13 (8–18)	– (5–9)	– (30–600)	– (1–4)
Abdominal angiography	29 (3–57)	<2	18 (2–112)	5 (2–11)
Cardiac catheterization + cineradiography	16 (2–40)	4 (0–34)	5 (2–16)	–
Cardiac catheterization	12 (2–33)	8	35	4
Percutaneous stone removal	18 (4–65)	10 (2–32)	27 (10–200)	4 (1–11)

Source: Data compiled and calculated from: Ardran, Fursdon 1973; Bush et al. 1985; Wold et al. 1971.

Table 10–7 Radiation Dose to Patient during Extracorporeal Shock Wave Lithotripsy

Area	Average Dose (mrem)
Entrance surface on stone side	10,000
Entrance surface on opposite side	5,500
Anterior abdominal surface at female gonad level	10
Female gonad (estimated from surface dose)	<100

Source: Bush et al. 1987.
Note: Average fluoroscopy time was 4.5 min (range, 1.3–11.5 min); average number of video spot films was 5 (range, 0–25).

Table 10–8 Radiation Dose to Personnel during Extracorporeal Shock Wave Lithotripsy

Personnel	Dose (mrem)
Urologist	<2
Anesthesiologist	<2
Nurse	<2

Source: Bush et al. 1987.
Note: Dose measured at collar level outside lead apron.

Minimizing Radiation Dose

All personnel working within the operating suite or radiology room must wear lead aprons. Personnel working adjacent to the main X-ray beam or patient should wear 0.5-mm lead-equivalent aprons, which allow only about 1% transmission of scattered radiation; whereas those working in the periphery of the room may wear 0.25-mm lead-equivalent aprons, which allow approximately 10% transmission of scattered radiation. The urologist and radiologist are advised to wear thyroid shields when they are close to the X-ray beam or patient, such as during cystoscopic surgery, percutaneous nephrostomy, or percutaneous nephrostolithotomy.

Eyeglasses are available that attenuate radiation, varying from heavy-duty 0.5-mm lead-equivalent glasses to the photography-type sunglasses. In laboratory testing, these glasses offer substantial protection. However, in clinical use, their effectiveness is limited if lateral eye shields are not used. Sterile gloves, which attenuate scattered radiation 15%–20%, also are available. These gloves are somewhat cumbersome and probably not necessary unless the radiologist or urologist is performing a procedure close to the X-ray beam.

Gonad shields should be placed on younger patients during uroradiologic tests or procedures, particularly when visualization of the distal ureter or bladder is not necessary. Two millimeters of lead-equivalent material will attenuate 90% of the primary radiation dose.

With knowledge of the equipment and procedure, it is possible to minimize radiation dosage to patients and personnel. Shielding techniques minimize the dose to critical areas during these procedures and make them safe for proper care of the patient.

References

Antoku S, Russell WJ: Dose to the active bone marrow, gonads, and skin from roentgenography and fluoroscopy. *Radiology* 101:669–678, 1971.

Ardran GM, Fursdon PS: Radiation exposure to personnel during cardiac catheterization. *Radiology* 106:517–518, 1973.

Bush WH, Brannen GE, Gibbons RP, Correa RJ, Elder JS: Radiation exposure to patient and urologist during percutaneous nephrostolithotomy. *J. Urol.* 132:1148–1152, 1984.

Bush WH, Jones D, Brannen GE: Radiation dose to personnel during percutaneous renal calculus removal. *Am. J. Roentgenol.* 145:1261–1264, 1985.

Bush WH, Jones D, Gibbons RP: Radiation dose to patient and personnel during extracorporeal shock wave lithotripsy. *J. Urol.* 138:716–719, 1987.

Cruikshank JG, Fraser GM, Law J: Finger doses received by radiologists during chiba needle percutaneous cholangiography. *Br. J. Radiol.* 53:584–585, 1980.

Finston RA: Radiation hazards and radiation protection. *In* Friedland GW et al. (eds.): *Uroradiology. An Integrated Approach.* New York: Churchill-Livingstone, 1983, pp. 179–192.

Gray JE, Ragozzino MW, Van Lysel MS, Burke TM: Normalized organ doses for various diagnostic radiologic procedures. *Am. J. Roentgenol.* 137:463–470, 1981.

Gustafason M, Lundquist A: Personnel exposure to radiation at some angiographic procedures. *Radiology* 140:807–811, 1981.

Hall EJ: *Radiation and Life.* Elmsford, NY: Pergamon Press, 1984.

International Commission on Radiological Protection. Recommendations of the International Commission on Radiological Protection (ICRP publication no. 26). *Ann ICRP* 1:3, 1977.

International Commission on Radiological Protection. Statement and recommendations of the 1980 Brighton meeting of the ICRP. *Ann ICRP* 4, 1980.

Judy PF, Zimmerman RE: Dose to critical organs. *In* McNeil BJ, Abrams HL (eds.): *Brigham and Women's Hospital Handbook of Diagnostic Imaging.* Boston: Little, Brown, 1986, pp. 318–322.

Kaude J, Svahn G: Absorbed gonad and integral doses to the patient and personnel from angiographic procedures. *Acta Radiol.* 15:454–458, 1974.

National Academy of Sciences: The Effects on Populations of Exposure to Low Levels of Ionizing Radiation: 1980. Washington, DC: National Academy Press, 1980, pp. 377–469.

National Regulatory Commission, Occupational Radiation Protection and Health Effects Branch, 1986.

Pavlicek W, Weinstein MA, Modic MT, Buonocore B, Duchesneau PM: Patient doses during digital subtraction angiography of the carotid arteries: Comparison with conventional angiography. *Radiology* 145:683–687, 1982.

Stacey AJ, Davis R, Kerr IH: Personnel protection during cardiac catheterization with a comparison of the hazards of undercouch and overcouch X-ray tube mountings. *Br. J. Radiol.* 47:16–19, 1974.

Whalen JP, Balter S: *Radiation Risks in Medical Imaging.* Chicago: Yearbook Medical Publishers, 1984, pp. 24–32, 96–97.

Wold GJ, Scheel RV, Agarwal SK: Evaluation of physician exposure during cardiac catheterization. *Radiology* 99:188–190, 1971.

Wyckoff HO: The international system of units (SI). *Radiology* 128:833–837, 1978.

CHAPTER

11

Pediatric Uroradiology: Unique Features

Jack S. Elder

Pediatric urology has evolved into an important subspecialty of urology, in large part because of the development of increasingly sophisticated radiologic technology. Whereas previously, only the voiding cystourethrogram and excretory urogram were utilized for diagnosis of many pediatric urologic diseases, ultrasonography now has emerged as an extremely important modality. Furthermore, images of the upper urinary tract obtained by nuclear medicine studies may be analyzed objectively to determine function, and also aid in determining whether an obstructive lesion is present. Since the majority of pediatric urology involves the management of congenital structural anomalies or their complicating features, the spectrum of these problems tends to be different from the adult population. Radiologic procedures in children must be tailored to the specific problem being studied; therefore, close communication between the pediatric urologist and radiologist is essential.

Uroradiologic Imaging

Excretory Urogram (IVP)

The indications for performing an IVP have changed considerably in recent years. This study is used primarily in children with urinary tract infections (UTI) who have an abnormality on voiding cystourethrogram or ultrasonography, suspected urolithiasis, a suspected structural basis for incontinence, hematuria, suspected renal trauma, and some patients with a neurogenic bladder. It is not necessary to perform an IVP in the routine evaluation of children with enuresis, hypospadias, or cryptorchidism.

Whether urography should be performed in a newborn is controversial. Since the renal concentrating ability does not reach adult levels until 2 to 3 months of age, many feel that an IVP does not image the renal cortex or collecting system sufficiently to allow its routine use in the newborn. Therefore, ultrasound and nuclear medicine studies of the kidney have been recommended as alternative imaging modalities. In reality, in most situations, the kidneys are visualized by urography quite satisfactorily in the neonate, and a child's age should not preclude obtaining this potentially important study. In general, a dose of 1.0 ml/lb of contrast, to a maximum of 50 ml, is utilized for the child with normal renal function. The incidence of hypersensitivity reactions in children appears to be significantly less than in the adult population (Gooding et al. 1975). The test should be monitored carefully to maximize the information with a minimum of filming to decrease radiation to the child.

Voiding Cystourethrogram (VCUG)

The VCUG should be the first study obtained in the complete radiographic evaluation of children with a urinary tract infection. In addition, it is obtained to assess boys with obstructive symptoms, boys 6 years of age or older with daytime incontinence, and any child with hydronephrosis demonstrated by IVP or ultrasonography (Fig. 11–1). In children with ureteropelvic junction obstruction, between 10% and 15% will have associated ipsilateral vesicoureteral reflux (Maizels et al. 1984); at times, there may be a suggestion of reflux on the IVP. The VCUG should be monitored fluoroscopically and, optimally, recorded on videotape for detailed review.

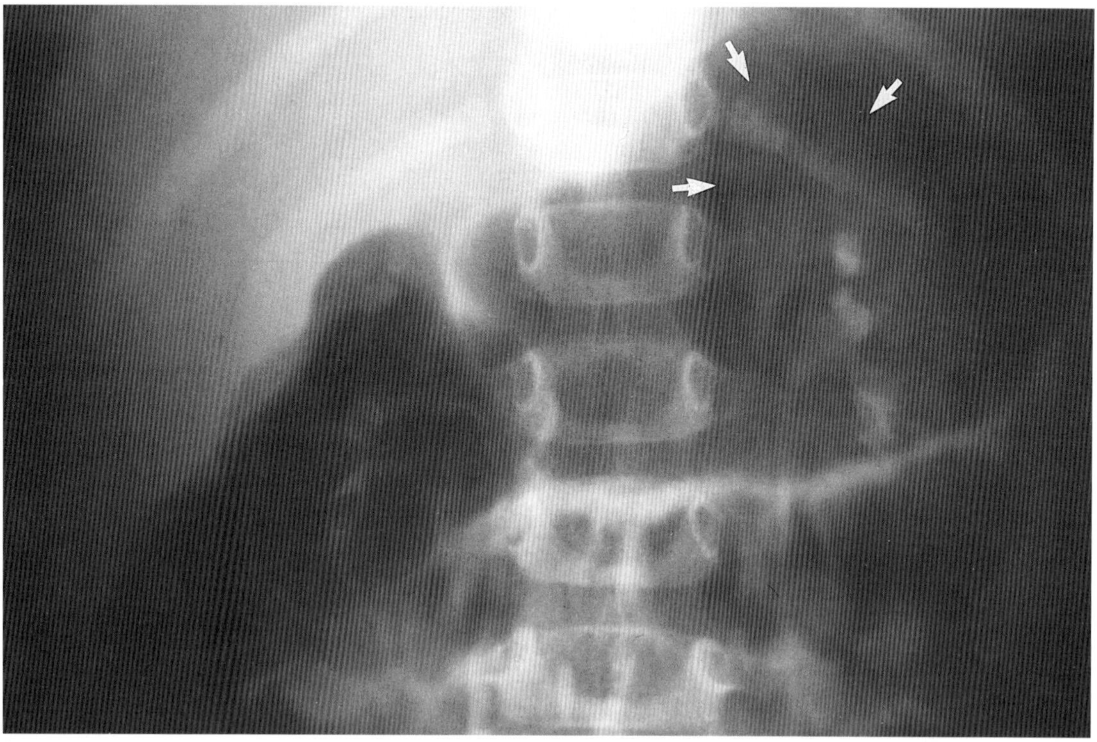

A

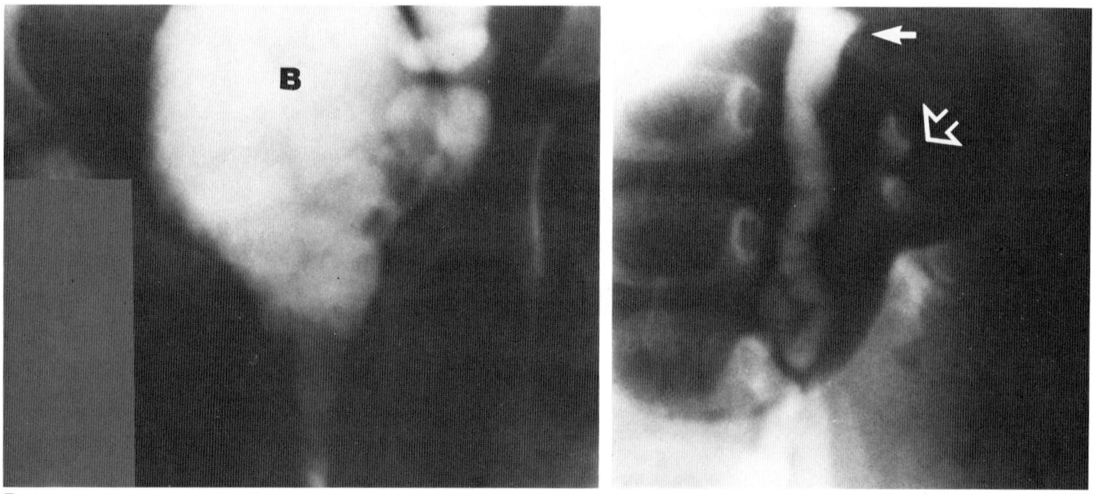

B

11–1 Two-year-old girl with duplicated collecting system and ectopic ureterocele. **(A)** IVP showing good excretion bilaterally, but there is excessive distance between uppermost calix and margin of upper left renal pole (arrows). **(B)** During VCUG, ureterocele was instrumented, resulting in reflux to upper pole (arrow) and grade-3 reflux to ipsilateral lower pole (open arrow). Patient was treated by excision of ureterocele and left common sheath and reimplantation of both upper and lower ureters with psoas hitch of bladder. (B = bladder.)

Vesicoureteral reflux may be inhibited by high rates of urine flow. Thus, in a child undergoing a VCUG who has had nothing by mouth because of a planned IVP, reflux is more likely. This may account for some variability in the reflux demonstrated in a given patient.

Nuclear Cystogram (NUC)

The NUC is performed in a manner similar to a voiding cystourethrogram. In this study, 1 mCi of ^{99m}Tc pertechnetate/500 ml isotonic sterile saline is instilled into the bladder under low pressure until the bladder is filled. The bladder and abdomen are imaged during filling, voiding, and post-void phases.

The two primary advantages of a NUC over a VCUG are: 1) radiation exposure is only 5%–10% of a standard cystogram, and 2) the NUC is more sensitive in detecting reflux, since the bladder and kidneys may be imaged continuously without concern for radiation exposure. On the other hand, the VCUG appears to be more sensitive in detecting reflux that extends only into the ureter.

The NUC is utilized primarily: 1) to follow patients with known vesicoureteral reflux; 2) to verify that reflux is not present following antireflux surgery; 3) to detect reflux in siblings of children with vesicoureteral reflux, which occurs in 45% (Van den Abbeele et al. 1987); and 4) to evaluate hydronephrosis detected by prenatal ultrasound.

The primary advantage of the VCUG over the NUC is in the initial evaluation of children with urinary tract infections or voiding disorders, in whom detailed anatomy of the bladder and urethra is necessary. For example, the NUC is unlikely to demonstrate a paraureteral diverticulum, bladder trabeculation or irregularity, or urethral valves. In addition, if reflux is present, current standards for the grading of reflux are based upon the VCUG.

Reflux is graded according to the International Grading System: I: Ureteral filling only; II: Ureteral and pelvicaliceal filling without dilatation; III: Ureteral and pelvicaliceal filling with mild caliceal blunting and mild dilatation of the pelvis and/or ureter, without caliceal clubbing; IV: Ureteral and pelvicaliceal filling with caliceal clubbing and moderate pelvic dilatation without ureteral tortuosity; V: Massive ureteral dilatation and tortuosity with loss of the papillary impression in the renal pelvis. These grades of reflux have tremendous value in terms of predicting whether vesicoureteral reflux will gradually resolve with linear growth of the child.

An indirect method of detecting reflux is the intravenous administration of ^{99m}Tc-DTPA for a renal scan. When the radionuclide reaches the bladder, it may be monitored continuously during voiding to determine whether reflux is present. Reliability is uncertain. Unfortunately, reflux is detected only during the voiding phase and not the filling phase. Furthermore, false-negative results may result from excessive background activity due to impaired renal function, and bladder and reflux volumes cannot be measured accurately. Consequently, this technique is not recommended for routine use.

The "champagne cystogram" is another method of detecting reflux that does not involve radiation exposure. A carbonated solution is instilled into the bladder with continuous sonography of the kidneys during bladder filling and voiding; the "bubbles" in urine refluxed to the kidneys are detected readily by ultrasound. In general, this is not felt to be as accurate as either the VCUG or NUC, nor does it demonstrate bladder anatomy or allow reflux to be graded accurately.

Radionuclide Scanning

The renal scan is used in pediatric urology for: 1) assessment of differential renal function; 2) detection of obstructive uropathy; 3) detection of renal scarring in a patient with pyelonephritis; 4) evaluation of renovascular hypertension; and 5) distinguishing pseudotumors (column of Bertin) from true renal masses (Velchik 1985).

Radionuclide renal imaging has multiple advantages over conventional urography. First, hypersensitivity reactions are extremely rare. Second, the radioisotope does not produce an osmotic diuresis. Third, images are generally satisfactory even in patients with renal failure and in the newborn. Finally, it is possible to quantify renal function or degree of functional impairment.

Glomerular function is evaluated primarily by ^{99m}technetium diethylenetriamine pentaacetic acid (^{99m}Tc-DTPA), which is filtered but not reabsorbed or secreted. This agent provides functional images similar to an IVP and is the best agent for estimating the glomerular filtration rate. ^{131}I-hippuran is used primarily to evaluate renal tubular function and excretion, but the disadvantage of its high radiation dose usually outweighs its functional advantage, especially in children.

Technetium dimercaptosuccinic acid (^{99m}Tc-DMSA) is an excellent parenchymal imaging agent and is used to quantitate differential renal function and renal tubular functional mass. Because of its cortical imaging property, DMSA is useful primarily in detecting renal scarring in children with a history of pyelonephritis, although most scars may be imaged by IVP or sonography. Technetium glucoheptanate (^{99m}Tc-GH) combines characteristics of the other agents and is a good general imaging agent.

Ultrasonography

Sonography is an excellent noninvasive screening modality for sepsis, microhematuria, dysuria, and abdominal or pelvic discomfort. A negative study gives reassurance to both family and physician that the urinary tract is normal. However, when an anomaly is detected, another method of upper tract imaging (IVP or renal scan) and assessment for vesicoureteral reflux are necessary.

Prenatal Ultrasonography

The overall incidence of detectable fetal anomalies is approximately 1%, and the incidence of urologic anomalies detected in utero is between 1 in 500 and 1 in 1,000 (Table 11–1) (Elder, Duckett 1987).

In the normal fetus, the bladder may be visualized by ultrasound at 14 weeks and the kidneys at 14–18 weeks. The fetal urinary bladder is an echo-free area at the base of the fetal trunk that varies in size as it fills and empties. The maximum bladder volume normally is 10 ml at 30 weeks and 50 ml at term. Nonvisualization of the urinary bladder, particularly if associated with oligohydramnios, suggests renal agenesis.

The fetal kidneys are seen in transverse section just below the level of the umbilical vein early in gestation. There are recognized standards for normal fetal renal size (Grannum et al. 1980), and the kidney circumference remains constant at one-third of the abdominal circumference throughout gestation. Normally, the fetal ureter is not seen. A renal pelvic diameter 10 mm or greater suggests that an obstructive anomaly or vesicoureteral reflux is present and necessitates postnatal evaluation with a VCUG and ultrasound or IVP (Arger et al. 1985).

Determination of fetal sex is important primarily when fetuses are at risk for X-linked genetic disorders such as chronic granulomatous disease and Lesch-Nyhan syndrome, and for suspected urethral valves (bilateral hydronephrosis with distended bladder, occurring exclusively in boys). A recent study by Birnholz (1983) demonstrated that 40% of fetuses less than 24 weeks were accurately identified, and 3% were misdiagnosed. In another study of second-trimester examinations, there was a 100% accuracy rate (Stephens, Sherman 1983). Determination of sex requires unequivocal visualization of the penis and scrotum, or of the labia majora. Nonvisualization of the genitalia during

Table 11–1 Genitourinary Anomalies Detectable by Prenatal Ultrasonography

Condition	Sex (Ratio)	Frequency	Kidney(s)	Ureter(s)	Bladder	Amniotic Fluid	Prognosis
Ureteropelvic junction obstruction (unilateral)	M:F (3–4:1)	1:2,000	Hydronephrosis	Not seen	Normal	Normal	Good after surgical correction
Multicystic kidney	M:F (1:1)	1:3,000	Large with cysts of variable size	Not seen	Normal	Normal	Normal
Primary obstructive megaureter	M:F (3:1)	1:10,000	Hydronephrosis	Dilated	Normal	Normal	Good after surgical correction
Ectopic ureterocele or ureter	M:F (1:6)	1:10,000	Large cyst; possible duplex kidney	Dilated	Normal or enlarged	Normal	Good after surgical correction
Posterior urethral valves	Male	1:8,000	Bilateral hydronephrosis; possible cortical cysts	Dilated	Enlarged	Variable; diminished or absent if severe	Usually good after surgical correction or drainage; poor if oligohydramnios present
Prune belly syndrome	Nearly always male	1:40,000	Bilateral hydronephrosis; possible cortical cysts	Dilated	Enlarged	Variable; diminished or absent if severe	Usually fair to good; may need surgical drainage; poor if oligohydramnios present
Infantile polycystic kidney disease	M:F (1:2)	1:6,000–1:14,000	Large, echogenic	Not seen	Small or not seen	Usually absent or severely diminished	Poor
Renal agenesis	M:F (2–2.5:1)	1:4,000 (bilateral)	Not seen	Not seen	Not seen	Severely diminished or absent	Stillbirth
		1:1,500 (unilateral)	Not seen	Not seen	Normal	Normal	Normal

Source: Data from Elder and Duckett (1987).

the second trimester generally is due to a prone or complete breech fetal position, or to impaired imaging from maternal obesity or oligohydramnios (Birnholz 1983).

Urinary Tract Infection

Clinical Features

Urinary tract infections (UTI) are the second most common bacterial infection in childhood, following pharyngeal and middle ear infections. Between 1.5% and 2% of children between the ages of 1 and 5 years develop a symptomatic UTI. In the newborn period, nearly 90% with a UTI are male, whereas beyond 6 months of age 90% with a UTI are female.

Most UTIs appear to occur in an ascending manner. In girls, nearly all bacterial infections involving the bladder originate from stool pathogens. The vast majority of males with a normal urinary tract who develop a UTI are uncircumcised neonates (Wiswell, Roscelli 1986), and in these cases the bacteria appear to originate from the unretracted prepuce. In general, pyelonephritis in childhood appears to occur when bacteria in the bladder reflux into the kidney, rather than from hematogenous infections.

Associated Vesicoureteral Reflux

The manner in which the ureter enters the bladder determines whether the ureterovesical junction is competent. Normally, the ureter travels in the submucosa of the bladder wall for approximately 2 cm before entering the lumen of the bladder in its trigone (base). The low pressure normally present in the resting bladder (8 mm Hg to 15 mm Hg) is sufficient to passively compress the roof of the intravesical ureter against the underlying detrusor and prevent reflux. Peristaltic pressure in the extravesical ureter, between 20 mm Hg and 35 mm Hg, propels urine into the bladder. Normal compliance and elasticity of the intravesical ureter are crucial, and inflammation of the overlying bladder mucosa may alter the ureterovesical junction and allow transient reflux. When the ureter enters the bladder superolateral to its normal position, the intramural ureter is shortened and reflux often results.

The presence of complete ureteral duplication predisposes to vesicoureteral reflux. When there is complete ureteral duplication, the upper pole ureter always enters inferomedial to the lower pole ureter (termed the Weigert-Meyer rule) (Fig. 11–1). Unless the upper pole ureter is ectopic, it almost always has a normal intramural ureteral length, whereas the tunnel of the lower pole ureter may be short because of its juxtaposition to the upper pole ureter. Indeed, as many as 50% of children with a complete duplication of the collecting system may have reflux.

Renal damage from reflux has one of three characteristic appearances: 1) focal pyelonephritic scarring, in which the contracted parenchyma is seen as a dimple on the outer perimeter of the renal shadow directly over a clubbed calix; 2) generalized caliceal dilatation and parenchymal atrophy; or 3) failure of renal growth with the kidney smaller than expected, often associated with focal scarring or generalized atrophy. The presence of one of these three findings associated with vesicoureteral reflux is termed reflux nephropathy. Long-term complications include hypertension, proteinuria, and reduced renal function.

While the vast majority of young patients with an appearance of renal scarring have true reflux nephropathy, in some cases it appears to be developmental. In a number of cases, vesicoureteral reflux is identified at birth in association with an atrophic kidney that has diminished function. In these cases, the ureteral orifice is almost always abnormally located in a superolateral position. Embryologically, the ureteral bud probably penetrates the metanephric blastema in an abnormal location, resulting in a small dysmorphic kidney that appears to be scarred.

Renal scarring seems to result from intrarenal reflux, that is, reflux of urine into the collecting tubules and parenchyma. In general, renal damage from vesicoureteral reflux occurs only if there is associated infection (i.e., pyelonephritis) or when the kidney is subjected to high pressures, as in dysfunctional voiding (e.g., detrusor-sphincter dyssynergia, voiding against a closed sphincter).

Pyelonephritis is most likely to produce scarring in children under age 2. However, it occasionally has been reported in older children. For example, Smellie et al. (1985) reported on 34 children over 5 years old who developed new renal

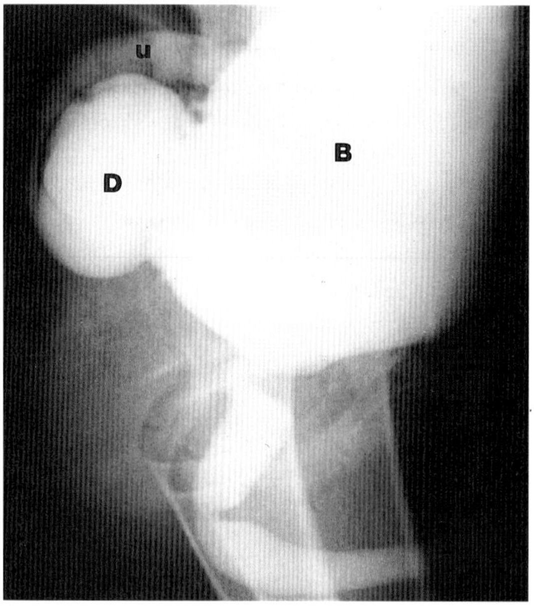

A

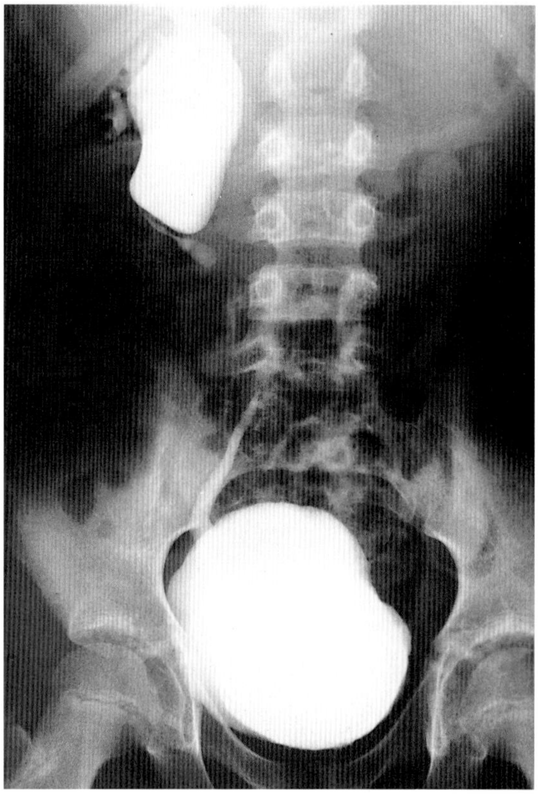

B

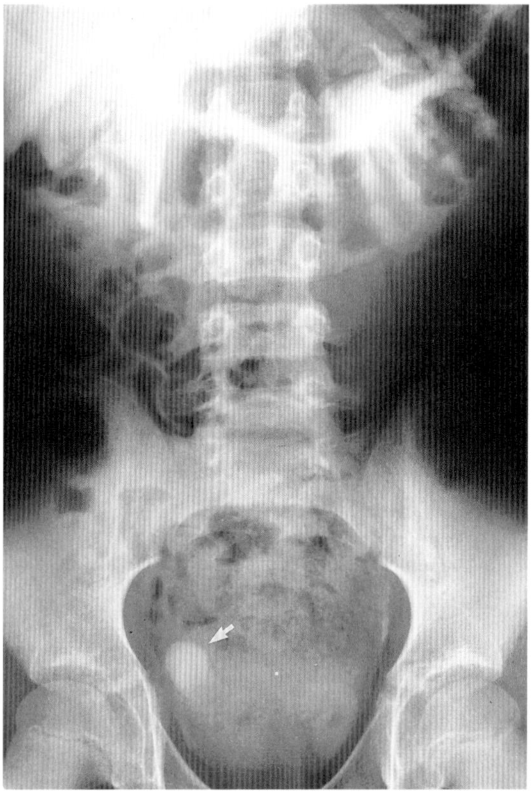

C

11–2 Eleven-year-old boy with febrile urinary tract infection and right flank pain. **(A, B)** VCUG lateral view shows normal urethra and large right paraureteral diverticulum (D); frontal view from VCUG shows grade-4 right vesicoureteral reflux and abnormal UPJ relationship with "high insertion" of ureter and secondary UPJ obstruction (arrow). (B = bladder; U = ureter.) **(C)** IVP shows normal collecting systems and bladder diverticulum (arrow). Renal ultrasonography in this boy would have been normal. He underwent right ureteral reimplantation and bladder diverticulectomy.

scars; 76% had normal kidneys on a previous IVP. All had experienced recurrent UTIs and nearly all had vesicoureteral reflux.

Radiographic Evaluation

The goal of radiographic studies is to identify features that could cause complications from the infection and anatomic factors that predispose one to a UTI. The most common finding is vesicoureteral reflux, identified in 20%–50% of children with UTIs (Spencer, Schaeffer 1986). Other findings include renal scarring, seen in approximately 25%, and obstructive uropathy, identified in 5%–10% of children with UTIs.

All girls less than 5 years old and all males should undergo radiographic evaluation following their first UTI. Girls over 5 years old should undergo evaluation if they have had two or more lower tract infections or one febrile UTI.

Radiographic evaluation generally begins with a VCUG to evaluate for reflux, a paraureteral diverticulum, ureterocele, or urethral abnormality (Fig. 11–2). Furthermore, the refluxing ectopic ureter has a characteristic appearance that can be distinguished from an orthotopic refluxing ureter.

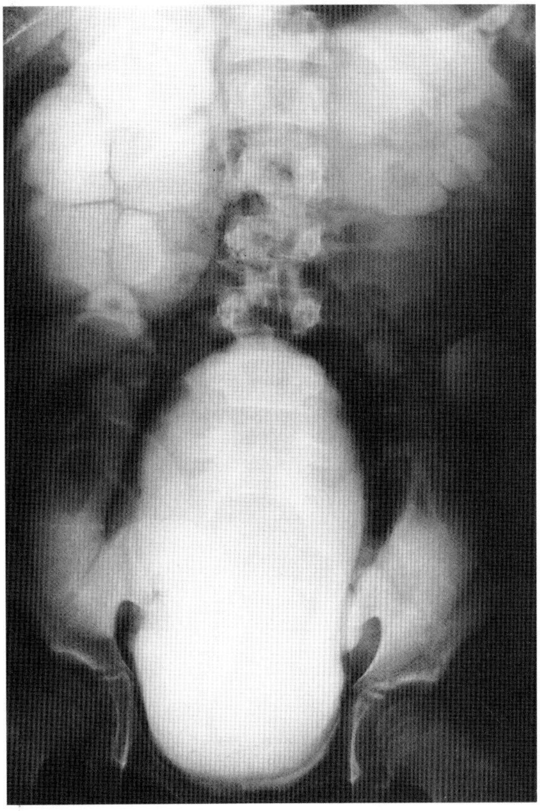

11–3 Ten-year-old boy with trisomy 18, incontinence, and renal insufficiency. Voiding cystourethrogram demonstrates grade-5 bilateral vesicoureteral reflux (it also showed normal urethra). He has megacystis-megaureter syndrome. Cutaneous vesicostomy was performed and renal function did not improve. There was no evidence of ureterovesical obstruction.

An extreme example of reflux is the megacystismegaureter syndrome in which massive reflux of urine occurs into the upper tracts (Burbige et al. 1984) (Fig. 11–3). The radiographic picture is that of a tremendously dilated collecting system and bladder. The back and forth churning of urine between the bladder and ureters results in considerable stasis, and the radiographic appearance may suggest obstruction. However, the bladder is smooth-walled and the urethra is normal.

If an abnormality is demonstrated on the VCUG, then an IVP should be performed. If the VCUG is normal, a renal ultrasound is sufficient. In this author's opinion, sonography or urography alone is not adequate to evaluate children with a UTI, as even in the presence of high-grade reflux, the upper urinary tract may be normal (Figs. 11–2, 11–4). If ultrasonography shows an abnormality of the upper urinary tract, then an IVP should follow. If the child is allergic to ionic contrast media, a radionuclide renal scan may be performed or premedication and nonionic contrast used.

Radiographic evaluation traditionally is performed 4 to 6 weeks after the acute UTI, for several reasons. Performing a cystogram during an acute infection may worsen the illness or introduce new infection. However, the VCUG is intended to be a sterile examination, and so long as the study is performed under physiologic pressures, this risk is mitigated. Another reason for delay is that reflux may be exacerbated by an acute UTI, with inflammation of the urinary bladder causing distortion of the ureterovesical junction, allowing reflux to occur (Kogan et al. 1986); knowing the status of reflux in a baseline uninfected state is more important than in the acutely infected condition. However, in the child hospitalized with a febrile UTI, this author believes that it is important to document whether the child is refluxing in the acutely infected state; if that is the case, a VCUG should be performed 1 or 2 days following hospital admission.

If reflux is demonstrated, the child is placed on a prophylactic dosage of antimicrobial medication, and periodic urine cultures are obtained to assure that the urine remains uninfected. In most children, reflux will resolve spontaneously as the ureterovesical junction "matures" with lengthening of the intramural ureter. The mean time for reflux to resolve spontaneously is 2 to 3 years.

Antireflux Surgery

Generally accepted indications for antireflux surgery include: 1) inability to take antimicrobial medication or noncompliance; 2) breakthrough UTIs while taking antimicrobial medication; 3) progressive renal scarring or lack of renal growth over time; 4) failure of reflux to resolve by puberty.

Open reimplantation surgery is performed by mobilizing the intramural ureter and creating a longer intramural bed or tunnel in which to place the ureter. In recent years, the most popular method has been the transtrigonal ("Cohen") technique, in which the ureter is advanced across the trigone to allow it to drain to the opposite side of the bladder.

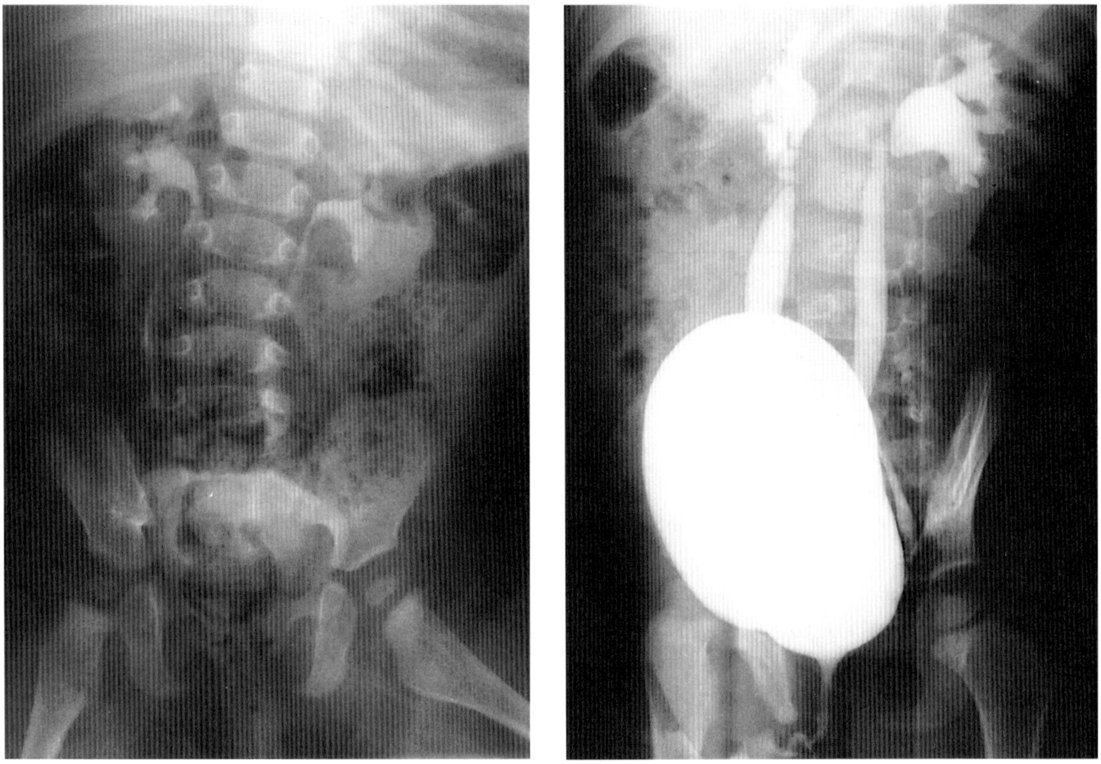

A

B

11–4 Fifteen-month-old girl with febrile urinary tract infections. **(A)** IVP is normal. **(B)** Voiding cystourethrogram demonstrating bilateral grade-4 vesicoureteral reflux with transient secondary ureteropelvic junction narrowing. This figure and Fig. 11–2 stress need for VCUG in evaluation of urinary tract infection, even if IVP or ultrasonography is normal.

Follow-up Imaging

Postoperative radiographic evaluation includes a VCUG and IVP 3 months following reimplantation. Renal ultrasound should not be substituted for an IVP, because it may not demonstrate ureteral dilatation suggestive of mild obstruction. Subsequently, at yearly intervals a follow-up urogram or sonogram should be performed to assure continued renal growth and lack of obstruction.

In the child with reflux who is not a surgical candidate, an annual NUC should be performed. If high-grade reflux is present, then an IVP should be performed also at follow-up evaluation. If low- or medium-grade reflux is present and previous urograms have been normal, then a renal ultrasound may be substituted.

Obstructive Uropathy

Fetus with Suspected Obstructive Uropathy

The amniotic fluid allows pulmonary development to proceed normally by providing a cushion for thoracic expansion and by directly inducing lung differentiation and growth. It is the most important prognostic feature in the fetus with bilateral hydronephrosis and a distended bladder. The combination of obstructive uropathy and oligohydramnios generally results in pulmonary hypoplasia, which is usually fatal. Renal dysplasia may be demonstrated by the presence of macroscopic cysts in the cortex. When a serious renal anomaly is detected, half of these fetuses will have associated anomalies. Work-up should include checking the fetal karyotype, obtaining maternal alpha-fetoprotein level, and careful imaging of the rest of the fetus.

A fetus with bilateral hydronephrosis should be monitored every few weeks to assess the hydronephrosis and to monitor the volume of amniotic fluid. If oligohydramnios develops, the cause must be determined; early delivery is advisable only if the amniotic fluid remains severely diminished. In the fetus with unilateral hydronephrosis, however, early delivery should not be undertaken.

The detection of presumed obstructive uropathy presents a dilemma, since prenatal drainage of the urinary tract could possibly salvage renal function and allow pulmonary development to proceed normally. In most cases, intervention has been used for presumed posterior urethral valves and associated oligohydramnios, with placement of a one-way shunt between the fetal bladder and amniotic sac. Recently, the International Fetal Surgery Registry reported 73 cases in which a vesicoamniotic shunt was placed; survival was 40% both in those with oligohydramnios and normal amniotic fluid (Manning et al. 1986). However, in 45% of the cases, the urologic diagnosis was unknown and the sonographic criteria for oligohydramnios were not defined. Although the authors did not conclude that such intervention was effective, further study was recommended.

In a review through 1985 of all 28 reported cases in which there was bilateral hydronephrosis, oligohydramnios, and an interventional procedure, survival was 21% (Elder et al. 1987). In no case did intervention improve renal function, although in 1 or 2 cases it may have allowed more normal pulmonary development. The complication rate has been approximately 40%, including failure of the shunt to function properly, migration of the shunt, perforation of bowel, induction of premature labor, and maternal chorioamnionitis.

Intervention is rarely effective because severe obstructive uropathy results in irreversible renal dysplasia. Thus, the fetus with urethral valves and associated anhydramnios identified at 18 to 20 weeks' gestation has little or no expectation of recoverable renal function. Intervention should be considered only in rare cases and by teams experienced in these techniques.

In the fetus with bilateral hydronephrosis or unilateral hydronephrosis in a solitary kidney, the baby probably should be delivered in a tertiary care center to allow an expeditious evaluation. On the other hand, if the fetus has one normal kidney, then it seems unnecessary to alter plans for delivery.

Ureteropelvic Junction Obstruction

The most common site of obstruction in the upper urinary tract is the ureteropelvic junction (UPJ). It usually occurs *in utero* and becomes apparent during infancy or childhood, although it occasionally does not manifest itself until adulthood. Obstruction is usually caused by a mechanical narrowing secondary to an intrinsic stenosis.

In some cases, the obstruction is functional, resulting from ureteropelvic incoordination secondary to abnormal development of the muscle fibers, with replacement of the normal spirals of muscle by longitudinal fibers. Increased distention elongates the longitudinal fibers without increasing their girth, resulting in luminal narrowing rather than widening that occurs with normal circular muscle fibers. The result is failure of the peristaltic wave to propagate from the renal pelvis to the ureter. In other cases, a kink, adhesion, extrinsic band, or accessory artery supplying the lower pole of the kidney may produce a sharp angulation of the ureter against the lower margin of the pelvis, resulting in obstruction during high rates of urine flow.

Evaluation of these patients usually consists of an IVP, diuretic renogram, and VCUG. Since 10% to 15% of children with a UPJ obstruction have ipsilateral reflux, a VCUG is recommended. Following the VCUG, delayed films are helpful by demonstrating whether contrast remains within the renal pelvis. With severe obstruction and associated reflux, contrast fills the ureter only to the ureteropelvic junction, and the IVP demonstrates hydronephrosis.

The diuretic renogram determines whether renal function is impaired and provides a baseline for following results of therapy. In patients with equivocal findings on other tests, a Whitaker antegrade perfusion study should be performed (Fig. 11–5). Although insertion of a percutaneous nephrostomy for temporary drainage is technically feasible, it is rarely necessary except in the presence of pyohydronephrosis or if the clinician is attempting to determine whether the patient has a nonfunctioning kidney.

Ureteropelvic junction obstruction usually is repaired by means of a dismembered pyeloplasty, in which the narrow segment is excised, the renal pelvis is trimmed to a normal size, and a ureteropyelostomy is performed. In general, the neonatal

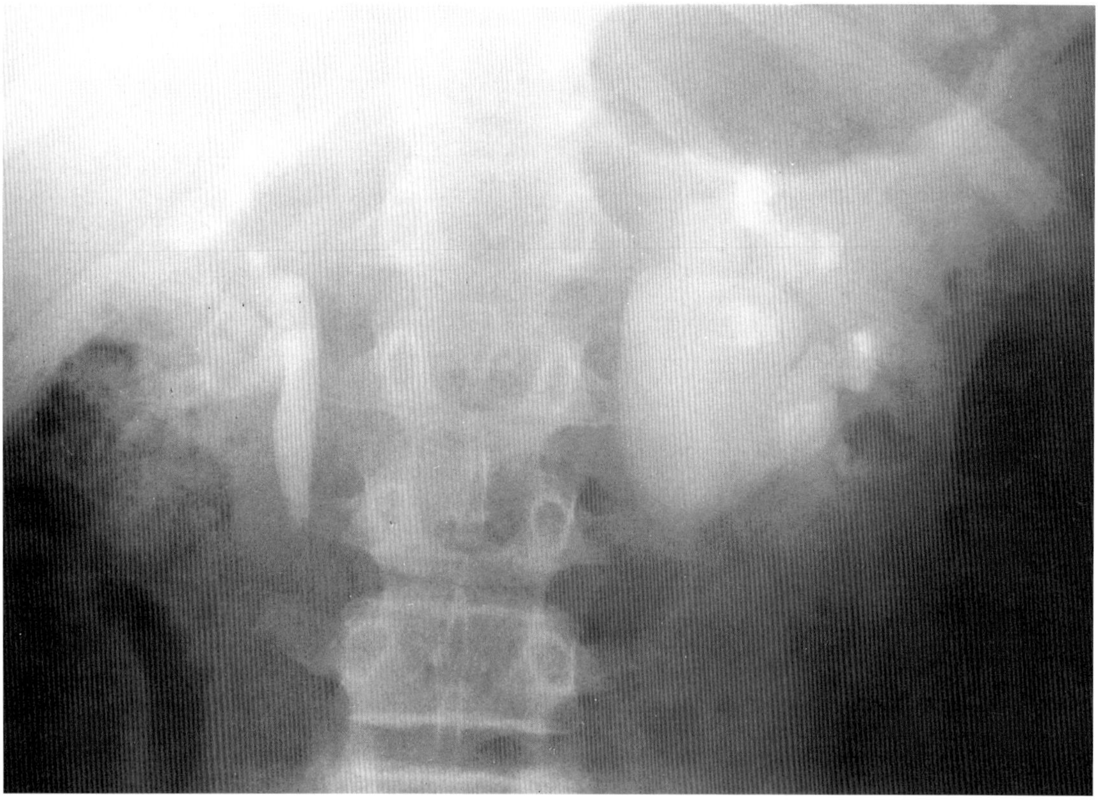

11–5A

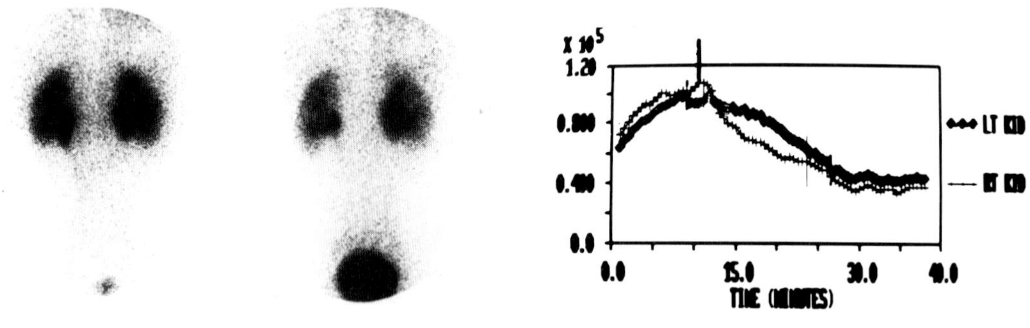

B

kidney with impaired function by UPJ obstruction has a much greater likelihood of improved function after surgery relative to the contralateral normal kidney than does the older child undergoing a pyeloplasty.

With the increased use of prenatal ultrasonography, cases of apparent UPJ obstruction have been recognized and followed into the newborn period. Although the washout curve following administration of furosemide indicates obstruction, the differential renal functions may be nearly equal, raising the dilemma as to whether there is a

11–5 Ten-year-old boy with nocturnal enuresis underwent ultrasonography, demonstrating left hydronephrosis. **(A)** IVP showing large renal pelvis on left side, but only mild caliectasis. Patient was asymptomatic. Diuretic renogram at this time showed no evidence of obstruction. **(B)** Radionuclide renogram (anterior view) 1 year later showing stasis in large left renal pelvis (images at 12 min and 27 min). Following administration of furosemide (Lasix), there is good "washout" bilaterally. **(C)** One year later, patient has intermittent left flank discomfort. IVP (supine) continues to suggest partial obstruction of left ureteropelvic junction (arrow). **(D)** Prone film in same study demonstrates patency of ureteropelvic junction. **(E)** Whitaker test demonstrated pressure differential between left renal pelvis and bladder of 40 cm H_2O during filling of renal pelvis at rate of 10 ml/min, indicating that UPJ obstruction is present.

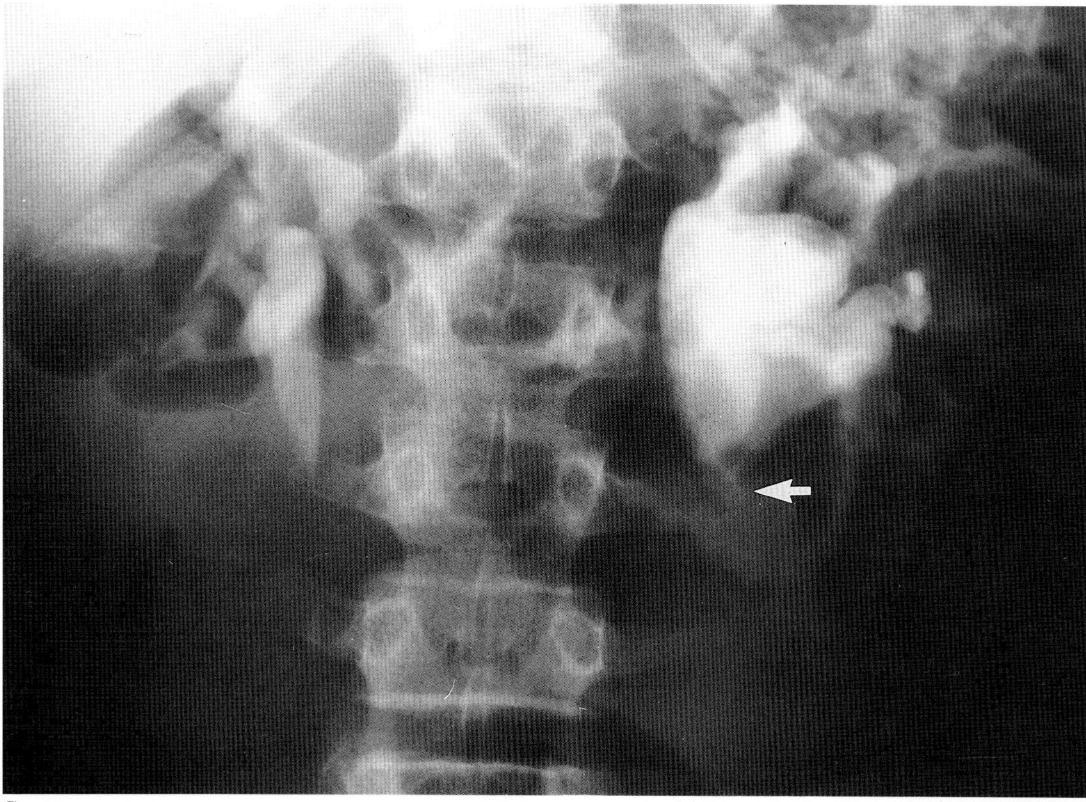

C

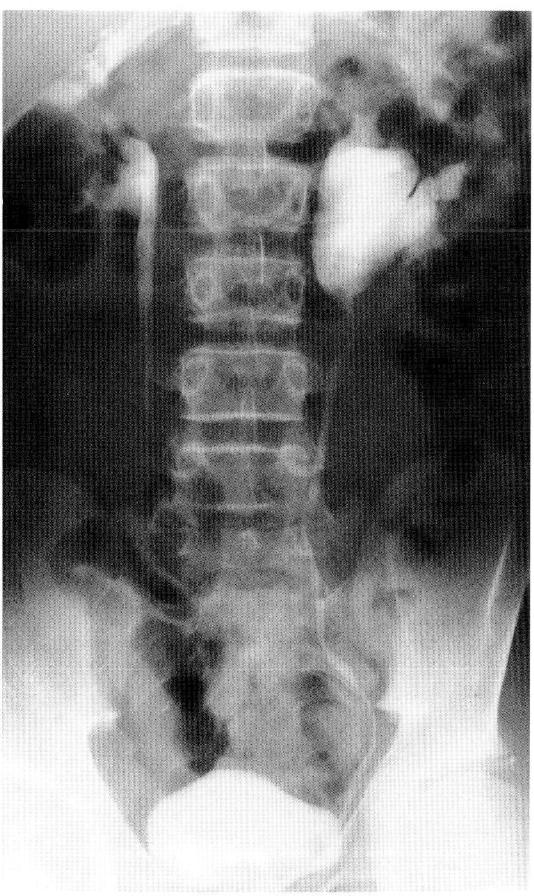

D

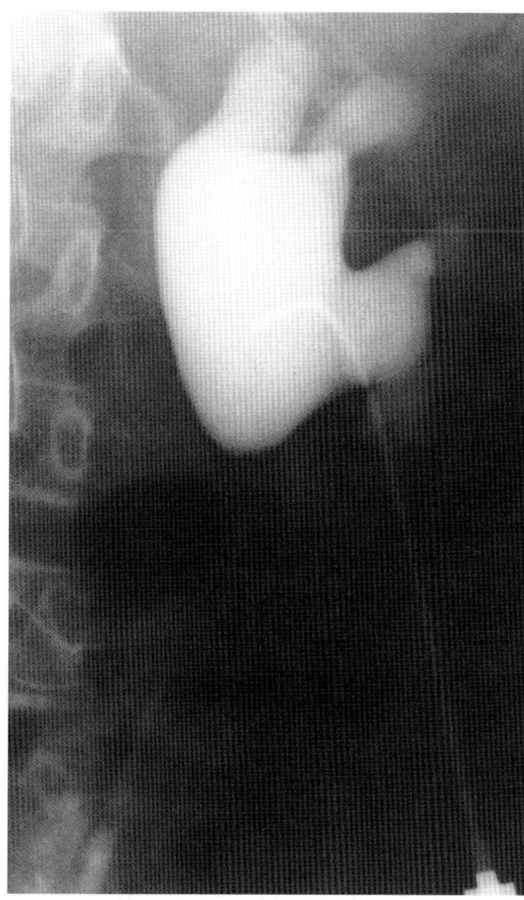

E

Table 11–2 Subclassifications of Megaureter

Refluxing		Obstructed		Nonrefluxing or Nonobstructed	
Primary	Secondary	Primary	Secondary	Primary	Secondary
Primary reflux Prune belly syndrome Ectopic ureter	Neuropathic bladder Urethral valves Bladder diverticulum Postoperative	Intrinsic (stenosis; adynamic segment) Ureteral valves Ectopic ureter Ectopic ureterocele	Neuropathic bladder Urethral valves Ureteral calculus Extrinsic (tumor; retroperitoneal fibrosis; vascular anomaly)	Nonrefluxing, nonobstructed	Polyuria Infection Persistent following relief of obstruction

true obstruction. In these cases, it is extremely unlikely that the kidney will show deterioration of renal function on differential renal function studies over 3 to 6 months, and therefore it seems prudent to follow such patients with serial DTPA diuretic radionuclide scans until renal function matures and the clinician can be more certain about obstruction.

Megaureter

Megaureter is subclassified based upon its various etiologies (Table 11–2). This classification is useful because most obstructed and refluxing megaureters require surgical correction.

With megaureter, there may be ineffective peristalsis if the walls of the dilated ureter are unable to come together to propel the urine downstream. In primary nonrefluxing megaureter with obstruction, the ureteral lumen at the site of apparent obstruction usually has a normal diameter. However, histologically there are disorganized muscle bundles causing an aperistaltic segment, resulting in a functional obstruction. Congenital nonobstructed megaureter often is associated with megacalycosis. Thus, ureteral dilatation with caliectasis is not an absolute indicator of ureterovesical obstruction.

The left ureter is involved two to three times as often as the right, and the incidence in males is approximately twice as high as in females. The incidence of contralateral renal agenesis is approximately 9%. Approximately 75% present with urinary tract infection, 45% with flank or abdominal pain, and 10% with hematuria or uremia.

Radiologic Evaluation of Upper Urinary Tract Obstruction

The diuretic renogram is used most commonly in the evaluation of suspected obstruction involving the upper urinary tract. It has been the topic of two recent reviews (Maizels et al. 1986; O'Reilly 1986). In the vast majority of cases of upper tract dilatation, the diuretic renogram provides sufficient information about renal function and dynamics to guide clinical management.

A diuretic renogram should probably not be done immediately after an IVP. The combination of preparation for the IVP, the osmotic diuretic effect of the radiographic contrast media, and the effect of furosemide administered during the renogram may cause postural hypotension and syncope, which will cause slowed parenchymal transit of the radionuclide.

In general, a 1-mg/kg dose of furosemide is sufficient, but children with preexisting renal insufficiency may require up to 4 mg/kg to induce satisfactory diuresis. Upright positioning can be used to facilitate drainage.

Severe renal insufficiency complicates interpretation. In general, if renal function is insufficient to provide a diuresis following furosemide administration, slow drainage may be secondary to obstruction, stasis, or simply renal insufficiency. Isolated renal tubular disorders may affect interpretation. For example, patients with Fanconi's syndrome or acute tubular necrosis may not have a diuresis after administration of furosemide. In patients with diabetes insipidus or a history of posterior urethral valves, delayed drainage of the upper urinary tract may be caused by bladder overdistention or inability to void completely, rather than ureterovesical obstruction. If the child has intermittently elevated intravesical pressure due to a spastic neurogenic bladder (as in myelomeningocele), posterior urethral valves, or following repeated bladder surgery, the bladder should be catheterized at the beginning of the study to allow satisfactory drainage of the upper urinary tract. Similarly, the bladder should be catheterized in children with vesicoureteral reflux.

Although many investigators routinely perform diuretic renograms on newborns with suspected obstruction of the upper urinary tract, in some cases the apparent obstruction improves or resolves by 3 months to 4 months of age, suggesting that newborns may have an impaired ability to respond to furosemide. The contralateral kidney may be used as a control.

The Whitaker antegrade pressure perfusion test is used when findings on the diuretic renogram are equivocal. With the patient prone, and a catheter in the bladder, a nephrostomy tube or a long needle is inserted percutaneously into the renal pelvis. A constant perfusion pump is used to perfuse the renal pelvis at rates up to 10 ml/min or 15 ml/min. A manometer is attached to the perfusion catheter and bladder outflow tubing. Constant perfusion is maintained until the renal pressure either reaches a plateau or increases far above the physiologic range indicating obstruction. Contrast is administered through the nephrostomy to visualize the urinary tract and better define the site and possibly the cause of obstruction. A maximum relative renal pressure (renal pelvic pressure minus needle resistance minus bladder pressure) less than 15 cm of water is normal; a pressure differential greater than 22 cm of water indicates obstruction; a maximum pelvic pressure between 15 cm and 22 cm of water is indeterminate. A disadvantage of the Whitaker test in children is that standards for the perfusion rate were established in adults. Another disadvantage is that the test is invasive and often requires general anesthesia or heavy sedation. However, in patients with intermittent UPJ obstruction, the test frequently provides evidence of impaired urinary flow (Fig. 11–5).

Posterior Urethral Valves

Posterior urethral valves are the most common cause of bladder outlet obstruction in children. In most cases, this condition is diagnosed either prenatally or, in the newborn period or infancy, because of a distended bladder, poor dribbling stream, urinary infection, vomiting, or failure to thrive. The effect on renal function is variable. Although nearly all such children have severe hydroureteronephrosis, the serum creatinine may return to a normal level following relief of obstruction. Although two or three types of urethral valves have been described, these cannot be distinguished radiographically and have little effect on management.

Posterior urethral valves are demonstrated radiographically by VCUG, with a dilated posterior urethra, hypertrophied bladder neck, and bladder trabeculation. The anterior urethra usually is not filled well. In some cases, the diagnosis of valves may be suggested by ultrasonography when the dilated posterior urethra is seen while imaging from the suprapubic or perineal positions (Elder, Duckett 1987).

Approximately one-half of these children also have vesicoureteral reflux, which carries a worse prognosis in terms of renal function. Patients with bilateral reflux tend to have the worst renal function. In approximately one-fourth of patients with reflux, the reflux resolves with linear growth of the child, usually within 1 to 2 years of valve ablation. In approximately 17% of patients with valves, there is persistent unilateral reflux. In two-thirds of these cases, the reflux is associated with a nonfunctioning kidney on the left side. This has been termed the vesicoureteral reflux and renal dysplasia (VURD) syndrome, since the kidney is severely dysplastic. Nephroureterectomy is recommended to establish more normal voiding dynamics and reduce the likelihood of infection.

In a few patients with urethral valves, the upper urinary tracts are surprisingly normal. This has been demonstrated primarily in boys with a large diverticulum of the bladder (Fig. 11–6). The diverticulum probably dissipates the high intravesical pressure, allowing normal drainage of the upper urinary tracts. Similarly, in the VURD syndrome, the right collecting system often appears nearly normal, particularly following valve ablation. Another potential protective factor in the newborn with valves is ascites, usually from forniceal extravasation of urine, which temporarily decompresses the obstructed urinary tract.

Ureteral dilatation and tortuosity often persist after valve ablation, falsely suggesting ureterovesical obstruction. In these cases, the dilatation improves significantly following drainage of the bladder, and there is rarely a true obstruction at the ureterovesical junction. This has been confirmed by Whitaker tests on these patients. In general, the ureteral dilatation improves over a long period of time. Some children have a poorly compliant bladder that results in persistent dilatation of the upper urinary tract ("valve bladder"). In these patients double and triple voiding may help drain the large volume of urine stored in the upper urinary tract.

Ureterocele

A ureterocele is a cystic dilatation of the distal end of the ureter that is obstructive. In children it is usually associated with the upper pole moiety of a duplicated system, and 85% of patients are female (Fig. 11–1). In such cases, the upper pole rarely functions and histologically demonstrates severe dysplasia or inflammatory changes with few glomeruli. Infrequently, the ureterocele may prolapse and be evident as an interlabial mass. Diagnosis is made by demonstrating a round filling defect in the base of the bladder on VCUG or IVP, in association with a "drooping lily" deformity of the affected kidney, representing distortion of the lower pole collecting system by the nonfunctioning hydronephrotic upper pole. Ultrasonography of the bladder also is an excellent modality for imaging the ureterocele. Reflux into the ipsilateral lower pole ureter and calices is common, and one-half of patients have a contralateral duplication. When a ureterocele occurs in boys, one-third to one-half have a single collecting system, and in such cases the obstructed kidney tends to function better than the typical obstructed upper pole system.

Ectopic Ureter

Ectopic ureter occurs primarily in girls in association with the upper pole of a duplicated collecting system. Approximately one-third drain into the bladder neck, one-third into the distal urethra or urethrovaginal septum, and one-fourth into the vagina. In boys, nearly one-half drain into the posterior urethra, one-third into the seminal vesicle, and the remainder into the prostatic utricle, ejaculatory duct, or vas deferens, all of which are above the external urinary sphincter. In girls, over one-half drain outside the external sphincter, and the typical presenting complaint is continuous incontinence or vaginal discharge; if the ectopic ureter drains inside the external sphincter, the diagnosis is usually made following a UTI.

When the ectopic ureter drains into the bladder neck, obstruction results in hydroureteronephrosis and variably diminished renal function. In many cases reflux into the upper pole moiety occurs during voiding, as a result of relaxation of the bladder neck. Demonstration of reflux may be difficult by VCUG if the contrast is diluted by the large amount of urine in the ureter. However, filling the bladder with contrast followed by voiding several times in a cyclical manner helps establish that reflux is present (Wyly, Lebowitz 1984).

Multicystic Kidney

The multicystic kidney has numerous cysts of varying size and no demonstrable parenchyma. Histologically, stroma between the cysts has only disorganized tubules and few or absent glomeruli. There is associated atresia of part or all of the ureter. In approximately one-third of cases, there is a contralateral structural renal anomaly.

Multicystic kidney is often detected prenatally by ultrasonography; occasionally, it is confused with hydronephrosis. In the newborn, multicystic kidney presents as an abdominal mass. The diagnosis may be made by sonography but should always be confirmed by a renal scan. If the kidney demonstrates any function on the renal scan, the child may instead have a severe UPJ obstruction. A VCUG also is recommended to detect vesicoureteral reflux.

The natural history of the multicystic kidney is unknown. In the past, nearly all of these were removed. There have been several reports of renal cell carcinoma or Wilms's tumor arising in a multicystic kidney. In one patient, nodular renal blastema (precursor of Wilms's tumor) was identified. Furthermore, there is evidence that hypertension may develop, which often resolves following nephrectomy. If the multicystic kidney is not removed, the patient should undergo long-term sonographic follow-up to detect possible malignant degeneration.

Prune Belly (Eagle-Barrett) Syndrome

The prune belly syndrome occurs almost exclusively in males. It is characterized by congenital absence, deficiency, or hypoplasia of the abdominal musculature, a large hypotonic bladder, dilated and tortuous ureters, and high intraabdominal undescended testicles. While the cause is unknown, there appears to be a diffuse mesenchymal abnormality. The diagnosis usually is obvious by the typical wrinkled abdominal wall. Associated skeletal anomalies are common. Renal development is variable, and while some boys have normal renal function, others have severe dysplasia with renal failure. A confusing feature in these patients is the tremendous hydroureteronephrosis and bladder distention, suggestive of obstructive uropathy. However, true anatomic obstruction rarely is present.

If renal function is normal or near normal, serial IVPs or renal scans are effective in confirming satisfactory renal growth, improvement in renal function, and satisfactory drainage of the kidneys and ureters. Occasionally a Whitaker antegrade perfusion test is needed to assure satisfactory drainage.

Abdominal Masses in the Newborn

Two-thirds of abdominal masses that are detected within the first months of life arise from the urinary tract, and 10% occur in the female genital system. Table 11–3 shows the distribution of abdominal masses based upon several large series. The most common abdominal mass is due to hydronephrosis. The most common solid renal tumor is a mesoblastic nephroma. Excluded are infants with distended bladders without hydronephrosis, isolated splenomegaly, pyloric stenosis, pelvic tumors palpable only by rectal examination, and babies with hydrocolpos in whom the diagnosis was obvious because of a bulging, imperforate hymen. Nearly all neonatal abdominal masses arising from the genitourinary tract may be diagnosed accurately based on history, physical examination, ultrasound, and renal scan. Ultrasonography should be the first imaging test.

Table 11–3 Distribution of Abdominal Masses in the Neonatal Period: 280 Cases

	Number
Kidney (65%)	
Hydronephrosis (UPJ obstruction, UVJ obstruction, ureterocele, etc.)	80 (28%)
Multicystic kidney	63 (22%)
Polycystic kidney disease	18
Renal vein thrombosis	5
Solid tumor	13
Ectopy	4
Total	183
Retroperitoneum (9%)	
Neuroblastoma	17
Teratoma	3
Hemangioma	1
Abscess	4
Total	25
Bladder (1%)	
Posterior urethral valves	2
Female genital system (10%)	
Hydrocolpos	16
Ovarian cyst	13
Total	29
Gastrointestinal (12%)	
Duplication	17
Giant cystic meconium ileus	4
Mesenteric cyst	3
Ileal atresia	2
Volvulus – ileum	2
Teratoma – stomach	1
Leiomyosarcoma – colon	1
Meconium peritonitis with ascites	1
Ascites	1
Total	32
Hepatic/biliary (3%)	
Hemangioma – liver	3
Solitary cyst – liver	2
Hepatoma	1
Distended gallbladder	1
Choledochal cyst	1
Adenomatoid malformation of lung	1
Total	9

Source: Data compiled from the following series: *Am J. Roentgenol.* 93:447, 1965; *Surgery* 63:514, 1968; *J. Urol.* 106:770, 1971; *Am. J. Dis. Child* 136:147, 1982; *Clin. Ped.* 7:529, 1968.

Note: Distended bladder, hepatomegaly, and splenomegaly excluded in most series.

Malignancies of the Genitourinary Tract

Wilms's Tumor

Wilms's tumor (nephroblastoma) is the most common malignant neoplasm of the urinary tract in children and is responsible for 8% of all childhood solid tumors. In approximately 75% of cases, the diagnosis is made between the ages of 1 and 5 years, with most cases presenting between ages 3 and 4 years. An equal number of boys and girls are affected. In 75% of cases, an abdominal mass or increasing abdominal girth is the presenting sign, and one-third have abdominal pain. While gross hematuria is uncommon, microhematuria is found in 25% of cases.

Wilms's tumor usually can be distinguished from nonrenal masses by IVP and ultrasonography. A neuroblastoma may be confused with Wilms's tumor if the tumor arises from the kidney, but a positive bone marrow aspiration or elevation of urinary catecholamines is conclusive for neuroblastoma. Although 5% of patients in the first National Wilms's Tumor Study were misdiagnosed preoperatively, today misdiagnosis is extremely uncommon because of improved imaging.

The IVP classically demonstrates distortion of the caliceal morphology by an intrarenal mass. Calcification is rarely present, but when found has a characteristic eggshell pattern resulting from old hemorrhage. If a stippled pattern of calcification is present, neuroblastoma is more probable. Nonvisualization of the affected kidney suggests renal vein invasion by the tumor, massive parenchymal replacement by tumor, or obstruction of the renal pelvis or ureter by tumor.

Ultrasonography demonstrates a solid renal mass and provides an assessment of the renal vein and inferior vena cava for intraluminal tumor. Furthermore, retroperitoneal lymphadenopathy and hepatic metastases may be demonstrated. Since 10% of patients have Wilms's tumor bilaterally, it is important to image the contralateral kidney.

Computed tomography (CT) scan and magnetic resonance (MR) imaging provide excellent anatomic delineation of the renal and retroperitoneal anatomy, but often require a general anesthetic in the small child. One of these studies is necessary if the mass is very large, if the contralateral kidney is abnormal, or if caval or hepatic invasion is suspected. A chest X ray should be routine.

Arteriography is recommended only if the mass is not clearly intrarenal or the tumor is suspected to be bilateral, particularly if partial nephrectomy is being considered. Inferior venacavography to evaluate renal vein or caval involvement may be necessary preoperatively with large tumors.

Other imaging studies for metastases generally are not performed until microscopic examination of the kidney is completed. If a clear cell carcinoma is present, a bone scan should be performed because of the high incidence of bony metastases with this variant of Wilms's tumor. When a rhabdoid tumor is found, a CT scan of the brain should be performed.

Neuroblastoma

Neuroblastoma is the most common malignant tumor of infancy and the second most common solid tumor of childhood. Although this tumor may arise anywhere along the sympathetic chain from the head to the pelvis, over one-half originate in the abdomen and two-thirds arise in the adrenal gland. If the tumor arises from an abdominal paravertebral sympathetic ganglion, there is a greater likelihood that it may grow through an intervertebral foramen to form a dumbbell-shaped tumor compressing the spinal cord. If the tumor arises in the presacral region, it may lead to urinary frequency or retention from extrinsic pressure on the bladder. Often, the first symptoms reflect involvement of the skull and long bones. At initial diagnosis, over 50% of children have bone marrow involvement.

When an abdominal tumor is present, ultrasonography and then, if necessary, an intravenous pyelogram should be performed. With urography the neuroblastoma arising from an adrenal gland characteristically is seen to displace the kidney inferiorly and laterally with maintenance of the normal caliceal pattern. This contrasts with the appearance of a Wilms's tumor, which distorts the collecting system. The abdominal paravertebral neuroblastoma may displace the ureter laterally. If ureteral obstruction is present, there may be delayed or absent visualization of the kidney. In 50% of cases, a stippled pattern of calcification is seen in the tumor. When a CT scan is performed, an additional 30% of tumors are found to have such calcification.

Ultrasonography is useful in locating the intraabdominal primary tumor. The inferior vena cava usually is well visualized and may be displaced anteriorly. Complete obstruction or tumor invasion of the vena cava is rare. CT scanning provides a more detailed image of the retroperitoneum and provides evaluation of the posterior mediastinum, as tumor extension may occur through the diaphragm. A skeletal survey should be performed routinely. Bony metastases occur most commonly in the skull and in the diaphyses of the femur and humerus. They usually are lytic and irregular with periosteal reaction. Metastases are rare distal to

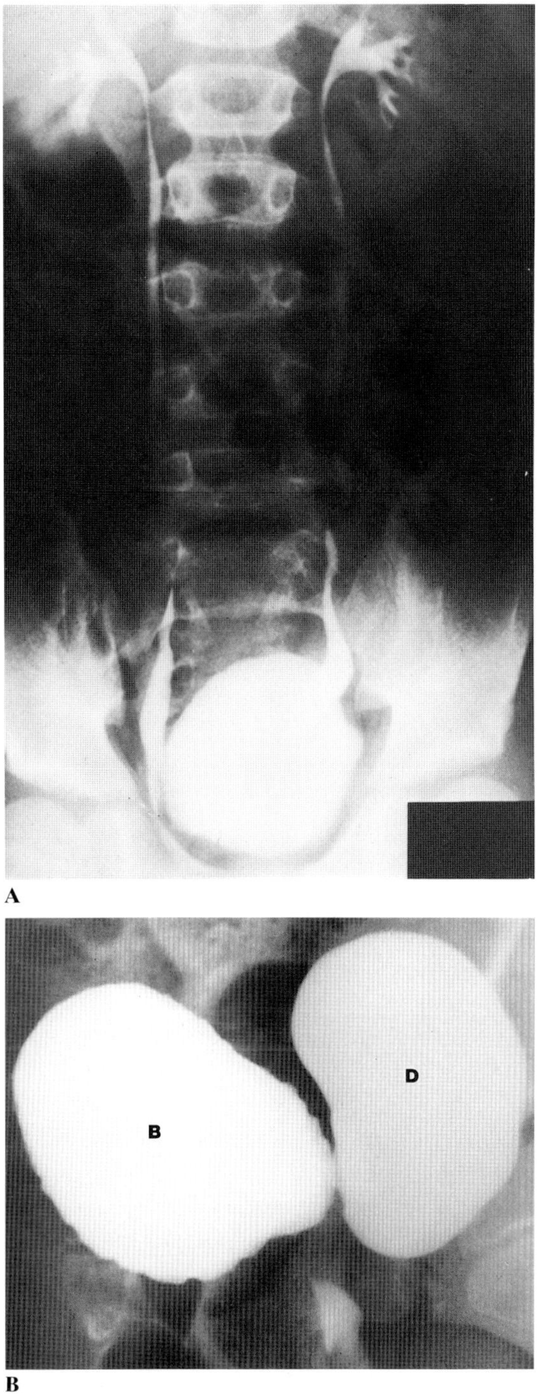

11–6 Four-year-old male with posterior urethral valves. **(A)** IVP performed prior to valve ablation shows normal upper urinary tracts with dilated lower ureters. Left ureter is deviated medially. **(B)** Oblique cystogram shows large vesical diverticulum (D) posteriorly. In patients with posterior urethral valves, vesical diverticulum acts as "pop-off valve," allowing upper urinary tracts to function relatively normally. (B = bladder.)

the knee and elbow. In general, arteriography and venography are not helpful unless the tumor is large and appears to involve the celiac axis or superior mesenteric artery.

Rhabdomyosarcoma

Rhabdomyosarcoma is the third most common solid tumor in childhood; approximately 20% arise in the genitourinary region. Incidence peaks during ages 2 to 6 years and between ages 15 to 19 years, with a slight male predominance. The most common genitourinary sites are the prostate, bladder (usually the trigone), vagina, and the paratesticular area. Rhabdomyosarcomas arising in the pelvis outside the bladder or prostate often have urologic consequences. These tumors are large before becoming symptomatic and have a worse prognosis than those arising in other genitourinary sites. Rhabdomyosarcoma is characterized by rapid growth with invasion of adjacent tissues.

Diagnosis and staging often are accomplished with an IVP, CT scan, and ultrasonography. Magnetic resonance imaging may replace CT for imaging the pelvis. When the tumor has a botryoid configuration, the appearance on imaging studies is strongly suggestive of rhabdomyosarcoma, but biopsy always is necessary for definitive diagnosis. Most of these tumors are managed initially by chemotherapy, and precise radiographic imaging is extremely important in follow-up. Occasionally, other diseases and tumors arising in the pelvis mimic a rhabdomyosarcoma. These include leiomyosarcoma, neurofibroma, lymphohemangioma, eosinophilic cystitis, and inflammatory pseudotumor of the bladder.

Bladder Abnormalities

Incontinence

In the child with day and nighttime wetting, a VCUG and renal ultrasound are part of the standard evaluation. The spine should be evaluated carefully for abnormalities, including spina bifida occulta or a missing vertebra. In the female, this evaluation may reveal evidence of an ectopic ureter.

Neuropathic (Neurogenic) Bladder

Myelodysplasia is the most common cause of a neurogenic bladder in children. In this condition, there are wide defects in the posterior neural arches caused by defective fusion of one or more of the posterior vertebral arches. The neural spines are absent, and the everted pedicles and laminae are well away from the midline, resulting in protrusion of the meninges and neural tissue through the bony defect. The distribution is: sacral, 20%; lumbosacral, 47%; lumbar, 26%; low thoracic, 5%; and cervical/high thoracic, 2%.

Associated anomalies of the genitourinary tract are relatively common in children with myelodysplasia. Nearly one-fourth of boys have cryptorchidism and 20% have structural renal anomalies. Fusion anomalies (horseshoe kidney) are the most common, with a significant incidence of multicystic kidney, renal agenesis, and ureteropelvic junction obstruction. Bladder function is thought to be normal in the fetus with myelodysplasia, with bladder dysfunction and secondary complications developing after birth.

The initial goal is to identify children at risk for upper urinary tract deterioration. Thus, a VCUG and renal ultrasound are performed following closure of the myelomeningocele. If either of these tests is abnormal, an IVP is performed.

Renal sonography shows hydronephrosis in approximately 25% of cases, and the VCUG demonstrates reflux in approximately 15% to 20%. When significant ureterectasis or hydronephrosis is demonstrated on the ultrasound, reflux is usually present. In patients with significant hydronephrosis or who demonstrate evidence of detrusor-sphincter dyssynergia, early urologic intervention is necessary. Following therapy, ultrasonography is used to verify that the upper urinary tract returns to normal. Infants who have mild-to-moderate hydronephrosis at birth are followed very closely with renal ultrasound or IVP at 3-month intervals. Some of these may return to normal without urologic treatment (Chiaramonte et al. 1986).

If the initial radiologic evaluation is normal, then a follow-up renal ultrasound usually is performed at 6 months and annually thereafter. In children with reflux, approximately one-half demonstrate spontaneous resolution, with the remainder requiring some form of antireflux surgery (Sidi et al. 1986).

In children or young adults who have undergone urinary diversion, close long-term radiographic follow-up is necessary, as 70% to 85% may develop complications, including stomal stenosis, fascial stenosis, ureterointestinal obstruction, stenosis of the ileal conduit, or urolithiasis (Schwarz, Jeffs 1975). An additional long-term complication this author has recently recognized in several patients is infundibulopelvic stenosis (Fig. 11–7), occurring primarily in patients with persistent bacteriuria or with recurrent pyelonephritis.

A variant of myelomeningocele is the lipomeningocele, in which a lipomatous tumor is embedded within the lumbar spinal cord, replacing the overlying dura. A soft mass may be palpable overlying the lumbar spine, or a small patch of hair, dermal sinus tract, or dimple may be evident overlying the sacrum. The lipomeningocele causes little if any early impairment but may produce a progressive neurologic deficit as the child grows, secondary to compression and stretching of the nerve roots.

"Nonneurogenic" Neurogenic Bladder

Older children with a normal neurologic examination and no anatomic obstruction may have symptoms and signs of bladder outlet obstruction, including hesitancy, a poor stream, urinary retention, incontinence, and hydronephrosis. The primary problem in this condition is detrusor-sphincter dyssynergia, that is, contraction of the external urinary sphincter during voiding. Because of the similarity to the neuropathic bladder, this condition is termed a "nonneurogenic" neurogenic bladder, or Hinman syndrome (Hinman 1986).

Urologic complications of this disease vary. While many children have little or no damage to the upper urinary tract, some develop vesicoureteral reflux, hydronephrosis, and renal scarring, secondary to the high bladder pressures that are generated.

A voiding cystourethrogram and IVP are performed during the initial evaluation. For the more severe cases, "videourodynamics" may be extremely helpful, which provides the most definitive assessment of a child's voiding pattern. This requires close cooperation between the urologist and radiologist. In these studies, cystometrogram, electromyogram, and assessment of abdominal

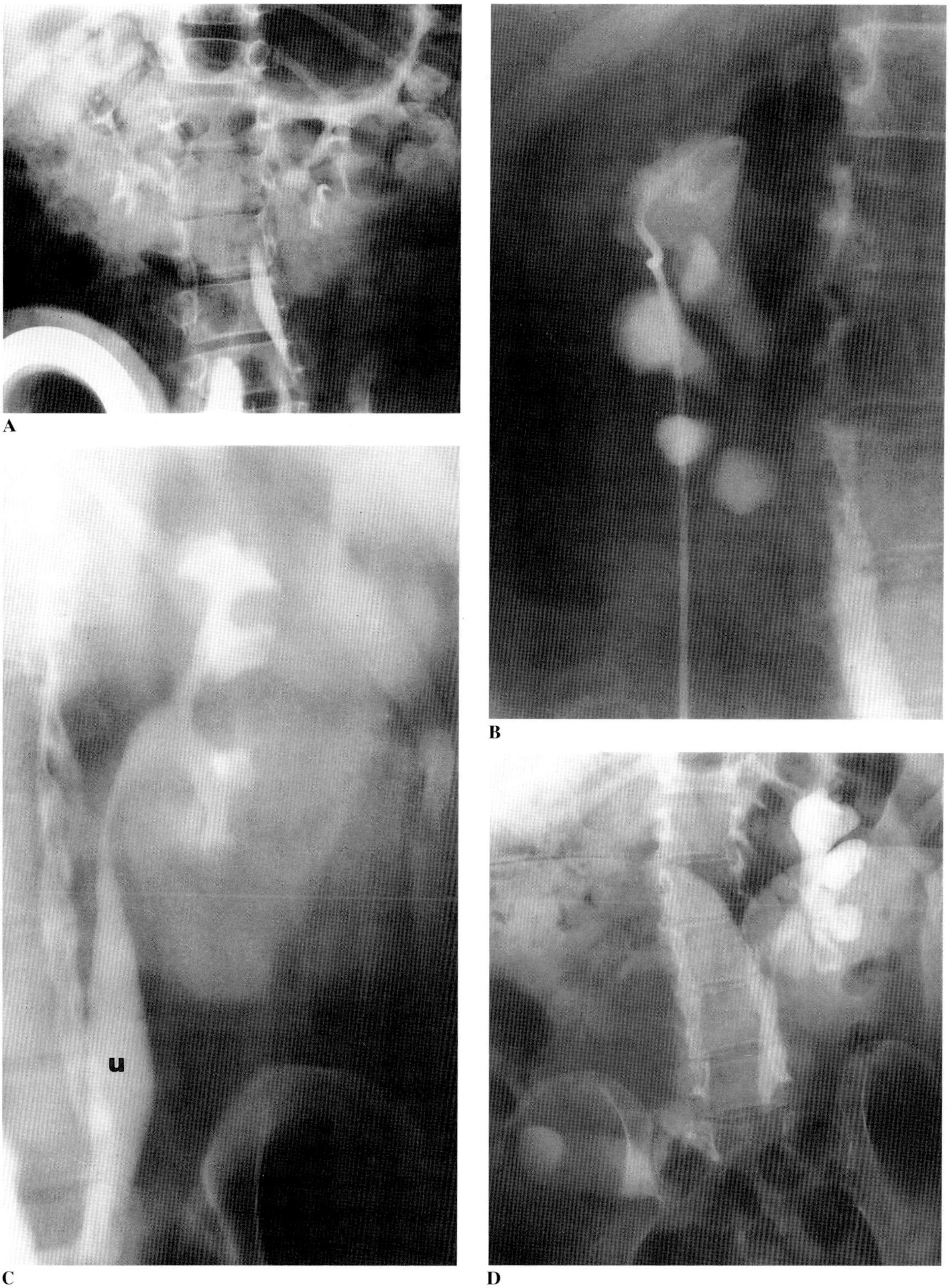

11–7 Girl born with myelodysplasia. **(A)** Seven-year-old patient with myelodysplasia has undergone ileal conduit. IVP shows normal upper urinary tracts. **(B, C)** Eleven years later, at age 18, antegrade nephrostogram through pigtail catheter demonstrates infundibulopelvic stenosis of right kidney. Left kidney was normal. She had unsuccessful reconstructive surgery on right kidney and subsequently underwent a right nephrectomy. (U = ureter.) **(D)** Three years later she presented with recurrent left pyelonephritis and had developed severe left infundibulopelvic stenosis and renal calculi.

pressure and a VCUG are performed simultaneously.

Urachal Disorders

The urachus is a fibrous cord arising from the anterior bladder wall and extending cranially to the umbilicus. A persistence of the entire tract or a portion of it may result in four anomalies: patent urachus, vesicourachal diverticulum, urachal sinus (also termed alternating sinus), or urachal cyst. With the exception of the patent urachus, most of these abnormalities are asymptomatic. However, if bacterial infection involves the urachal cyst, then fever, suprapubic pain, dysuria, frequency, or a palpable suprapubic mass may result. These signs and symptoms are also suggestive of a variety of inflammatory pelvic and abdominal diseases, including severe cystitis, pelvic inflammatory disease, appendicitis (with or without abscess), inflammatory bowel disease, and tumor. In a recent series from this author's institution, 10 patients had an infected urachal cyst; 5 were less than 3 years of age and 5 were young adults (Goldman et al. 1988). Ultrasonography, barium enema, CT scan, and cystography were most helpful in the diagnosis (Fig. 11–8). Treatment generally has involved initial percutaneous drainage followed by interval excision of the infected cyst.

Disorders of the Genitalia

Interlabial Masses

The differential diagnosis of a mass between the labia includes prolapsed ectopic ureterocele, urethral prolapse, sarcoma botryoides (rhabdomyosarcoma) arising from the vagina, paraurethral cyst, and imperforate hymen. Examination of the mass and, occasionally, ultrasound usually provide the diagnosis.

Undescended Testis

Approximately 3% to 4% of boys are born with an undescended testis, with the incidence decreasing to 0.8% by 1 year of age. In general, or-

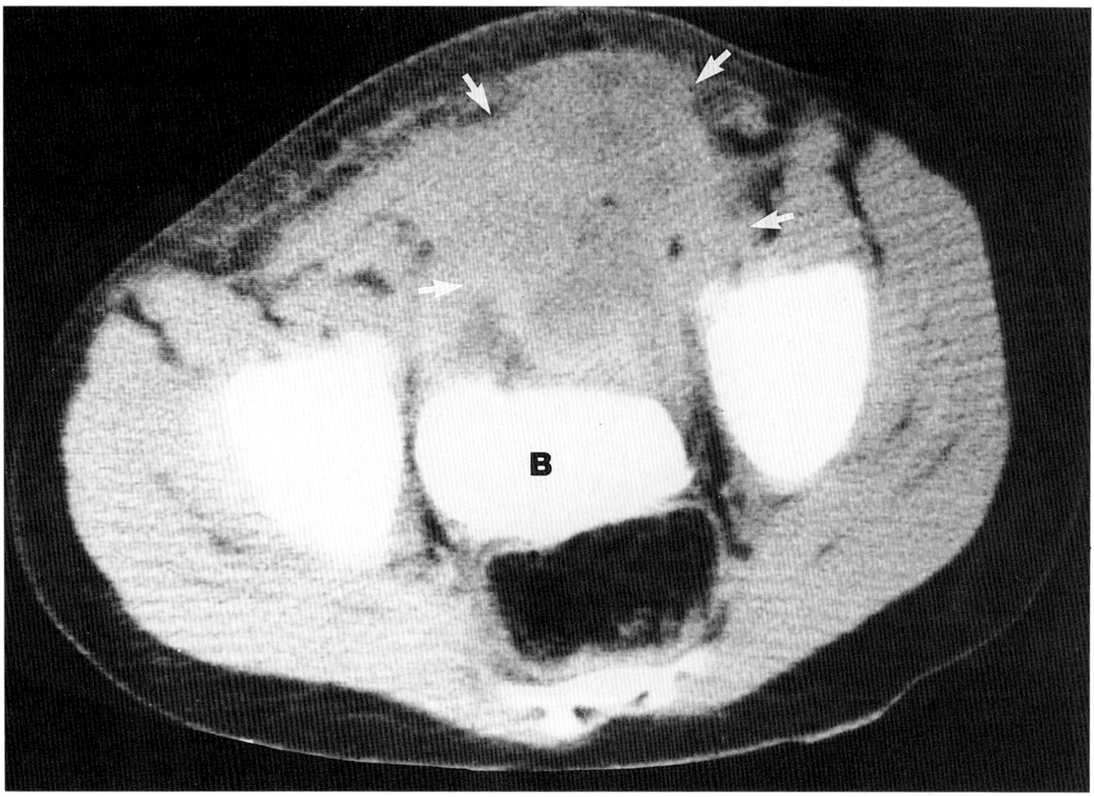

11–8 Five-year-old girl with infected urachal cyst. CT scan demonstrates loculated mass (arrows) of mixed density anterior to bladder (B). Treatment was drainage and excision of mass.

chiopexy is recommended between 12 and 18 months of age in order to maximize chances for ultimate fertility (Elder 1987). Approximately 20% of boys with cryptorchidism have an impalpable testis. Half of these are located in the inguinal canal, while 20%–25% are intraabdominal, 15% are at the external inguinal ring, and 10% are absent.

Imaging techniques to localize the nonpalpable testis include ultrasound, gonadal venography, MRI, and computed tomography. Of these modalities, ultrasound seems the least useful. In one recent series, an impalpable testis was localized by ultrasound in only 13% of patients (Weiss et al. 1986). Gonadal venography is difficult in children less than 3 years old and often requires anesthesia or heavy sedation. In one-fourth of patients, the internal spermatic vein cannot be identified at all. The CT scan reliably localizes a nonpalpable testis that is present but cannot prove that a testis is absent. Perhaps the most useful application of CT scanning is in the child who has had a previous inadequate surgical exploration. This author and colleagues have found magnetic resonance imaging helpful in localizing the nonpalpable testis. The advantages of MR imaging are that it requires no radiation to the patient, no contrast media, and is painless. In the T2-weighted image, the testes appear as very bright images, clearly differentiated from blood vessels and lymph nodes. However, further experience is necessary. Any form of radiologic evaluation for localizing an impalpable testis is discouraged unless it is expected to influence surgical management.

In the past, many boys with cryptorchidism as an isolated abnormality have undergone an IVP. However, in a compilation of five series with a total of 526 asymptomatic patients, in only 1% was an asymptomatic abnormality of the urinary tract detected that required operative correction (Marshall, Elder 1982). Thus, routine urography seems unwarranted, even in boys with bilateral cryptorchidism. Only if a significant epididymal abnormality is detected at the time of orchiopexy might a renal abnormality be suspected, since the kidney and the Wolffian duct have a common embryologic origin.

Varicocele

Approximately 15% to 20% of adolescent and adult men have a varicocele. This occurs almost exclusively on the left side and is the most commonly identified correctable abnormality in infertility clinics. In adults, parameters of semen analysis improve in the majority of cases following internal spermatic vein ligation. This author and colleagues' current practice in the adolescent with a varicocele is to measure testicular size by ultrasound and repeat the study annually. If there is failure of ipsilateral testicular growth or if there is a significant disparity in size between the testes, then varicocelectomy is recommended, which has been demonstrated to result in substantial improvement in ipsilateral testicular growth (Kass, Belman 1987).

Testicular Torsion

Testicular torsion is one of the most critical surgical emergencies in urology. Onset is most common between 10 and 16 years of age and usually is characterized by sudden severe testicular pain, nausea, and vomiting. There may be a history of recent minor testicular trauma. Similar episodes may have subsided spontaneously in the past. Detorsion must be accomplished within 4 to 6 hours to preserve spermatogenesis, and within 8 to 12 hours to preserve Leydig cell function (i.e., testosterone production). The differential diagnosis includes torsion of the appendix testis, epididymitis, hematoma secondary to trauma, testicular tumor, and idiopathic scrotal edema.

The definitive method of diagnosing testicular torsion is a radionuclide testicular flow scan using ^{99m}technetium pertechnetate. When the clinical findings are unclear, or a decision about urgent surgery is uncertain, the radionuclide study should be performed on an emergency basis.

Imperforate Anus

Anorectal malformations occur at a rate of 1 in 5,000 live births. These lesions are classified according to whether the end of the rectum is supralevator (high), fully translevator (low), or partially translevator (intermediate).

The most common associated abnormality of the genitourinary system is a fistulous tract between the rectum and the urinary tract in the male, and between the rectum and the vagina in the female. These fistulas are usually associated with supralevator lesions. Approximately 80% of such males have a rectourethral fistula and 7% have a rectovesical fistula, whereas rectovaginal fistulas are present in 80%–94% of females with intermediate or high lesions and in whom a rectovesical fistula is rare. The rectourinary fistula is usually demonstrable by VCUG.

Genitourinary anomalies are more common with supralevator lesions. Nearly one-third of these patients have structural renal anomalies, nearly 50% have reflux, and 25% have cryptorchidism. Conversely, with infralevator lesions, approximately 7% have a structural renal anomaly, 20% to 25% have reflux, and 7% have cryptorchidism. Finally, some patients have evidence of a neuropathic bladder, secondary either to sacral agenesis, which is present in 15% of these patients, or to the extensive pelvic dissection during the definitive surgical pull-through procedure. In these patients, anomalies of other organ systems also may be present. The presence of vertebral defects (V), anal anomalies (A), cardiac anomalies (C), tracheoesophageal fistula (T, E), renal anomalies (R), and limb deformities (L) is termed the VACTERL syndrome.

Initial evaluation of the neonate with suspected imperforate anus includes: 1) determination of the level of the blind rectal pouch, 2) identification of a rectourethral or rectovaginal fistula, and 3) a search for associated anomalies. Accordingly, the initial step generally is the Wangensteen-Rice "invertogram." In addition, a film of the lumbosacral spine is taken to detect vertebral anomalies.

In patients with suspected high imperforate anus, an abdominal ultrasound should be performed prior to colostomy, because the information obtained may alter the type of procedure. For example, males with structural renal anomalies or reflux are at risk for pyelonephritis, and a divided colostomy is recommended to minimize the chance that feces may drain into the mucous fistula and contaminate the urinary tract through the rectourinary fistula.

A VCUG should be performed before the neonate leaves the hospital. If reflux is demonstrated, the infant should be placed on a regimen of prophylactic antimicrobials.

Hematuria

The most common causes of hematuria in children are glomerulonephritis, focal nephritis, hemolytic-uremic syndrome, and Alport's disease, as well as a bleeding diathesis and sickle cell disease or trait. Bacterial or viral URI, stone disease, hypercalciuria, foreign body, trauma, tumor, and urinary tract obstruction are urologic causes. During infancy, renal vein thrombosis, renal artery occlusion, and sepsis are the most common causes of hematuria.

Urologic evaluation for hematuria depends on the presumptive diagnosis. Even if a nephrologic cause is suspected, imaging of the upper urinary tract is desirable. Ultrasonography is recommended either to detect the occasional tumor associated with glomerulonephritis or to demonstrate the urinary tract obstruction associated with nephrotic syndrome and to verify that two kidneys are present if renal biopsy is contemplated. If a urologic cause for hematuria is suspected, both a VCUG and an IVP should be performed.

References

Arger PH, Coleman BA, Mintz MC, Snyder HM, Camardese T, Arenson RL, Gabbe SG, Aquino L: Routine fetal genitourinary tract screening. *Radiology* 156:485–489, 1985.

Birnholz JC: Determination of fetal sex. *N. Engl. J. Med.* 309:942–944, 1983.

Burbige KA, Lebowitz RL, Colodny AH, Bauer SB, Retik AB: The megacystis-megaureter syndrome. *J. Urol.* 131:1133–1136, 1984.

Chiaramonte RM, Horowitz EM, Kaplan GW, Brock WA: Implications of hydronephrosis in the newborn with myelodysplasia. *J. Urol.* 136:427–429, 1986.

Elder JS: Cryptorchidism: Isolated and associated with other genitourinary defects. *Ped. Clin. North Am.* 34:1033–1053, 1987.

Elder JS, Duckett JW: *Perinatal urology. In* Gillenwater JY, Grayhack JT, Howards SS, Duckett JW (eds.): *Adult and Pediatric Urology.* Chicago, Yearbook Medical Publishers, 1987, pp. 1512–1603.

Elder JS, Duckett JW, Snyder HM: Intervention for fetal obstructive uropathy: Has it been effective? *Lancet* 2:1007–1010, 1987.

Goldman IL, Caldamone AA, Gauderer MWL, Hampel N, Wesselhoeft CW, Elder JS: Infected urachal cysts: A review of ten cases. *J. Urol.* 140:375–378, 1988.

Gooding CA, Berdon WE, Brodeur AE: Adverse reactions to intravenous pyelography in children. *Am. J. Roentgenol.* 123:802–804, 1975.

Grannum P, Bracker M, Silverman R, Hobbins JC: Assessment of fetal kidney size and normal gestation by comparison of ratio of kidney circumference to abdominal circumference. *Am. J. Obstet. Gynecol.* 136:249–254, 1980.

Hinman F, Jr.: Nonneurogenic neurogenic bladder (Hinman syndrome) – 15 years later. *J. Urol.* 136:769–777, 1986.

Kass EJ, Belman AB: Reversal of testicular growth failure by varicocele ligation. *J. Urol.* 137:475–476, 1987.

Kogan SJ, Sigler L, Levitt SB, Reda EF, Weiss R, Greifer I: Elusive vesicoureteral reflux in children with normal contrast cystograms. *J. Urol.* 136:325–328, 1986.

Maizels M, Firlit CF, Conway JJ, King LR: Troubleshooting the diuretic renogram. *Urology* 28:355–363, 1986.

Maizels M, Smith CK, Firlit CF: Management of children with vesicoureteral reflux and ureteropelvic junction obstruction. *J. Urol.* 131:722–727, 1984.

Manning FA, Harrison MR, Rodeck C, Members of the International Fetal Medicine and Surgery Society: Catheter shunts for fetal hydronephrosis and hydrocephalus: Report of the International Fetal Surgery Registry. *N. Engl. J. Med.* 315:336–340, 1986.

Marshall FF, Elder JS: *Cryptorchidism and Related Anomalies.* New York, Praeger Publishers, 1982.

O'Reilly PH: Diuresis renography 8 years later: Update. *J. Urol.* 136:993–999, 1986.

Schwarz GR, Jeffs RD: Ileal conduit urinary diversion in children: Computer analysis of follow-up from 2–16 years. *J. Urol.* 114:285–288, 1975.

Sidi AA, Pang W, Gonzalez R: Vesicoureteral reflux in children with myelodysplasia: Natural history and results of treatment. *J. Urol.* 136:329–331, 1986.

Smellie JM, Ransley PG, Normand ICS, Prescod N, Edwards D: Development of new renal scars: A collaborative study. *Br. Med. J.* 290:1957–1960, 1985.

Spencer JR, Schaeffer AJ: Pediatric urinary tract infections. *Urol. Clin. North Am.* 13:661–672, 1986.

Stephens JD, Sherman S: Determination of fetal sex by ultrasound. *N. Engl. J. Med.* 309:184, 1983.

Van den Abbeele AD, Treves ST, Lebowitz RL, Bauer S, Davis RT, Retik A, Colodny A: Vesicoureteral reflux in asymptomatic siblings of patients with known reflux: Radionuclide cystography. *Pediatrics* 79:147–153, 1987.

Velchik MG: Radionuclide imaging of the urinary tract. *Urol. Clin. North Am.* 12:603–631, 1985.

Weiss RN, Carter AR, Rosenfield AT: High resolution realtime ultrasonography in the localization of the undescended testis. *J. Urol.* 135:936–938, 1986.

Wiswell TE, Roscelli JD: Corroborative evidence for the decreased incidence of urinary tract infections in circumcised male infants. *Pediatrics* 78:96–99, 1986.

Wyly JB, Lebowitz RL: Refluxing urethral ectopic ureters: Recognition by the cyclic voiding cystourethrogram. *Am. J. Roentgenol.* 142:1263–1267, 1984.

Suggested Reading

Blane CE, Koff SA, Bowerman RA, Barr M, Jr.: Nonobstructive fetal hydronephrosis: Sonographic recognition and therapeutic implications. *Radiology* 147:95, 1983.

Chrispin AR, Gordon I, Hall C, Metrewek C: *Diagnostic Imaging of the Kidney and Urinary Tract in Children.* Berlin, Springer International, 1980.

Glick PL, Harrison MR, Golbus MS, Adzick NS, Filly RA, Kallen PW, Mahony BS, Anderson RL, DeLorimier AA: Management of the fetus with congenital hydronephrosis. II: Prognostic criteria and selection for treatment. *J. Ped. Surg.* 20:376–387, 1985.

Grignon A, Filion R, Filiatrault D, et al.: Urinary tract dilatation in utero: Classification and clinical applications. *Radiology* 160:645–648, 1986.

Lebowitz RL: *Postoperative Pediatric Uroradiology.* New York, Appleton-Century-Crofts, 1981.

Lebowitz RL, Ben-Ami T: Trends in pediatric uroradiology. *Urol. Radiol.* 5:135–147, 1983.

Magill HL, Clarke EA, Fitch SJ, et al.: Excretory urography with iohexol: Evaluation in children. *Radiology* 161:625–630, 1986.

Pollack HM, Banner MP: Current status of excretory urography: A premature epitaph? *Urol. Clin. North Am.* 12:585–601, 1985.

Romero R, Cullen M, Jeanty P, Grannum P, Reese EA, Venus I, Hobbins JC: The diagnosis of congenital renal anomalies with ultrasound II. Infantile polycystic kidney disease. *Am. J. Obstet. Gynecol.* 150:259–262, 1984.

Roodhooft AM, Birnholz JC, Holmes LB: Familial nature of congenital absence and severe dysgenesis of both kidneys. *N. Engl. J. Med.* 310:1341–1345, 1984.

Teele RL: Pediatrics. *Semin. Ultrasound* 5(March):1–101, 1984.

CHAPTER

12

Sonography of the Pediatric Urinary Tract

Henrietta Kotlus Rosenberg

During the past decade, sonography has emerged as the preferred imaging modality for examination of the pediatric urinary tract. Exquisite detail may be demonstrated without dependency on renal function, ionizing radiation, or intravenous contrast material (Rosenberg 1986). Preparation for routine sonography of the urinary tract includes adequate hydration and a full bladder if possible. Fasting is required for a complete abdominal and pelvic sonogram to evaluate suspected neoplasm and for duplex Doppler evaluation of the renal arteries and veins. Sedation is rarely needed. Colorful wall posters, mobiles, and a VCR to show movies and cartoons helps maximize the child's comfort and confidence. The patient's cooperation is generally enhanced by having family members present during the sonogram.

Ultrasound examinations are routinely performed with real-time in-line multifrequency scanheads; additional static scanning is used when an organ or lesion is too large to demonstrate on a single real-time image. Static scanning shows a more global relationship of a mass or other abnormality to the remaining anatomy.

The bladder is evaluated first, since an untrained child tends to inadvertently empty the bladder with very little stimulation. If voiding occurs, infants will rapidly refill the bladder when given a bottle while the upper tracts are being examined. The bladder wall should be thin, not more than 2 mm, and smooth in the distended state. Depending on the size of the child, a 3-, 5-, 7.5-, or 10-MHz transducer may be used to obtain the routine transverse and sagittal scans. The bladder also provides a sonic window for evaluation of the distal ureters, uterus, ovaries, and prostate gland.

Appearance of Normal Anatomy

Kidney

The kidneys are imaged in the following positions: sagittal imaging of the right kidney in the supine position; coronal transverse and sagittal imaging in both decubitus positions; transverse and sagittal planes in the prone position. Scanheads of 3 MHz, 5 MHz, or 7.5 MHz are used, depending on the size of the child. Size, configuration, texture, and position of the kidneys are recorded. If serial measurements are available, adequacy of growth should be determined (Rosenbaum et al. 1984).

The appearance of the kidney in a newborn differs greatly from that of the older infant and child (Fig. 12–1 A) (Hayden et al. 1984). The renal cortex is isoechoic with the liver in a full-term infant, but may be hyperechoic in a premature infant. There is accentuation of the corticomedullary junctions. During the first 6 months of life, these findings gradually change, and the renal cortical echogenicity becomes hypoechoic compared with the liver (Fig. 12–1 B). The parenchyma is evaluated for thinning and diffuse or focal scarring.

Collecting System

The ureters are not normally visualized unless they are dilated, in which case they should be traced to their distal insertion so that obstruction, reflux, or ectopia may be demonstrated. The ureterovesical junction should be evaluated for evidence of obstruction or reflux by carefully observing the orifice and the presence and direction of peristalsis. When the bladder is distended

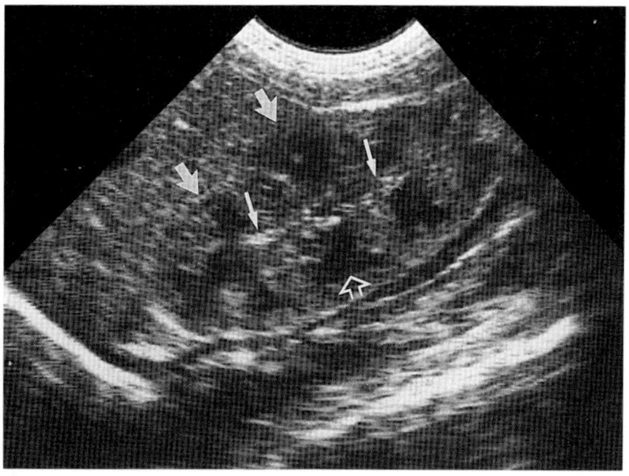

A

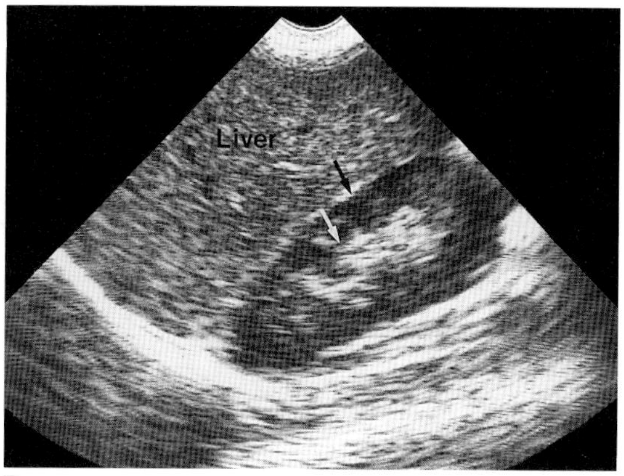

B

12–1 Normal kidney. **(A)** Normal kidney in newborn. Coronal scan demonstrating hypoechoic medullary pyramids (open white arrow), renal cortex (large white arrows), which is isoechoic with adjacent liver, and accentuation of corticomedullary junctions. Renal sinus echoes (small white arrows) are inconspicuous, due to paucity of peripelvic fat in newborn. **(B)** Normal kidney in 6-year-old. Coronal scan demonstrating hypoechoic appearance of renal parenchyma (large black arrow) in comparison with adjacent liver. Corticomedullary junction is no longer accentuated. Renal sinus echoes (small white arrow) are more prominent, owing to more peripelvic fat in child this age.

and the collecting systems appear prominent, the child should be rescanned following bladder emptying by micturition, Credé, or catheterization to assess the degree of emptying and to look for subsequent decompression of the collecting systems. If bladder wall thickening is observed in a male child, the posterior urethra should be examined for an obstructing lesion such as posterior urethral valve, polyp, or anterior duplication. The posterior urethra can also be examined using the perineal approach.

Uterus, Ovary, and Prostate

The normal uterus varies considerably in size and configuration during stages of development (Fig. 12–2A–C). In the newborn female, the uterus measures approximately 3.5 cm in length, with a fundus to cervix ratio of 1:2. The prominence of the uterus and the brightly echogenic endometrial lining are a result of *in utero* hormonal stimulation. After approximately 2 months, the uterus regresses and measures approximately 2.5 cm in length, with a fundus to cervix ratio of 1:1. At this time, the endometrial lining is no longer accentuated. This configuration is maintained until puberty begins, when the uterus gradually changes its configuration and develops a length of 5–7 cm, with a fundus to cervix ratio of 3:1. The size and echogenicity of the endometrial lining then fluctuate according to the phase of the menstrual cycle, just as in adult females.

The ovaries in newborns and very young children may not be visible because they are less than 1 cm in size. Not uncommonly, multiple small cysts measuring less than 5 mm are seen in one or both ovaries, despite the prepubertal state of the patient.

The prostate gland in children has the same configuration as in adults, but is smaller, with the largest anteroposterior diameter 1–2.5 cm, depending on the age of the child (Fig. 12–2D, E).

Indications for Ultrasonography

Renal Failure

Sonography is indispensable for evaluating pediatric patients with renal failure and in determining a cause for nonvisualization of one or both kidneys on excretory urography. Rapid differentiation can be made between unilateral or bilateral renal agenesis, renal dysplasia, congenital or acquired obstruction, medical renal disease, multicystic dysplastic kidney, or renal vein thrombosis. Duplex Doppler ultrasound, particularly color Doppler, has added a new dimension by enabling the sonographer to assess the patency and flow in the major abdominal vessels (aorta and inferior vena cava), renal arteries, and veins. Ultrasound evaluation of the urinary tract in the ill newborn has obviated the need for excretory uro-

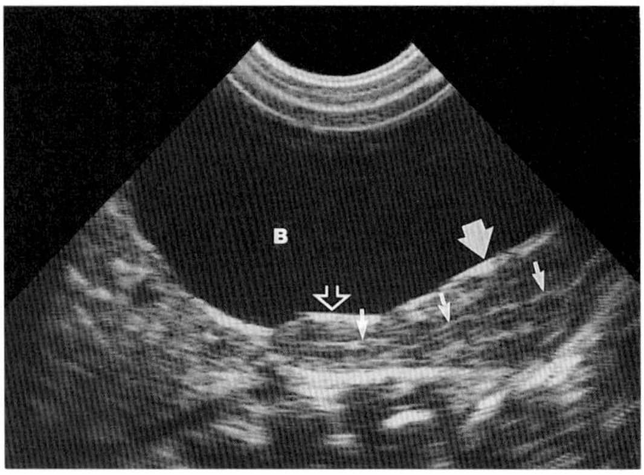

A

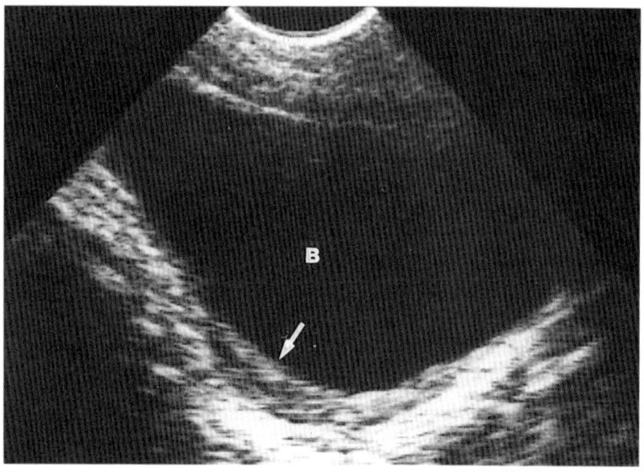

B

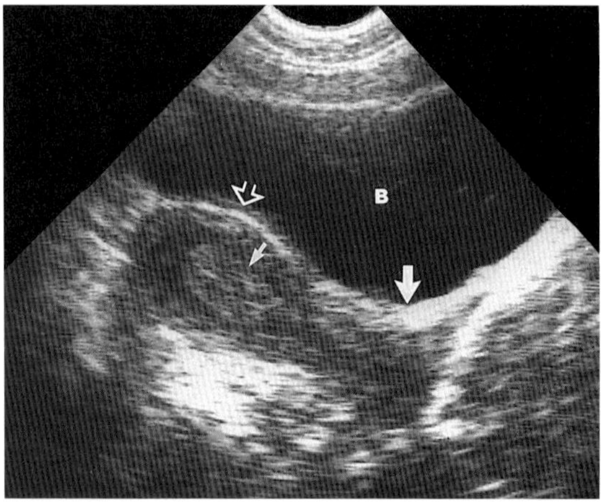

C

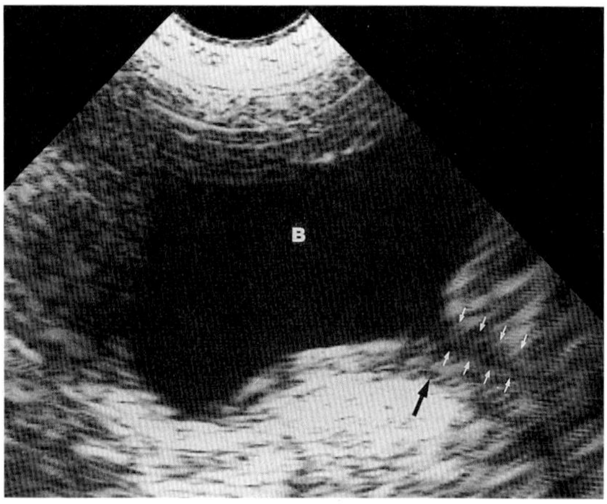

D

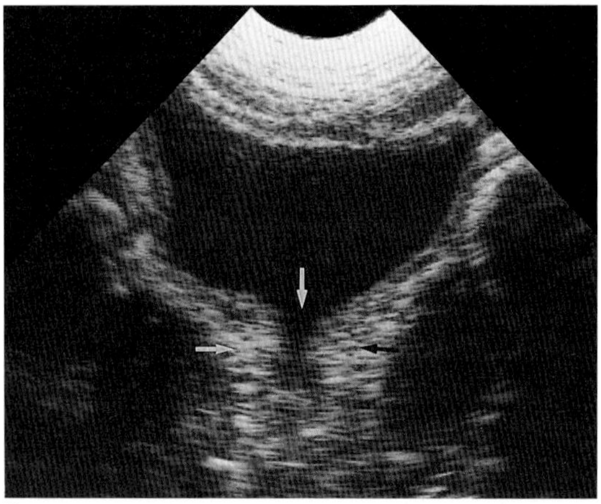

E

12–2 Normal uterus. **(A)** Sagittal scan of uterus in newborn female. Bladder (B) has smooth thin wall. Uterine length is 3.5 cm, with a fundus to cervix ratio of 1:2. Endometrial lining is slightly thickened and echogenic, owing to *in utero* maternal hormonal stimulation. (Open arrow = fundus; large arrow = cervix; small arrows = endometrial lining.) **(B)** Sagittal scan of bladder (B) and uterus (arrow) in prepubertal female. Uterus (arrow) is 2.5 cm long, with the fundus to cervix ratio 1:1 and no stimulation of the endometrial lining. **(C)** Sagittal scan of uterus in mature female. Uterus is 7 cm long with a fundus to cervix ratio of 3:1. Patient is premenstrual, evidenced by thick bright endometrial lining (small arrow). (B = bladder; open arrow = fundus; large arrow = cervix.) (Reprinted, by permission, from Rosenberg HK: Sonography of the pediatric urinary tract. *In* Coleman B. (ed.): *Genitourinary Ultrasound*. © 1988 Igaku-Shoin, New York, NY.) **(D)** Sagittal scan of bladder in prepubertal male child. At base of bladder (B), a relatively anechoic channel is identified (white arrows), representing posterior urethra as it courses through prostate (black arrow). **(E)** Transverse view of bladder in prepubertal male demonstrating posterior urethra (white arrow) as it courses through prostate gland (black arrows).

graphy and the risk of evoking congestive heart failure or dehydration due to the high osmolality of intravenous contrast. In the neonate particularly, glomerular filtration is normally markedly reduced, owing to the immaturity of the outer cortical nephrons. This limits the ability of the neonatal kidney to filter contrast material through the glomeruli and concentrate it, making excretory urography a suboptimal imaging modality in this age group.

In the neonate with renal agenesis, the adrenal gland occupies the renal fossa and assumes a very slender, reniform configuration (Fig. 12–3A). The medullary stroma appears as slender echogenic linear densities within the diffusely hy-

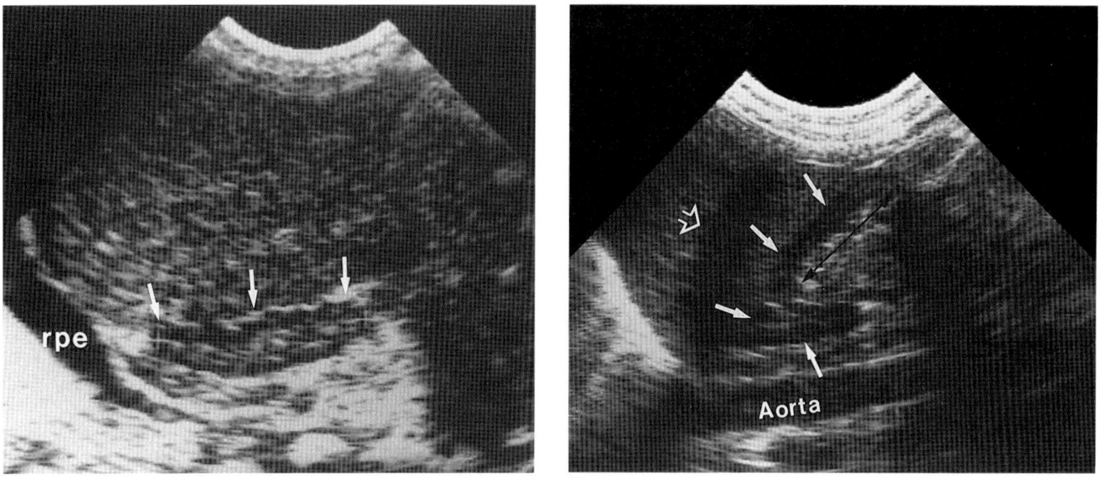

A B

12–3 Renal agenesis. **(A)** Newborn infant with no urine output. Coronal view of right renal fossa shows absence of kidney. Adrenal gland (white arrows) assumes a longitudinal orientation and appears as a slender reniform structure with generally hypoechoic parenchyma and echogenic linear medullary stripes. (rpe = right pleural effusion.) **(B)** Rudimentary kidney. Newborn infant with no urine output. Coronal view of left kidney; double-headed black arrow indicates small (2-cm length) echogenic nondescript kidney flanked by normally positioned adrenal gland (white arrows). (Open arrow = rib artifact.) (Reprinted, by permission, from Rosenberg HK, Sherman NH, Boyle G: Sonography in the neonate. *Ultrasound Quarterly* 16(2):91–150, © 1988, Raven Press, New York, NY.)

poechoic adrenal parenchyma. Occasionally, infants with renal failure have tiny echogenic rudimentary kidneys flanked by the adrenal glands superiorly and anteriorly (Fig. 12–3B). Poorly functioning kidneys may be due to renal dysplasia in which the kidneys may be small, normal, or enlarged with diffusely increased bright echogenicity, and often containing scattered cysts.

In the older child with renal failure due to diffuse medical renal disease that is glomerular, interstitial, or infiltrative, nonspecific types of parenchymal abnormalities are seen with ultrasound. Medical renal disease is usually manifested by enlarged kidneys, increased cortical echogenicity, and accentuated corticomedullary junctions. Interstitial nephritis in children causes enlarged kidneys with overall increased parenchymal echogenicity. Occasionally, bright echogenicity in the medullary pyramids of patients with medical renal disease is observed. This may be due to precipitation of Tamm-Horsfall protein or other material such as calcium in the tubules, renal tubular acidosis, acute tubular necrosis, medullary sponge kidney, or nephrocalcinosis (Fig. 12–4). When renal failure is due to obstruction, excretory urography and nuclear scanning may not visualize the kidney, even on delayed images. Sonography usually can identify the level of obstruction (ureteropelvic junction, ureteral, ureterovesical junction, bladder neck, or urethral). Although urinary tract obstruction in children is usually secondary to congenital anomalies, ultrasound can reveal other etiologies such as stones and neoplasms.

Congenital Anomalies

Infants with multiple congenital anomalies, such as Potter's facies, imperforate anus, hypo-

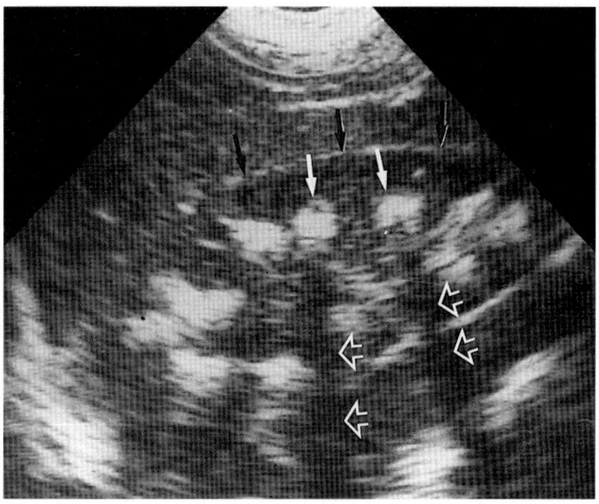

12–4 Nephrocalcinosis. Nineteen-year-old male with lifetime history of renal tubular acidosis. Renal cortex shows normal hypoechoic appearance (small black arrows). The medullary pyramids are diffusely and brightly echogenic (white arrows), with shadowing of ultrasound beam (open arrows) consistent with nephrocalcinosis.

spadias or epispadias, and exstrophy have a higher incidence of congenital anomalies and should be screened with ultrasound. In babies with ambiguous genitalia, ultrasonography can identify a uterus and aid in gender assignment.

Abdominal and Renal Masses

Sonography should be the first step in evaluating infants and children with clinical suspicion of an abdominal mass. Overdistension of the bladder and renal ectopia may masquerade as a neoplasm, but can easily be identified with ultrasound. In the newborn, an abdominal mass is most frequently due to either hydroureteronephrosis or multicystic dysplastic kidney (Potter type II); ultrasound can easily differentiate one from the other and from suprarenal or paravertebral masses. If a mass is caused by ureteropelvic junction obstruction, the pelvocaliceal system will be dilated. All of the dilated calices can be shown to communicate with the renal pelvis, which is the largest and most medially located cystic structure (Fig. 12–5A) (Pope et al. 1980). Renal parenchyma, even when extremely thin, can be identified.

Multicystic Dysplastic Kidney

The ultrasonic features of multicystic dysplastic kidney include nonmedial location of the largest cyst; multiple oval or round cysts of varying sizes, most of which do not communicate; no identifiable renal sinus; tissue between the cysts that is often echogenic and may contain tiny cystic spaces; and the absence of parenchymal renal tissue (Fig. 12–5B). An anomaly develops in the contralateral kidney in 25% of cases, most often a form of hydronephrosis.

Classic multicystic kidney disease (Potter type II) results from complete ureteral obstruction, usually before the first 8–10 weeks of fetal life. Because there is interference with ureteral branching, the division of the collecting tubules is decreased, and induction and maturation of the nephrons are inhibited. The terminal portions of the enlarged collecting tubules develop into cysts, which are joined by small connective tissue cords.

Incomplete obstruction occurring after the 36th gestational week, when nephrogenesis is complete, causes internal hydronephrosis with dilatation of the pelvocaliceal system, a form of ureteropelvic junction obstruction. Nephrons and ducts are normally developed in this situation, and there is no evidence of dysgenesis. However, when incomplete obstruction occurs between the 10th and 36th gestational weeks, the results are variable, with different degrees of cyst formation, pelvocaliceal dilatation, and dysplastic parenchymal changes. This combination of abnormalities is referred to as the hydronephrotic form of multicystic dysplastic kidney (Fig. 12–5C).

Solid Masses in the Newborn

Solid renal masses are rare in the newborn and, when present, are most likely due to congenital mesoblastic nephroma, a predominantly mesenchymal benign renal neoplasm (Fig. 12–5D). This tumor has also been referred to as fetal renal hamartoma, fibroma, leiomyomatous hamartoma, and leiomyoma. Mesoblastic nephroma is generally a solid infiltrating mass, but a cystic variant has been reported. There is an increased incidence of maternal polyhydramnios and premature delivery.

Unlike Wilms's tumor, no capsule exists between the tumor and the compressed normal kidney. Typically, there is no lobulation, hemorrhage, or necrosis. Histologically, mesoblastic nephroma consists of whorled sheets of connective tissue cells. The tumor cells are elongated and spindle shaped without nuclear pleomorphism. The cytoplasm is eosinophilic, and nests of abnormal tubules (often cystic and dysplastic) and glomeruli are present within the depths of the tumor. Mitotic figures may be seen. Vascular spaces of variable size are present within the neoplasm. Mesoblastic nephroma is usually a benign tumor and is cured by nephrectomy.

Cysts

Benign renal cysts are rare in children, especially in the neonate, but may present as a mass (Fig. 12–6). The following sonographic criteria must be met to make a correct diagnosis: observation of an anechoic mass with a smooth posterior wall, posterior wall enhancement, and good transmission of sound waves. The simple renal cyst is usually solitary and unilocular, and does not communicate with the renal collecting system. There is generally no family history of renal cystic disease. Conservative management is recommended.

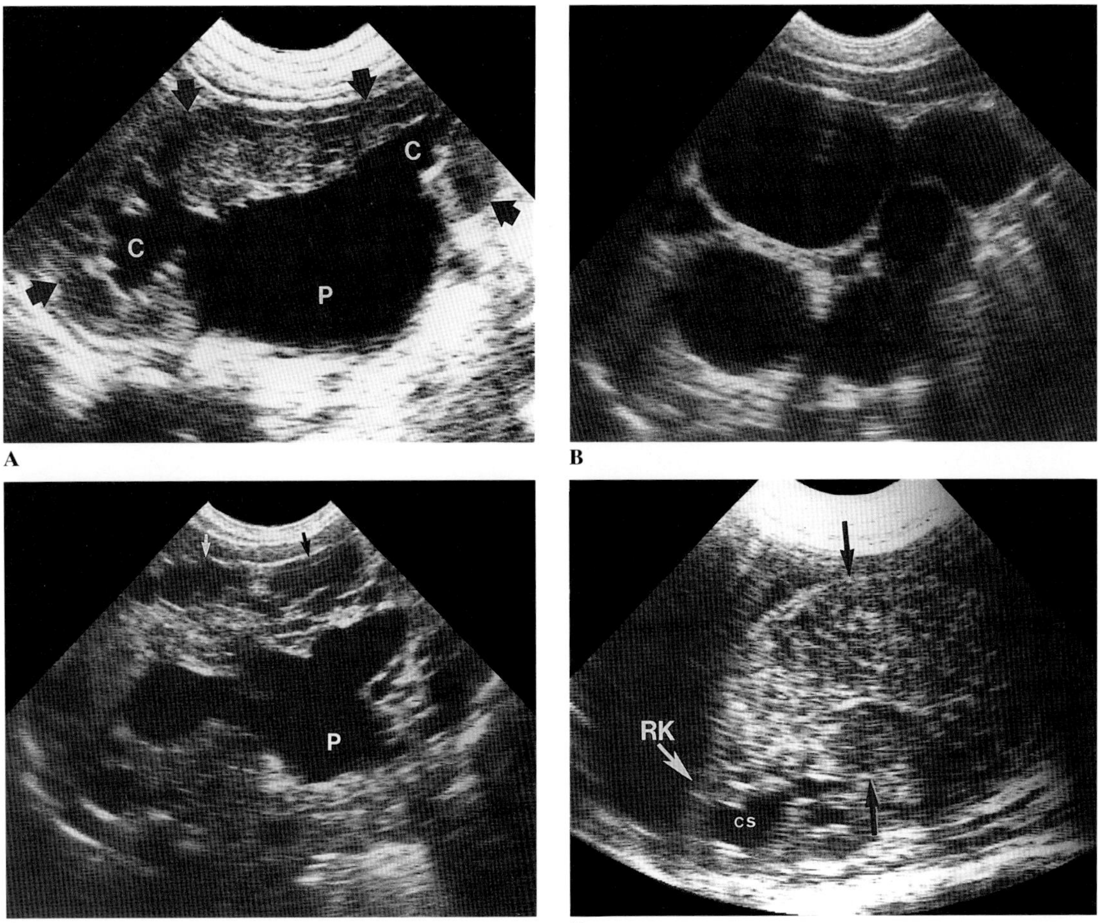

12–5 Renal mass in infant. **(A)** Ureteropelvic junction obstruction. Infant with left flank mass: moderate dilation of intrarenal collecting system with all of the cystic structures communicating with the medially located dilated renal pelvis, which is the most medially located cystic structure. Definite renal parenchyma is present (black arrows). (C = calices; P = pelvis.) **(B)** Multicystic dysplastic kidney. Newborn with flank mass: no normal renal parenchyma is identified. Multiple, variable-sized cysts are present throughout kidney, most of which do not communicate. Brightly echogenic septa are interspersed between cysts, consistent with dysplastic tissue. **(C)** Hydronephrotic form of multicystic dysplastic kidney. Dilated pelvocaliceal system (P) is surrounded by multicystic dysplastic renal parenchyma (small arrows). **(D)** Mesoblastic nephroma (fetal renal hamartoma). Newborn with flank mass: large solid echogenic mass (black arrows) arises from midpole of right kidney (RK), causing dilation and splaying of intrarenal collecting system (cs). (**D** reprinted, by permission, from Rosenberg HK: Sonography of pediatric urinary tract abnormalities: Part I. *AUA Update Series 5* [Lesson 35], © 1986.)

However, if the child has discomfort due to the size of the cyst, ultrasound guided percutaneous puncture can be accomplished safely. It is important to differentiate simple cysts from the cystic mass caused by an obstruction of a duplicated collecting system to the upper pole.

A parapelvic cyst arising in the hilus of the kidney is rare; it does not communicate with the

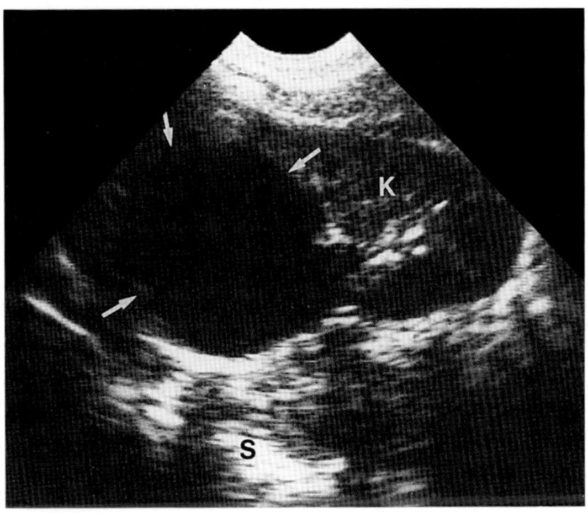

12–6 Simple renal cyst. Prone view of kidney shows rounded anechoic area (arrows) occupying upper pole with strong back wall echoes and good through-transmission of sound waves (S); these are characteristic features of simple renal cyst.

collecting system. It may be an incidental finding, may present as an abdominal mass, or be associated with urinary tract infection. Parapelvic cysts are usually medially placed cystic masses with an echogenic wall. The pelvocaliceal echo complex is displaced and, on rare occasions, may be dilated as a result of a mass effect and partial obstruction due to the location of the cyst.

Urinoma/Bladder Obstruction

Urinoma is an unusual cause of abdominal mass in a neonate or young child. This echo-free fluid collection around the kidney most often results from severe urinary tract obstruction, although occasionally from trauma.

Posterior urethral valve is the most common cause of severe urinary tract obstruction in male infants (McAlister 1984). It is usually due to fusion of the normal urethral folds and consists of a flap of mucosa in the anterior urethral wall of the posterior urethra that has a slitlike opening below the verumontanum. Fifty percent of patients with posterior urethral valve present with symptoms before 3 months of age and 75% within the first year.

Urinary tract infection is the most common presenting sign at all ages. Urinary dribbling (poor stream), failure to thrive, respiratory distress, urinary ascites, and acute urinary retention have been noted in affected children less than 1 year old. Between ages 1 and 5, additional symptoms of acute epididymitis or perinephric abscess may occur. Sonographic findings in posterior urethral valve patients include bilateral hydroureteronephrosis with tortuous ureters; abnormal renal texture in most patients (loss of corticomedullary junction due to reflux or obstructive nephropathy or diffusely echogenic parenchyma due to renal dysplasia); thick-walled, trabeculated bladder; and dilated posterior urethra observed either with suprapubic or perineal sonography. Voiding cystourethrography is necessary to confirm the diagnosis, evaluate for reflux, and exclude other types of obstructing urethral lesions.

Polycystic Kidney Disease

Bilateral flank masses in the neonate, in the presence of poor renal function, are most often due to infantile polycystic kidney disease (Potter type I), a genetic disorder with autosomal recessive inheritance (Fig. 12–7 A). The kidneys maintain their reniform configuration and have brightly increased echogenicity throughout both renal cortex and medulla (Metreweli, Garel 1980). The calyceal systems and renal margins are poorly delineated. Because the cysts are so small, the fluid-filled spaces cannot usually be seen individually, but provide a myriad of reflecting surfaces resulting in the hyperechoic appearance. The cysts are usually 1–8 mm, although occasionally larger. Characteristically, there is cystic dilation and hyperplasia of the collecting tubules. In addition,

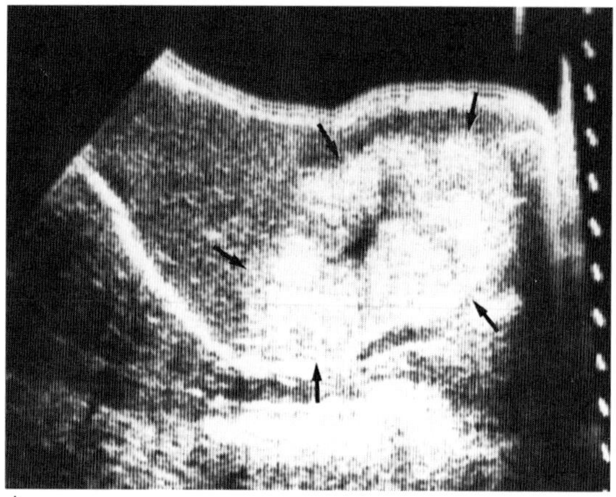

A

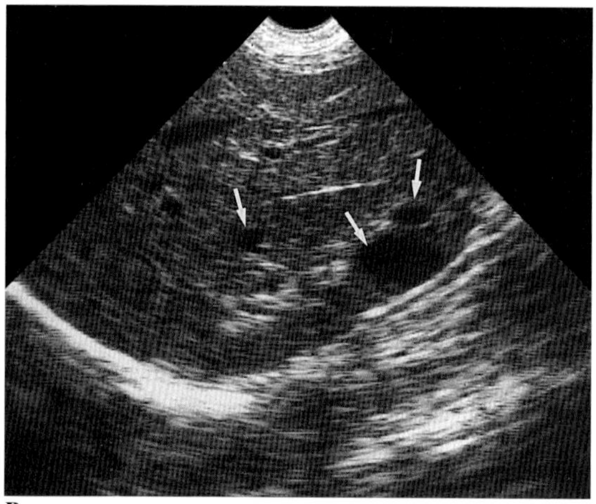

B

12–7 Polycystic disease. **(A)** Infantile polycystic kidney disease. Newborn with bilateral flank masses and poor urine output: coronal view of right kidney (arrows) demonstrating diffusely echogenic renal parenchyma, indistinct renal outline, and normal-size intrarenal collecting system. Overall increased echogenicity is due to a myriad of reflecting surfaces secondary to multiple tiny cysts. **(B)** Adult-type polycystic kidney disease. Coronal view of kidney screened in child with family history of adult-type polycystic disease demonstrates several small intraparenchymal cysts (arrows). (**D** reprinted, by permission, from Rosenberg HK: Sonography of pediatric urinary tract abnormalities: Part II. *AUA Update Series 5* [Lesson 35], © 1986.)

there may be periportal fibrosis of the liver with increased hepatic parenchymal echogenicity and decreased visualization of peripheral portal venous vasculature. Splenomegaly due to portal hypertension may occur. Cysts may also be identified in the liver and pancreas.

Juvenile polycystic kidney disease is part of the spectrum of the infantile form of polycystic disease. Infants most often present with renal failure, whereas the older children develop systemic hypertension or portal hypertension with esophageal varices. As with infantile polycystic kidney disease, the kidneys are diffusely echogenic due to ectatic tubules.

Nephromegaly due to Potter type–III adult-type polycystic kidney disease is not usually evident until late childhood or mid-adulthood. The inheritance pattern of this type–III cystic kidney disease is autosomal dominant. Cysts may occur at any point along the nephrons or collecting ducts. Sonography can be used to detect small cysts in asymptomatic patients, to provide information for genetic counseling, and to identify patients who require frequent monitoring (Fig. 12–7B). Clinical symptoms such as hypertension and urinary tract infection usually do not occur until ages 50 or 60, with renal failure usually appearing 10 years after the initial symptoms.

Vascular Thrombosis

Renal vein thrombosis should be considered when enlargement of one or both kidneys occurs in the presence of hematuria and thrombocytopenia. Infants of diabetic mothers and infants with diarrhea and dehydration, congenital heart disease, acute blood loss, sepsis, asphyxia, or shock have a higher incidence of renal vein thrombosis. Varying renal parenchymal appearances have been described, including hyperechoic, hypoechoic, and a patchwork-type echogenicity.

A clot in the inferior vena cava and renal vein is difficult to see in a small infant, although duplex Doppler scanning can be helpful in assessing the presence and pattern of blood flow in these vessels. Doppler ultrasound is equally important in the evaluation of infants with suspicion of renal ischemia (Fig. 12–8A–C). As a result of decreased renal arterial blood flow, the kidneys will enlarge initially, owing to swelling and edema. The parenchymal echogenicity may be hyperechoic or hypoechoic, or have a heterogeneous appearance. A clot in the aorta and renal artery may be seen better when occlusion is incomplete because anechoic blood surrounds the clot. With complete thrombosis, the vessel and clot appear isoechoic in comparison with the surrounding structures, and visualization is difficult. Nuclear renal flow studies are especially helpful in corroborating the duplex Doppler impression. Follow-up sonograms may show renal shrinkage after significant ischemia.

Nephroblastomatosis

Nephroblastomatosis is caused by the persistence of immature renal tissue beyond the cessation of nephrogenesis. It is rarely the underlying etiology for unilateral or bilateral nephromegaly. There are two patterns of nephroblastomatosis: diffuse and multifocal.

Diffuse nephroblastomatosis occurs in infancy and early childhood. In the pancortical (pannephric) form, nephroblastomatosis completely replaces renal parenchyma, and death occurs early. In the superficial form, a rind of nephroblastomatosis surrounds the normal renal cortex and medulla. This type is purely epithelial, but it may also contain blastemal and stromal elements.

The multifocal form of nephroblastomatosis is found in the subcapsular cortex and along the column of Bertin. These lesions may occur in children of all ages and may not be associated with enlargement of the kidney. Wilms's tumor, including multifocal or bilateral tumor, is frequently associated with multifocal nephroblastomatosis.

Wilms's Tumor

Wilms's tumor (nephroblastoma) is the most common malignant renal and intra-abdominal tumor in childhood and often presents as an asymptomatic abdominal mass in children ages 2–5 years (Fig. 12–9A). Many patients have hypertension and hematuria. Wilms's tumor is an embryonal tumor that consists of neoplastic blastemal tissue differentiating toward epithelial and stromal derivatives in its classic triphasic form. Heterotopic stromal elements, including cartilage and striated muscle, may develop. The monomorphic Wilms's tumors may be either epithelial or stromal in nature, with a low local invasive and metastatic tendency.

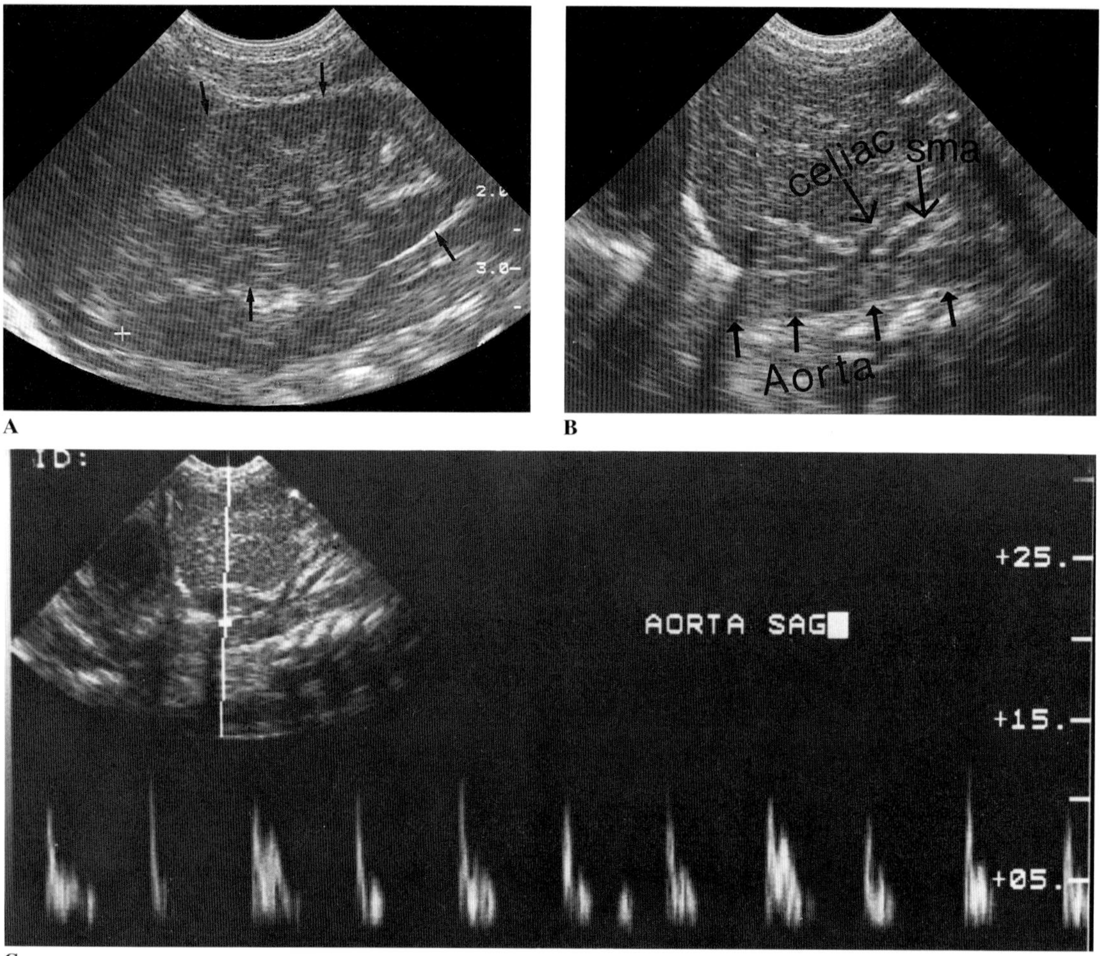

12–8 Renal ischemia. **(A)** Newborn with history of umbilical artery catheter, decreased urine output, and decreased perfusion to lower extremities. Left kidney (arrows) is enlarged (length = 5.37 cm), with diffusely abnormal heterogeneous texture suggesting ischemia. **(B)** Sagittal scan of aorta demonstrating echogenic material within aorta, consistent with intravascular clot. **(C)** Duplex/Doppler sonogram with signal obtained in upper abdominal aorta, showing no diastolic flow, consistent with increased resistance due to intravascular clot. There was no flow into left kidney. (**A, B,** and **C** reprinted, by permission, from Rosenberg HK, Sherman NH, Boyle G: Sonography in the neonate. *Ultrasound Quarterly* 6(2):91–150, © 1988, Raven Press, New York, NY.)

Ultrasound can be used reliably to establish the kidney as the organ of origin, by observing synchronous motion of the mass with the remaining normal parts of the kidney during real-time scanning (Jaffe et al. 1981). Although Wilms's tumor is essentially a solid mass, sonography often demonstrates small cystic areas due to hemorrhage or necrosis. The tumor is bilateral in 5%–10% of patients, and the opposite kidney should be carefully scanned with a high-resolution technique to look for small tumors. Ultrasound can evaluate for regional adenopathy, hepatic metastases, and tumor thrombus in the renal vein, inferior vena cava, and right atrium (Fig. 12–9B, C). Duplex Doppler ultrasound plays an important role in the evaluation of vessels prone to tumor thrombus. Sonography can monitor response to therapy.

There is a higher incidence of Wilms's tumor in children younger than 6 years old who are born with aniridia, hemihypertrophy, Beckwith-Wiedemann syndrome, or nephroblastomatosis. These high-risk patients should be screened with ultrasound at regular 3-month intervals until age 6, and then yearly.

Other Renal Masses

The nonhereditary multilocular cyst is a rare renal mass seen in children less than 2 years old (Fig. 12–10). As with Wilms's tumor, the patients

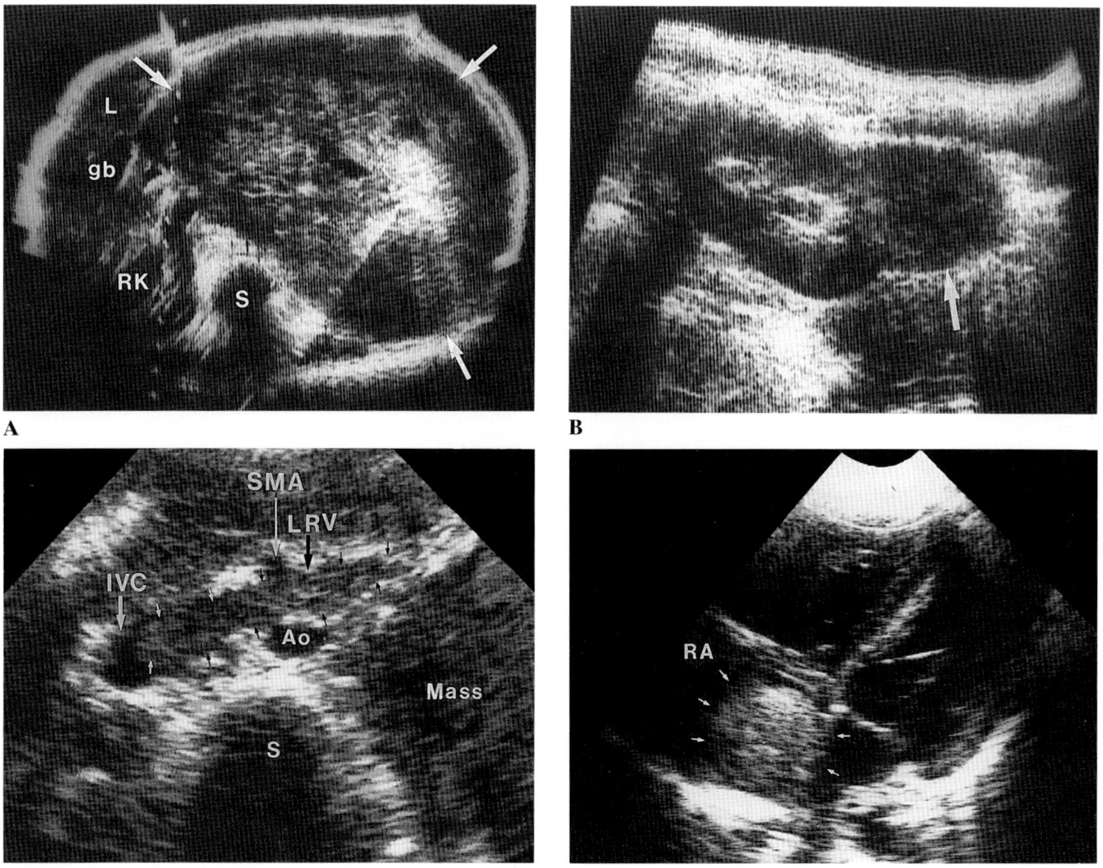

A B C D

12–9 Wilms's tumor. **(A)** Four-year-old child with large asymptomatic abdominal mass. Transverse static image demonstrates complex, mainly solid mass occupying left renal fossa (white arrows) extending across midline, causing shift of the liver (L) and gallbladder (gb) to the right. Mass contains anechoic areas suggesting hemorrhage and necrosis as well as more echogenic areas suggesting hemorrhage. S = spine; RK = right kidney. **(B)** Exophytic Wilms's tumor. Five-year-old female with bilateral Wilms's tumor. Prone sonogram shows relatively hypoechoic, exophytic solid mass (arrow) arising from lower pole of right kidney. (**A** and **B** reprinted, by permission, from Rosenberg HK, Sonography of the pediatric urinary tract. *In* Coleman B (ed.): *Genitourinary Ultrasound.* © 1988, Igaku-Shoin, New York, NY.) **(C)** Five-year-old female, with Wilms's tumor thrombus in left renal vein and inferior vena cava. Transverse view of left renal vein shows large left renal mass with tumor extension (tiny arrows) into left renal vein (LRV) and inferior vena cava (IVC). Left renal vein passes between aorta (Ao) and superior mesenteric artery (SMA). (S = spine.) **(D)** Subxyphoid view of heart in 8-year-old with large left-sided Wilms's tumor. Extension of intracaval tumor thrombus (arrows) is noted in right atrium (RA). (**C** and **D** reprinted, by permission, from Rosenberg HK: Sonography of pediatric urinary tract abnormalities: Part II. *AUA Update Series 5* [Lesson 36], © 1986.)

often present with an abdominal mass, abdominal pain, hematuria, or hypertension. The well-encapsulated mass is multiseptated, cystic, bulky, and sharply separated from the surrounding normal tissue. It consists of multiple noncommunicating cysts with brightly echogenic septations and solid tissue interspersed between the cysts. Usually the normal renal tissue and the displaced, splayed collecting system can be identified. A multilocular cyst is generally benign, although some may contain partially differentiated Wilms's tumor.

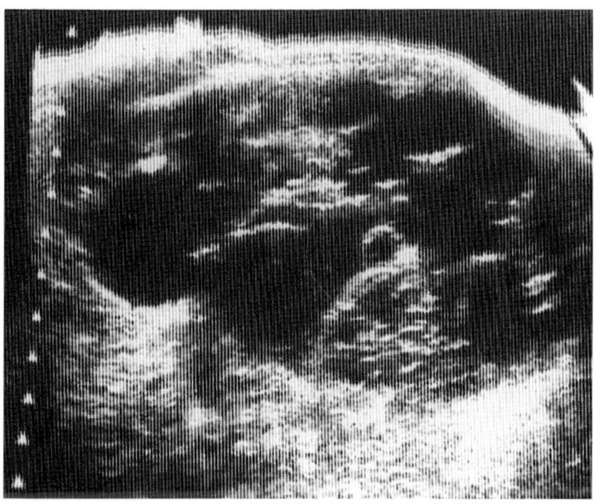

12–10 Multilocular renal cyst. Prone view of renal fossa in 6-month-old male with rapidly growing flank mass shows multiseptated cystic mass virtually replacing left kidney.

Hypernephroma (renal cell carcinoma, adenocarcinoma) is rare in patients less than 10 years of age. The patients may present with a palpable mass, pain, or hematuria. Typical sonographic appearance is an ill-defined, slightly hyperechoic intrarenal mass, occasionally containing calcifications and distorting the intrarenal collecting system (Fig. 12–11). It may be confused with other entities, such as ischemia, inflammation, or swelling following trauma. Contrast-enhanced computed tomography can help confirm the sonographic impression. In the clear-cell type of renal carcinoma, the cells are large and round with a strikingly clear or vacuolated cytoplasm due to the presence of cholesterol and glycogen. The cellular arrangement may be a cystic papillary form, an alveolar arrangement of solid cords, or tubular. Renal cell carcinoma is less responsive than Wilms's tumor to multimodal therapy.

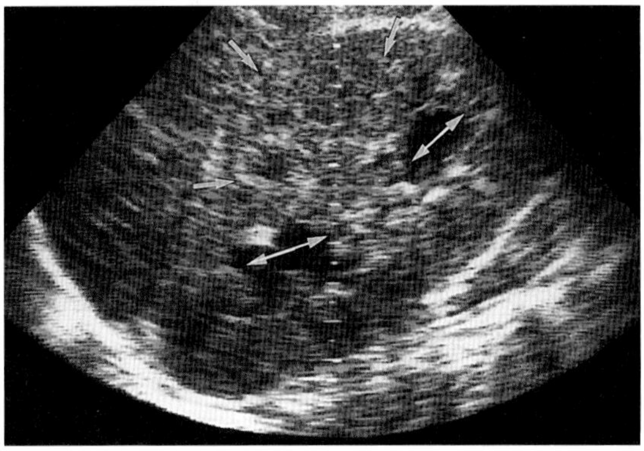

12–11 Hypernephroma. Thirteen-year-old male with right flank pain, hematuria, malaise, weight loss, and weakness. Ill-defined relatively echogenic mass (black arrows) in midpole of right kidney, causing dilation of intrarenal collecting system (double-headed white arrows).

Multiple renal masses due to angiomyolipomas are common in children with tuberous sclerosis. They are usually echogenic, owing to a high fat content. Hemorrhage and necrosis within the tumors may cause symptoms. Computed tomography can confirm the fat content of these benign tumors.

Children with leukemia or lymphoma may present with, or subsequently develop, bilateral renomegaly due to diffuse infiltration. Often, the kidneys are diffusely echogenic and may demonstrate accentuated corticomedullary junction due to leukemic infiltration or associated uric acid nephropathy. With lymphoma, especially Burkitt's, hypoechoic masses within the renal parenchyma may be seen (Fig. 12–12).

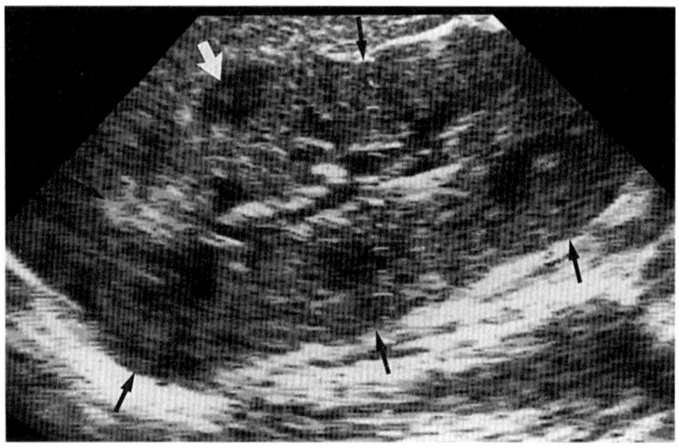

12–12 Lymphoma/leukemia syndrome. Six-year-old with bilateral flank masses in presence of acute lymphoblastic leukemia. Coronal view of right kidney showing renomegaly (black arrows), overall increased cortical echogenicity with accentuation of corticomedullary junctions due to leukemic infiltration and uric acid nephropathy, and a focal hypoechoic mass (white arrow) in anterior portion of midpole due to lymphomatous infiltration.

Urinary Infection

Infection is the most frequent urinary tract problem seen in pediatrics. Between 1.5% and 2% of children ages 1–5 years will develop a symptomatic urinary tract infection, most often beginning with infection of bladder urine via the urethra. The introitus of little girls is regularly colonized with bacteria of the colon (especially *E. coli*). One percent of asymptomatic girls ages 2–5 have bacteriuria. Urinary tract infection is less common in males, most likely because of the greater length of the male urethra.

If a child is acutely ill with urosepsis, sonography should be done immediately (Ben-Ami 1984). Renal sonography can help differentiate hydronephrosis, pyonephrosis, focal lobar nephronia, renal abscess, perinephric abscess, or xanthogranulomatous pyelonephritis. Pyonephrosis can be suspected when the urine in the collecting system and bladder appears echogenic. Proteinuria and hematuria can have the same appearance, but urinalysis differentiates these. Clumped areas of bright echogenicity within the collecting system can indicate fungus balls such as candidiasis. Focal lobar nephronia usually appears as a fairly well-defined hypoechoic mass without cavitation.

Renal abscess is generally a complex, mainly cystic mass that may contain septations or a fluid-debris level. With perinephric abscess, a cystic or complex mass containing debris and septations is seen adjacent to the kidney. Xanthogranulomatous pyelonephritis appears as a complex mass with or without calcifications.

A voiding cystourethrogram should be postponed until the acute infection has subsided. In a child with an uncomplicated urinary tract infection without evidence of urosepsis, nuclear cystography is recommended. Although the use of sonography in the presence of vesicoureteral reflux is controversial, in the author's experience sonography alone is sufficient to evaluate renal size, configuration, position, texture, focal or diffuse scarring, the size and configuration of the collecting systems, bladder size, thickness and smoothness of the bladder wall, degree of bladder emptying, and evidence of dilatation of the posterior urethra. In patients who are candidates for ureteroneocystostomy procedures, conventional voiding cystourethrography and excretory urography may be needed.

During real-time sonography, evidence of significant vesicoureteral reflux may be obtained when the ureterovesical junction is patulous and reversed ureteral peristalsis is observed (Fig. 12–13 A, B). The use of sterile saline for cystography during real-time observation of the renal pelvis has been advocated as a means of identifying significant (grade III or higher) vesicoureteral reflux without X-ray filming or nuclear scintigraphy. The microbubbles in the water can be observed as they reflux from the bladder via the ureter into the renal pelvis. Following surgical correction for vesicoureteral reflux, sonography can be used for follow-up evaluation of the urinary tract.

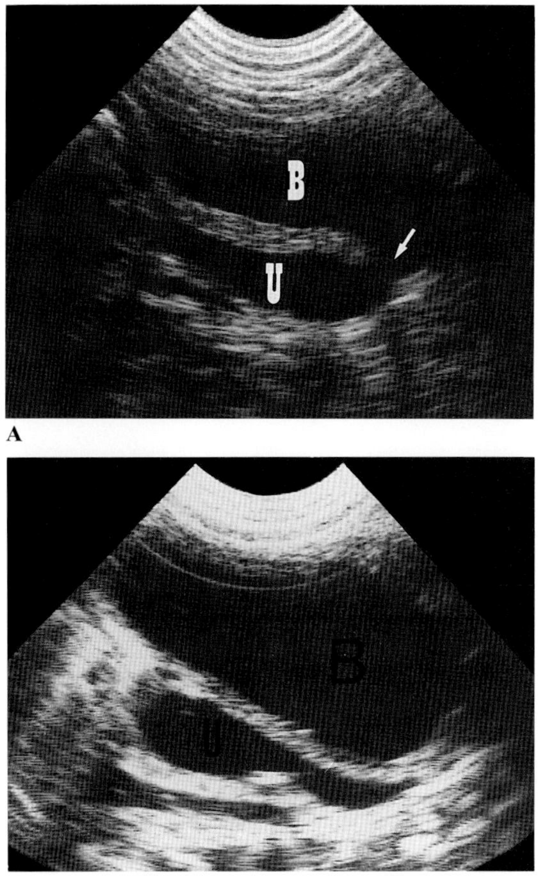

A

B

12–13 Urinary tract infection. **(A)** Sagittal view of bladder (B), demonstrating patulous ureterovesical junction (arrow) with dilation of distal right ureter (U) consistent with reflux. **(B)** Ureterovesical junction obstruction. Sagittal view of bladder (B) showing tapered distal dilated right ureter (U). (**A** und **B** reprinted, by permission, from Rosenberg HK, Sherman NH, Boyle G: Sonography in the neonate. *Ultrasound Quarterly* 6(2):91–150, © 1988, Raven Press, New York, NY.)

Duplication Anomalies

Duplication of the collecting systems is the most common major anomaly of the genitourinary tract, occurring in 2.7%–4.2% of children (Fig. 12–14 A–C). Duplication is often demonstrated by sonography. This anomaly most often presents with urinary tract infection. The lower pole ureter enters the bladder at the trigone, and vesicoureteral reflux into the lower pole system frequently occurs. The upper pole ureter enters the bladder inferior to the trigone (Fig. 12–14 D). Ectopic insertion of the upper pole ureter is more common in girls, with the ureter draining into the vesical neck or beyond the sphincter into the urethra, vagina, or uterus; hence, urinary dribbling is a frequent complaint.

Urinary incontinence does not occur in males because the ectopic ureter ends proximal to the external urinary sphincter, in the vesical neck, prostatic portion of the urethra, seminal vesicle, vas deferens, or ejaculatory duct.

Ureterocele

Ureterocele is the cystic dilation of the submucosal segment of the intravesical portion of the ureter, due to stenosis of the orifice. Ureterocele

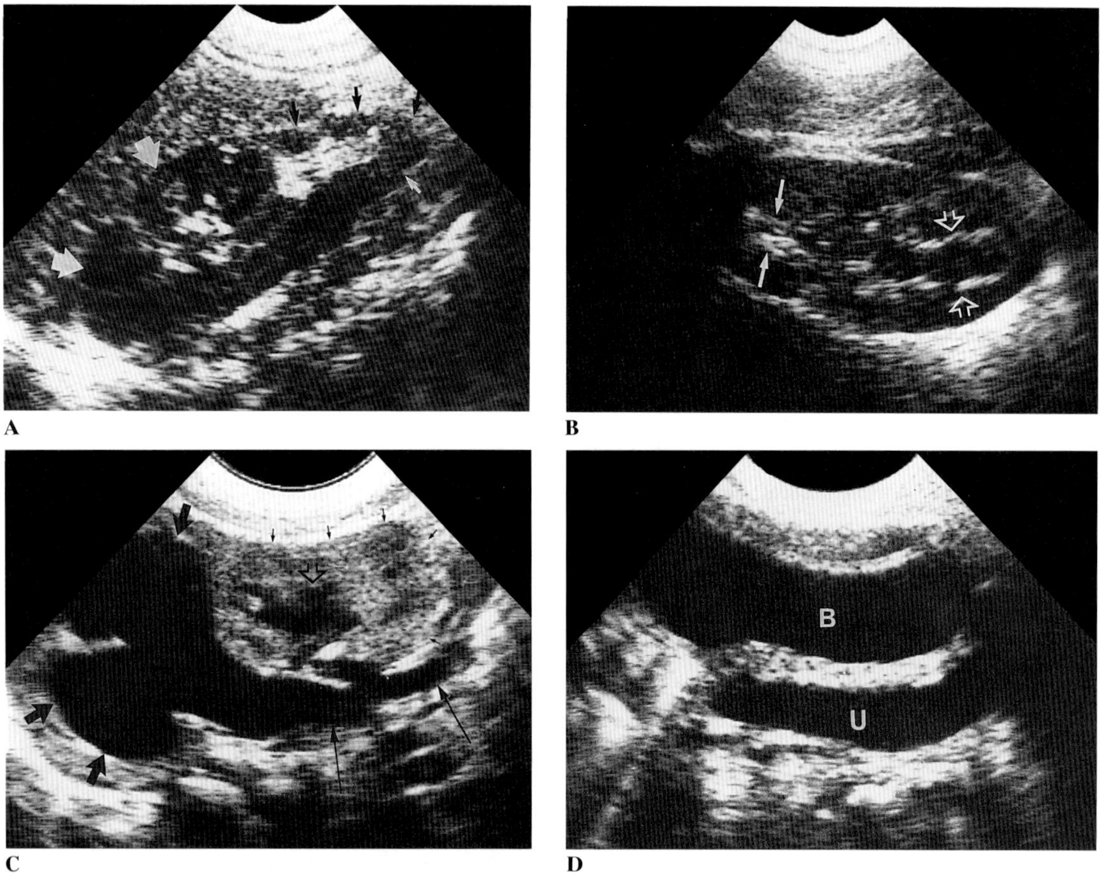

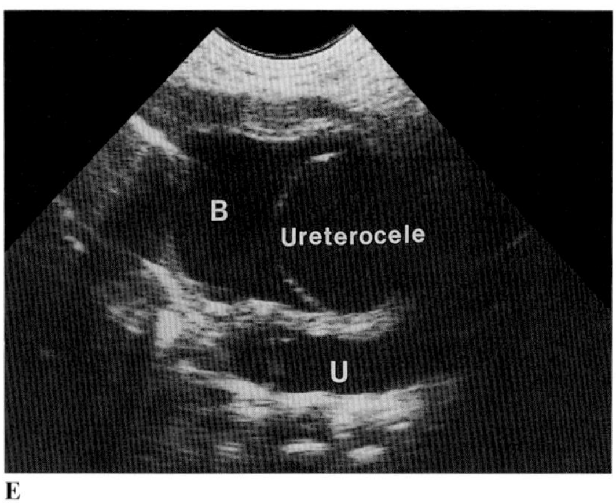

12–14 Urinary tract infection/duplication anomalies. **(A)** Parenchymal scarring. Coronal view of right kidney in young child, showing duplicated collecting systems with normal upper pole parenchyma (white arrows) and scarring and contraction of lower pole (black arrows) due to reflux. **(B)** Duplication anomaly: Prone view of right kidney in young child with normal right upper pole collecting system (solid arrows) and separation of renal sinus echoes in lower pole (open arrows) in child with known vesicoureteral reflux into lower pole moiety. **(C)** Coronal view of left kidney in infant demonstrating massive dilation of left upper pole moiety (medium-size black arrows) communicating with tortuous dilated upper pole ureter (long-tailed black arrows). There is no definite identifiable left upper pole parenchyma. Left lower pole shows mild dilatation of intrarenal collecting system (open arrow), either secondary to pressure from upper pole moiety or vesicoureteral reflux. Lower pole parenchyma is normal (smallest arrows). **(D)** Baby with duplication anomaly showing dilated distal ureter (U) inserting ectopically below bladder (B) neck. **(E)** Sagittal view of bladder in baby with duplication anomaly showing dilated distal upper pole ureter (U) communicating with intravesical ureterocele. (B = bladder.) (Reprinted, by permission, from Rosenberg HK, Sonography of the pediatric urinary tract. *In* Coleman B (ed.): *Genitourinary Ultrasound.* © 1988, Igaku-Shoin, New York, NY.)

may occur in the ureter that drains the upper pole of the duplex system and cause marked dilation of the upper pole collecting system (Fig. 12–14E).

Ectopic ureteroceles are most frequently encountered during evaluation of a child for urinary tract infection. Occasionally, a child may present with sepsis, failure to thrive, abdominal pain, or difficulty voiding. A flank or suprapubic mass, flank tenderness, or a perineal mass caused by a prolapsed ureterocele may be found. Sonography can rapidly determine the level of obstruction and obviate the need for excretory urography in patients whose renal function may be abnormal. Nuclear renal scan provides quantitative functional information.

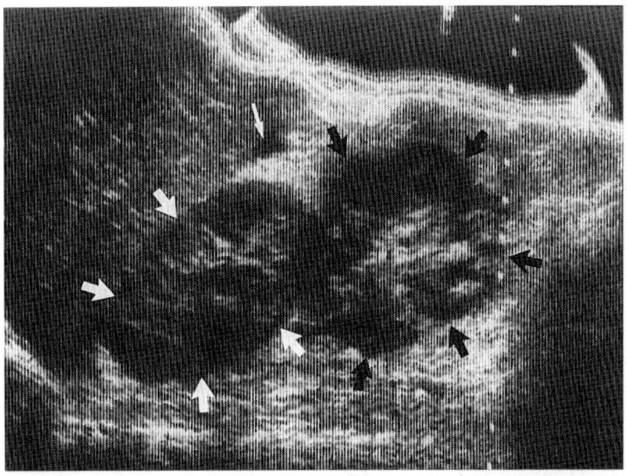

A

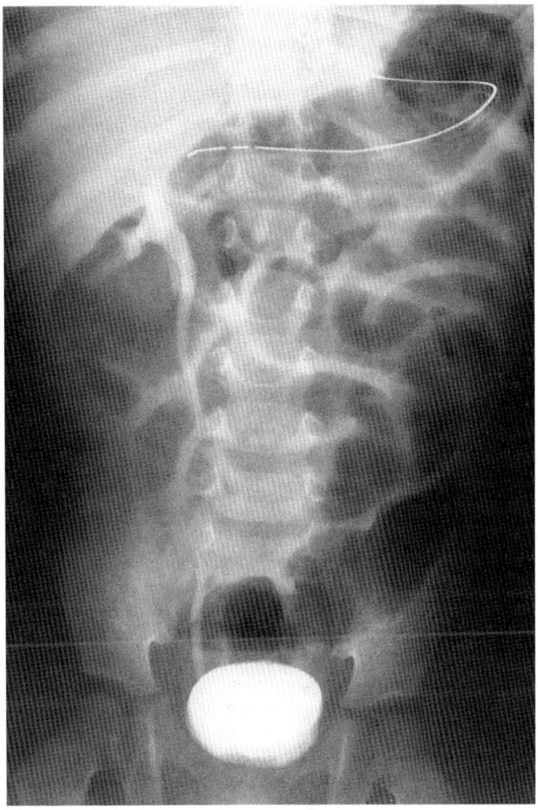

B

12–15 **(A)** Trauma. Coronal view of right abdomen demonstrates normal-appearing kidney in right renal fossa (large white arrows); a crossed unfused renal ectopia (black arrows) is present with evidence of hypoechoic parenchyma; there is also a small amount of ascites (small white arrow). **(B)** Excretory urogram showing function in the normal-sized kidney occupying right renal fossa (arrows). Lack of function in crossed unfused ectopic kidney suggested avulsion of vascular pedicle, which was confirmed at surgery. (**A** and **B** reprinted, by permission, from Rosenberg HK: Traumatic avulsion of the vascular supply of a crossed unfused ectopic kidney: Complementary roles of ultrasonography and intravenous pyelography. *J. Ultrasound Med.* 3 (Feb.):89–91, © 1984, American Institute of Ultrasound in Medicine.)

Hematuria

For children with hematuria not clinically suspected to have resulted from trauma, this author uses sonography as the screening modality. In a traumatized child, excretory urography is recommended as the imaging modality for assessing both structure and function. If a kidney or portion of a kidney fails to visualize on excretory urography, sonography can differentiate a nonfunctioning kidney from unilateral renal agenesis (Fig. 12–15 A, B). If there is clinical suspicion that trauma has occurred to other abdominal and pelvic structures, CT with contrast is recommended; thereafter, this can be followed up with sonography.

Neurogenic Bladder

Patients with spina bifida require yearly surveillance of the urinary tract to identify sequelae of a neurogenic bladder. Sonography is a reliable and accurate replacement for routine excretory urography. The following assessments can be made: renal size and growth; evidence of hydroureteronephrosis due to obstruction or reflux; presence of bladder wall thickening; trabeculation; diverticula formation in the neurogenic bladder; degree of bladder emptying – either spontaneously, with Credé, or with intermittent catheterization; and stones.

Enuresis

In patients with dysfunctional voiding, the bladder wall often appears thickened and trabecu-

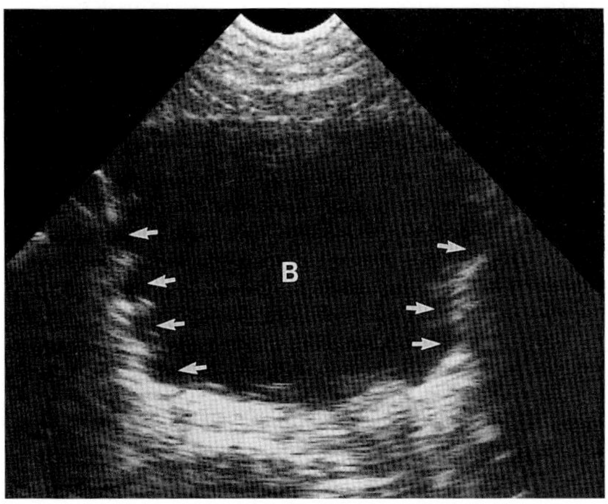

12–16 Dysfunctional voiding. Transverse view of thick-walled trabeculated bladder (B) in a child with dysfunctional voiding. White arrows indicate multiple diverticula.

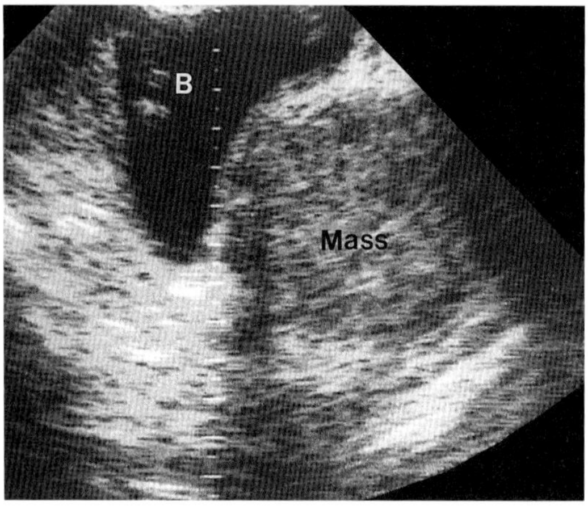

12–17 Rhabdomyosarcoma of the prostate. Sixteen-year-old male with urinary retention. Sagittal view of pelvis demonstrates solid mass arising in prostate gland, causing an indentation on posteroinferior aspect of the urinary bladder (B). (Reprinted, by permission, from Coleman B (ed.): Genitourinary Ultrasound. © 1988, Igaku-Shoin, New York, NY.)

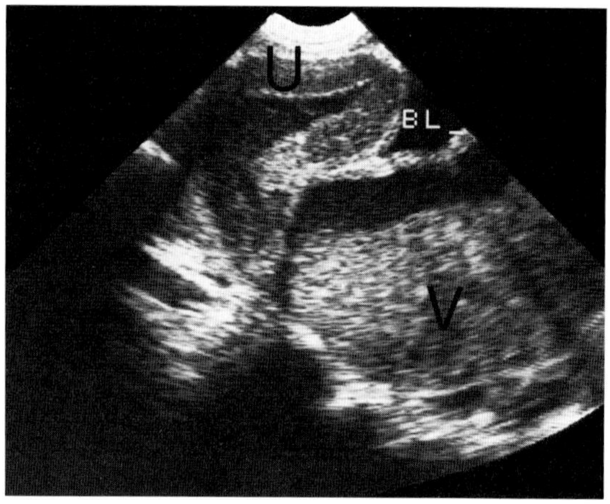

12–18 Hydrometrocolpos. 16-year-old girl with amenorrhea and cyclic pelvic pain. Sagittal view of pelvis demonstrating bladder (BL), obstructed uterus (U), and massively dilated vagina (V). Vagina contains large echogenic fluid debris level consistent with menstrual blood products and mucus. Uterus contains echogenic fluid as well.

lated with diverticula (Fig. 12–16). Following several attempts to void, moderate to large postvoid residuals are demonstrated. The kidneys may be normal in the young child, but without treatment such as intermittent catheterization, patients may develop hydroureteronephrosis and scarring. Occasionally, an ectopic ureter from the upper pole moiety of a duplicated collecting system inserting below the bladder neck or into the vagina may be identified.

Pelvic Masses

Sonography is recommended for evaluation of pelvic masses in infants and children (Kangarloo et al. 1980). The urine-filled bladder acts as a sonic window for the evaluation of the pelvis, bladder wall, uterus, ovaries, vagina, rectum, and prostate. Ultrasound-guided water vaginography and water enema techniques may be necessary.

Pelvic masses are uncommon in the neonate; an overdistended bladder should first be excluded. The differential diagnosis of a neonatal cystic pelvic mass includes ovarian cyst, cystic lymphangioma, hydrocolpos, hydrometrocolpos, anterior meningocele, and rectal duplication. Sarcomas and other solid masses are rare. Teratomas are generally complex, but mainly cystic, and may contain calcifications.

In the older child, rhabdomyosarcoma is the most common tumor of the bladder and prostate (Fig. 12–17). Other solid pelvic masses in the older infant and child are neuroblastoma, chordoma, endodermal sinus tumors, and lymphoma, particularly Burkitt's. Cystic masses include, as in the young infant, a distended bladder, bladder diverticulum, hydrocolpos, hydrometrocolpos (Fig. 12–18), ovarian cysts, and seminal vesicle cysts. Complex masses may be due to endometriosis, teratoma, complex ovarian tumors, and in the sexually active child or teenager, a tubo-ovarian abscess or ectopic pregnancy. In addition, a pelvic kidney and an intrauterine pregnancy can present as a pelvic mass.

Summary

Sonography is the imaging modality of choice for the evaluation of the urinary tract in infants and children. It is cost-effective, noninvasive, does not require ionizing radiation or intravenous contrast material, rarely requires sedation of the child, and is an effective, portable technique.

References

Ben-Ami T: The sonographic evaluation of urinary tract infections in children. *Semin. Ultrasound* 5:19–34, 1984.

Hayden CK, Santa-Cruz FR, Amparo EG: Ultrasonographic evaluation of the renal parenchyma in infancy and childhood. *Radiology* 152:413–417, 1984.

Jaffe MH, White SJ, Silver TM, et al.: Wilms's tumor: Ultrasonic features, pathologic correlation, and diagnostic pitfalls. *Radiology* 140:147–152, 1981.

Kangarloo H, Sarti DA, Sample WF: Ultrasound of the pediatric pelvis. *Semin. Ultrasound* 1:51–60, 1980.

McAlister WH: Demonstration of the dilated prostatic urethra in posterior urethral valve patients. *J. Ultrasound Med.* 3:189–190, 1984.

Metreweli C, Garel L: The echographic diagnosis of infantile renal polycystic disease. *Ann. Radiol.* 23:103–107, 1980.

Pope TL, Alford BA, Buschi AJ, et al.: Nuclear scintigraphy and ultrasound in the diagnosis of congenital ureteropelvic junction obstruction. *J. Urol.* 124:917–918, 1980.

Rosenbaum DM, Korngold E, Teele RL: Sonographic assessment of renal length in normal children. *Am. J. Roentgenol.* 142:467–469, 1984.

Rosenberg HK: Sonography of pediatric urinary tract abnormalities: Part I. *AUA* [American Urological Association] *Update Series 5* (Lesson 35):1–8, 1986.

Rosenberg HK: Sonography of pediatric urinary tract abnormalities: Part II. *AUA [American Urological Association] Update Series 5* (Lesson 36):1–8, 1986.

CHAPTER

13

Integrated Use of Imaging Modalities in the Upper Urinary Tract

Peggy J. Fritzsche, Linda D. Mulder, and Pauline K. Chu

A selective approach to imaging disease of the upper urinary tract can expedite patient care and, at the same time, reduce costs. Certain conditions can be specifically diagnosed by a single test. Others require a more algorithmic sequence. The goal of imaging is to assist the clinician in caring for the patient. This chapter reviews the major applications of excretory urography, ultrasonography, computed tomography (CT), and magnetic resonance (MR) imaging to the upper urinary tract.

Excretory urography is often the first procedure. However, it is not specific and requires iodinated contrast material and ionizing radiation. Ultrasonography is used to differentiate cystic lesions from solid lesions in patients with oliguria and anuria and in the pediatric age group. The limitations of ultrasonography are related to body habitus and technique. Computed tomography effectively characterizes renal and retroperitoneal masses, tumor extent, and renal obstruction. The primary disadvantages of CT are the need for iodinated contrast material and ionizing radiation. Magnetic resonance is useful in tissue characterization and tumor staging.

The cause of the presenting signs and symptoms can usually be determined by integrated use of several imaging modalities. A testing sequence expedites the diagnosis of renal disease (Fig. 13–1).

Anomalies

Agenesis

Renal agenesis is often an incidental radiologic finding. A major clue is the characteristic compensatory hypertrophy of the contralateral kidney. A

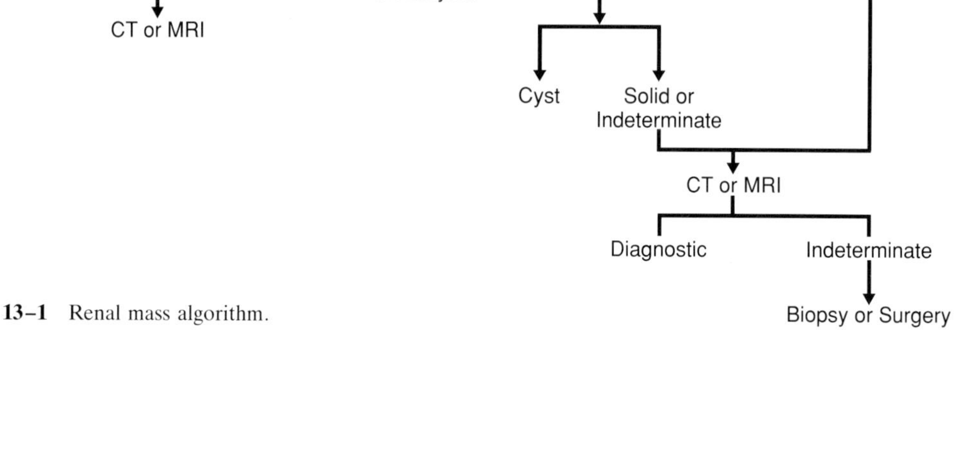

13–1 Renal mass algorithm.

nonvisualizing kidney on urography caused by renal agenesis can be confirmed by ultrasound or CT. Ultrasonography can evaluate the renal fossae, but CT is more effective in evaluating the lower abdomen or pelvis for a small ectopic kidney.

Several anatomic variations are found with renal agenesis or ectopy and are readily demonstrated on CT. The empty renal bed on the right allows posterior displacement of the second portion of the duodenum. On the left side, the splenic flexure, small intestine, and perhaps even the spleen and pancreatic tail may migrate into the unoccupied space. In addition, left-sided renal agenesis may be associated with an abnormally shaped left adrenal gland, either a slender linear shape or possibly elongation of one limb.

Duplication

Duplication of the renal collecting system is easily diagnosed on urography when renal function of both the upper and lower segments is preserved. Reflux into the lower collecting system commonly occurs, and an ectopic ureter with associated ureterocele usually obstructs the upper collecting system. Obstructed duplication may be suspected on the urogram when there is downward displacement of the calices and fewer than the normal number of calices, the so-called drooping lily sign (Fig. 13–2A). Ultrasound is the best method to demonstrate the dilated upper collecting segment, which is seen as a cystic structure just medial to the normal renal parenchyma (Fig. 13–2B). Duplication of the collecting system of the contralateral kidney is a helpful sign, since renal duplication is bilateral in 15% of the cases, and partial duplication is even more frequent.

The correct preoperative diagnosis of a duplicated system with ectopic ureterocele helps the urologist plan the appropriate surgical approach. Therefore, indirect signs of duplication must be evaluated even in a small kidney. The kidney is frequently small, since the parenchyma of the lower collecting moiety may be dysplastic or atrophic secondary to reflux nephropathy. The ureterocele, which occurs in conjunction with the upper collecting moiety, may be visualized as a mass effect on the contrast-filled bladder film of an excretory urogram and as a "cyst within a cyst" on pelvic ultrasound.

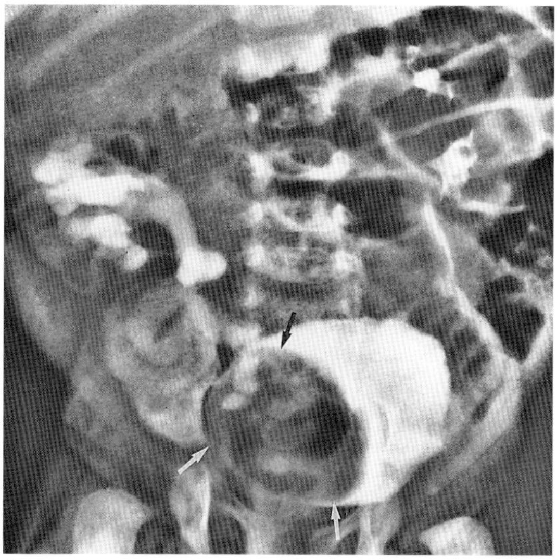

A

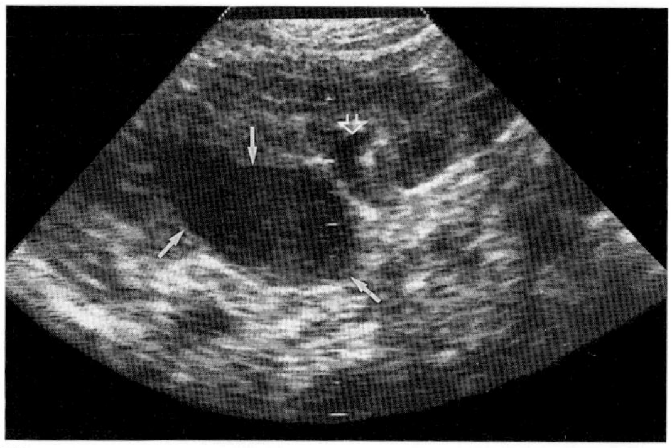

B

13–2 Obstructed duplication. **(A)** Urogram. Note downward displacement of calices on right and large ureterocele (arrows), characteristic of obstructed duplication. **(B)** Longitudinal sonogram in same patient reveals dilated collecting system of obstructed upper moiety as a cystic structure (arrows). Note nondilated lower collecting moiety (open arrow).

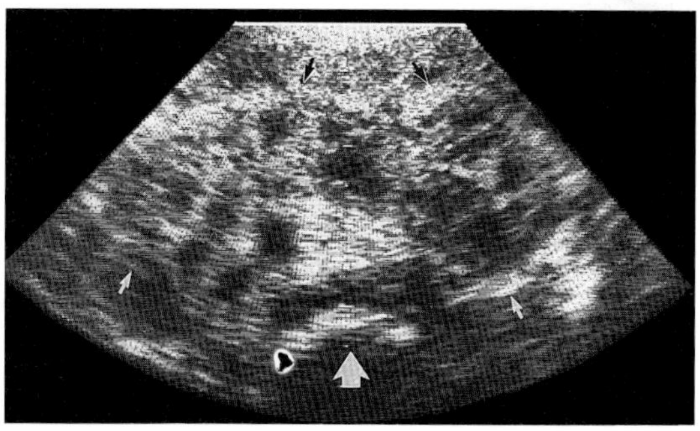

13–3 Horseshoe kidney. Transverse sonograms demonstrating renal parenchyma (arrows) and overlying spine (large arrow).

Fusion

Fusion anomalies of the kidneys are often asymptomatic. Urography will show the abnormal axis of fusion variations and delineate the ureters.

Horseshoe kidneys are recognized on ultrasound by the extension across the spine (Fig. 13–3). CT and MR readily identify both horseshoe kidneys and renal ectopy.

Dysplasia

Renal dysplasia is nonfunctional and thus not seen by urography. CT can identify the variation of renal dysplasia that does not display multicystic changes as a small mass of tissue in the renal fossa. Ultrasonography will show absence of a normal kidney and will identify a typical multicystic dysplastic kidney. However, ultrasound is limited in separating a small noncystic dysplastic kidney from agenesis and ectopy.

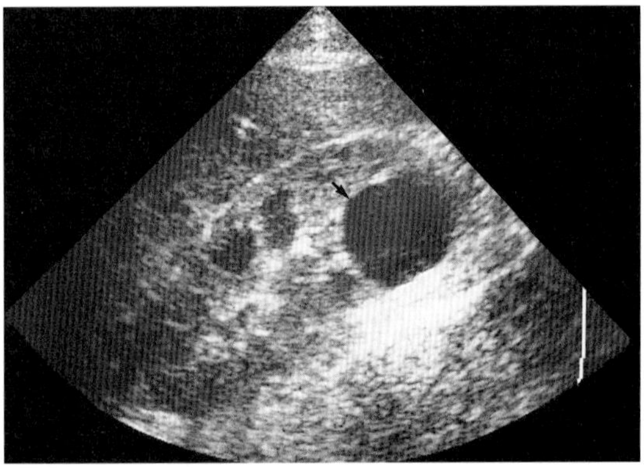

13–4 Simple cyst. Supine longitudinal sonogram clearly shows large sharply defined mass in lower pole of right kidney (arrow), demonstrating wave transmission.

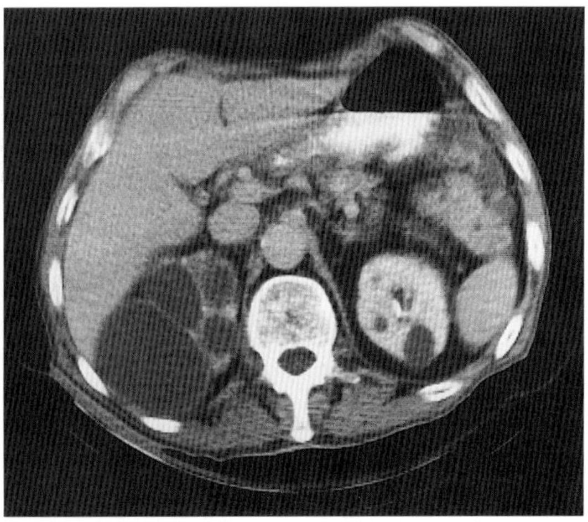

13–5 Multiple simple cysts. Postcontrast CT scan demonstrates multiple nonenhancing, water-density cysts involving both kidneys. Note homogeneous appearance of cysts, imperceptible cyst wall, and sharp interface between cyst and renal parenchyma.

Cystic Renal Masses

Simple Cysts

Renal cysts have been detected more readily since the advent of ultrasound and CT. The ultrasound criteria for a benign cyst include the absence of internal echoes; smooth, sharply defined walls; and acoustic enhancement beyond the posterior wall proportional to the fluid content (Fig. 13–4) (McClennan et al. 1979).

The CT criteria for a benign cyst include homogeneous attenuation value near the density of water; imperceptible cyst wall; smooth interface with the renal parenchyma; and lack of enhancement following intravenous contrast infusion (Fig. 13–5) (Sagel et al. 1977). When these criteria are met, the diagnosis of a simple cyst is accurate in 93%–98% of cases (Pollack et al. 1982). In those cases not meeting the strict criteria for ultrasound or CT, needle aspiration or MR imaging should be considered to establish the final diagnosis (Amis et al. 1987; Marotti et al. 1987).

Excretory urography remains the basic screening examination for renal pathology; often, a renal cyst is first suspected on this examination. In most cases, urography and ultrasonography together will provide enough information for accurate diagnosis of a simple renal cyst. A simple cyst must be differentiated from a sonolucent mass in the upper pole of the kidney representing a hydrocalix, or the dilated portion of a duplicated collecting system. On the urogram, a hydrocalix is easily identified, but both an upper pole cyst and obstructed duplication will displace the calices. Duplication is suggested on ultrasound by a bilobed appearance of the renal parenchyma and identification of a dilated upper pole ureter and an associated ectopic ureterocele. Simple renal cysts do occur in children, and approximately 50% of these cysts are located in the upper pole of the kidney, emphasizing the importance of distinguishing these cysts from obstructed duplication.

Multicystic Dysplastic Kidney

Abdominal masses in neonates are commonly of renal origin, usually secondary to either hydronephrosis or multicystic renal dysplasia. Multicystic renal dysplasia must be differentiated from surgically correctable obstruction, in order to pre-

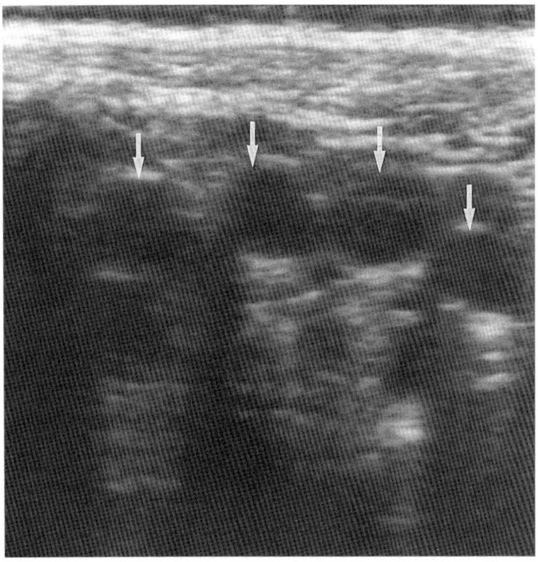

13–6 Multicystic dysplastic kidney. Prone longitudinal sonogram through right kidney shows several noncommunicating cystic masses (arrows). No identifiable normal renal sinus complex or parenchymal rim.

serve renal function. Ultrasonography has replaced urography in evaluating the neonate, because it does not depend on renal function or require ionizing radiation.

Severe hydronephrosis may be difficult to differentiate from multicystic dysplastic kidney because of the large cystic structures that occur in both entities. Some characteristics of multicystic dysplastic kidneys that help in differentiation are the lack of communication between cystic structures; clawlike appearance between cysts secondary to septa; larger cysts being eccentric; lack of renal sinus and pelvis; and lack of parenchymal rim (Stuck et al. 1982). Using these criteria, multicystic dysplastic kidneys will usually differ enough from hydronephrosis for accurate diagnosis (Fig. 13–6). If the ultrasound findings are indeterminate, additional studies, such as a retrograde ureteropyelogram or antegrade puncture with opacification, may be indicated. Radionuclide studies are useful because there is little, if any, function in multicystic dysplastic kidneys, whereas salvageable renal parenchyma can be identified in hydronephrosis.

Occasionally, urography may be necessary to supplement the evaluation of the contralateral kidney and ureter, since 16% of cases with multicystic dysplastic kidney have associated ureteropelvic junction obstruction on the contralateral side.

Polycystic Renal Disease

In infantile polycystic renal disease, the morphological abnormality is tubular ectasia identified as increased echogenicity in the renal pyramids of neonates (Fig. 13–7). The ectatic tubules enlarge and can later be discerned as discrete cystic structures throughout the renal parenchyma. When the disease manifests in the neonatal period, the major abnormality is in the kidneys rather than the liver, and there is often renal failure. However, when the disease is manifested in an older child, periportal fibrosis becomes the dominant abnormality. Esophageal varices and hepatic malfunction then become the major clinical problems with less abnormality in renal function, even though the kidneys may be enlarged and show the characteristic findings of tubular ectasia on imaging examinations. Opacification of the ectatic tubules is responsible for the striated appearance in the pyramids (Fig. 13–8).

In adult polycystic renal disease, the cysts may occur anywhere along the nephron. Patients often present in their fifties or sixties with clinical symptoms of hypertension and increasing abdominal girth. The adult type of polycystic renal disease is also known to occur in children. Ultrasonography is the examination of choice for evaluating patients suspected of having the disease and for evaluating the asymptomatic family members. The cysts are easily detected by ultrasound, CT, and MR imaging, using the criteria for cysts (Fig. 13–9). It is also important to evaluate the liver because of the associated hepatic cysts, which occur in approximately 33% of patients. Hemorrhage within one or more of the cysts occurs in two-thirds of patients

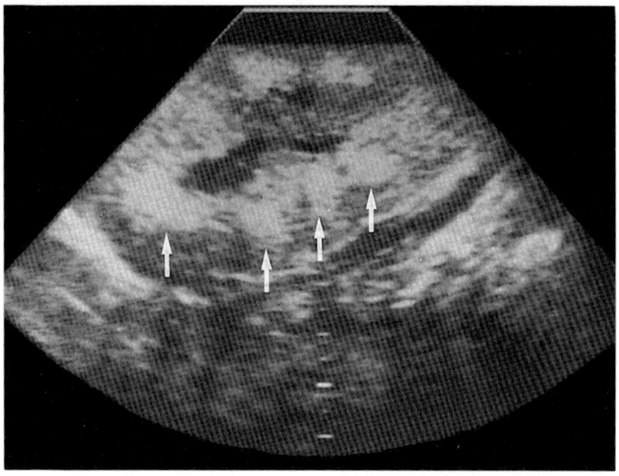

13–7 Infantile polycystic renal disease (neonate). Longitudinal sonogram demonstrates increased echogenicity in renal pyramids (arrows).

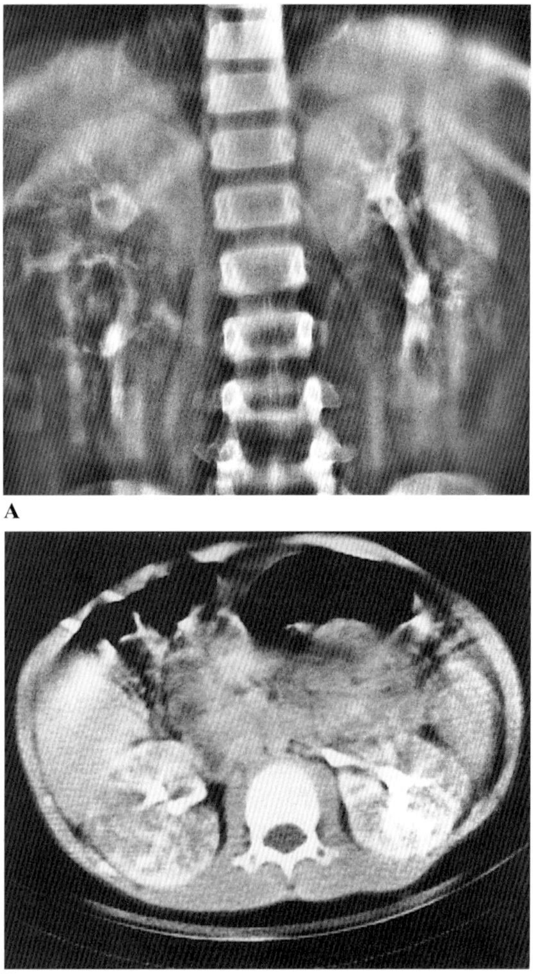

A

B

13–8 Infantile polycystic renal disease (age 5). **(A)** Tomogram during excretory urography demonstrates bilateral large kidneys with opacification of dilated tubules responsible for "brush border" appearance of pyramids. **(B)** CT scan through both renal hila demonstrates nonuniform contrast enhancement, predominantly in medullary zone of kidney. Note streaks of contrast medium in dilated collecting tubules.

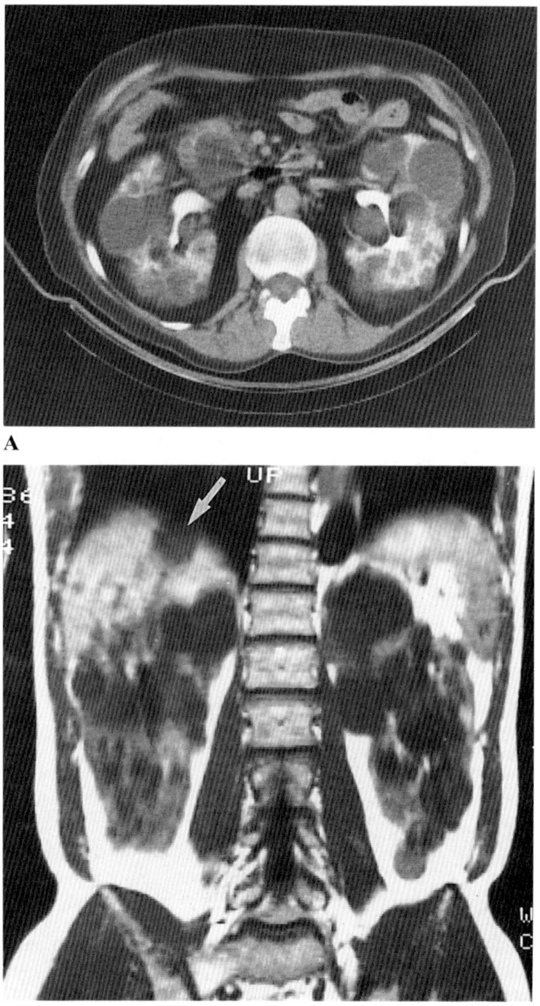

A

B

13–9 Adult polycystic renal disease. **(A)** Postcontrast CT scan through renal hila demonstrates bilateral functioning kidneys with cysts in both medullary and cortical zones of kidneys grossly distorting the renal contours. **(B)** Coronal MR scan of kidneys shows cysts with decreased signal on short TR/TE (500/17) sequence compatible with simple fluid content. Note liver cyst (arrow).

with polycystic renal disease and is best evaluated by MR imaging.

Solid Renal Masses

Benign Masses

Benign solid lesions are difficult to differentiate preoperatively from malignant neoplasms unless there is a specific imaging characteristic present such as fat.

Pseudotumors

One of the most common space-occupying lesions in the kidney is the hypertrophied column of Bertin, which is normal renal parenchyma, most characteristically separating the superior from middle pole calices. Other so-called pseudotumors include the prominence of the lateral renal margin secondary to the splenic impression and the hilar lip, which often occurs superior to the hilus, secondary to focal hypertrophied parenchyma. Focal parenchymal hypertrophy adjacent to an area of

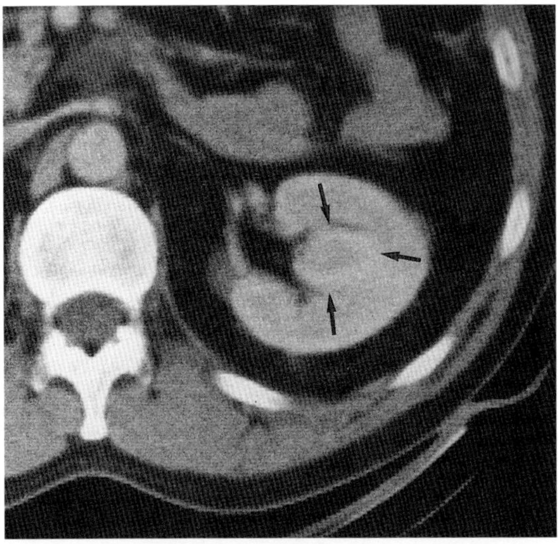

A

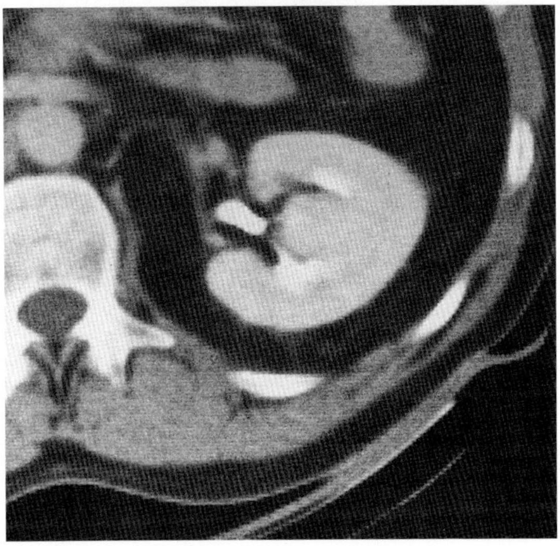

B

13–10 Column of Bertin. **(A)** Dynamic CT scan made during vascular nephrogram phase shows well-defined area of enhancement (arrows) in midportion of left kidney. Note corticomedullary demarcation within column of Bertin. **(B)** CT scan during the tubular nephrogram made a few minutes after **(A)** reveals that so-called mass has become isodense with adjacent parenchyma characteristic of a Bertin's column.

scarring from previous inflammation is another cause for pseudotumor.

Characteristically, the diagnosis of pseudotumor is established with ultrasound or radionuclide studies. On ultrasound, the echogenicity of the pseudomass will be similar to normal renal parenchyma. Because all of the described pseudotumors contain normal functioning renal parenchyma, they will show uniform uptake on radionuclide studies. CT is rarely needed to establish the diagnosis except in indeterminate cases. On CT, the

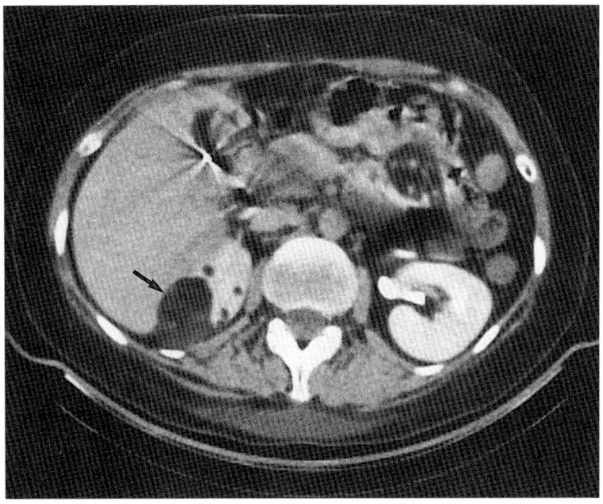

13–11 Angiomyolipoma. Postcontrast CT scan reveals large mass at posterior border of right upper pole, with low attenuation values consistent with fat (arrow) and several smaller fatty spherical masses within the parenchyma.

pseudotumor will appear isodense with the normal renal parenchyma prior to administering intravenous contrast. During dynamic CT scanning, the mass will enhance uniformly like normal renal cortex, and occasionally a low-density pyramid within the enhancing septum will be seen (Zeman et al. 1986; Fig. 13–10 A). This mass of normally functioning renal tissue should not be mistaken for a hypervascular renal tumor, because it will become isodense with normal renal parenchyma on the later scans (Fig. 13–10 B). The most specific test is a nuclear scintigram using a parenchymal agent such as ^{99m}Tc-DMSA. The column of Bertin shows normal activity; all other masses appear as a defect on the kidney.

Angiomyolipoma

Angiomyolipomas contain varying amounts of smooth muscle, blood vessels, and mature fat cells. It is the presence of the fat cells that allows the most accurate preoperative diagnosis of this tumor by CT (Fig. 13–11). CT is able to differentiate tissues by their attenuation values. The diagnosis can be established without surgery if the fat content is visible on the section selected. However, some tumors contain only small amounts of fat, which may be undetectable. In addition, angiomyolipomas commonly are associated with hemorrhage, which can mask the areas of fat and preclude accurate evaluation. CT is superior to ultrasound in establishing the diagnosis of angiomyolipoma, since some renal cell carcinomas will also

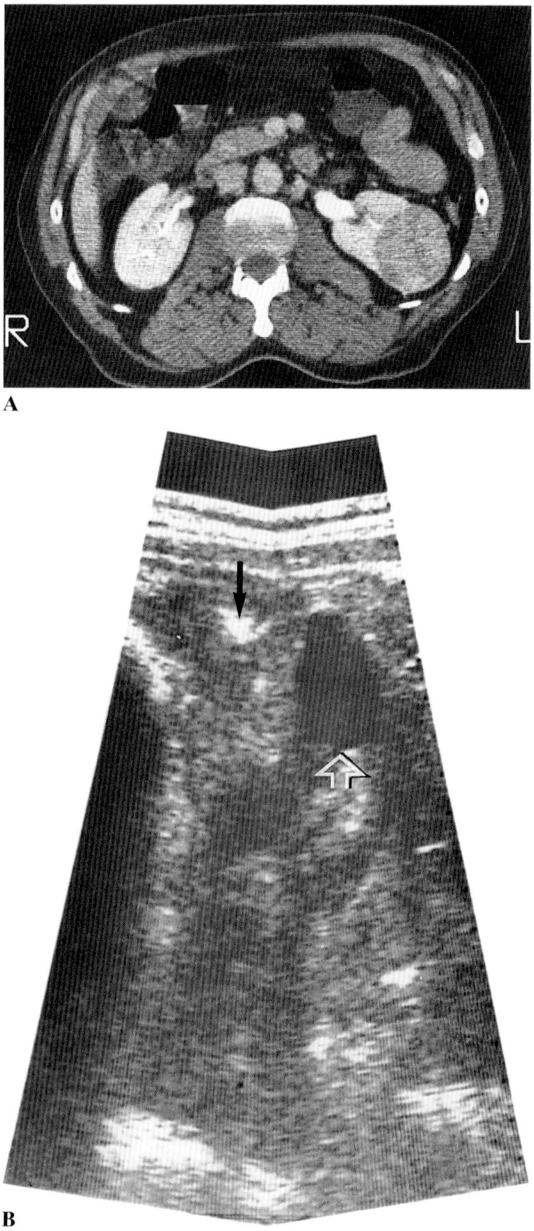

A

B

13–12 Oncocytoma. **(A)** Contrast-enhanced CT scan through hila of both kidneys reveals an enhancing, nonhomogeneous spherical (L) renal mass with sharp demarcation from normal kidney. **(B)** Longitudinal sonogram through left kidney shows oncocytoma as solid mass with central scarring (arrow) and an incidental simple cyst inferiorly (upon arrow).

demonstrate increased echogenicity (Hartman et al. 1987). In a series of patients evaluated by MR imaging, without fast imaging, angiomyolipomas could not be accurately separated from hemorrhage and renal cell carcinomas (Marotti et al. 1987).

Oncocytoma

Oncocytomas are epithelial neoplasms believed to originate from the proximal collecting tubules. These tumors are characteristically benign, but because of their solid nature cannot be definitely categorized as benign prior to surgery. However, there are some clues to separate oncocytoma from renal cell carcinoma. Specifically, ultrasound, CT, and MR imaging may show central scarring; a suggestive angiographic appearance of a spoke-wheel pattern has been described (Weiner, Bernstein 1977) (Fig. 13–12A, B). However, similar-appearing changes on CT, MR, and angiography can be found with renal cell carcinoma (Ball et al. 1986). An enucleation may be considered rather than radical surgery if the suggestive patterns are found and if there is a compelling reason to spare parenchyma – for example, in a solitary kidney.

Malignant Masses

Renal neoplasms accounted for 2% of all new malignancies in the United States in 1985. Many masses are first detected on an initial imaging exam sometimes obtained for nonrenal indications, and require further evaluation by at least one other imaging study. Currently, CT and MR imaging are used for staging malignant neoplasms. Indeterminate masses can be evaluated by MR for tissue and fluid characterization (Fig. 13–13). More recently, MR with gradient echo imaging permits depiction of the varying stages of hemorrhages (Fig. 13–14).

Renal Cell Carcinoma

Magnetic resonance imaging, CT, and ultrasonography can all be used in diagnosing the nature of renal cell carcinoma (Figs. 13–15, 13–16). The CT criteria for renal malignancy are: heterogenous tissue with attenuation coefficient close to that of renal parenchyma; contrast enhancement, usually less than that of normal parenchyma following intravenous injection of iodinated contrast medium; irregular interface with surrounding parenchyma; and secondary characteristics such as enlargement of the renal vein and regional lymph nodes (Levine et al. 1979); (Fig. 13–17). Areas of calcification may not be appreciated unless CT images are obtained initially without intravenous contrast.

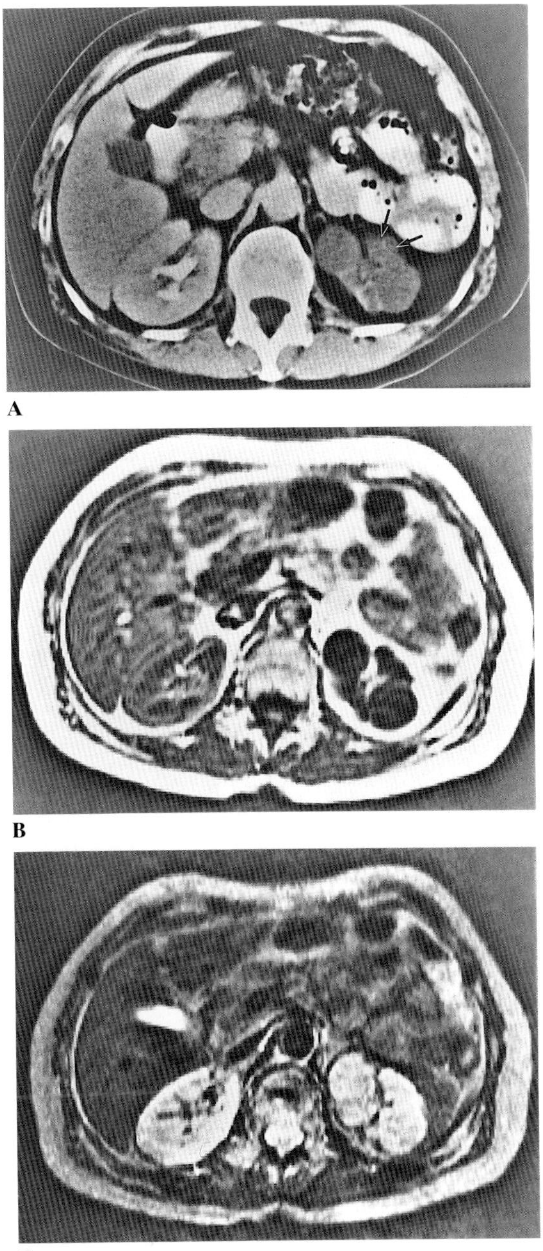

13–13 Multiloculated renal cysts. **(A)** Contrast-enhanced CT scan at level of both kidneys shows lobulated mass with questionable nodularity and enhancement on anterior midsurface (arrows). **(B)** Transverse abdominal MR image (SE TR500/TE17) shows upper pole renal lesion to have long T1 similar to urine. **(C)** Transverse abdominal MR image (SE TR2000/TE70) shows T2 lengthening in left upper pole renal lesion consistent with simple fluid, confirming diagnosis of multiloculated benign cysts.

Hypovascular renal masses, such as papillary cell-type carcinomas, are best evaluated by ultrasound, CT, and MR imaging. Complex renal masses are more difficult to categorize as benign or malignant. A septated benign renal mass with partial liquefaction may be indistinguishable from a necrotic renal cell carcinoma, particularly since both of these lesions may be hypovascular. Some cystic lesions may have a solid component easily identified by CT (Fig. 13–18). Fine-needle aspiration biopsy with cytology can be helpful if confirmation is needed before nephrectomy (Amis et al. 1987); tract seeding is not the problem with fine-needle aspiration (less than 20 gauge) as it is with large bore needles. A limitation of MR is the nonspecific pattern of a malignant neoplasm, which can mimic a benign lesion containing fat or pus. Very long spin echo sequences (TR 3000/TE 120 msec) help to characterize mass content and delineate the mass from adjacent normal parenchyma.

Accuracy of staging renal tumors with CT has been reported in 80%–95% of cases (Jaschke et al. 1982). In 1985, staging of renal tumors with MR had a reported accuracy of 95%, especially useful for neoplasm stages II–IV (Hricak et al. 1985). Reassessment of MR capabilities in 1988 by Hricak et al. showed that accurate staging was possible in 82% of all detected renal tumors (106 lesions), with a negative predictive value of 98% for renal vascular extension and 99% for tumor spread into adjacent structures.

Staging requires detailed evaluation of the renal vein and inferior vena cava, demonstration of hilar and perivascular extension, and detection of tumor invasion into adjacent organs. MR has the advantage over CT of multiplanar imaging, which allows better delineation of renal tissue from the liver and other retroperitoneal structures (Fig. 13–19). A disadvantage is inability to evaluate other areas in the same scanning sequence as used for evaluation of the kidney itself.

Venous invasion is usually identified on CT, but there are some false positives due to flow phenomenon (Marks et al. 1978) and false negatives if there is not good filling of the vascular structures with dynamic scanning. Therefore, ultrasound and MR are more accurate in precise evaluation of venous involvement (Figs. 13–20, 13–21).

Angiography is generally not necessary, except in special situations such as inconclusive evaluation of venous involvement; planned embolization; or a need to define vascular supply, especially when renal-sparing surgery is planned.

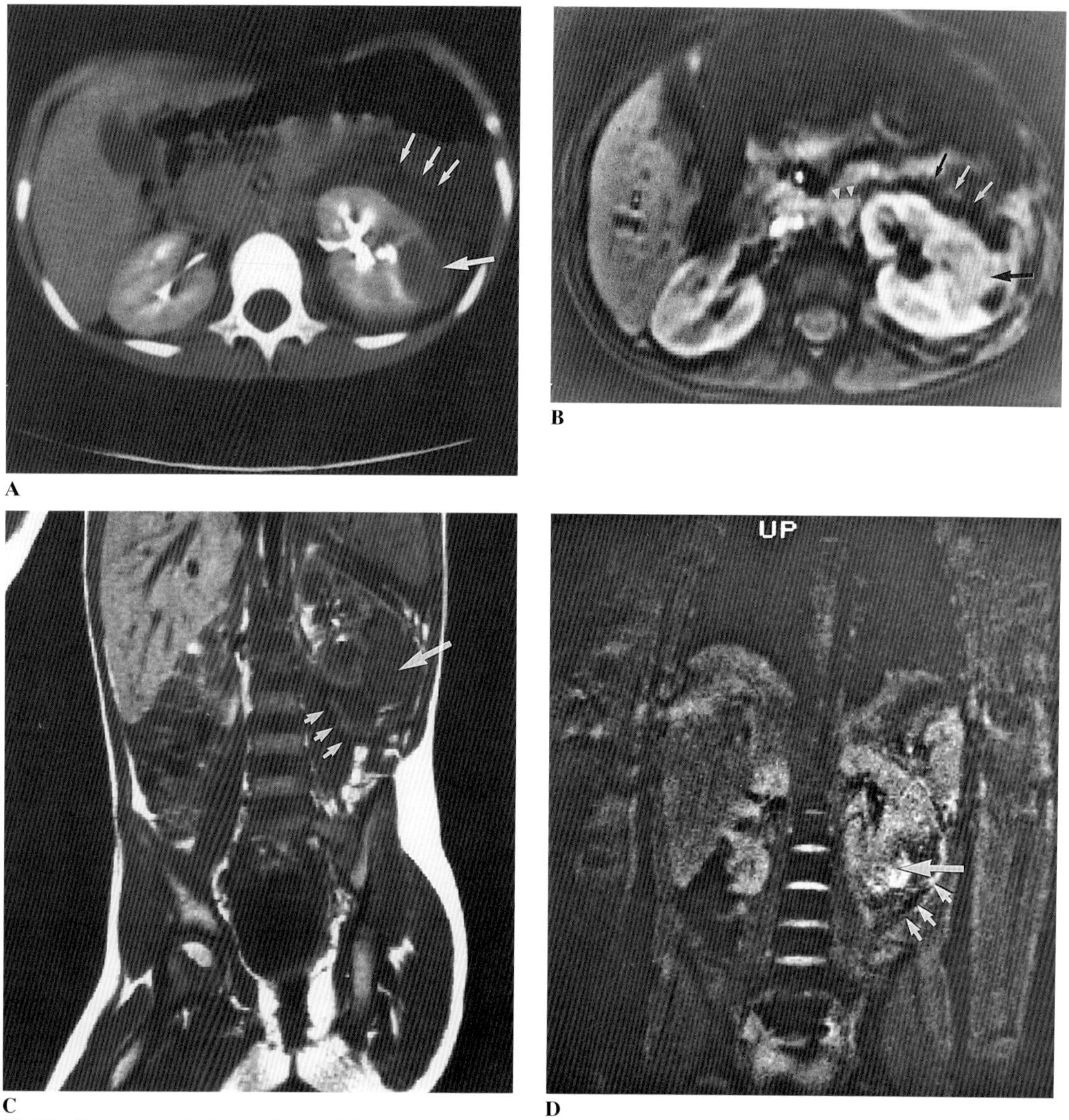

13–14 Posttraumatic hemorrhage with Wilms's tumor. **(A)** CT scan obtained initially following traumatic event. The postcontrast CT scan at level of both kidneys shows low attenuation mass (arrow) in periphery of left kidney, with evidence of fluid extending along anterior perinephric space (small arrows). **(B)** Transverse abdominal MR image (FISP 20° TR600/TE35) shows intrarenal component to have a mixed signal characteristic of a solid mass (arrow). The anterior perinephric component (arrows) shows decreased signal characteristic of hemorrhage on fast imaging because of the magnetic susceptibility. Note peri-aortic lymphadenopathy (arrowhead). **(C)** Coronal MR abdominal image (SE TR500/TE17) shows slight signal differentiation of tumor (arrow) and perinephric hemorrhage (small arrows). **(D)** Coronal MR abdominal image (FLASH 20° TR300/TE30) shows nonspecific intermediate-high signal of left lower pole intrarenal neoplasm and low signal of the recent hemorrhage (arrowheads). Note small area of long T2 (long arrow) interposed between hemorrhage and the kidney, representing necrotic tumor. Surgery confirmed a ruptured Wilms's tumor with hemorrhage and retroperitoneal lymphadenopathy.

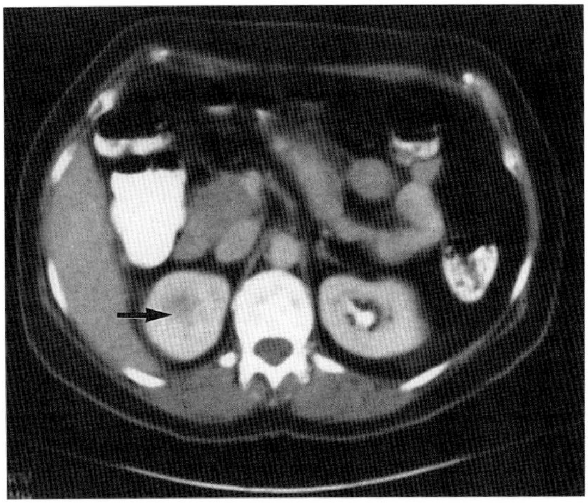

A

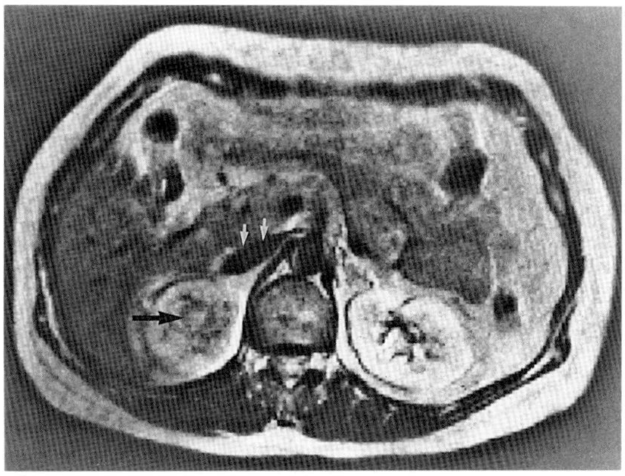

B

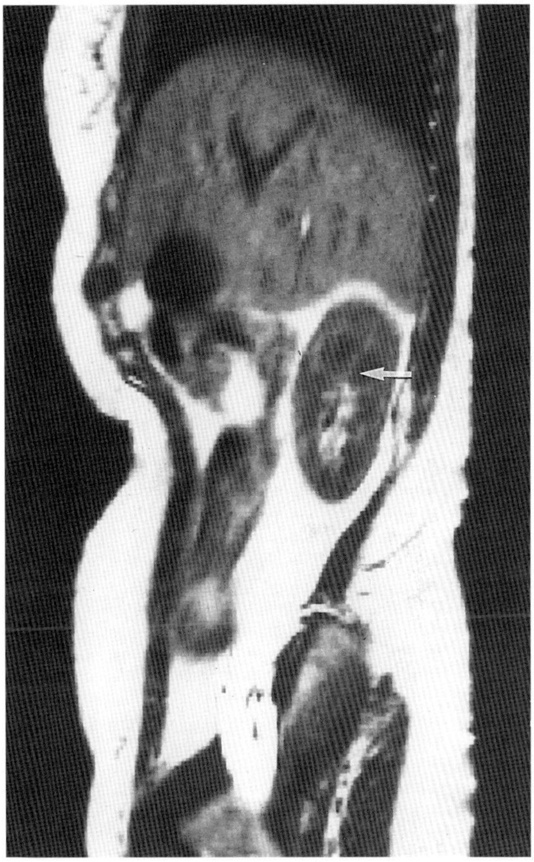

C

13–15 Renal cell carcinoma. **(A)** CT examination obtained because of vague abdominal pain. Postcontrast scan through both kidneys shows vague area of decreased attenuation (arrow) in upper pole of right kidney. **(B)** Transverse abdominal MR image (SE TR2000/TE70) showing nonspecific signal but disturbance of central intrarenal architecture on right (arrow). The inferior vena cava shows normal signal void (short arrows), confirming no tumor thrombus. **(C)** Sagittal MR abdominal image (SE TR500/TE17) demonstrates expansion of upper pole with extension of solid tissue into upper renal sinus (arrow).

Wilms's Tumor

Wilms's tumor is the most common renal neoplasm of childhood and is generally solitary and quite large at the time of detection. The tumor can often be correctly diagnosed on the urogram based on displacement of the collecting system and its intrarenal characteristics. The other intrarenal tumors occurring in children are mesoblastic nephroma (the most common intrarenal tumor in neonates) and multilocular cystic nephroma, occurring in a slightly older age group than Wilms's tumor. One of the hallmarks of the multilocular cystic nephroma is herniation of the tumor into the pelvis, which is best visualized during examinations with contrast filling of the pelvis such as urography or CT.

The other tumor of childhood that must be differentiated from Wilms's tumor is neuroblastoma. It is primarily adrenal in origin, although it can arise from the sympathetic nervous system. It shows the characteristics on imaging examinations of an extrarenal mass that will contain calcifications in 60% of cases and a propensity to extend across midline.

Ultrasonography is not highly specific for Wilms's tumor, but commonly shows relatively uniform echogenicity except for small echo-free spaces and a pseudocapsule (Fig. 13–22A). A large exophytic tumor may resemble an extrarenal mass with little caliceal displacement, which limits the diagnosis by urography and occasionally even by CT and ultrasound, but should not interfere with the diagnosis by MR imaging.

Computed tomography is superior to urography in demonstrating multicentric Wilms's tumors and also in evaluating the contralateral kidney. Precontrast CT usually demonstrates Wilms's

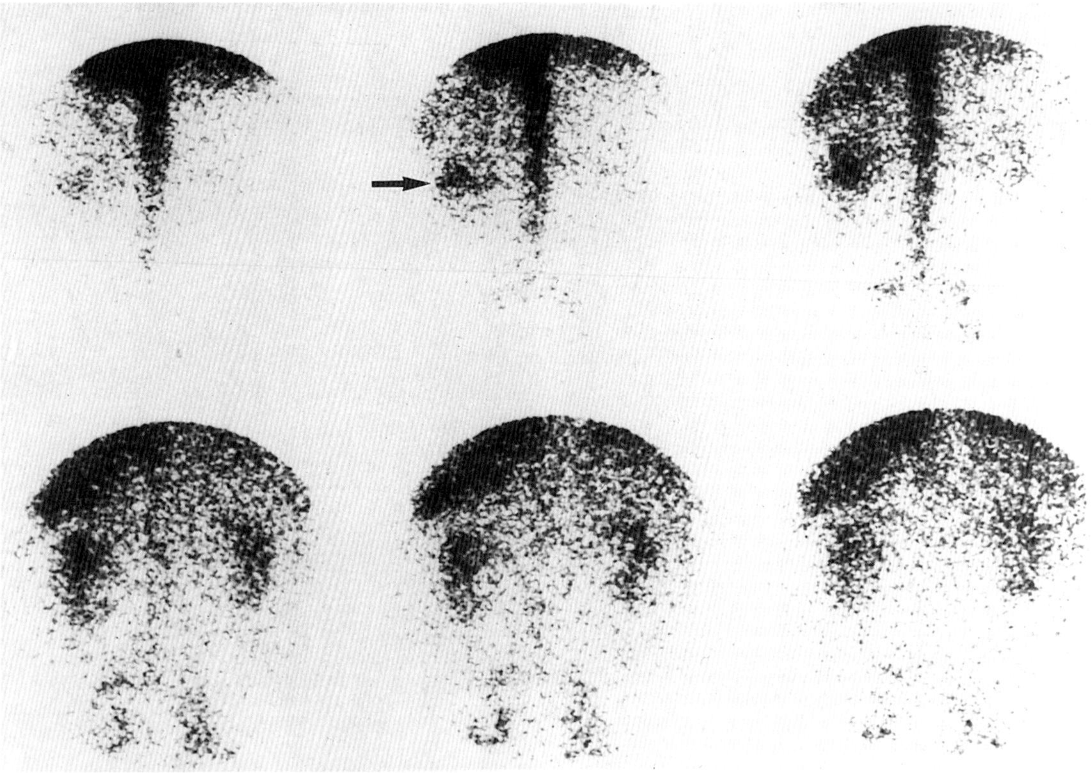

A

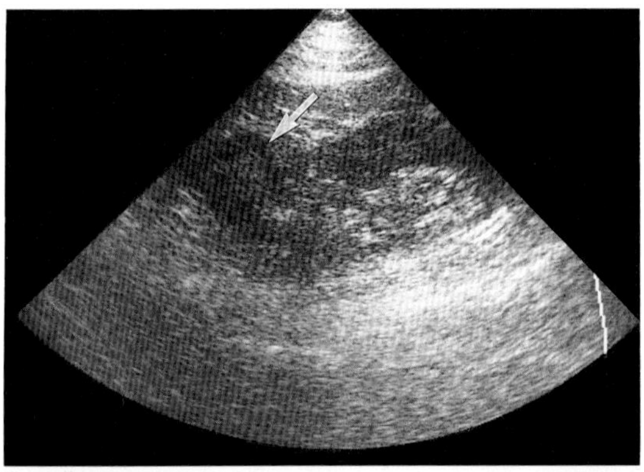

B

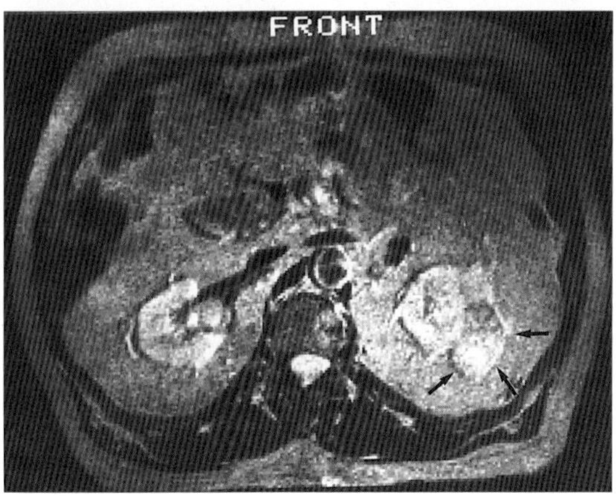

C

13–16 Renal cell carcinoma. **(A)** Renogram obtained with ^{99m}Tc for hypertension. Early sequential images (posterior view) of renogram show increased uptake of a hypervascular mass in upper pole of left kidney (arrow). **(B)** Longitudinal sonogram of left kidney demonstrates solid mass (arrow) extending from the periphery of left upper pole. **(C)** Axial MR abdominal image (long TR/TE) shows mixed and high signal intensity in the left renal mass (arrows).

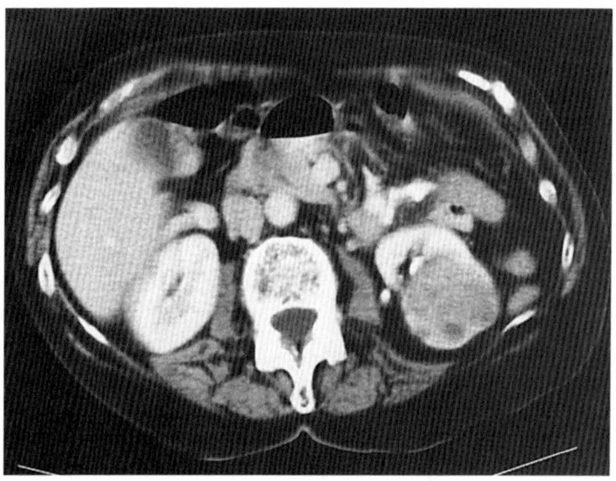

13–17 Renal cell carcinoma. Postcontrast CT scan through both kidneys reveals nonhomogeneous, enhancing mass in left kidney posteriorly that has indistinct interface with normal renal parenchyma.

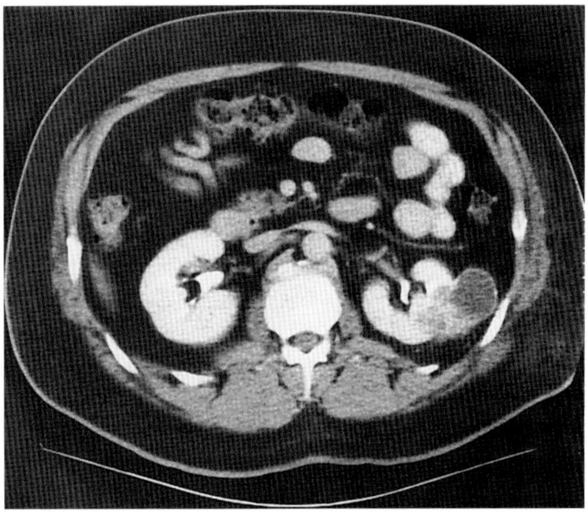

13–18 Renal cell carcinoma. Postcontrast CT shows thick-walled cystic mass peripheral to irregular solid tumor.

tumor as a mass with less attenuation than the surrounding renal parenchyma; 10% have calcifications. Following contrast there is nonhomogeneous enhancement with a persistent area of increased attenuation at the normal parenchymal interface, which apparently represents compressed normal renal parenchyma and corresponds to the pseudocapsule. Magnetic resonance imaging is superior to CT in predicting tumor origin and also for evaluation of extension into the adjacent organs such as the liver and retroperitoneum (Fig. 13–22C, D).

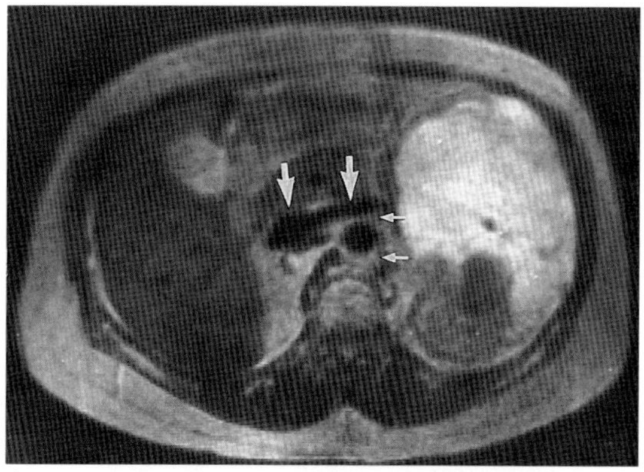

A

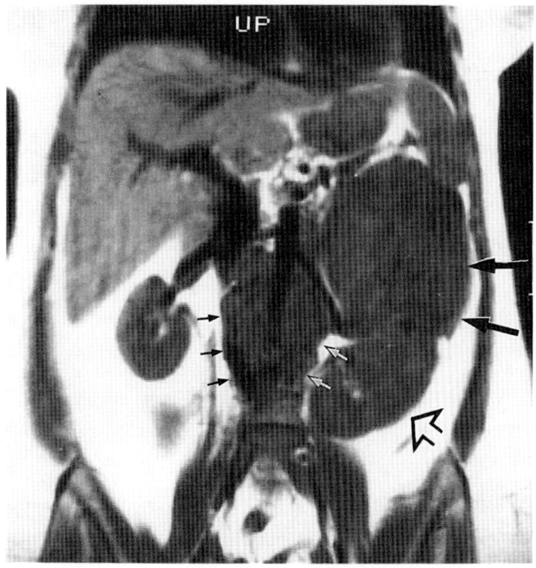

B

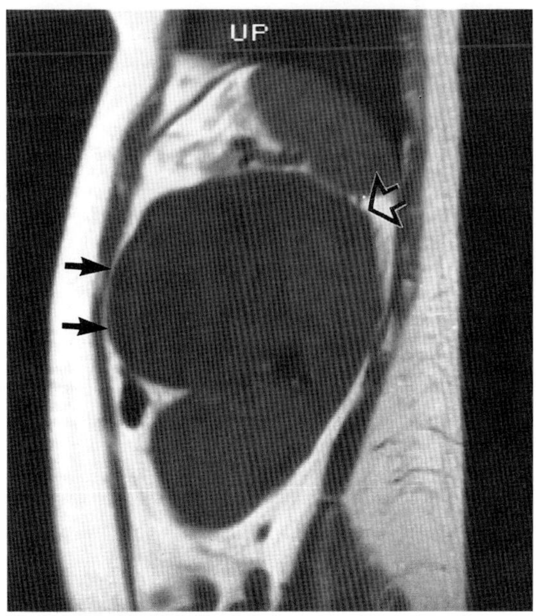

C

13–19 MR staging of renal cell carcinoma. **(A)** Transverse abdominal MR image (SE TR2000/TE70) showing stage-III disease. Left renal vein and inferior vena cava show normal signal void (arrows), indicating no tumor involvement. Note retroperitoneal lymphadenopathy (small arrows). Large renal neoplasm shows nonspecific areas of both high and low intensity secondary to various amounts of vascularity and necrosis. **(B)** Coronal MR abdominal image (SE TR500/TE17) shows low signal intensity of renal neoplasm (arrows) similar to intensity of adjacent renal parenchyma (open arrow). Note extensive retroperitoneal lymphadenopathy encircling vascular structures (small arrows). **(C)** Sagittal MR abdominal image (SE TR500/TE17) demonstrates low signal intensity of large renal cell carcinoma (arrows). There is a distinct fatty perimeter around tumor, indicating no violation invasion of perinephric space and a defined margin (open arrow) between renal neoplasm and adjacent spleen .

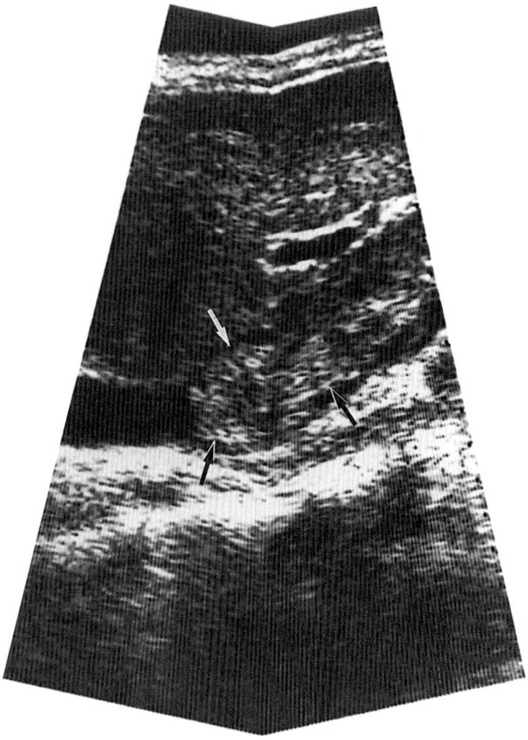

13–20 Renal cell carcinoma with tumor thrombus. Longitudinal sonogram of patient with renal cell carcinoma demonstrates tumor extension (arrows) into inferior vena cava.

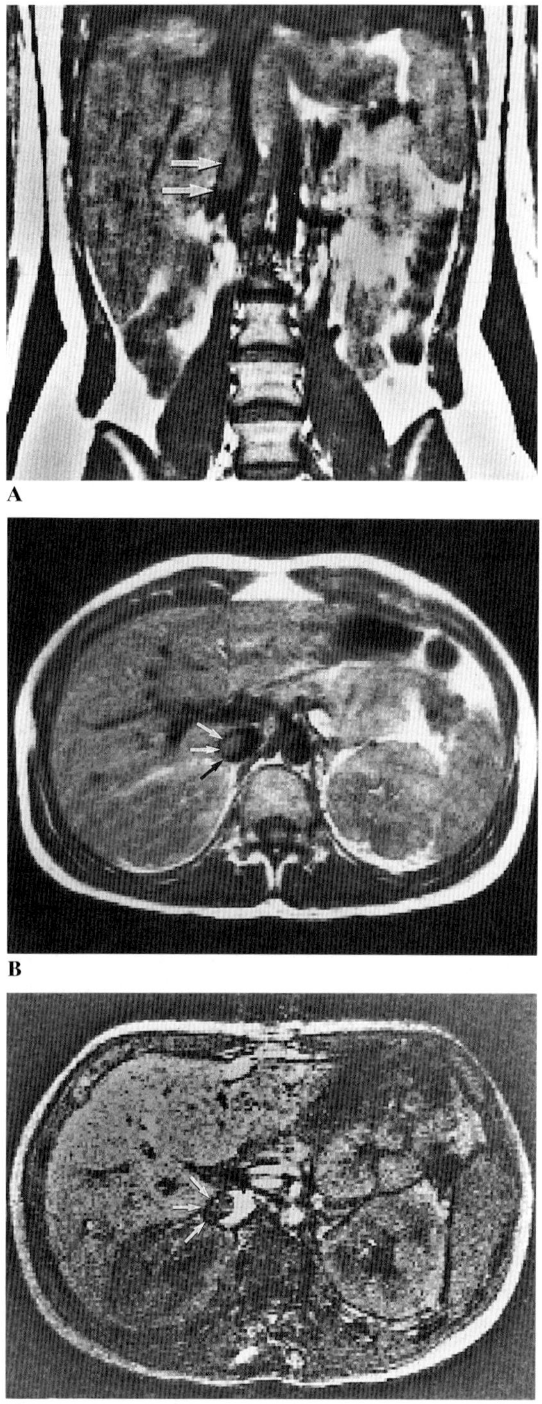

A

B

C

13–21 Inferior vena cava thrombus. **(A)** Coronal MR abdominal image (SE TR500/TE28) in patient with acute glomerulopathy shows intermediate signal of thrombus (arrows) extending from right renal vein orifice into inferior vena cava. **(B)** Transverse abdominal MR image (SE TR500/TE28) shows intraluminal filling defect (arrows) surrounded by normal signal void of flowing blood in inferior vena cava. **(C)** Transverse abdominal fast MR image (FLASH 70° TR700/TE12) shows intraluminal clot (arrows) to remain intermediate in signal, while flowing blood shows a bright signal because of accentuation of entry slice phenomena.

Lymphoma

Lymphoma is a likely diagnosis when an intrarenal mass is present with associated extrarenal adenopathy. The ultrasound findings of a hypoechoic homogenous mass with little or no wave transmission and lack of a sharply defined margin are characteristic of uniform small-cell tumors such as lymphoma. On CT, renal lymphoma appears as a homogenous mass with minimal, but uniform, contrast enhancement. The main differential diagnosis includes renal infarction, focal infection, hypovascular carcinomas such as papillary cell carcinoma, transitional cell carcinoma, and metastatic lesions. A retroperitoneal mass that invades the renal fossa is sometimes difficult to differentiate from a lymphoma, but most primary retroperitoneal tumors displace the kidney rather than invade it like a lymphoma does. In renal masses where lymphoma is suspected, biopsy of a peripheral node or percutaneous biopsy of the mass itself may be necessary for accurate diagnosis.

Azotemia in patients with lymphoma is usually secondary to obstruction of the ureter. Other

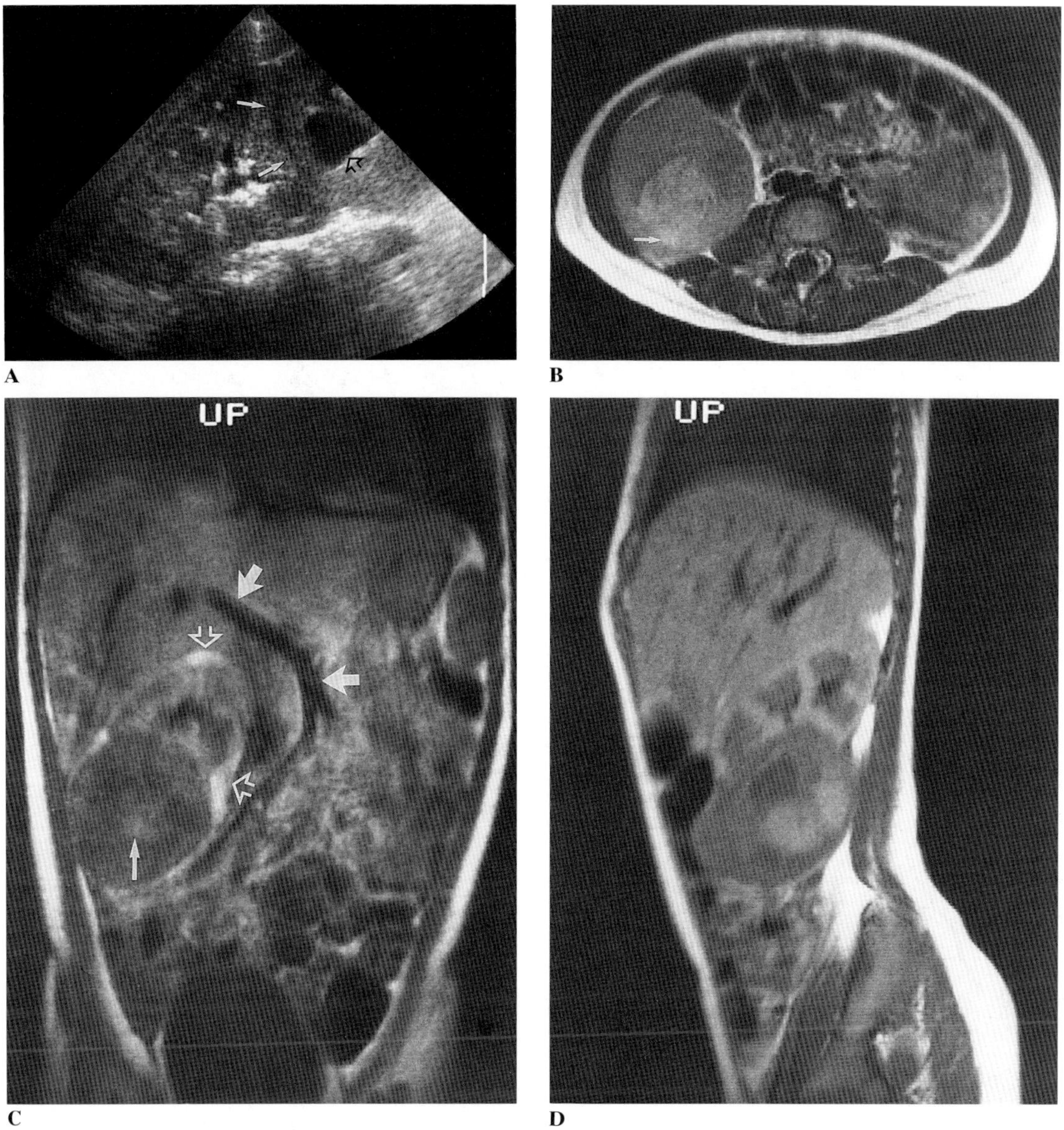

13–22 Wilms's tumor. **(A)** Longitudinal supine sonogram reveals intrarenal mass in right lower pole with uniform echogenicity peripherally and echo-free spaces (open arrow). Note curvilinear hypoechoic rim of pseudocapsule at parenchymal interface (arrows). **(B)** Axial MR abdominal image at TR1700/TE30 shows nonhomogeneous tissue character of this tumor. Note relatively bright signal representing hemorrhage (arrow) posteriorly in the mass, corresponding to anechoic spaces on ultrasound. **(C)** Coronal MR abdominal image at short TR/TE (700/30) shows bright signal centrally in the lower pole mass, consistent with hemorrhage (arrow). Note distinct perinephric fat (open arrows) and displaced IVC (large arrows). **(D)** Sagittal MR abdominal image at short TR/TE (700/30) again shows nonhomogeneous character of this tumor. Note that intrarenal tumor origin and lack of extension are easily identified.

etiologies for failure related to the lymphoma are vascular compromise secondary to lymphadenopathy, and replacement of renal parenchyma by lymphomatous tissue. Tubular or ureteral obstruction by calculi may occur secondary to the hyperuricemia that accompanies the treatment of lymphoma.

Urothelial Tumors

Transitional cell carcinoma is a relatively rare neoplasm of the upper urinary tract and tends to be recurrent. The common imaging techniques of urography and retrograde pyelography are used to detect intraluminal lesions, but are limited by their

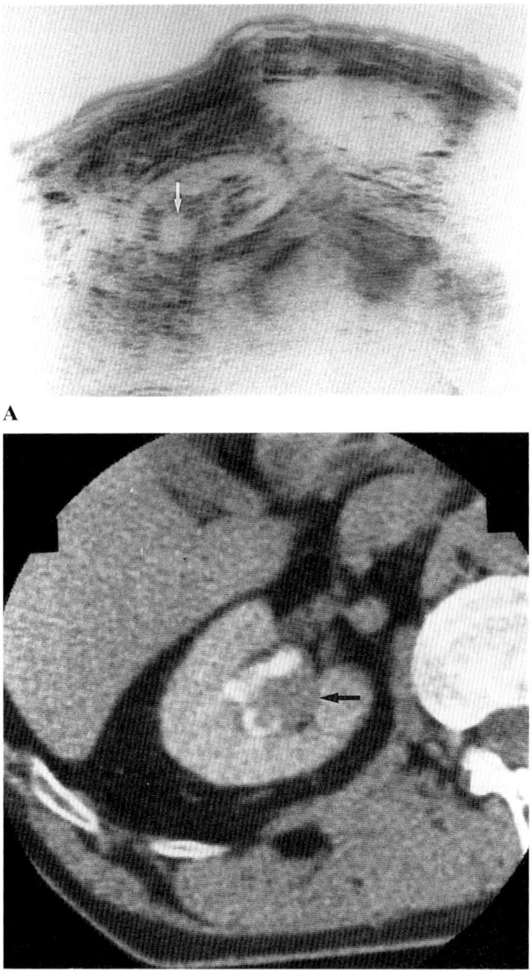

A

B

13–23 Transitional cell carcinoma. **(A)** Longitudinal ultrasound shows hypoechoic mass (arrow) in right upper pole, which partially replaces central renal echoes. **(B)** Contrast-enhanced CT scan through upper pole of right kidney shows soft tissue filling defect (arrow) within contrast-filled collecting system.

inability to detect extension into the periureteral regions or metastasis to lymph nodes. Therefore, CT has become the examination of choice in staging transitional cell carcinoma of the upper urinary tract.

The main differential of an intraluminal defect of the collection system detected by urography or retrograde pyelography is tumor versus calculus. Ultrasonography can demonstrate shadowing from a calculus, whether opaque or nonopaque; there will be no shadowing from tumor (Fig. 13–23A). Differentiation of tumor from nonopaque calculus by careful evaluation of the CT attenuation numbers is also possible. Transitional cell carcinoma has attenuation values that approach soft tissue density and will show detectable enhancement following iodinated intravenous contrast media (Fig. 13–23B). Nonopaque calculi have much higher attenuation values than soft tissue, but less than calcified stones (Hillman et al. 1984). Precontrast studies should be obtained to verify the attenuation values and to prevent contrast from obscuring a small mass associated with the calculus. The postcontrast scans are useful for enhancement evaluation of a soft-tissue lesion and for confirming extent of the disease. Although approximately 2% of transitional cell carcinomas may calcify, the amount of calcification and density should not approach that of opaque or nonopaque calculi.

Because CT can determine lymphadenopathy and extent of tumor beyond the urothelial wall, it is possible to accurately stage tumors preoperatively. However, CT cannot accurately differentiate stages I and II because it is virtually impossible to separate mucosa from muscle wall invasion of the ureter and pelvis. The possibility of overstaging exists when lymphadenopathy is actually due to inflammatory change rather than to the tumor metastasis. Understaging also occurs because CT is unable to detect metastasis within normal-size lymph nodes.

Metastasis to Kidney

Metastatic tumors to the kidney have been discovered more commonly since the use of CT, and are often asymptomatic. The kidney is the fifth most common site of metastasis after lung, liver, bone, and adrenals. A solid hypovascular lesion of the kidney in a patient with primary carcinoma, especially lung carcinoma, should be considered metastatic. If the lesions are multiple and bilateral, metastatic disease is more likely than a primary renal tumor. Confirmation can be obtained with fine-needle aspiration biopsy.

The differential diagnosis of a hypovascular lesion on CT includes metastatic lesions, other solid renal masses such as lymphoma, focal renal infarction, focal inflammation, and papillary-cell-type renal cell carcinoma. A history of heart disease without a known primary tumor would be more suggestive of renal infarction than metastasis. No vascular enhancement on CT is expected in the infarcted area, which is quite different from the enhancement occurring with neoplasms. The shape of the lesion may be helpful, since most infarctions are peripheral and elongated rather than masslike. Focal renal inflammation occurs in patients with clinical symptoms and signs of infection, which are helpful in differentiating inflammation from renal metastasis. Thickening of the renal fascia is commonly associated with renal infections and is best visualized with CT. Follow-up CT examinations are also helpful in differentiating inflammation and infarctions from metastatic lesions, since the latter will show gradual enlargement; infarctions and inflammation will show resolution.

Papillary-cell-type renal cell carcinoma is a problem in differentiation from metastasis, particularly if the lesion is unilateral. Metastases are usually contained within the kidney margin, whereas renal cell carcinoma is often exophytic as it increases in size.

Indeterminate Renal Masses

An estimated 7% of renal masses remain indeterminate even after careful ultrasound and CT. Some of the features that preclude accurate evaluation are irregular or thickened walls, indistinct margins, numerous septa of variable thicknesses, calcifications, internal low-level echoes, or increased attenuation. An indeterminate mass by CT is commonly indeterminate by angiography, since most of these masses are hypovascular.

Using ultrasound or CT, Rosenberg and colleagues (1985) found 26 primarily cystic lesions with 1 or more septa to be benign when all the other criteria of a simple cyst were fulfilled. Malignancy must always be suspected when hemorrhage or a solid component is present. Hemorrhage seldom occurs in benign multilocular cysts.

MR imaging can further clarify renal masses identified as indeterminate or complex by CT (Marotti et al. 1987). Magnetic resonance imaging separates lesions containing simple fluid similar to urine from complicated cysts containing blood, protein, or both. All of the lesions in the series that contained simple fluid were benign. Aspiration is an alternative method to evaluate the mass labeled indeterminate by CT.

Etiologies of the hyperdense renal cyst found on CT include hemorrhage and increased protein or calcium content. CT can reliably differentiate hyperdense renal cysts from other renal lesions if the following criteria are used: smooth contours sharply demarcated from the kidney, homogeneous internal content with precontrast density over 40% greater than kidney, and persistent postcontrast internal homogeneity with insignificant enhancement relative to the renal parenchyma. Hyperdense renal cysts that meet these criteria are considered benign and require no further evaluation (Zirinsky et al. 1984).

Hydronephrosis

Acute urinary tract obstruction is commonly evaluated by urography or ultrasound. Ultrasonography is independent of renal function and has high diagnostic accuracy in identifying moderate and severe hydronephrosis, but is limited in evaluating the level of obstruction within the ureter. Distal obstruction is suggested when the ureter is dilated in the region of the urinary bladder. Increased hydration may produce fullness of the collecting system secondary to diuresis – rather than true obstruction – giving a false-positive reading, as can an extrarenal pelvis. Patients with minimal dilation may require further evaluation for more accurate diagnosis, since a completely intrarenal collecting system may dilate very little in spite of ureteral obstruction, giving a false-negative report. Since ultrasound usually cannot follow the entire course of the ureter, CT is helpful when the cause of the obstruction is in doubt after retrograde ureteropyelography.

Multiple parapelvic cysts may mimic pelvicaliectasis, since the ultrasound appearance is similar. A coronal view of the kidney is helpful in differentiating the branching calices in pelvicaliectasis from the nonbranching and septated appearance of multiple parapelvic cysts. Furthermore, a fluid challenge may be helpful in distinguishing hydronephrosis from parapelvic cysts, since hydronephrosis will show increased dilatation with the fluid challenge. Occasionally, urography or CT with intravenous contrast media will be necessary for further differentiation.

Computed tomography obtained for other reasons in the abdomen may be the first examination to detect hydronephrosis. In these cases, images should be obtained to determine the level and cause of obstruction. On CT, an obstruction caused by periureteral tumor invasion versus periureteral fibrosis cannot be reliably distinguished, but CT is excellent for detecting adjacent periureteral masses and other causes such as aneurysm, urinoma, and extensive retroperitoneal fibrosis. Computed tomography without intravenous contrast is also able to differentiate between intraluminal calculi and primary urothelial tumors because of the increased attenuation occurring with both opaque and nonopaque calculi.

Real-time ultrasound is routinely used in the preliminary evaluation of the urinary tract in children, particularly in conjunction with the voiding cystourethrogram. If the ultrasound is abnormal or indeterminate in these patients, urography is indicated.

Calculi

Renal calculi vary in their radiodensity on conventional radiographs because of the differences in their calcium content. However, the plain radiograph or urography cannot distinguish nonopaque calculi from other filling defects such as blood clots, tumor, necrotic papillae, or fungus balls.

Evaluation of intraluminal filling defects by ultrasound depends on size and echogenicity. The calculus matrix will demonstrate a dense echo pattern with pronounced distal shadowing, regardless of whether it contains calcium or has another chemical composition. The differential diagnosis of acoustic shadowing within the kidney is limited to renal calculi and intrarenal gas, which are easily distinguished on the plain radiograph. The detection of blood clots, fungus balls, and urothelial tumors in the renal pelvis depends on the size of the defect, since they do not produce a shadow effect.

The use of CT to diagnose nonopaque calculi has been well established in all parts of the urinary tract, since CT can detect the increased attenuation seen in any calculus regardless of chemical composition. The attenuation of nonopaque calculi is much greater than that of intraluminal soft tissue defects such as neoplasm, blood clots, sloughing debris, and fungus balls. In an *in vitro* setting, CT is also able to differentiate among the 90% of calculi common to the clinical setting – for example, calcium oxylate, struvite, and uric acid.

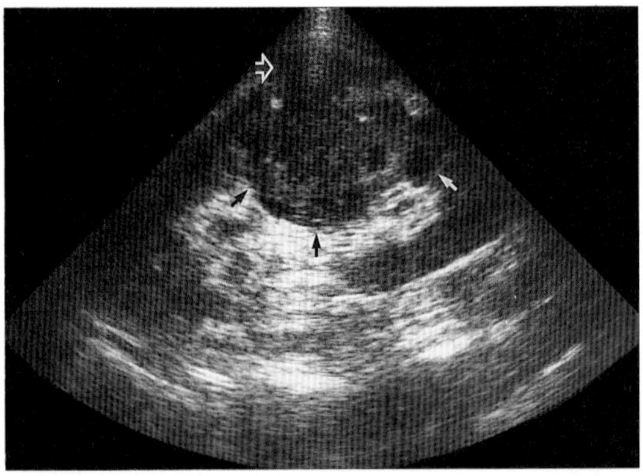

A

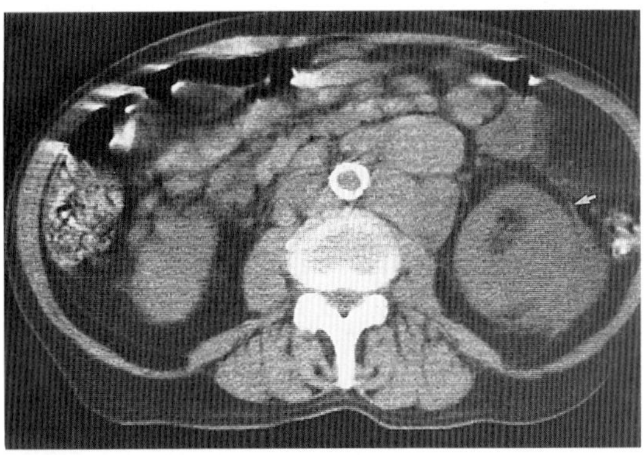

B

13–24 Renal abscess. **(A)** Longitudinal supine sonogram demonstrates poorly defined complex mass (arrows) with variable echogenicity. Note extension into retroperitoneum (open arrow). **(B)** Noncontrast CT scan shows nonhomogeneous enlargement of left lower pole with infiltration of adjacent peri-/paranephric fat and thickening of Gerota's fascia (arrow). There is retroperitoneal lymphadenopathy consistent with known lymphoma. No intravenous contrast was used because of renal failure.

Intrarenal Infections

Focal Infections

Focal acute bacterial nephritis, also known as acute lobar nephronia or carbuncle, is a localized form of pyelonephritis without liquefaction, midway in the spectrum from acute pyelonephritis to abscess. By ultrasound, an interstitial infection such as a carbuncle may appear as a solid, hypoechoic mass disrupting the corticomedullary junction. A renal abscess will show an irregular, thick-walled, hypoechoic mass with increased wave transmission proportional to the amount of liquefaction (Fig. 13–24 A). Small intrarenal lesions are sometimes difficult to identify by ultrasound, since there is echogenicity similar to the adjacent renal parenchyma and no definite demarcation.

Computed tomography is more sensitive than either urography or ultrasound in detecting focal areas of interstitial infection and is the most sensitive evaluation for perirenal extension. Focal bacterial nephritis appears as an ill-defined low-attenuation area in a lobar distribution (Fig. 13–24B). A renal abscess is usually well demarcated and rounded and does not follow the lobar distribution of focal bacterial nephritis. The attenuation of a renal abscess is related to the amount of liquefaction present, usually 20 HU to 30 HU. The central portion of the mass does not enhance after intravenous contrast, whereas the thick walls often do.

Aspiration of a suspected abscess for culture can be directed by ultrasound or CT. Focal infections of the kidney may be monitored with either ultrasound or CT to check response to antibiotic therapy. Up to 20% of patients with renal abscess will have a negative urinalysis and culture. Focal infection must be differentiated from other causes of focal defect, such as renal infarct, lymphoma, renal abscess, and hypovascular tumors such as papillary cell carcinoma and metastatic carcinoma.

The genitourinary tract is second only to the respiratory system as a site of tuberculosis infection. Renal tuberculosis is hematogenously spread from the lung, although radiographic evidence of pulmonary tuberculosis is present in less than 50% of patients. The urinalysis characteristically shows "sterile" pyuria, but may be normal if the disease is focal or if the affected calix is obstructed. Urine cultures for acid-fast organisms are notoriously negative in spite of active disease. Therefore, renal tuberculosis often presents a diagnostic dilemma.

Renal tuberculosis may be first visualized on the urogram as focal papillary necrosis, which is secondary to parenchymal infection. CT is the ideal method for determining the extent of renal involvement. Periureteral and peripelvic fibrosis occur with renal tuberculosis in response to healing and can be best evaluated by CT. Obstruction associated with focal or diffuse pyelonephritis due to tuberculosis may be difficult to differentiate from xanthogranulomatous pyelonephritis and infected hydronephrosis secondary to either a tumor or calculus. Tuberculosis will eventually cause parenchymal destruction by infection or obstruction from ureteral strictures.

Diffuse Infections

Acute pyelonephritis is generally diagnosed clinically from a symptom complex of fever, flank pain, and dysuria associated with positive urine cultures. Radiographic imaging with urography or ultrasound is used to exclude urinary tract obstruction and renal abscess.

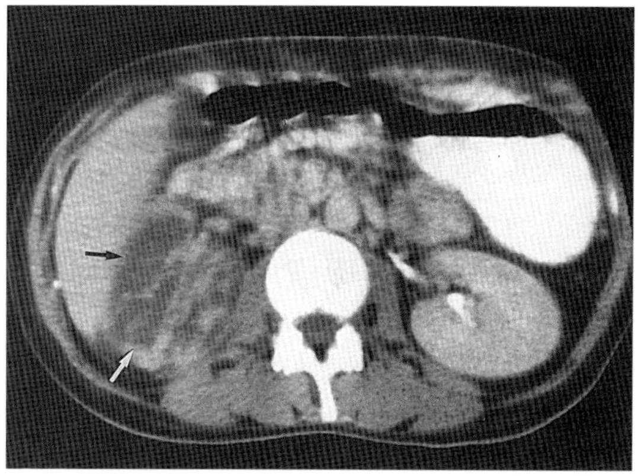

13–25 Diffuse pyelonephritis. Post-contrast CT scan demonstrates diffuse enlargement of right kidney with irregular, variable enhancement (arrows).

In diffuse pyelonephritis, the affected kidney may be enlarged, and, after IV contrast, there is often a nonhomogeneous nephrogram with segmental or diffuse areas of variable attenuation resulting in macrostriations. This pattern may be visible with urography, angiography, or CT (Fig. 13–25). Progression of acute pyelonephritis to abscess or extension beyond the renal capsule is most easily evaluated by CT.

Xanthogranulomatous pyelonephritis is an uncommon granulomatous inflammation characterized by destruction of the renal parenchyma and the presence of lipid-laden macrophages. The disease occurs predominately in middle-aged women and is associated with obstruction, chronic urinary tract infection, and calculi. The most common bacteria are *E. coli* and *Proteus*. Usually the entire kidney is involved; however, this condition can manifest as a focal disease and must be differentiated from other causes of hypovascular parenchymal masses.

Commonly, this pyelonephritis presents on the urogram as an enlarged nonfunctioning kidney with associated calculi. On ultrasound, the findings include pelviscaliectasis with medium amplitude echoes corresponding to the xanthomatous tissue and debris. Evaluation by CT shows dilated calices filled with debris having attenuation values from −15 to +15.

The contrast-enhanced CT scan will show a "blush" of the dilated calices, due to the abundant vascularity within the granulomatous tissue and the compressed normal renal parenchyma. This blush is responsible for the accentuation of the cystic areas following intravenous contrast material. The hallmark of xanthogranulomatous pyelonephritis by retrograde pyelography is pelvicaliectasis filled with destroyed parenchyma and debris; this differs from the retrograde appearance of infected hydronephrosis where the caliceal architecture is preserved.

Urothelial Infections

By urography or retrograde pyelography, urothelial infections commonly demonstrate mucosal irregularity and submucosal edema, or deposits such as are found with ureteritis cystica. Fungal infections, such as *Candida albicans*, more typically involve the urothelium than the renal parenchyma and are commonly associated with diabetes mellitus or with chronically ill or immunologically suppressed patients. The hallmark of a fungal infection in the urinary tract is the fungus ball or a castlike mass in the ureter.

Extrarenal Infections

Perinephric abscesses are readily demonstrated by both CT and ultrasound when they are well-defined fluid collections. However, when gas-forming organisms are present, the perinephric abscess will be more easily shown on CT and may be undetected by ultrasound.

References

Amis ES, Jr, Cronan JJ, Pfister RC: Needle puncture of cystic renal masses: A survey of the Society of Uroradiology. *Am. J. Roentgenol.* 148:297–299, 1987.

Ball DS, Friedman AC, Hartman DS, Radecki PD, Caroline DF: Scar sign of renal oncocytoma: Magnetic resonance imaging appearance and lack of specificity. *Urol. Radiol.* 8:46–48, 1986.

Hartman DS, Davis CJ, Sanders RC, Johns TT, Smirniotopoutos J, Goldman SM: The multiloculated renal mass: Considerations and differential features. *Radiographics* 7:29–52, 1987.

Hillman BJ, Drach GW, Tracey P, Gaines JA: Computed tomographic analysis of renal calculi. *Am. J. Roentgenol.* 142:549–552, 1984.

Hricak H, Demas BE, Williams RD, McNamara MT, Hedgcock MW, Amparo EG, Tanagho EA: Magnetic resonance imaging in the diagnosis and staging of renal and perirenal neoplasms. *Radiology* 154:709–715, 1985.

Hricak H, Thoeni RF, Carroll PR, Demas BE, Marotti M, Tanagho EA: Detection and staging of renal neoplasms: A reassessment of MR imaging. *Radiology* 166: 643–649, 1988.

Jaschke W, Van Kaick G, Peter S, Palmtag H: Accuracy of computed tomography in staging of kidney tumors. *Acta Radiol. (Diagn.)* 23:593–598, 1982.

Levine E, Rak Le K, Weigel J: Preoperative determination of abdominal extent of renal cell carcinoma by computed tomography. *Radiology* 132:395–398, 1979.

Marks WM, Korobkin M, Callen PW, Kaiser JA: CT diagnosis of tumor thrombosis of the renal vein and inferior vena cava. *Am. J. Roentgenol.* 131:843–846, 1978.

Marotti M, Hricak H, Fritzsche P, Crooks LE, Hedgcock MW, Tanagho EA: Evaluation of complex renal cysts by magnetic resonance imaging. *Radiology* 162:679–684, 1987.

McClennan BL, Stanley RJ, Melson GL, Levitt RG, Sagel SS: CT of the renal cyst: Is cyst aspiration necessary? *Am. J. Roentgenol.* 133:671–675, 1979.

Pollack HM, Banner MP, Arger PH, Peters J, Mulhern CH, Jr., Coleman BG: The accuracy of gray-scale renal ultrasonography in differentiating cystic neoplasms from benign cysts. *Radiology* 143:741–745, 1982.

Robson CH, Churchill BM, Anderson W: The results of radical nephrectomy for renal cell carcinoma. *J. Urol.* 101:267–301, 1969.

Rosenberg ER, Korobkin M, Foster W, Silverman PM, Bowie JD, Dunnick NR: The significance of septations in a renal cyst. *Am. J. Roentgenol.* 144:593–595, 1985.

Sagel SS, Stanley RJ, Levitt RG, Geisse G: Computed tomography of the kidney. *Radiology* 124:359–370, 1977.

Stuck KJ, Koff SA, Silver TM: Ultrasonic features of multicystic dysplastic kidney: Expanded diagnostic criteria. *Radiology* 143:217–221, 1982.

Weiner SN, Bernstein RG: Renal oncocytoma: Angiographic features of two cases. *Radiology* 125:633, 1977.

Zeman RK, Cronan JJ, Rosenfield AT, Choyke PL, Paushter DM, Clark LR, Jaffe MH, Schiebler ML: Computed tomography of renal masses: Pitfalls and anatomic variants. *Radiographics* 6:351–372, 1986.

Zirinsky K, Auh YH, Rubenstein WA, Williams JJ, Pasmantier MW, Kazam E: CT of the hyperdense renal cyst: Sonographic correlation. *Am. J. Roentgenol.* 143:151–156, 1984.

Suggested Reading

Daniel WW, Jr, Hartman GW, Witten DM, Farrow GM, Kelalis PP: Calcified renal masses: A review of 10 years of experience at the Mayo Clinic. *Radiology* 103:503–508, 1972.

Drach GW: Urinary lithiasis. *In* Harrison JH, et al. (eds.): *Campbell's Urology.* Philadelphia, W. B. Saunders, 1978.

Elkin M: Renal cyst and renal abscess. *Curr. Probl. Diagn. Radiol.* 5:1–56, 1975.

Goldberg BB: *Abdominal Grey Scale Ultrasonography.* New York, John Wiley & Sons, 1977.

Griscom NT, Vawter GF, Fellers FX: Pelvoinfundibular atresia: The usual form of multicystic kidney: 44 unilateral and two bilateral cases. *Semin. Roentgenol.* 10:125–132, 1975.

Gross M, Beach PD: The simultaneous occurrence of renal carcinoma and cyst: Problems in management. *South. Med. J.* 64:1059–1062, 1971.

Kramer SA, Hoffman AD, Aydin G, Kelalis PP: Simple renal cysts in children. *J. Urol.* 128:1259–1261, 1982.

Levine E, Grantham JJ: High-density renal cysts in autosomal dominant polycystic disease demonstrated by CT. *Radiology* 154:477–482, 1985.

Madewell JE, Goldman SM, Davis CJ, Jr., Hartman DS, Feigin DS, Lichtenstein JE: Multilocular cystic nephroma: A radiographic pathologic correlation of 58 patients. *Radiology* 146:309–321, 1983.

Murphy DM, Zincke H, Furlow WL: Primary grade 1 transitional cell carcinoma of the renal pelvis and ureter. *J. Urol.* 123:629–631, 1980.

Privett JTJ, Jeans WD, Roylance J: The incidence and importance of renal duplication. *Clin. Radiol.* 27:521–530, 1976.

Silverberg E: Cancer statistics, 1985. *CA-A Cancer Journal for Clinicians* 35:26, 1985.

Snyder HM, Lebowitz RL, Colodny AH, Bauer SB, Retik AB: Ureteropelvic junction obstruction in children. *Urol. Clin. North Am.* 7:273–290, 1980.

Thorley JD, Jones SR, Sanford JP: Perinephric abscess. *Medicine* 53:441–451, 1974.

CHAPTER

14

Correlative Imaging of the Lower Genitourinary Tract

John Stassi and Matthew D. Rifkin

This chapter summarizes the major benefits of several imaging modalities used to diagnose lower genitourinary pathology.

Plain Film and Contrast Radiography

Plain film radiography of the bladder is limited by the inherent low contrast of the soft-tissue and fluid-containing structures within the pelvis. While plain film is useful for detection of calcifications, gas collections, and radiodense foreign bodies, it is often difficult to identify these as intravesical (either intraluminal or intramural) or extravesical.

Iodinated contrast can be instilled in a retrograde fashion as a primary examination (cystography), or radiographs of the bladder can be obtained following an intravenous urogram. This allows limited definition of the mucosal surface of the bladder, which is tangential to the radiographic beam. Oblique and lateral images, in addition to anteroposterior views, are therefore necessary for a complete examination. Intraluminal filling defects may be detected, but their appearance is nonspecific. Small mural or luminal masses may be obscured by contrast.

Computed Tomography

The benefits of computed tomography (CT) are its improved contrast resolution and ability to produce cross-sectional images. Thus, CT scanning can routinely differentiate the urine-filled bladder lumen and its contents from the bladder wall and perivesical fat. The attenuation coefficient of some intraluminal filling defects may be diagnostic. The adjacent perivesical space, which includes bowel, reproductive organs, lymph nodes, surrounding fascial planes, and the bony pelvis, can also be imaged. In evaluating these adjacent structures, opacification of bowel with oral contrast is necessary; rectal contrast is often helpful. In some cases, the use of intravenous contrast will aid in the evaluation, allowing differentiation of blood vessels from lymph nodes and definition of enhancing neoplasms.

Images are usually limited to the transaxial plane. Direct coronal and sagittal imaging have been employed by some investigators to better evaluate adjacent organs in several scan planes, but these techniques are limited by gantry size and agility of the patient (van Waes et al. 1986). Mathematical algorithms can be used to reformat axial data into coronal and sagittal images. However, image quality is degraded, and diagnostic information may be diminished.

Ultrasound

Delineation of anatomy and detection of pathology by ultrasound depend on an acoustic mismatch of adjacent tissues. Fluid and soft tissues have characteristic echo patterns and, if the ultrasound examination is performed in real-time, dynamic studies can be undertaken. Bladder wall pliability can be assessed with this technique.

Transabdominal ultrasound is the conventional approach. Adequate distension of the bladder with urine is required for an optimal study. The transducer is placed on the anterior abdominal wall just superior to the symphysis pubis, and images can be obtained in sagittal, axial, and oblique planes. Unless overlying bowel gas obscures information, adjacent perivesical structures can be imaged, including the seminal vesicles.

The techniques of endorectal and endourethral sonography allow for the use of higher-frequency transducers, as there is less tissue intervening between the bladder and the probe. This provides greater axial resolution and increases the ability to detect subtle infiltrative processes. However, both field of view and scan plane are limited with these techniques. Endourethral scanning is performed at the time of cystoscopy while the patient is sedated. Images are usually obtained in an axial scan plane. The dome of the bladder is seen segmentally by angulating the sonocystoscope. The prostate and seminal vesicles may also be imaged.

Endorectal scanning does not require patient preparation or anesthesia. Images can be obtained in the transverse or sagittal planes. The seminal vesicles can also be seen. Since both of these orientations have a limited field of view, the entire bladder and all the perivesical structures may not be visualized. Complete examination may require both transabdominal and endorectal approaches.

Magnetic Resonance Imaging

The use of various pulse sequences in magnetic resonance (MR) imaging allows clear differentiation of the bladder wall and intra- and extravesical contents and structures; the seminal vesicles can also be seen. Direct sagittal, transverse, coronal, and various oblique images can be obtained. Imaging is based on the changes in applied magnetic field forces of the hydrogen ion within the tissue and subsequent relaxation of these forces. Currently, the major limitations are expense and the time needed to obtain a diagnostic study.

Abnormalities of the Bladder and Perivesical Region

Bladder Neoplasia

Transabdominal sonography detects many bladder cancers with the exception of stage-0 and small stage-A tumors. The transabdominal technique accurately distinguishes stages B1 and B2 from stage-C and stage-D disease up to 80% of the time. However, this is limited to larger lesions (Fig. 14–1) (Abu-Yousef et al. 1984; Singer et al. 1981).

Although conventional transabdominal ultrasound may define and accurately stage large lesions, it has limited benefit for small tumors. Transurethral sonoendoscopy is the more sensitive examination for small lesions. Papillary lesions as small as a few millimeters can be identified (Fig. 14–2). Although the depth of penetration

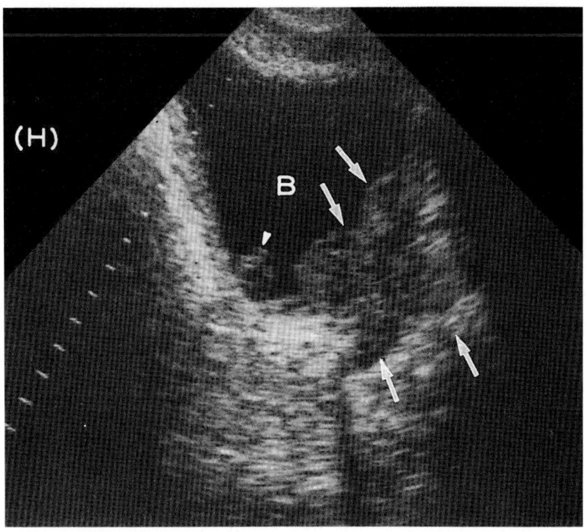

14–1 Bladder cancer – ultrasound. Longitudinal image of urinary bladder demonstrates large tumor mass with infiltration into prostate and seminal vesicles (arrows). A smaller secondary mass (arrowhead) is also identified. (B = bladder; H = toward patient's head.)

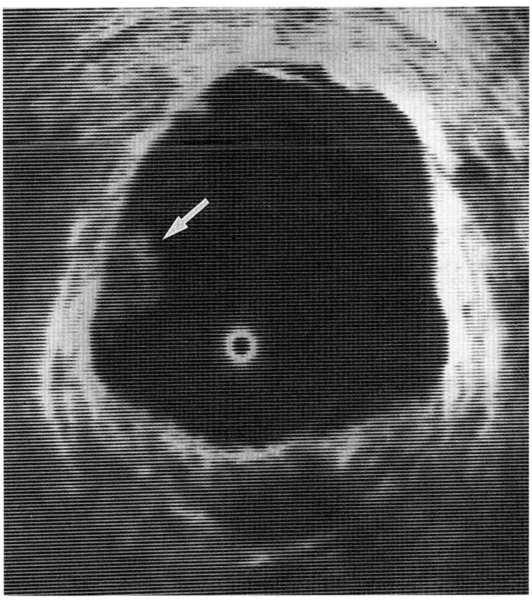

14–2 Transurethral ultrasound demonstrates small, noninvasive bladder carcinoma (arrow). (Reprinted, by permission, from Rifkin MD: *Diagnostic Imaging of the Lower Genitourinary Tract.* © 1985, Raven Press, New York, NY.)

and transvesical extension cannot be determined with conventional cystoscopy, the simultaneous use of the sonoendoscope raises accuracy of staging to nearly 100% (Schuller et al. 1982). Endorectal sonography can be almost as accurate and does not require anesthesia. However, it cannot reliably diagnose stage-A tumors, and some areas near the dome of the bladder may not be imaged (Watanabe et al. 1983).

CT is useful for evaluating extravesical spread of disease in a patient with known bladder carcinoma. The accuracy of CT in detecting perivesical and seminal vesicle involvement in these patients is between 65% and 85%. However, CT cannot distinguish between stage-0, stage-A, stage-B1, and stage-B2 lesions (Frodin et al. 1980; Hodson et al. 1979). Microscopic invasion of the perivesical fat and metastases to nonenlarged nodes will not be detected.

MR imaging may be superior to CT in defining the extent of bladder neoplasia. Early results suggest that MR imaging is not as sensitive as endourethral sonoendoscopy (Amendola et al. 1986; Lee, Rholl 1986).

Inflammatory Disease

Imaging has limited application in inflammatory bladder disease. Transurethral endosonography may be the most helpful in visualizing the trigone and distal ureters. Useful information may be obtained by imaging cystitis if causative factors or complications, such as intravesical foreign bodies, blood clots, and calculi, can be demonstrated.

Plain films can be diagnostic in emphysematous cystitis; gas is seen in the bladder wall, bladder lumen, or both. These findings can be demonstrated with CT as well. The appearance of air, which causes acoustic shadowing, can be confusing during ultrasonography. Since it may be introduced into the bladder wall or lumen during instrumentation, accurate clinical history is required.

Bladder Diverticula

Bladder diverticula are best demonstrated on conventional cystograms or excretory urograms. Some diverticula opacify only on the postvoid film. Oblique projections are usually necessary to demonstrate the neck of the diverticulum. If the neck is obstructed because of tumor, blood clot, stone, or stricture, the diverticulum may not fill with contrast.

Ultrasound, CT, or MR demonstrate a fluid density mass adjacent to the bladder. While a soft tissue mass protruding from the bladder may be seen on noncontrast CT, the diagnosis is confirmed with the administration of intravenous contrast if the diverticulum fills. Ultrasound can be diagnostic if a discontinuity between the adjacent walls of the diverticulum and the bladder is seen (Rifkin et al. 1984). A study done during voiding may show the neck more clearly and document emptying or enlargement of the diverticulum.

There is increased incidence of malignancy developing within urinary diverticula; consequently, if the diverticulum fills on contrast studies, a distortion of the wall or an associated mass should be sought. Transabdominal ultrasound and CT are most helpful in instances where the diverticulum cannot be filled on contrast studies. Regardless of the imaging study, the differentiation between intradiverticular hematoma, debris, and tumor can be difficult, and cystoscopy will be necessary. Magnetic resonance imaging may eventually offer more tissue-specific information in cases of complicated diverticula.

Miscellaneous Bladder Lesions

Contrast studies can visualize foreign bodies, blood clots, and calculi as filling defects within the bladder lumen. All may mimic a tumor. Radiopaque stones and foreign bodies can usually be diagnosed on the plain film. Ultrasound can demonstrate calculi regardless of mineral composition. They appear as brightly echogenic areas with acoustic shadowing. All calculi appear as high density on CT.

Intravesical hematomas examined over a period of time with ultrasound may demonstrate a characteristic appearance that allows differentiation from tumor. Blood clots will usually decrease in size over several days and change in echogenicity on follow-up examinations; some will liquefy.

Bladder Outlet Obstruction

The estimation of urine volume before and after voiding can be performed without catheterization as part of an intravenous urogram or cystogram. However, relatively accurate measurements of clinically significant post-void residual can only be obtained by sonography. The transabdominal approach is accurate and easier to use than other techniques. Derived formulas have an accuracy within about 25% of the actual urine volume in the clinically significant range (Griffiths et al. 1986).

In cases of outlet obstruction, the plain film may reveal a large soft-tissue density in the pelvis or low abdomen, representing the distended bladder. The trabeculations, cellule formation, and diffuse wall thickening associated with bladder outlet obstruction are demonstrated by radiographic contrast studies. CT and ultrasound are more sensitive in detecting early stages of wall thickening. The trabeculated appearance of the urine-filled bladder on coronal MR images may be as informative as a radiographic contrast study.

Congenital Lesions

Ureteroceles

Ectopic termination of a ureter within the bladder has a characteristic appearance on intravenous contrast examinations; the contrast-filled distal ureter protrudes into the lumen (cobra head) and is surrounded by a radiolucent rim of mucosa. This is not seen with ectopic ureteroceles terminating in the seminal vesicles, urethra, or vagina. Ultrasound, CT, and MR can detect ureteroceles as cystic intravesical structures. However, the appearance will not be as characteristic as that seen with the intravenous urogram. CT scans performed with intravenous contrast can define the ectopic termination, either within the bladder or a more distal portion of the genital tract. For ureters terminating within the bladder, ultrasound may offer a specific diagnosis, if, under real-time examination, a stream or jet of urine arises from the ectopic orifice.

Urachal Cysts

Urachal cysts (allantoic duct remnants) may be situated in the midline of the lower abdomen from the anterior-superior aspect of the bladder to the umbilicus. CT, ultrasound, and MR imaging will define these cysts as midline fluid-filled structures. If the cyst is small or does not communicate with the bladder, it will not be seen with contrast radiography. When cysts are large, they can compress and displace the bladder and sometimes be mistaken for it. Filling the bladder with water through a Foley catheter during the ultrasound examination will clarify the findings.

Infection, tumor, or hemorrhage can complicate a urachal cyst. CT (Fig. 14–3), transabdominal ultrasound, and MR imaging demonstrate irregularity and thickening of the wall. The mass appears solid. Ultrasound may show internal

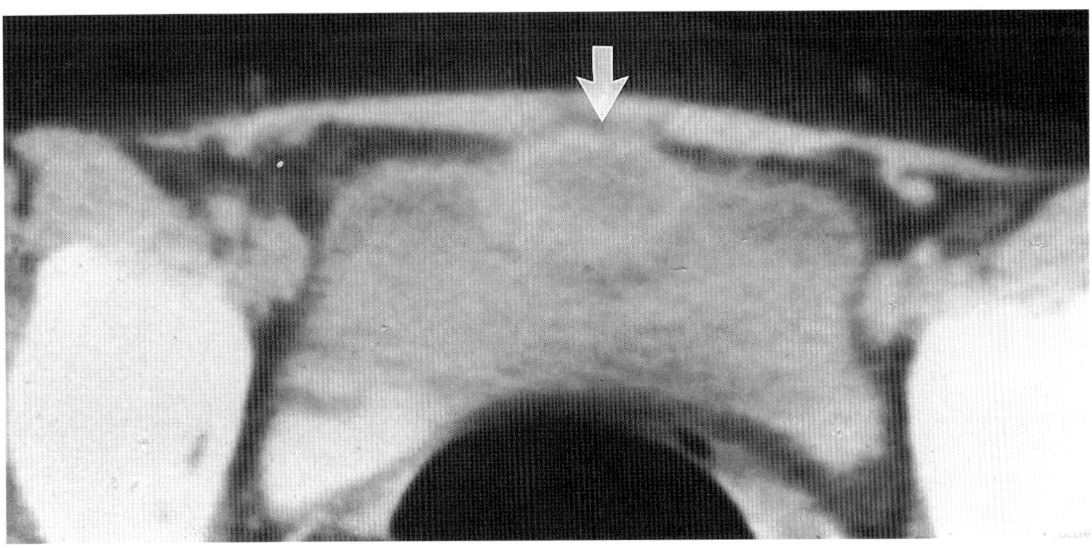

14–3 Infected urachal cyst. Contrast-enhanced computed tomography demonstrates extrinsic mass adjacent to superior aspect of bladder in midline (arrow). Thickened walls posteriorly are suggestive of a complicated cyst, in this case, infection.

echoes suggesting hemorrhage or purulent debris. Ultrasound or CT-guided drainage and biopsy can be performed easily.

Extravesical Abnormalities

A variety of extravesical abnormalities, such as lipomas, fibromas, and metastatic deposits from prostate or other organs, can compress and distort the urinary bladder. In general, conventional ultrasound, CT, and MR imaging show these lesions better than conventional intravenous urography. While the latter examination may demonstrate a mass effect, the cross-sectional imaging studies frequently define differences in soft-tissue density more accurately. For example, a lipoma will have negative CT numbers, but highly reflective echogenic characteristics by sonography. A lymphoma will be seen as a solid mass on CT; it will be anechoic, yet attenuate the sound waves on sonographic examination (Fig. 14–4).

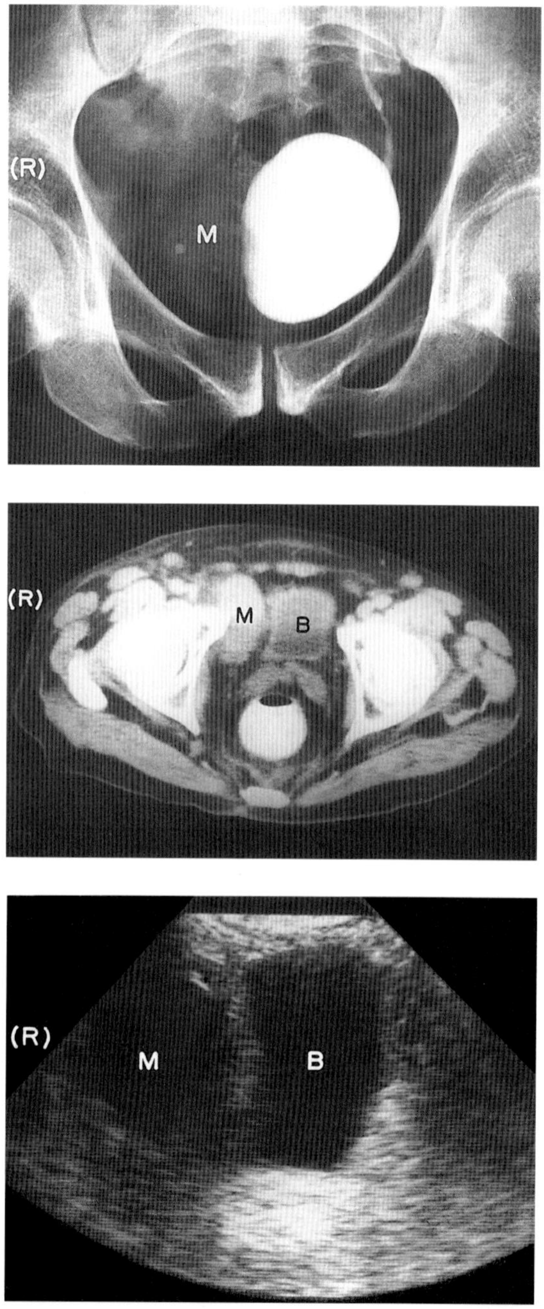

14–4 Lymphoma. **(A)** Intravenous pyelogram demonstrates extrinsic mass (M) compressing bladder. **(B)** Contrast-enhanced computed tomography again demonstrates mass (M) compressing bladder (B). **(C)** Ultrasound image is more diagnostic. This mass (M) is anechoic, but attenuates sound findings highly suggestive of lymphoma. B = bladder; R = right side. (Reprinted, by permission, from Rifkin MD et al.: Sonography of nongynecological cystic masses of the pelvis. *Am. J. Roentgenol.* 142:1169–1174, © 1984, American Roentgen Ray Society.)

Abnormalities of the Prostate

Enlarged Prostate

Accurate estimation of prostate size helps the clinician plan therapy for bladder outlet obstruction. Enlarged glands of less than 60 g to 75 g can usually be resected transurethrally. Larger glands may require open prostatectomy.

The estimation of size by contrast studies is based on displacement of the bladder. This technique presupposes symmetric enlargement of the prostate, which is often not the case. The simplest and most accurate method for assessing size is transabdominal ultrasound, which can obtain measurements of length, width, and height. Since the specific gravity of prostatic tissue is close to 1, an accurate estimation of weight is obtained by calculating size in cubic centimeters. A useful formula is: Weight = $4/3\ \pi\ r^3$ (Henneberry et al. 1979). These dimensions can also be obtained with MR imaging and endorectal ultrasound. Estimating size with CT requires multiple images and more complicated planimetric calculations.

Focal Abnormalities

CT cannot distinguish focal benign from malignant lesions unless extension of malignant tumor

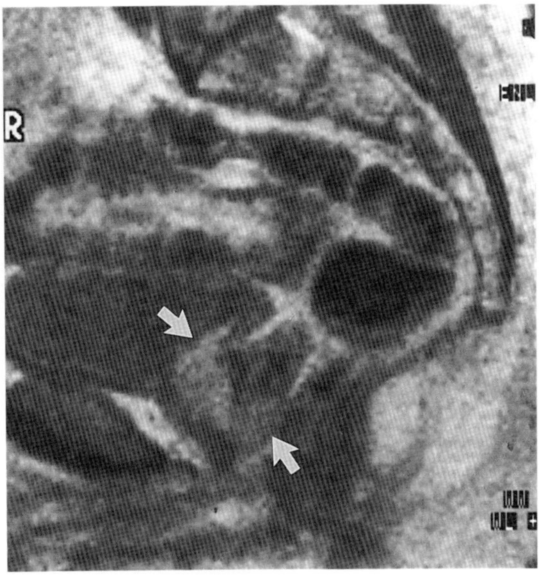

14–5 Prostate carcinoma – MR imaging. A direct sagittal magnetic resonance image, spin echo technique with TR of 1 sec and TE of 50 msec demonstrates nonspecific inhomogeneous changes in prostate (arrows), in this case due to carcinoma.

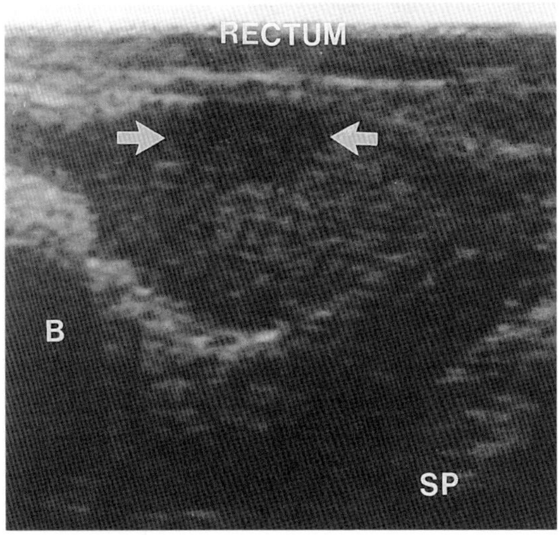

14–6 Prostate cancer – endorectal ultrasound. Longitudinally oriented linear array examination of prostate demonstrates 1-cm hypoechoic area (arrows) caused by small noninvasive prostatic carcinoma. (B = bladder; SP = symphysis pubis.)

beyond the capsule is identified. Recent studies have revealed the nonspecific appearance of focal benign and malignant lesions on MR studies (Fig. 14–5) (Bryan et al. 1986). As yet, there is no capability to biopsy prostatic lesions under MR guidance.

Transrectal sonography is the most sensitive technique in the detection of focal prostatic abnormalities. Subtle alterations in echotexture can be seen with the use of high-frequency transducers. Small carcinomas usually appear hypoechoic and ill-defined (Fig. 14–6). While the irregular margin of a lesion suggests malignancy, a necrotic adenoma may have this appearance; when calcified, it causes shadowing. Benign and malignant focal lesions cannot be reliably distinguished by acoustic criteria alone (Dahnert et al. 1986; Rifkin et al. 1986). Any peripheral, asymmetrically situated, or irregular focus, regardless of echogenicity, is suspicious, as is any lesion that distorts the capsule. Invasion and extension beyond the capsule are associated with malignant disease.

Endorectal ultrasound evaluates the prostate by detecting focal nonpalpable abnormalities, which, in most cases, will require a tissue diagnosis. An additional benefit of endorectal ultrasound is the ability to perform guided biopsy of any visualized lesion. Ultrasound guidance has

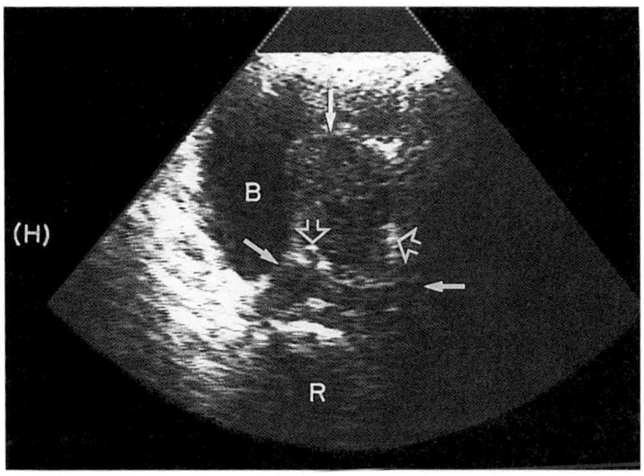

14–7 Prostatic enlargement and calculi – ultrasound. Longitudinal transabdominal ultrasound image demonstrates large prostate (arrows) impinging upon base of bladder (B). Prostatic calculi (open arrows) appear as bright echogenic areas. (R = rectum; H = toward patient's head.)

been shown to be more accurate than conventional digital guidance for biopsy of all lesions, even palpable ones (Lidell et al. 1986). Imaging in the longitudinal plane allows the needle to be guided throughout the biopsy procedure.

Suprapubic ultrasound may demonstrate larger focal lesions and some calculi (Fig. 14–7), but is of limited use for small abnormalities.

Prostate Carcinoma

Endorectal ultrasonography and perhaps MR imaging are the only tests with sufficient resolution to define subtle malignant invasion. The axial scan is most useful in detecting subtle asymmetry. Only large, invasive lesions will be detected by conventional suprapubic ultrasound (Abu-Yousef, Narayana 1985).

Extension of tumor into the seminal vesicles can be seen with endorectal ultrasound and on some transabdominal studies. Defining further extension of disease in the pelvis is best accomplished with CT; MR imaging will likely emerge as the most accurate modality for this. The CT study should be performed following administration of oral and rectal contrast in order to distinguish bowel loops from a neoplastic process. Intravenous contrast helps to separate vascular structures from lymph nodes. In addition to defining pelvic and retroperitoneal adenopathy, CT can demonstrate liver and lung metastases as well as pleural and ascitic fluid, mesenteric and peritoneal implants, and bone metastases. CT cannot distinguish nonneoplastic causes of lymph node enlargement from metastases. Metastatic foci in nonenlarged nodes cannot be detected.

CT cannot always distinguish inflammatory or postsurgical infiltration of soft tissues from neoplastic infiltration. Suspicious areas detected with CT can be biopsied easily under CT guidance. Soft-tissue characterization using MR imaging may yield more specific information in such cases. CT may have difficulty in defining the inferior surface of the prostate, owing to poor imaging of the cleavage plane between the prostate and the bladder base in axial scans. MR images in the coronal and sagittal planes overcome this problem (Hricak et al. 1987).

Lymphography, unlike CT, can define architectural changes within nodes that are not enlarged. Lymphography, if combined with fine-needle aspiration biopsy, can distinguish neoplastic from fatty or granulomatous change. One drawback is the inability of lymphography to image obturator and hypogastric nodal chains, which are often the first sites of nodal spread.

Radionuclide scans are more sensitive than plain film radiography or CT for bone metastases, and allow study of the entire skeleton with a single injection. The appearance or distribution of an abnormality on the scan may not always be typical for metastatic disease; plain film radiographic correlation is required.

Treatment planning in radiation therapy of prostatic malignancy can be performed using CT-acquired data (Pilepich et al. 1980).

Radium seed implants can be placed percutaneously via the transperineal route during endorectal ultrasound scanning using a specially designed guide. Seeds are inserted during axial ultrasonographic guidance and can be placed in a predetermined location with respect to the neoplastic focus being treated (Holm et al. 1983). This technique provides for more exact dosimetry calculations and theoretically reduces the risks of local radiation damage to surrounding genitourinary structures.

Contrast radiography, CT, transabdominal ultrasound, and endorectal ultrasound may be used to monitor therapeutic response (Carpentier, Schroder 1984). Serial bone scans can be used to monitor osseous metastases. The region of the bladder neck may be a site of recurrence in men who have undergone radical prostatectomies. This area is not accessible to clinical evaluation, but is well imaged by transrectal ultrasound (Rifkin 1984; Spirnak, Resnick 1984). Recurrence in the pelvis and abdomen is best ascertained by CT. MR imaging may replace CT because of its potential to obtain more tissue-specific information (Bryan et al. 1986).

Abnormalities of the Scrotum

Extratesticular Fluid Collections

Fluid collections of less than 1 ml can be detected with ultrasound. Sonographic differentiation between hydrocele, hematocele, and pyocele cannot be made, but the skin thickening accompanying chronic hydroceles can be detected (Fig. 14–8). When a fluid collection is reactive or secondary to trauma, ultrasound may demonstrate inflammatory or posttraumatic changes in the epididymis or testis (Fig. 14–9).

If the collection is large enough, a CT examination will demonstrate fluid separate from solid scrotal structures. Radionuclide studies will show a crescentic halo or floating testicle in a sizable collection. However, other cystic extratesticular processes may have this appearance. Reactive hydrocele suggests an underlying epididymitis, orchitis, or other process.

MR imaging might be expected to detect extratesticular fluid; however, no study has been reported detailing the specificity or sensitivity of such an examination.

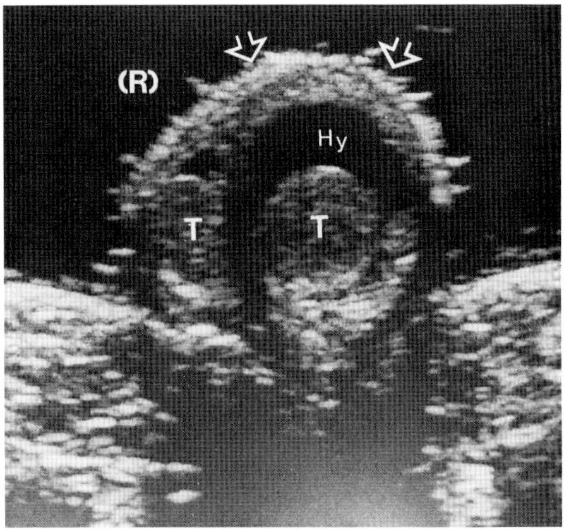

14–8 Chronic hydrocele – ultrasound. Water bath ultrasound demonstrates two normal testes (T), a hydrocele on left side (Hy) and thickened skin (open arrows). Thickened skin is highly suggestive of a chronic hydrocele. (Reprinted, by permission, from Rifkin MD: Ultrasonography of the lower genitourinary tract. *Urol. Clin. North Am.*, ©1985, W. B. Saunders Co., Philadelphia.)

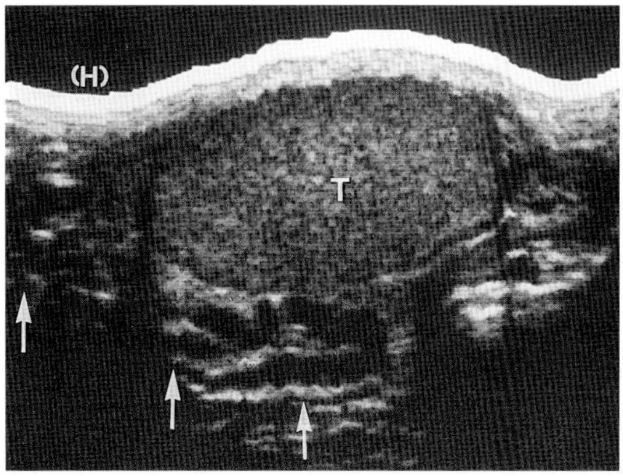

14–10 Varicocele – ultrasound. Longitudinally oriented ultrasound examination demonstrates dilated veins (arrows) posterior to normal testis (T) draining into region of spermatic cord. (H = toward patient's head.) (Reprinted, by permission, from Rifkin MD: Ultrasonography of the lower genitourinary tract. *Urol. Clin. North Am.* 12(4), © 1985, W. B. Saunders Co., Philadelphia.)

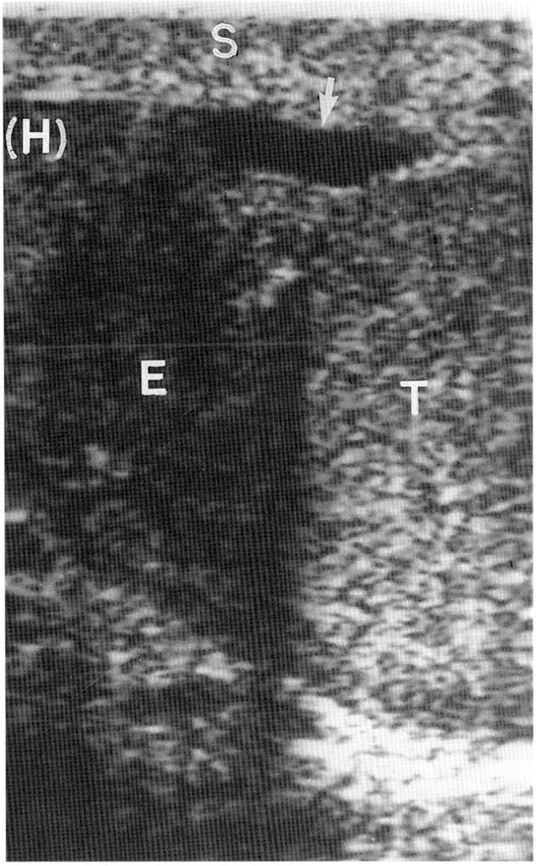

14–9 Epididymitis – ultrasound. Longitudinally oriented ultrasound examination demonstrates normal testis (T), thickened scrotal skin (S), small hydrocele (arrow), and enlarged hypoechoic epididymal head (E), diagnostic of epididymitis. (H = toward patient's head.)

Varicoceles

Since varicoceles, regardless of size, can be the cause of male infertility, the detection of subclinical lesions is important. Ultrasound is the most sensitive noninvasive imaging modality to define such lesions. Doppler analysis can detect venous stasis, reversals of flow, and thrombosis. With real-time high-resolution imaging, dilated vessels of the pampiniform plexus can be identified (Fig. 14–10). Real-time studies also allow imaging during maneuvers such as Valsalva.

Venous angiography, although sensitive, is invasive and uncomfortable; it is no longer routinely used. Radionuclide red blood cell studies may demonstrate venous stasis in large varicoceles. Thermography will be able to detect large lesions and some less obvious varicoceles. However, if venous reflux is intermittent or absent at the time of study, the lesion will be missed by this technique (Gold et al. 1977).

If surgical intervention is planned, a contrast study is performed to define vascular anatomy. As an alternative to open surgical ligation, percutaneous techniques, such as sclerotherapy or embolization with detachable balloons or stainless steel coils, can be performed at the time of the vascular study. The recurrence rates for percutaneous and open surgical techniques are comparable (Hamm et al. 1986).

Epididymal Masses and Spermatoceles

The cystic nature and anatomic location of epididymal cysts and spermatoceles can be accurately defined by ultrasound (Fig. 14–11). MR studies may eventually contribute to the diagnosis of cystic masses (Baker et al. 1987). Solid epididymal neoplasms are most often benign, but no available modality can distinguish benign from malignant or primary from metastatic disease. Ultrasound is the most accurate examination for epididymal masses.

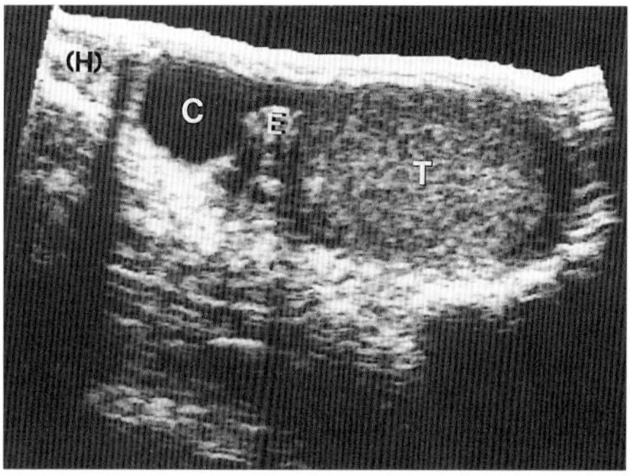

14–11 Epididymal cyst – ultrasound. Longitudinally oriented ultrasound demonstrates normal testicle (T). Extending from epididymal head (E) is an epididymal cyst (C). (H = toward patient's head.) (Reprinted, by permission, from W. B. Saunders Co, Philadelphia.)

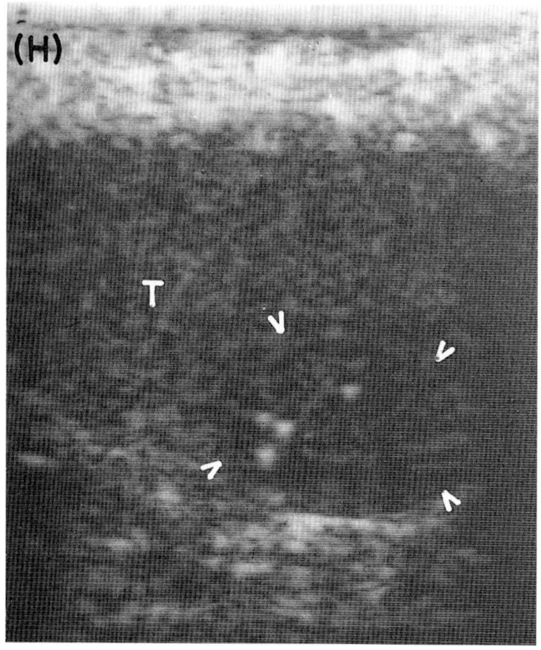

14–12 Nonpalpable testicular carcinoma – ultrasound. High-resolution ultrasound demonstrates infiltrating area (arrowheads) in posterior inferior aspect of testicle (T). This was a nonpalpable seminoma in patient who presented clinically with metastatic disease to mediastinum. (H = toward patient's head.)

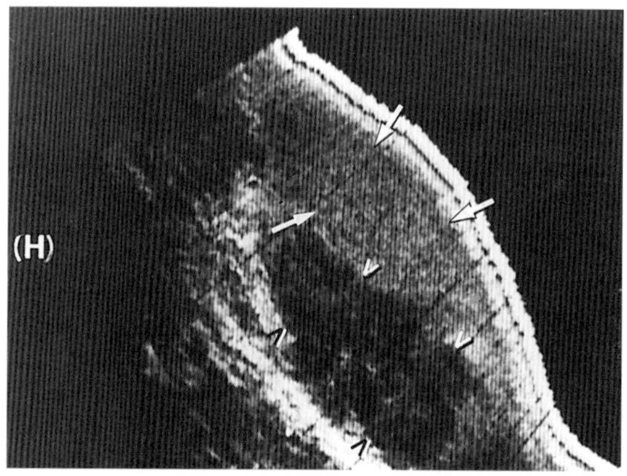

14–13 Seminoma – ultrasound. Longitudinally oriented sonogram demonstrates hypoechoic infiltrating area (arrowheads) in inferior posterior aspect of testicle. There is a residual portion of normal testicle (arrows). (H = toward patient's head.)

Testicular Masses

Sonography is the most useful modality in the evaluation of intratesticular masses (Rifkin 1985). It can detect small, nonpalpable lesions (Fig. 14–12) as well as larger lesions (Fig. 14–13). The examination can accurately differentiate cystic from solid masses. However, primary and secondary malignant lesions cannot reliably be distinguished from most benign processes (Rifkin et al. 1985; Tackett et al. 1986).

While most malignancies appear as focal hypoechoic masses, diffuse infiltration by tumor may simulate abscess, infarction, or hemorrhage. Clinical correlation is mandatory. Areas of previous hemorrhage within a malignancy can present as echogenic areas with calcification and fibrosis. Other benign intratesticular lesions that can mimic carcinoma include benign stromal tumors, sarcoidosis, and adrenal rests. The tunica albuginea, or testicular cyst, is one benign entity that can be accurately diagnosed sonographically without the need for surgical confirmation (Rifkin, Jacobs 1983).

Radionuclide studies will show evidence of increased flow if the mass is vascular; however, distinction between inflammatory and neoplastic lesions may be difficult. Early reports of MR imaging of benign and malignant scrotal pathology

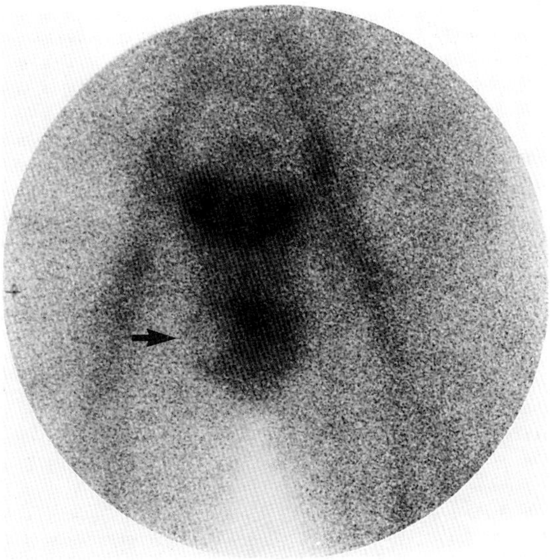

14–14 Torsion – radionuclide study. Static image in patient with torsion demonstrates no radioisotope activity in right testicle (arrow), diagnostic of torsion.

suggest that MR is as sensitive as, but no more specific than, ultrasound (Baker et al. 1987). Computed tomographic evaluation of testicular masses is best applied to the detection of extrascrotal spread of disease, particularly to retroperitoneal lymph nodes in cases of malignant testicular neoplasms.

The staging of testicular malignancy is currently best accomplished by CT. Mediastinal and retroperitoneal adenopathy as well as hepatic and pulmonary parenchymal metastases can be seen. Serial CT scans can be performed to follow response to therapy.

Respiratory, cardiac, and peristaltic motion may degrade MR images of the chest and abdomen. Nevertheless, in one study the accuracy of MR imaging approached that of CT in detecting retroperitoneal adenopathy. In that study, which evaluated 25 patients with nonseminomatous germ cell carcinoma, CT established the presence or absence of adenopathy in 88% of patients, and MR imaging established it in 84% (Ellis et al. 1984). With further refinements in technique, MR studies may surpass the accuracy of CT.

Lymphography has been shown to be insensitive in detecting metastases within nonenlarged nodes in patients with nonseminomatous tumors (Lien et al. 1983). Lymphography also opacifies poorly the first echelon of nodal spread from left testicular tumors, that is, to the left renal vein area.

Acute Scrotum

There is much overlap in the clinical presentation of epididymitis, orchitis, and testicular torsion. Ultrasound and radionuclide studies currently provide the basis for diagnostic imaging in all three entities.

Rapid clinical diagnosis and differentiation of testicular torsion from other acute scrotal processes is essential. When a study is needed, radionuclide imaging is the best choice. With torsion, a "nubbin" sign may be seen on flow images in both the acute and more chronic stages. Delayed images will show a lack of flow to the affected testicle (Fig. 14–14).

When an imaging study is needed for epididymitis, ultrasound is the preferred diagnostic examination. Although a radionuclide study may demonstrate increased uptake by the epididymis, subtle lesions may not be identified. On ultrasound, the epididymis is generally of decreased echogenicity and is enlarged (Fig. 14–9). Skin thickening may be seen in all inflammatory processes such as epididymitis and orchitis. Reactive hydroceles may be present, but are not associated with any specific cause.

Orchitis is usually a diffuse process secondary to epididymitis; however, some cases of orchitis are blood-borne and unrelated to the epididymis. In severe cases the radionuclide study will generally demonstrate increased uptake in the hemiscrotum or testicle (Fig. 14–15); subtle abnormalities may not be identified. Ultrasound (Fig. 14–16) may demonstrate enlargement and a diffuse inhomogeneous texture of the entire testicle. Because tumors may involve the testicle similarly, further differentiation is necessary. Ultrasound may reveal skin thickening, suggesting an inflammatory process. On the isotope study, tumors usually show less uptake than the inflammatory conditions. Clinical correlation is helpful; tumors are not painful, whereas inflammatory processes are.

CT does not demonstrate inflammatory processes in the scrotum unless an abscess develops. If the infection is gas forming, diagnostic lucencies will be detected within the scrotum. Ultrasound shows gas as bright echogenic areas with acoustic shadowing.

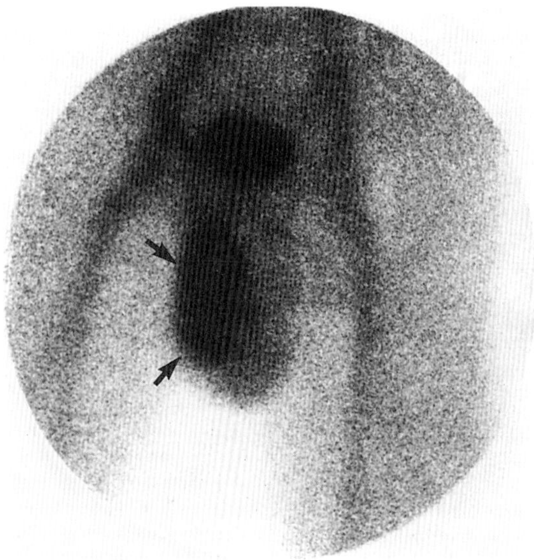

14–15 Orchitis – radionuclide study. Static radionuclide image demonstrates increased activity in right testicle (arrows), as compared to left. This indicates an inflammatory process instead of neoplasia, which in general will demonstrate less activity.

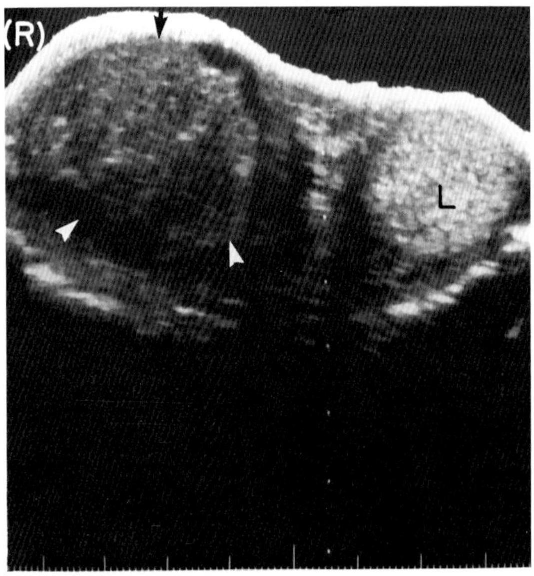

14–16 Orchitis – ultrasound. Right testis (arrowheads) is diffusely enlarged with an inhomogeneous pattern compared to the left testis (L). There is surrounding hydrocele fluid on the right. This orchitis was a diffuse inflammatory process, but a diffuse malignant infiltrative process can have a similar appearance. Skin thickening, present on right side in this case, suggests inflammation.

Cryptorchidism

The undescended testicle may be located within the inguinal canal, the abdomen, low pelvis, or high scrotum, in order of decreasing frequency. Ultrasound identifies testes located at the scrotal base or in the inguinal canal, usually with high reliability. Diagnosis is based on finding an ovoid soft tissue mass. The undescended testicle will be smaller than the normal testis unless malignant degeneration has occurred.

Ultrasound will be less successful in locating some small inguinal and most intra-abdominal testes (Wolverson et al. 1983). Computed tomography of the abdomen and pelvis is currently performed following a negative ultrasound. It is necessary to opacify the entire small and large bowel prior to scanning. Dynamic scanning with bolus injection of intravenous contrast is done to opacify the vascular structures of the pelvis and abdomen. A soft-tissue mass along the course of testicular descent is diagnostic. MR imaging is likely to replace CT for detecting an undescended testis and requires no radiation.

If CT, ultrasound, and MR imaging prove negative, gonadal venography may be indicated. However, testicular venography is invasive and not always successful. Defining the pampiniform plexus does not always indicate the presence of a gonad, and, in some cases, no testicular tissue is found with surgical exploration (Wolverson et al. 1983).

References

Abu-Yousef MM, Narayana AS: Prostatic carcinoma: Detection and staging using suprapubic US. *Radiology* 156:175–180, 1985.

Abu-Yousef MM, Narayana AS, Brown RC, Franken EA, Jr.: Urinary bladder tumors studied by cystosonography. *Radiology* 153:227–231, 1984.

Amendola MA, Glazer GM, Grossman HB, Aisen AM, Francis IR: Staging of bladder carcinoma: MRI-CT-surgical correlation. *Am. J. Roentgenol.* 146:1179–1183, 1986.

Baker LL, Hajek PC, Burkhard TK, Dicapua L, Landa HM, Leopold GR, Hesselink JR, Mattrey RF: MR imaging of the scrotum: Pathologic conditions. *Radiology* 163:93–98, 1987.

Bryan PJ, Butler HE, Nelson AD, LiPuma JP, Kopiwoda SY, Resnick MI, Cohen AM, Haaga JR: Magnetic resonance imaging of the prostate. *Am. J. Roentgenol.* 146:543–548, 1986.

Carpentier PJ, Schroder FH: Transrectal ultrasonography in the follow-up of prostatic carcinoma patients: A new prognostic parameter. *J. Urol.* 131:903–905, 1984.

Dahnert WF, Hamper UM, Eggleston JC, Walsh PC, Sanders RC: Prostatic evaluation by transrectal sonography with histopathologic correlation: The echopenic appearance of early carcinoma. *Radiology* 158:97–102, 1986.

Ellis HH, Bies JR, Kopecy KK, Klatte EC, Rowland RG, Donohue JP: Comparison of NMR and CT imaging in the evaluation of metastatic retroperitoneal lymphadenopathy from testicular carcinoma. *J. Comput. Assist. Tomogr.* 8:709–719, 1984.

Frodin L, Hemmingsson A, Johansson A, Wicklund H: Computed tomography in staging of bladder cancer. *Acta Radiol.* 21:763–767, 1980.

Gold RH, Ehrlich RM, Samuels B: Scrotal thermography. *Radiology* 122:129–132, 1977.

Griffiths CJ, Murray A, Ramsden PD: Accuracy and repeatability of bladder volume measurement using ultrasonic imaging. *J. Urol.* 136:808–812, 1986.

Hamm B, Fobbe F, Sorensen R, Felsenberg D: Varicoceles. Combined sonography and thermography in diagnosis and post-therapeutic evaluation. *Radiology* 160:419–424, 1986.

Henneberry M, Carter MF, Neiman HL: Estimation of prostatic size by suprapubic ultrasonography. *J. Urol.* 121:615–616, 1979.

Hodson NJ, Husband JE, Macdonald JS: The role of computed tomography in recurrent rectal tumors. *Clin. Radiol.* 30:389–395, 1979.

Holm HH, Juul N, Pedersen JF, Hansen H, Stroyer I: Transperineal ^{125}Iodine seed implantation in prostatic cancer guided by transrectal ultrasonography. *J. Urol.* 130:283–286, 1983.

Hricak H, Dooms GC, Jeffrey RB, Avallone A, Jacobs D, Benton WK, Narayan P, Tanagho EA: Prostatic carcinoma: Staging by clinical assessment, CT and MR imaging. *Radiology* 162:331–336, 1987.

Lee JKT, Rholl KS: MRI of the bladder and prostate. *Am. J. Roentgenol.* 147:732–736, 1986.

Lidell HT, McDougal WS, Burk DD, Fleischer AC: Ultrasound versus digitally directed prostatic needle biopsy. *J. Urol.* 135:716–718, 1986.

Lien HH, Fossa SD, Ous S: Lymphography in retroperitoneal metastases in non-seminoma testicular tumor patients with normal CT scan. *Acta Radiol. (Diagn.)* 4:319–322, 1983.

Pilepich MV, Perez CA, Prasad S: Computed tomography in definitive radiotherapy of prostatic carcinoma. *Int. J. Radiat. Oncol. Biol. Phys.* 6:923–926, 1980.

Pollack HM, Banner MP, Martinez LO, Hodson NJ: Diagnostic considerations in urinary bladder wall calcification. *Am. J. Roentgenol.* 136:791–797, 1981.

Rifkin MD: Sonourethrography: Technique for evaluation of prostatic urethra. *Radiology* 153:791–792, 1984.

Rifkin MD: *Diagnostic Imaging of the Lower Genitourinary Tract.* New York, Raven Press, 1985.

Rifkin MD, Friedland GW, Shortliffe L: Prostatic evaluation by transrectal endosonography: Detection of carcinoma. *Radiology* 158:85–90, 1986.

Rifkin MD, Jacobs JA: Simple testicular cyst diagnosed preoperatively by ultrasound. *J. Urol.* 129:982–983, 1983.

Rifkin MD, Kurtz AB, Pasto ME, Goldberg BB: Diagnostic capabilities of high-resolution scrotal ultrasonography. *J. Ultrasound Med.* 4:13–19, 1985.

Rifkin MD, Needleman L, Kurtz AB, Fornage BD, Pasto ME, Cole-Beuglet C, Goldberg BB: Sonography of nongynecological cystic masses of the pelvis. *Am. J. Roentgenol.* 142:1169–1174, 1984.

Schuller J, Walther V, Schmiedt E, Staehler G, Bauer HW, Schilling A: Intravesical ultrasound tomography in staging of bladder carcinoma. *J. Urol.* 128:264–266, 1982.

Singer D, Itzchak Y, Fischelovitch Y: Ultrasonographic assessment of bladder tumors. II. Clinical staging. *J. Urol.* 126:34–36, 1981.

Spirnak JP, Resnick MI: Transrectal ultrasonography. *Urology* 23:461–467, 1984.

Tackett RE, Ling D, Catalona WJ, Melson GL: High-resolution sonography in diagnosing testicular neoplasms. Clinical significance of false-positive scans. *J. Urol.* 135:494, 1986.

van Waes PFGM, Feldberg MAM, Goldberg HI, Herve P, Zonneveld FW, Cann CE: Direct coronal and direct sagittal CT of abdomen and pelvis: An approach to staging of malignancies. *Radiographics* 6:213–244, 1986.

Watanabe H, Mishina T, Ohe H: Staging of bladder tumors by transrectal ultrasonotomography and U.I. octoson. *Urol. Radiol.* 5:11–16, 1983.

Wolverson MK, Houttuin E, Heiberg E, Sundaram M, Shields JB: Comparison of computed tomography with high-resolution real-time ultrasound in the localization of the impalpable undescended testis. *Radiology* 146:133–136, 1983.

CHAPTER
15
Percutaneous Nephrostomy

Andrew J. LeRoy

Percutaneous puncture of cystic renal masses was originally performed using measurements from standard radiographs. Antegrade pyelography was developed in the early 1950s to better delineate the renal collecting systems and to complement retrograde ureteral procedures. The first series of interventional percutaneous renal decompression procedures was reported in 1955 (Goodwin et al.). Subsequent developments occurred primarily in Europe until the early 1970s. Since Stables and colleagues' classic 1978 review, thousands of percutaneous nephrostomy procedures have been performed, and the field of interventional uroradiology has been created.

Indications

Initially, percutaneous nephrostomy was limited to use on critically ill patients or as a temporary procedure prior to surgical therapy. However, due to its clinical effectiveness and the need for only local anesthetics, there are now numerous applications for its use (Table 15–1).

An obstructed collecting system is usually decompressed via a cystoscopic transurethral retrograde approach, but if that approach is unsuccessful, percutaneous nephrostomy placement is done.

Table 15–1 Indications for Percutaneous Nephrostomy

1. Decompression of obstructed urinary tracts
2. Functional assessment of a kidney (Whitaker test)
3. Diversion of urine flow
4. Collecting system access prior to endourologic procedure:
   a. Stricture dilation/incision
   b. Stent placement
   c. Removal of calculi or foreign bodies
   d. Biopsy/endoscopy
   e. Chemotherapy instillation

Since permanent loss of function of an obstructed kidney takes several weeks, treatment can be delayed for several days following a failed retrograde procedure if other serious medical problems coexist. However, infection occurring with the obstruction and causing urosepsis usually requires immediate drainage.

Percutaneous renal drainage together with chemical and volumetric urine studies and radionuclide scans permit assessment of recoverable renal function prior to surgery. In some cases, ultrasound or computed tomography (CT) will show only a thin, nonfunctional rim of renal cortex and preclude the need for percutaneous nephrostomy (Fig. 15–1).

Diversion of urine allows healing of postoperative edema or of urinary fistulas. Within several days after nephrostomy placement, swelling at anastomoses or incisions will resolve. Most benign urinary fistulas will heal with proximal urinary

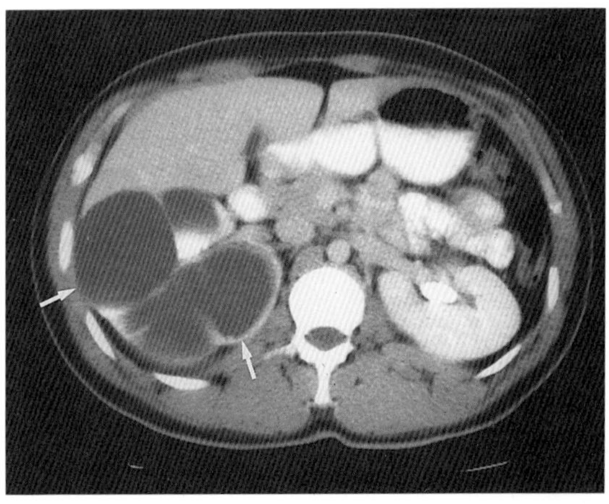

15–1 Abdominal CT scan at renal level shows abnormal right kidney with marked collecting system dilation (arrows) and almost no residual renal parenchyma. Contrast material present on right is from a previous retrograde pyelogram documenting a ureteropelvic junction obstruction. This nonfunctioning kidney was removed rather than repaired.

diversion and stenting. Urinary fistulas due to malignancies are more difficult to treat and rarely respond completely to percutaneous nephrostomy drainage.

Safe and reliable access to the urinary collecting systems has made possible interventional techniques such as stricture dilation, endopyelotomy, stent placement, removal of upper tract calculi, and diagnostic endoscopy. Accurate percutaneous nephrostomy placement is essential to those techniques.

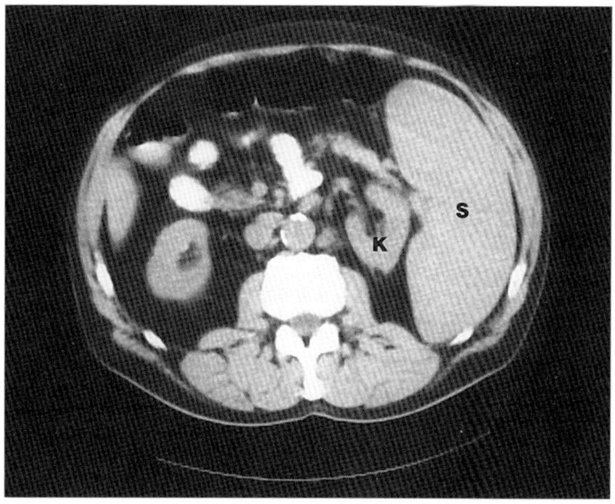

15–2 CT scan in a patient with lymphoma shows marked splenomegaly (S) displacing left kidney (K) anteriorly and medially. The usual percutaneous access tract to left kidney must be modified to avoid splenic puncture.

Contraindications

Clinical factors influence the appropriateness of percutaneous nephrostomy. Uncorrectable bleeding diathesis must be considered a contraindication except when percutaneous nephrostomy drainage is needed to reverse a coagulopathy, such as in urosepsis. Collecting system puncture and subsequent intrarenal manipulation of catheters in the presence of an untreated urinary tract infection often result in sepsis; preprocedural antibiotic administration lessens this risk. In the clinical situation of sepsis due to infection and urinary obstruction, percutaneous nephrostomy placement often facilitates adequate urine flow for effective urinary antibiotic levels.

Hyperkalemia, which occurs with acute urinary obstruction, may cause cardioplegia refractory to therapy. It is best to defer percutaneous nephrostomy placement in this situation until after emergency hemodialysis or intravenous therapy corrects the most serious metabolic abnormalities. Subsequent nephrostomy placement is safe and allows renal mechanisms to reverse serum biochemical alterations gradually. Surgical excision is the accepted therapy for renal mass lesions or urothelial neoplasm. Nephrostomy placement in those situations delays the definitive surgical procedure and may seed the tumor along the nephrostomy tract.

Severe deformities such as scoliosis may alter the normal position of intra-abdominal organs. In those cases, there is the risk of major injury to other organ systems. CT defines organ position and helps determine an appropriate entry; CT is also necessary in cases of splenomegaly prior to left renal percutaneous nephrostomy. Since the spleen displaces the kidney anteriorly in this situation, the usual flank percutaneous nephrostomy tract must be modified or abandoned to avoid splenic puncture (Fig. 15–2).

Infants and extremely obese patients present technical problems but are not excluded from nephrostomy placement due to size alone. Complex percutaneous manipulations, such as rigid nephroscopy, may be impossible in grossly obese adults.

The mere presence of a reversible renal collecting system obstruction does not mandate decompression. In cases of terminal malignancy, relief of ureteral obstruction may be a disservice to a uremic patient because the time gained is often filled with unrelieved pain. Occasionally, nephrostomy placement is necessary despite serious contraindications in the extremely ill patient. These situations require honest discussions between physicians and patient prior to intervention.

Percutaneous Nephrostomy Procedure

Preparation

Patients should be told the risks and goals of the procedure. Laboratory examination should include a hemostasis evaluation. Anticoagulant drugs, including aspirin, should be discontinued to allow normal blood clotting at the time of percutaneous nephrostomy placement.

In cases of calculus disease, urography usually shows stone location, collecting system anatomy, and extent of renal function. Ultrasound and CT facilitate accurate identification of the level and cause of obstruction in nearly all patients. Use of these imaging modalities helps avoid both inappropriate percutaneous nephrostomy placement and potential complications such as splenomegaly.

Imaging

The use of fluoroscopy, ultrasound, and CT permits accurate and safe percutaneous nephrostomy. The ideal guidance system for percutaneous decompression of urinary tract obstruction combines portable real-time ultrasound scanning for initial renal localization and puncture with immediate continuation of the needle, guide-wire, and catheter manipulations under fluoroscopic guidance (Fig. 15–3). The use of ultrasonic guidance alone is limited to decompression of the dilated systems, since the necessary intrarenal manipulations cannot be adequately observed by ultrasound. The initial localization and puncture of dilated collecting systems may be slightly less efficient without ultrasound, but subsequent intrarenal guide-wire and catheter manipulations require fluoroscopic precision.

Percutaneous nephrostomy placement in complex endourologic cases is often done only with fluoroscopy because precision is required both in the initial puncture and in the subsequent manipulations within normal-sized or stone-filled collecting systems. The use of C-arm or biplane fluoroscopic units facilitates percutaneous access, particularly in complex cases; however, standard tube-under-table fluoroscopic units are adequate for most applications.

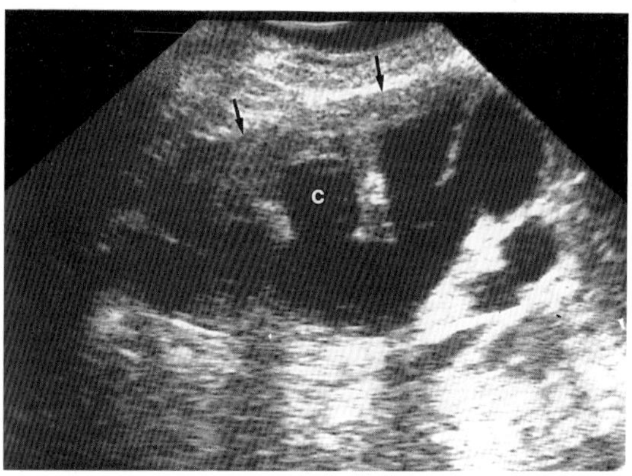

15–3 Real-time ultrasound examination of right kidney shows collecting system dilation but adequate residual renal parenchyma (arrows). Percutaneous nephrostomy access needle was accurately directed into dilated middle calix (C) using ultrasonic guidance.

In patients with splenomegaly, anomalous colon position, scoliosis, or extensive postoperative changes, CT scanning shows the available access tract and allows initial needle placement to avoid injury to adjacent organs. Subsequently, the drainage catheter can be positioned with CT verification or further manipulated in a fluoroscopic suite.

Anesthesia

Percutaneous nephrostomy placement requires only local anesthesia, an advantage over surgical nephrostomy. Infiltration of the flank area with generous doses (30–50 ml) of local anesthetics such as lidocaine or bupivacaine (Marcaine) is usually sufficient. Intravenous sedation, using incremental doses of fentanyl and diazepam, further facilitates patient comfort. Medications must be monitored carefully in severely uremic patients because, in these cases, drug metabolism is altered and sedative requirements are minimal.

Percutaneous nephrostomy placement in infants and pediatric patients is facilitated by preprocedural sedation in the nonemergency situation. Rare cases of extreme agitation or anxiety may require a general anesthetic.

Instrumentation

Originally, percutaneous nephrostomy was performed using cannula or trocar systems. While these sets may be useful in decompression of obstructed kidneys, they are not compatible with further endourologic manipulations. Needle, catheter, guide-wire percutaneous nephrostomy systems based on angiographic techniques are most widely used because they are adaptable, relatively inexpensive, and compatible with commercially available endourologic equipment (Banner, Pollack 1984).

Several similar angiographic-type percutaneous nephrostomy systems are available that provide opacification and access needles, guide wires, and fascial dilators, but the final nephrostomy tube is different in each system. The tube is usually 6–14 F in diameter in a variety of pigtail, self-retaining, Malecot, or balloon-tip styles.

Two initial access techniques are widely used. In one, a 22-gauge needle is inserted initially to define the route and inject contrast media to opacify the renal pelvis and calices. Subsequent puncture of a specific calix with an 18-gauge needle allows direct introduction of standard (0.89 mm or 0.97 mm, 0.035 in. or 0.038 in.) angiographic guide wires into the collecting systems before tract dilation and catheter placement.

The alternative access needle is the Cope Catheter Introducing System, in which a 21-gauge needle puncture may be converted to a percutaneous tract via a series of guide-wire and catheter exchanges. The additional equipment needed to adapt these sets to the demands of complex percutaneous nephrostomy placement consists of various angiographic guide wires and catheters.

Collecting System Opacification

The renal collecting systems must be outlined prior to the definitive puncture in order to choose the proper percutaneous tract. Adminstration of intravenous contrast media is of little value in subsequent fluoroscopic visualization of obstructed systems.

Direct antegrade pyelography through a 22-gauge needle provides good collecting system delineation and is easily and safely done in most kidneys. In normal-sized nonobstructed collecting systems, however, accurate antegrade pyelography needle placement is more difficult. Initial cystoscopic placement of a retrograde transurethral ureteral catheter into those undilated systems permits excellent opacification and distention of the renal pelvis and calices using contrast media, air, or CO_2 (Fig. 15–4). In percutaneous nephrostomy for decompression of obstructed kidneys, however, this retrograde route of opacification is unavailable. Preliminary opacification of the collecting system is not needed for many stone-containing kidneys, especially those with large branched stones. In these situations, the stone itself accurately displays caliceal anatomy. The use of real-time ultrasonic guidance for direct caliceal puncture with the access needle eliminates the need for initial opacification in obstructed kidneys, but is difficult to perform in nondilated systems.

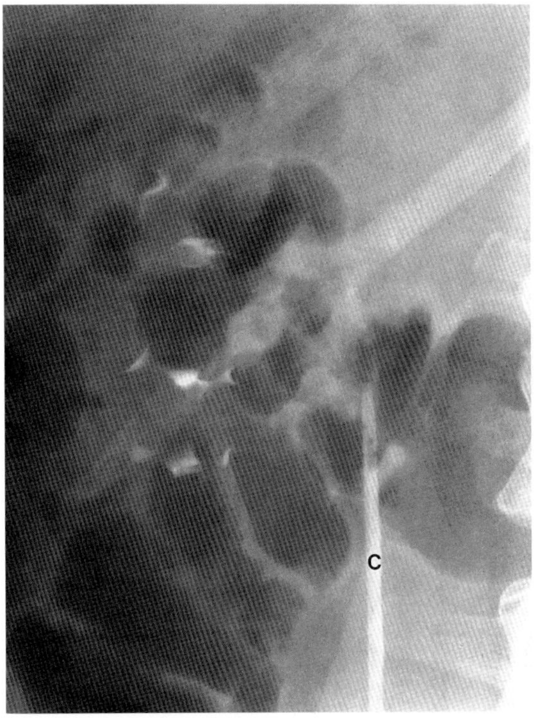

A

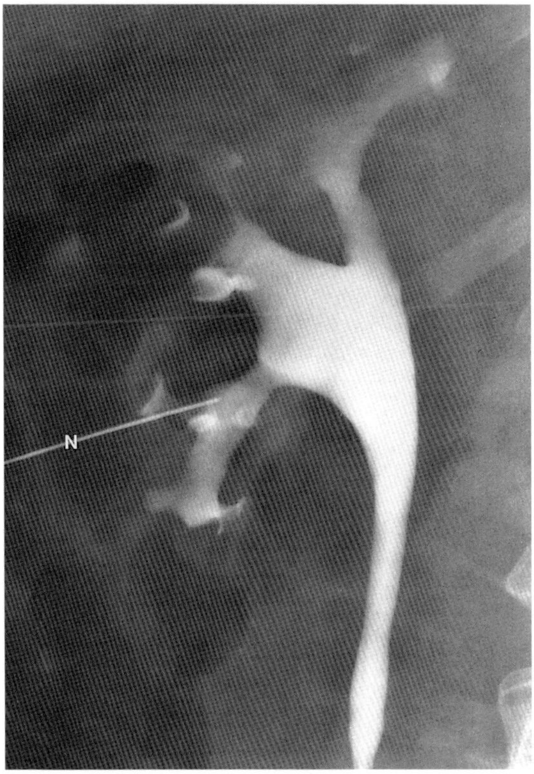

B

15–4 **(A)** Retrograde ureteral catheter (C) has been inserted to ureteropelvic junction level prior to placement of nephrostomy tube in nonobstructed kidney. **(B)** Injection of contrast material through ureteral catheter gives excellent collecting system opacification and distention, and facilitates access needle placement into lower pole calix. (N = needle)

Whitaker Test

Antegrade pyelography performed before anticipated nephrostomy placement may be ex-

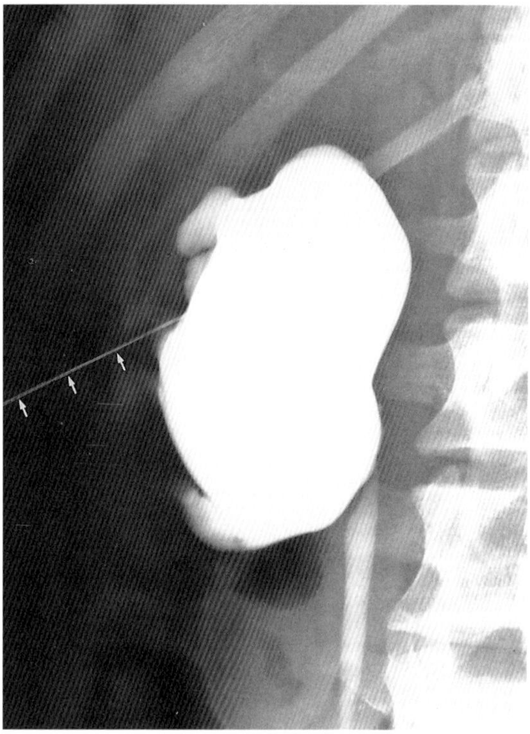

15–5 Antegrade pyelogram through 22-gauge needle (arrows) was done as the initial procedure in a Whitaker test to evaluate persistent pyelocaliectasis 8 months after surgical repair of ureteropelvic junction obstruction. Recurrent obstruction was diagnosed by pressure-flow studies, leading to percutaneous nephrostomy and subsequent percutaneous endopyelotomy.

tended to help define anatomic abnormalities (Pfister 1986). The Whitaker test is an examination that monitors pressure within the renal pelvis while well-defined flow rates are injected through a 22-gauge antegrade pyelography needle. Pressure measurements are modified by subtracting urinary bladder pressure obtained from an indwelling catheter; the numbers are then compared to established standards. This technique evaluates persistent pyelocaliectasis after surgery to repair the ureteropelvic junction or ureterovesical junction (Fig. 15–5). In general, initial renal pelvic pressures over 15 cm of H_2O with 10- to 15-ml/min flow into the renal pelvis indicate obstruction. Decompressive percutaneous nephrostomy may begin immediately, followed by therapeutic endourologic intervention.

Location of the Percutaneous Nephrostomy Tract

Two important considerations in locating the nephrostomy tract are its purpose and the patient's anatomy. Generally, the tract enters the flank near the posterior axillary line, courses subcostally to avoid pleural injury, courses through renal parenchyma, and enters a calix (Fritzsche 1986). This provides a stabilizing renal parenchymal seal around the catheter, avoids the large central renal blood vessels, and permits good access to the remaining renal collecting system. Entry through a middle or lower pole calix is adequate for short- or long-term drainage. Renal pelvic calculi can be extracted through a similar tract, but caliceal stone removal usually requires entry through the stone-containing calix.

Access to the ureter for endourologic procedures can be achieved from nearly any caliceal entry site, but may be simpler if a middle to upper pole calix is punctured. Direct entry into the collecting systems by puncture into the upper pole calices often necessitates a relatively high intercostal approach with an increased risk of complications. Modification of this ideal tract is needed in cases of renal malrotation or anomalous position of intraabdominal organs.

A renal transplant in the iliac fossa is entered percutaneously through the lateral lower abdominal wall extraperitoneally into a middle or upper pole calix. The skin puncture site is near the palpable anterior iliac spine of the bony pelvis. Ultrasound guidance can be very helpful in achieving percutaneous access to the transplant kidney.

Catheter Placement

Percutaneous nephrostomy placement requires access to the posterior flank for needle placement through the retroperitoneum into the kidney. This is most easily done with the patient prone or prone-oblique, depending on operator preference and the type of guidance system being used. Although needle placement into the proper calix is probably easier to perform with the patient prone-oblique, the prone position is more comfortable and minimizes radiation exposure to the operator. If a C-arm or multidirectional fluoroscope is not available, needle position within the patient can be determined by rolling the patient obliquely. In extremely ill patients, these prone positions may be impossible, necessitating nephrostomy placement with the patient supine-oblique or lateral (Barbaric 1984). Multidirectional fluoroscopy is invaluable when a complicated approach for tube placement is required.

Placement of the access needle from the tract origin site on the skin into the desired calix requires continuous needle advancement and reorientation based on the fluoroscopic or ultrasonic display. Intraluminal position of the needle tip within the calix is confirmed by aspiration of urine and injection of contrast material.

If an 18-gauge access needle system is used, a 0.89-mm or 0.97-mm (0.035-in. or 0.038-in.) guide wire is advanced through the needle, into the calix, and then into the renal pelvis. Teflon-coated J-tip guide wires are used for this because they are relatively atraumatic and deflect off caliceal walls rather than perforate, as straight-tip or stiffer wires often do. When a J-tip guide wire cannot be advanced easily out of the calix, gentle angulation of the needle or slight retraction of the needle tip away from the far wall of the calix may help. In patients with excessive stone material or intrarenal strictures, torquable guide wires may be necessary to gain access from the calix into the renal pelvis.

If the Cope system is used for access, a specially designed stiff-bodied 0.46-mm (0.018-in.) guide wire is placed through the lumen of the 21-gauge access needle. Usually, the soft tip of this fine wire passes directly or buckles out of the punctured calix into the renal pelvis and then often into the upper ureter (Fig. 15–6). A conversion catheter is inserted over this initial wire, allowing exchange for a 0.97-mm (0.038-in.) J-tip, which becomes the working guide wire. The major problem with either system is accurate initial placement to allow free guide-wire entry from the needle into the calix, and then into the renal pelvis. In minimally or nondilated collecting systems, precision is required to prevent excursion of the guide wire into the pericaliceal and peripelvic tissues with subsequent extravasation of urine and contrast media.

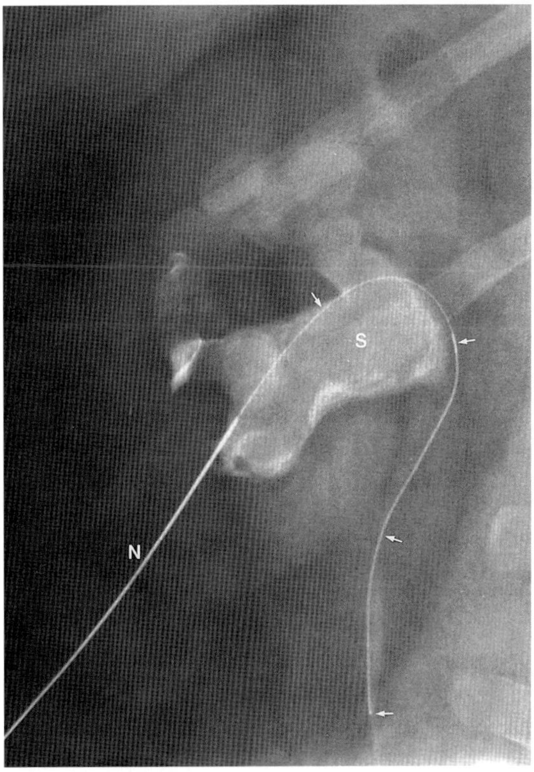

15–6 Percutaneous nephrostomy access is created with the Cope System. After lower pole caliceal puncture with 21-gauge access needle (N), the 0.046-mm (0.018-in.) guide wire (arrows) has passed around a large staghorn calculus (S) outlined by contrast and has entered upper ureter.

Tract dilation is performed after the guide wire is successfully coiled in the renal pelvis or advanced across the ureteropelvic junction and down the ureter. Successively larger fascial dilators, usually 6 F to 10 F, are serially advanced over the guide wire into the calix and pelvis. Fluoroscopic monitoring in this procedure is necessary to prevent guide-wire buckling, kinking, or dislodgement; or trauma to the medial wall of the renal pelvis or ureteropelvic junction by the dilators. Steady backward traction of the guide wire as each catheter or dilator is inserted, plus a spinning or "boring" of the dilator, help prevent buckling of the retroperitoneal segments of the guide wire, which occurs frequently in obese patients.

The extent of tract dilation depends on the final drainage catheter but, in general, the tract should be dilated 2 F larger than the nephrostomy tube for passage through the flank. If a catheter larger than 10 F is introduced, tract dilation from 7 F to the desired size can be performed in a single setting with serial fascial dilators or with the single inflation of a long angioplasty-type high-pressure balloon catheter. The final nephrostomy tube is then inserted through the acutely dilated tract.

Usually, adequate urinary drainage can be achieved with a 7- or 8-F catheter. Larger catheters are occasionally needed if considerable viscous or particulate debris is in the collecting system. Polyethylene pigtail, self-retaining, or other simple drainage catheters are introduced over the guide wire under fluoroscopic guidance, permitting accurate catheter placement and limiting the risk of perforation or catheter dislodgement.

If desired, stable external drainage can be established by advancing a catheter down the ureter so that its tip is in the bladder. Custom-placed extra drainage holes added to this type of drainage catheter should be located throughout the length of the ureter and the renal pelvis. Larger long-term drainage catheters, such as Foley-type or Councill balloon catheters, are most easily introduced through appropriate-sized tear-away sheaths in the acute tract.

Complex indications for percutaneous nephrostomy often require modification of these basic drainage techniques. Intrarenal maneuvering around a large staghorn calculus often requires substitution of torquable guide wires such as the Lunderquist-Ring, Wholey wires, or preformed angiographic catheters to establish a secure tract into the collecting system (LeRoy et al. 1984). Cobra-shaped or angle-tipped torquable angiographic catheters are the most useful for intrarenal manipulations or for crossing the ureteropelvic junction (Fig. 15–7).

In most intrarenal endourologic procedures, advancing the guide wire and catheter across the ureteropelvic junction and down the ureter helps establish a stable tract for subsequent manipulations. These same operator skills and equipment are necessary for complex manipulations in the ureter.

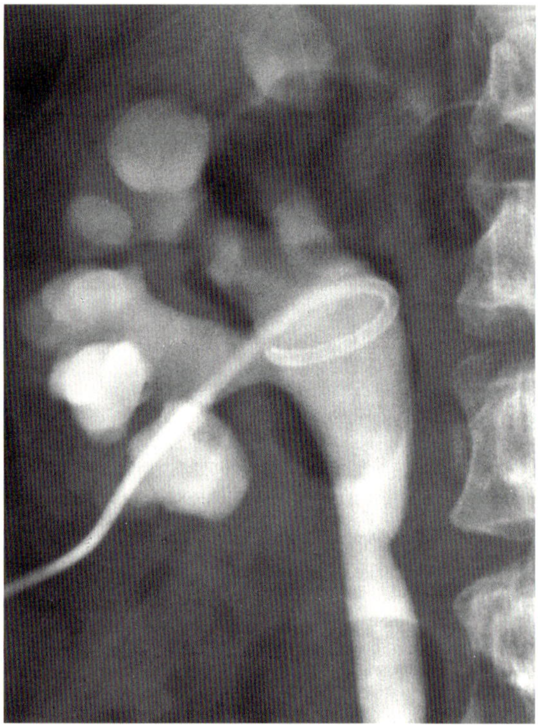

15–8 An 8-F pigtail nephrostomy catheter has been positioned appropriately in renal pelvis after lower pole access puncture. After obstructive postoperative lower ureteral edema resolved, catheter was easily removed. Stiffer pigtail catheters should be removed over a guide wire.

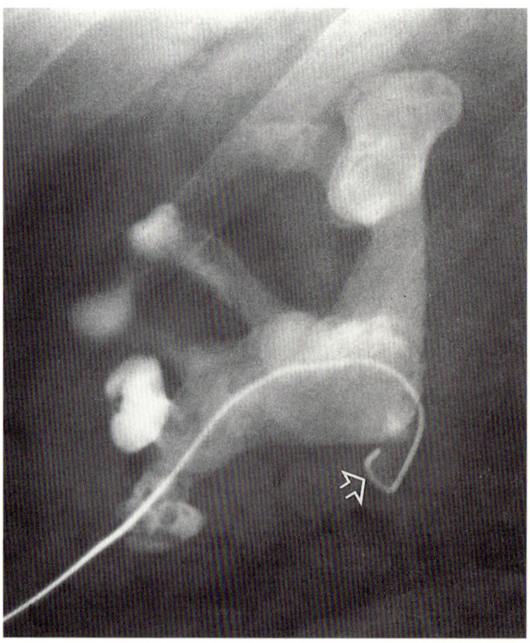

15–7 Percutaneous nephrostomy tract around large staghorn calculus outlined by contrast has been extended across ureteropelvic junction by using cobra-shaped torquable catheter and soft J-tip guide wire (open arrow).

Postprocedural Care

Numerous catheter fixation techniques using self-retaining catheters, rings, or disks applied to the catheter, as well as extensive suture or adhesive attachments, are available (Saxton 1981). Patient instruction and attentive nursing care are important to prevent catheter dislodgement. Patients are hospitalized overnight and monitored for potential bleeding or septic complications. A udden cessation of urine flow is usually due to nephrostomy dislodgement rather than to catheter occlusion. Polyethylene pigtail angiographic-type nephrostomy tubes are easily inserted and provide good initial drainage, but are poorly suited to long-term drainage because of their rigidity, ease of dislodgement, and complex fixation requirements (Fig. 15–8). Reliable long-term external nephrostomy drainage is better achieved after converting to a Foley type, Malecot, or self-retaining loop catheter.

Complications

Complications from percutaneous nephrostomy placement occur at an acceptably low rate. All patients have hematuria following percutaneous nephrostomy, but this clears in 24–48 hr. Hematuria may be prominent in profoundly uremic patients until renal function improves (Fig. 15–9). Less than 1% of patients will develop severe hemorrhage due to arterial pseudoaneurysm or arteriovenous fistula formation caused during needle or tube placement; angiographic embolization is the best treatment in those situations.

Percutaneous nephrostomy placement in pyohydronephrosis leads to overt clinical sepsis in a few patients, but this usually resolves rapidly with aggressive medical therapy. Limiting collecting system distention, minimizing catheter manipulation, and providing adequate external drainage help reduce septic occurrences.

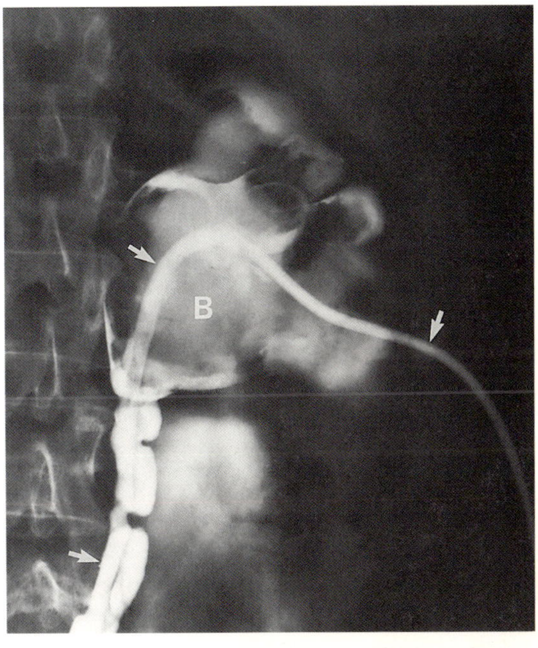

15–9 Renal pelvic blood clot formation (B) outlined by contrast in profoundly uremic patient after percutaneous nephrostomy placement. This clot cleared within 48 hr with adequate urine flow. Percutaneous nephrostomy catheter (arrows) was placed with its tip in bladder across a lower ureteral obstruction with catheter drainage holes positioned in renal pelvis and ureter.

Other major complications involve injury to adjacent organ systems. Inadvertent punctures of the colon, liver, spleen, duodenum, and lung have occurred with potentially serious sequelae requiring surgical intervention.

Catheter dislodgement is minimized by proper initial fixation and the use of self-retaining or balloon-type catheters for long-term external drainage situations. Perforation of the collecting system during percutaneous nephrostomy placement may occur around large renal calculi in chronically distended systems or during the course of extensive catheter and guide-wire manipulations. With adequate urinary drainage, nearly all of these localized perforations heal in 1–2 days without further intervention.

Urinomas are rare, usually resulting from inadequate urinary drainage after a collecting system puncture. Subcapsular renal hematomas may result from nephrostomy placement in chronically obstructed kidneys or in situations requiring extensive catheter and guide-wire exchanges. These cases generally resolve without long-term effects.

Conclusion

Successful percutaneous nephrostomy placement can be achieved in nearly all patients, and clinical results are excellent. This procedure relieves ureteral obstruction and allows the return of renal function with occasional postobstructive diuresis. In cases of malignancy, this improved renal function permits higher doses of chemotherapeutic drugs. Percutaneous drainage of pyohydronephrosis usually reduces fever within 48 hr and permits further therapy in a more stable clinical situation.

The rapid growth in the numbers, complexity, and success rates of endourologic procedures over the past decade is directly related to the excellent results in establishing reliable and safe percutaneous nephrostomy access.

References

Banner MP, Pollack HM: Percutaneous antegrade renal drainage techniques. *In* Carson CC, Dunnick NR (eds.): *Endourology.* New York, Churchill Livingstone, 1984, pp. 127–157.

Barbaric ZL: Percutaneous nephrostomy for urinary tract obstruction. *Am. J. Roentgenol.* 143:803–809, 1984.

Fritzsche P: Antegrade pyelography: Therapeutic applications. *Radiol. Clin. North Am.* 24:573–586, 1986.

Goodwin WE, Casey WC, Woolf W: Percutaneous trocar (needle) nephrostomy in hydronephrosis. *J.A.M.A.* 157:891–894, 1955.

LeRoy AJ, May GR, Bender CE, Williams HJ, Jr., McGough PF: Percutaneous nephrostomy for stone removal. *Radiology* 151:607–612, 1984.

Pfister RC: Obstruction and percutaneous ureteral urodynamics: The Whitaker test. *In* Lang EK (ed.): *Percutaneous and Interventional Urology and Radiology.* Berlin, New York, Springer-Verlag, 1986, pp. 19–54.

Saxton HM: Percutaneous nephrostomy: Technique. *Urol. Radiol.* 2:131–139, 1981.

Stables DP, Ginsberg NJ, Johnson ML: Percutaneous nephrostomy: A series and review of the literature. *Am. J. Roentgenol.* 130:75–82, 1978.

Suggested Reading

Cope C: Percutaneous nephrostomy drainage procedures: Single-stick percutaneous nephrostomy. *Semin. Intervent. Radiology* 1:1–4, 1984.

Curry NS, Cochran S, Barbaric ZL: Interventional radiologic procedures in the renal transplant. *Radiology* 152:647–653, 1984.

Pollack HM, Banner MP: Percutaneous nephrostomy and related pyeloureteral manipulative techniques. *Urol. Radiol.* 2:147–154, 1981.

Reznek RH, Talner LB: Percutaneous nephrostomy. *Radiol. Clin. North Am.* 22:393–406, 1984.

Stanley P, Diament MJ: Pediatric nephrostomy: Experience with 50 patients. *J. Urol.* 135:1223–1226, 1986.

Zegal HG, Pollack HM, Banner MP, et al.: Percutaneous nephrostomy: Comparison of sonographic and fluoroscopic guidance. *Am. J. Roentgenol.* 137:925–927, 1981.

CHAPTER 16

Placement of Percutaneous Ureteral Stents

Gregory P. Lewis

Ureteral stents are used to maintain continuity and function of the injured or obstructed ureter. Most stents are placed to avoid or relieve ureteral obstruction due to malignancy, renal calculi, or benign strictures (Mitty et al. 1983). A smaller number of patients have stents placed to maintain continuity and to facilitate healing of the injured or postsurgical ureter (Bettman et al. 1983; Lang 1984; Smith 1984).

Stents can be placed cystoscopically, surgically, or percutaneously. Cystoscopic placement is the favored method, due to its technical ease, safety, and high success rate, the latter of which can be further increased with the use of special catheters and guide wires for difficult cases.

Percutaneous stent placement, the procedure of choice when cystoscopic techniques fail, requires a nephrostomy access to the collecting system (Barbaric 1984; Pfister 1986). Percutaneous antegrade stent placement is the preferred method in patients with a preexisting nephrostomy and in those where retrograde placement has failed (for example, owing to a large prostate or because such placement is not feasible, as in an ileal loop).

Preliminary Considerations

Many problems will be averted if the interventional radiologist and urologist review the clinical problem and therapeutic goals before beginning the procedure. Obstruction and sepsis should be treated with a drainage nephrostomy and appropriate antibiotics before placing a percutaneous stent. Trauma to the urothelium, inadvertent elevation of collecting system pressure, and manipulations in the setting of obstruction or sepsis predispose to complications and should be minimized.

A delay between nephrostomy and stent placement is technically advantageous. An established nephrostomy, even one less than 24 hr old, will usually bleed less than an acute tract, and therefore will minimize stent occlusion. Moreover, ureteral edema at the point of obstruction and ureteral tortuosity are frequently reduced after nephrostomy drainage, simplifying stent placement. Even apparently complete ureteral occlusions can at times be traversed following several days of decompression.

Ultrasound or single plane fluoroscopy is adequate for placing a decompressing nephrostomy; however, multidirectional fluoroscopy is useful when stent placement is anticipated. Multidirectional fluoroscopy simplifies stent placement by improving the nephrostomy access to the collecting system with selective caliceal puncture and avoidance of unnecessary angles. Contrast opacification of the collecting system for fluoroscopic guidance can be achieved by using 100 ml 60% intravenous contrast injection if excretory function is adequate. The timing of the injection should anticipate excretion delays due to reduced renal function or obstruction. Direct opacification of the collecting system with a 22-gauge Chiba needle using ultrasound or fluoroscopic guidance is an effective alternative, particularly in cases with high-grade obstruction or impaired renal function.

Ultrasound-guided puncture of the collecting system using the ultrasound biopsy guide is increasingly used in this author's practice, owing to the elegant needle control this offers, successful even in nonhydronephrotic systems. Fluoroscopy still remains the preferred imaging modality for the actual nephrostomy tube placement after successful ultrasound-guided needle puncture.

Patient Preparation

Prophylactic antibiotic coverage prior to nephrostomy placement is warranted in all settings of potential urinary tract infection. Coagulation studies are not necessary, unless the patient is on anticoagulation medication, including high-dose aspirin, or has evidence of a bleeding diathesis.

Adequate sedation and analgesia are important in any percutaneous procedure. This author has found that 0.25% bupivacaine hydrochloride (Marcaine, 30–60 ml) supplemented with intravenous analgesia (fentanyl, 0.5–1.0 ml or Demerol, 75–100 mg) are usually adequate. Sedation with intravenous diazepam (Valium, 3–5 mg) is a useful adjuvant to analgesia. Analgesia given in anticipation of pain is more effective than attempting to "catch up."

The optimal patient position for percutaneous nephrostomy and stent placement is a prone oblique position with the side of interest elevated approximately 30°. This facilitates three-dimensional (two-plane) imaging and provides good exposure to the puncture area. The patient should be in a comfortable position before the procedure begins. Occasionally, clinical conditions such as recent surgery or kyphosis may require alternative prone or decubitus positions.

Percutaneous Access

A straight line is the ideal course over which to advance a catheter or stent. Anatomic constraints prevent achieving this ideal, and, as a result, angles and curves are introduced. Angles create a point of resistance to the advancement of the catheter or stent over the guide wire. When the angle is large enough, the catheter or guide wire will buckle or deflect rather than advance to the desired location (Fig. 16–1). This effect is not usually seen unless the deviation is greater than 120° (Fig. 16–2). The larger the angle, the greater the deflecting tendency; sequential angles produce cumulative effects. Angles may occur not only in the familiar coronal plane but also in the sagittal plane. Limiting the size and number of angles requires multiplanar imaging (Fig. 16–3). A nephrostomy access that minimizes angles will simplify stent placement.

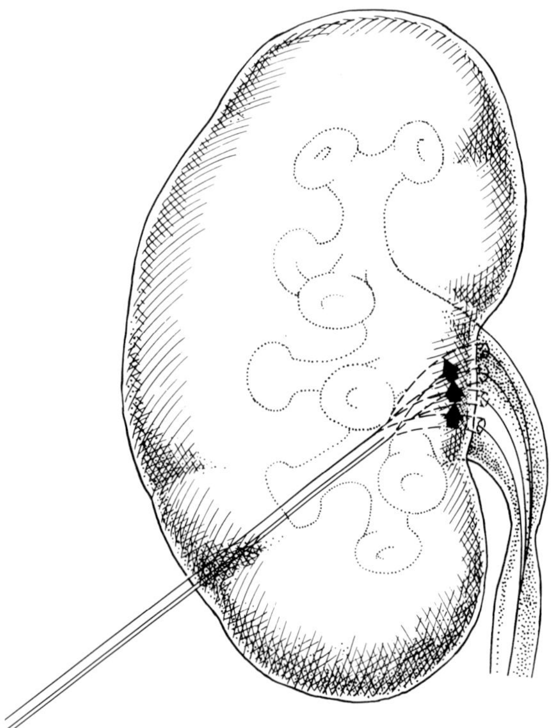

16–1 Catheter deflecting into renal pelvis at angle made by nephrostomy access tract and ureter, rather than following guide wire down ureter.

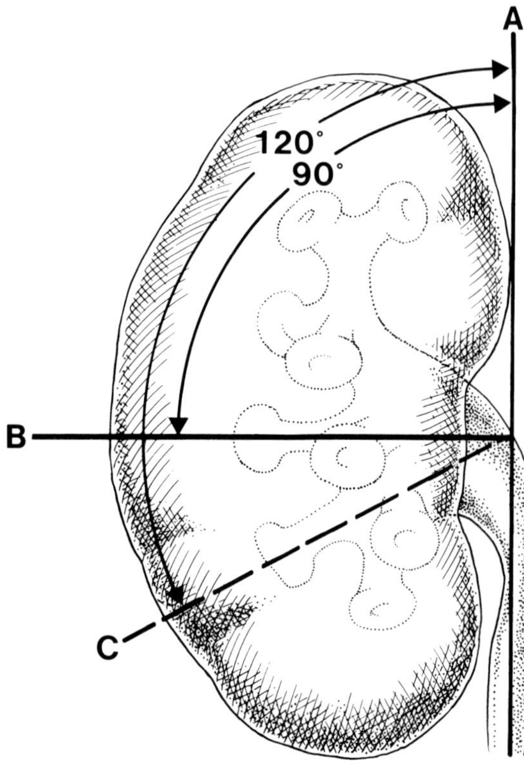

16–2 Increasing approach angle from theoretical straight line (0°) down ureter A, 90°; satisfactory angle B; undesirable 120° angle C.

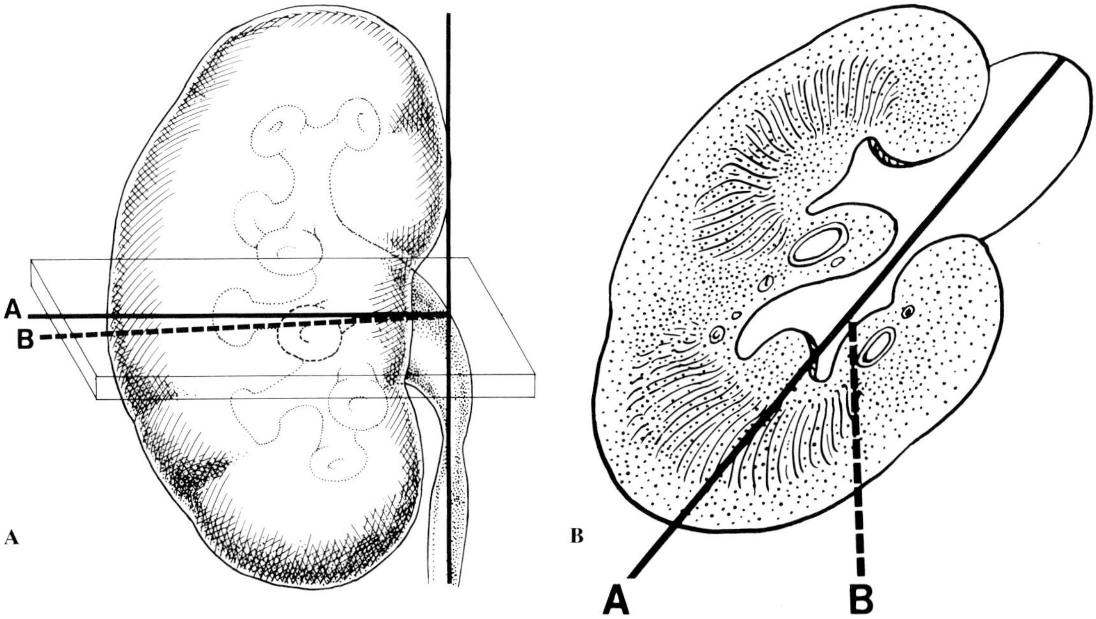

16–3 **(A)** Access approaches A and B to right kidney in coronal plane appear to have identical straight line courses. **(B)** Access approaches A and B to right kidney when viewed in axial plane show approach B has introduced an unnecessary angle, while A maintains ideal straight line approach in both axial and coronal planes.

Nephrostomy access through a posterolateral puncture between the twelfth rib and iliac crest avoids the strong fascia of the erector spinae muscles and minimizes tube discomfort when the patient is supine. The intercostal approach, although reducing the access angle, increases the risk of pneumothorax or hydrothorax and is often uncomfortable to the patient. The lowest calix should be avoided when stent placement is anticipated, because of the large angle this creates at the ureteropelvic junction (Fig. 16–2); a middle or, occasionally, upper-lateral calix should normally be selected. The change in kidney position with breathing may be useful in lowering the middle and upper calices below the level of the twelfth rib for puncture.

The ideal puncture axis is down the long axis of the infundibulum leading from the target calix to the renal pelvis, avoiding a curve (Fig. 16–3). Multiplanar fluoroscopy is required with both sagittal-oblique and coronal plane projections. A relatively lateral position often allows a straight line approach to the renal pelvis along the target infundibulum, eliminating any angle in this axis. However, the more lateral the puncture, the greater the risk of inadvertent colon puncture.

The colon is normally anterolateral to the kidney, but may be lateral or even posterior to it. Its position can usually be determined by multiplanar fluoroscopic visualization of gas relative to the puncture axis. Fluoroscopic observation while administering local anesthesia with a 22-gauge 15-cm needle can be helpful in questionable cases by demonstrating displacement of the colon gas by the advancing needle. When the location of the colon cannot be determined, the puncture should be medial to the posterior axillary line.

After nephrostomy drainage has been established and obstruction and infection treated, the ureter can be traversed with a guide wire and a stent placed. The nephrostomy tube is removed over a guide wire, and a catheter is inserted into the collecting system over the guide wire.

It is wise to place an additional safety guide wire

Table 16–1 Tubes and Stents

Name	Description	Size	Guide Wire	Length	Company
Pigtail	Nephrostomy Pigtail Catheter	5 F, 8.3 F, 10 F	.038 in.	30 cm	Cook
10 F Sheath	Amplatz Renal Dilator	10 F	–	–	Cook
Peel-Away Sheath	Peel-Away Sheath Introducer Set	8 F–12 F	–	–	Cook
Nephrostent	Nephro-ureteral Stent System	8 F, 10 F	.038 in.	28 cm	Cook
Double J Stent	Percutaneous Antegrade Double-J Stent	7 F, 8.5 F	.038 in.	18–26 cm	Surgitek

either through the nephrostomy tube at the time of removal or through a 10-F sheath (Table 16–1) introduced over the access guide wire. The safety guide wire is coiled and clamped to the sterile drapes while using the catheter and guide wire combination to traverse the ureter. If the combination is inadvertently dislodged from the collecting system, then the safety guide wire can be used for reentry.

Negotiating the Urinary System

All percutaneous stents are passed over a guide wire using the Seldinger technique (Fritzsche 1986; Mitty et al. 1986). This requires placement of a guide wire from the skin through the collecting system into the bladder, traversing any strictures, fistulas, or perforations. This can be accomplished in most cases by using a catheter and guide wire combination. The collecting system anatomy can be determined from a nephrostogram; the appropriate catheter and guide wire combination can then be selected.

Catheters provide torque control to point and direct the guide wire as it is gently advanced down the ureter and past strictures or injured areas. Usually, the guide wire should lead, to minimize the risk of inadvertent perforation. The catheters, although designed for visceral angiography, work equally well in the urinary system and come in a variety of sizes, shapes, and flexibilities. However, a cobra-shaped catheter in either a 5-F or 6.5-F size with a 3-cm straight taper tip or a C-shaped guide wire is usually sufficient (Tables 16–2, 16–3).

Particular problems that may require the use of other catheters or guide wires include: eccentric stenosis, the tortuous ureter, and sequential curves. The anatomy can be assessed by removing the guide wire and injecting contrast. Eccentric stenoses often can be crossed with the aid of a torque or steerable guide wire, such as the Wholey or Coudé (Fig. 16–4). The recently introduced

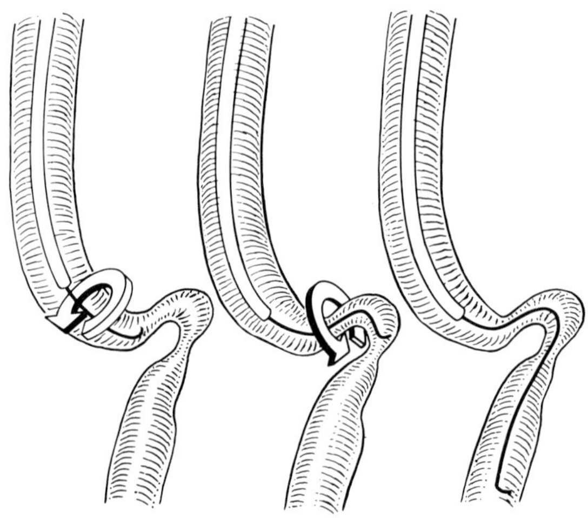

16–4 Use of catheter to direct torque guide wire throughout eccentric stenosis.

Table 16–2 Guide Wires

Name	Diameter (in./mm)	Length (cm)	Curve	Company	Description
Rosen	.035/.89	145	J	Cook	Teflon coated heavy duty curved
Movable Core J	.035/.89	145	J	Cook	Teflon coated curved movable Tefcor
Movable Core C	.035/.89	145	C	Cook	Teflon coated curved movable Tefcor
Lunderquist	.035/.89	125	THG	Cook	Teflon coated Lunderquist
Lunderquist-Ring	.038/.97	125	THG	Cook	Lunderquist-Ring Torque HSF
Wholey Wire	.035/.89	145	120°	A.C.S.	Wholey-Hi-Torque modified J guide wire
Straight	.035/.89	145	straight	Cook	4-cm taper guide wire
Coudé	.038/.97	100	Coudé tip	Cook	–
Glidewire™	.035/.89	120, 150	angled	Medi-Tech	–
Glidewire™	.038/.97	150	angled	Medi-Tech	–

Table 16–3 Catheters

Name	Size	Length	Tip Curve	Company	Description
Cobra	5–6.5 F	65 cm	C2	Cook	Cobra Visceral Torcon Blue
RC	5–6.5 F	65 cm	RC1–3	Cook	Rösch Celiac

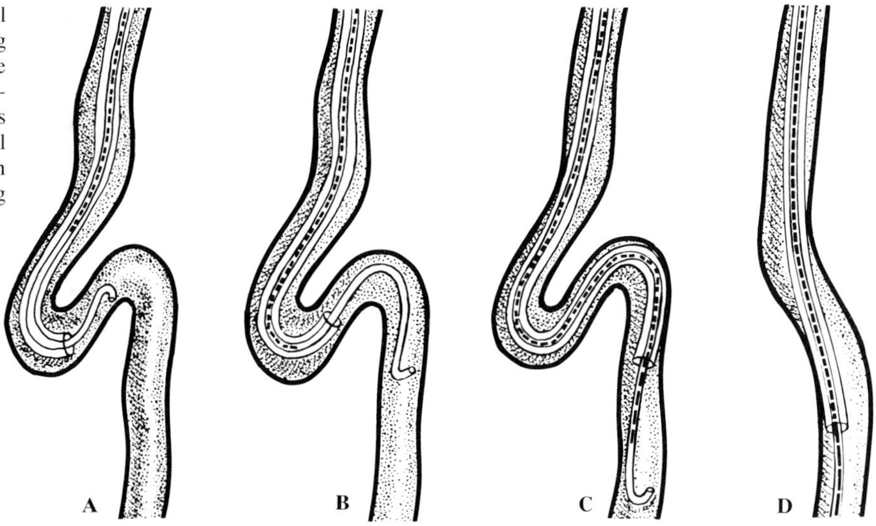

16–5 **(A)** Stiff mandril pulled back, softening guide wire tip. **(B)** Guide wire with softened tip advanced through tortuous ureter. **(C)** Mandril readvanced to stiffen guide wire, allowing catheter to follow **(D)**.

Glidewire™ (Table 16–2) has excellent torque and slip characteristics that are useful in many ureteral problems.

Stiffer torque guide wires such as the Lunderquist (Table 16–2) should be used with caution, owing to the risk of perforation. Movable-core guide wires such as C- and J-shaped tips are useful in the tortuous ureter when standard guide wires will not advance through a curve.

The movable-core guide wires have a central core that can be withdrawn. With the stiffening mandril (core) partially withdrawn, the tip is flexible and will often advance through a tortuous ureter. The mandril can then be replaced, causing the guide wire to be stiff enough to allow the catheter to traverse the area (Fig. 16–5). When multiple curves limit directional control of the catheter tip, a stiffening of the catheter at the proximal curve with a coaxial 10-F Teflon introducer sheath (Table 16–1) may improve distal force and directional control enough to traverse the ureter (Fig. 16–6). Whenever difficulty is encountered, a reevaluation of the anatomy and the tools being used is always in order.

Most fistulas and perforations can be crossed if the distal ureter segment can be identified. This can usually be done with gentle probing and contrast injections. In the unusual situation where the

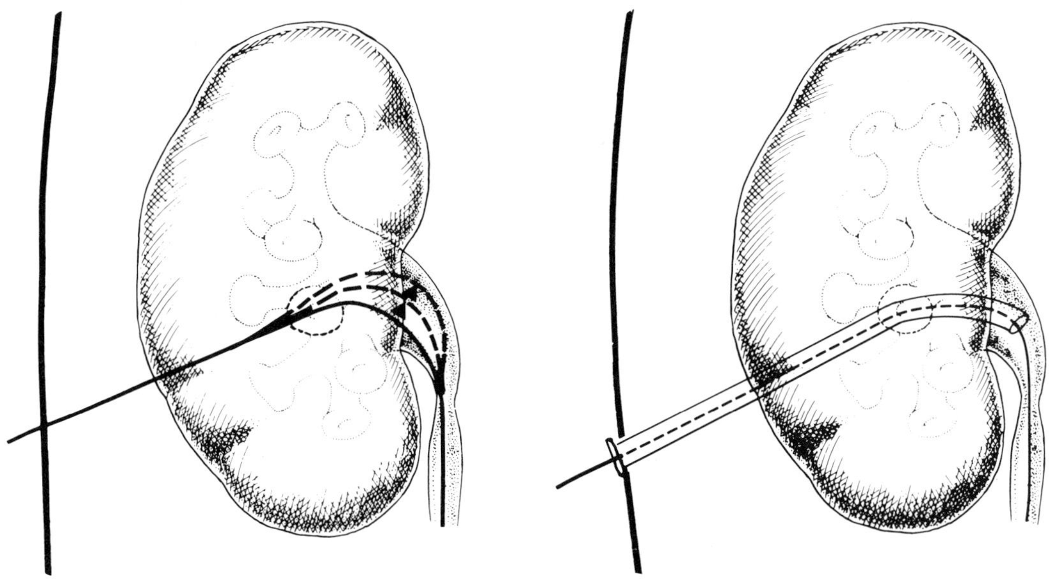

16–6 Peel-Away Sheath (Cook) is used to stiffen angle between nephrostomy tract and ureter, to allow placement of ureteral stent through sheath without deflection of stent into renal pelvis. After stent is in place, sheath is "peeled away."

distal segment cannot be identified, a retrograde ureteral stent injection may be useful.

Once the guide wire has crossed the stenosis or fistula into the bladder or ileal loop, the catheter is advanced over the guide wire into the bladder. This action assesses the tightness of any stenosis and gives some estimation of the likelihood of successful stent placement. If the 6.5-F catheter cannot be advanced into the bladder, there is no point in attempting to pass a 7-F stent. If a stenosis was difficult to traverse, leaving the catheter in place for a few days often causes enough dilation for subsequent stent placement or passage of a balloon dilation catheter. With the catheter in the bladder, a much stiffer guide wire can be exchanged for the traversing one, which will make stent placement (Rosen or Lunderquist) easier (Table 16–2). Moreover, the required stent length can be measured, if necessary.

Stent Selection and Placement

Size

Selection of stent size depends on the expected duration of the stenting and technical safety considerations. In general, the largest stent easily placed is preferred; this is usually an 8-F stent, with the 7-F used less often (Table 16–1). Most percutaneous stents have a double-J configuration, which minimizes irritation and dislodgment. The leading end is tapered to facilitate passage. Newer stent materials such as Percuflex™ (Medi-Tech) attempt to balance softness and comfort with the rigidity and smoothness necessary for easy placement (Table 16–1).

Nephrostent (Cook), a one-piece nephrostomy and ureteral stent combination, is also available (Table 16–1). This stent tapers from a 10-F nephrostomy loop to a 7-F ureteral stent. In the author's practice, this stent is used in patients having percutaneous endopyelotomy and balloon dilation of the ureteropelvic junction stenosis. It preserves nephrostomy access, stents the ureter, and can be easily removed in the office.

Stent length ranges from 16–28 cm. A 24-cm stent will be adequate in an average adult, with 2–3 cm of stent in the bladder and upper system. The guide wire is inserted into the catheter to the desired distal location. A crimp is placed in the guide wire at the point it enters the catheter, and the guide wire is withdrawn to the desired proximal stent location, where a second crimp is placed. The distance between the crimps corresponds to the desired stent length. A stent that is too long will leave either an excessive loop in the bladder, which may cause irritation, or will make it difficult to get the entire proximal end of the stent into the collecting system.

The distal end of stents in an ileal loop should reach nearly to the stoma, to facilitate subsequent retrograde stent change or removal. The length of a left stent to an ileal loop should be longer than the right because of the longer distance to the stoma. Some radiologists favor making ileal loop stents long enough to protrude through the stoma, in order to minimize mucous plugging and to better assess function (Pfister 1986).

Placement Technique

The variables governing stent placement are: angles, guide-wire stiffness, and stent friction over the guide wire and through the ureter. Overcoming difficulties is primarily a matter of addressing these variables (Pfister 1986).

Once the 6.5-F catheter has traversed the stenosis, the guide wire is replaced with a more rigid one, such as a Rosen or Lunderquist (Table 16–2). If measurement for stent selection is required, it should be done prior to placement of the stiffer guide wire. A safety thread loop is located on the proximal end of most stents, to allow retrieval if the stent is advanced too far. A suture can be secured to those without a safety loop. The stent is placed tapered end first over the guide wire and is followed with the pusher.

Fluoroscopy is used to monitor progress and to watch for the development of buckles at any of the angles, which can dislodge the guide wire from the bladder into the ureter. If this happens, the stent has to be removed and the guide wire repositioned. A small amount of traction on the guide wire is often useful in overcoming the initial sliding inertia of the stent. Sterile mineral oil, provided with some Silastic stents, can be useful in reducing friction.

Buckling of the wire just outside the capsule of the kidney is usually a result of an excessive skin, calix, or infundibulum angle. This can often be overcome by using a metal stiffening cannula inserted over the wire and inside either the stent or pusher to prevent the buckling. The problem of cephalad buckling of the loaded guide wire and stent combination into the renal pelvis can be corrected with several techniques: 1) the guide wire may be exchanged for a stiffer one; 2) a smaller stent may be used; 3) varied inspiratory levels may reduce the curve enough to allow the stent to be advanced; 4) the stent may be inserted through a peel-away Teflon sheath (10-F, 12-F, 14-F) (Table 16–1).

If use of stiffening cannulas, guide wires, and sheaths is unsuccessful, a new access route to minimize angles should be considered. If a stricture creates resistance, then dilation may be necessary. Occasionally, despite all efforts, the stent cannot be advanced over the guide wire. In this case, cystoscopic retrieval of the guide wire in the bladder will allow fixation of both ends for either retrograde or antegrade stent placement.

When the stent is properly positioned, the safety loop is removed. This should be done while the guide wire and pusher are in place, to prevent unwanted retraction on the stent. The guide wire is then removed, leaving the pusher in place to resist the retraction force of the guide wire on the stent. A guide wire can then be advanced back through the pusher catheter to allow placement of a 5-F or 8.3-F pigtail nephrostomy catheter (Table 16–1). This diverts bloody urine away from the stent and provides confirmation of the stent function with a nephrostomy still in place.

In renal transplants, antegrade stent placement uses the same principles already described (Barbaric, Thompson 1978). The access approach should remain extraperitoneal, by using a puncture just anterior to the innominate bone near the anterior superior iliac spine. Ultrasound guidance is particularly useful in transplants.

For patients with ileal loop diversion, it has not been difficult, in the author's experience, to achieve successful retrograde stent placement through the ileal loop, using a guide wire and catheter combination with fluoroscopic guidance.

References

Barbaric ZL: Percutaneous nephrostomy for urinary tract obstruction. *Am. J. Roentgenol.* 143:803–809, 1984.

Barbaric ZL, Thompson KR: Percutaneous nephropyelostomy in the management of obstructed renal transplants. *Radiology* 126:639–642, 1978.

Bettmann MA, Murray PD, Perlmutt LM, et al.: Ureteroileal anastomotic leaks: Percutaneous treatment. *Radiology* 148:95–100, 1983.

Fritzsche PJ: Antegrade and retrograde ureteral stenting. *In* Lang EK (ed.): *Percutaneous and Interventional Urology and Radiology.* Berlin, Heidelberg, New York, Springer-Verlag, 1986, pp. 91–111.

Lang EK: Antegrade ureteral stenting for dehiscence, strictures, and fistulae. *Am. J. Roentgenol.* 143:795–801, 1984.

Mitty HA, Train JS, Dan SJ: Antegrade ureteral stenting in the management of fistulas, strictures, and calculi. *Radiology* 149:433–438, 1983.

Mitty HA, Train JS, Dan SJ: Placement of ureteral stents by antegrade and retrograde techniques. *Radiol. Clin. North Am.* 24(4):587–600, 1986.

Pfister RC: Percutaneous nephrostomy. *In* Lang EK (ed.): *Percutaneous and Interventional Urology and Radiology.* Berlin, Heidelberg, New York, Springer-Verlag, 1986, pp. 1–27.

Smith AD: Percutaneous ureteral surgery and stenting. *Urology* 23 (Special Issue): 5, 1984.

CHAPTER

17

Percutaneous Endopyelotomy

George E. Brannen

Obstruction of the ureter at its junction with the renal pelvis may become clinically apparent at any age. The resulting distention and dilation of the renal pelvis and calices, especially after large fluid intake, may cause intermittent flank pain that mimics ureteral colic. In addition, with the relative stagnation of urine in the renal pelvis, there is risk of infection (pyelonephritis) or of formation of calculi.

The standard approach to correcting an obstruction at the ureteropelvic junction has been surgical reconstruction through a flank incision (Anderson, Hynes 1949; Culp, DeWeerd 1951; Foley 1937; Scardino, Prince 1953). Recent technical advances in instruments and lens optics have enabled a percutaneous approach through a nephroscope, a method initially developed for the removal of kidney stones. Percutaneous incision of stenosis of the ureteropelvic junction is a natural evolution of this technology. This chapter describes the procedure that has been used at the Virginia Mason Medical Center in Seattle.

Pathology

Obstruction of the ureteropelvic junction is a consequence of anomalous arrangement of otherwise normal tissues. Abnormal conduction by deformed smooth muscle bundles of the ureteral wall may prevent adequate peristalsis of urine through the obstruction. A band of fibrous tissue or an aberrant lower pole renal artery may cause extrinsic compression (Figs. 17–1 and 17–2). An intrinsic stenosis may cause mechanical narrowing, and a high insertion of the ureter into the renal pelvis may cause stagnation of urine in the dependent portion of the renal pelvis, preventing adequate urinary drainage.

Percutaneous repair is possible because a full-thickness longitudinal incision of a stenotic ureter will generally heal when stented for a period of 4–6 weeks.

Technique

The method of percutaneous access to the renal collecting system has been reported (Brannen, Bush 1984; Brannen et al. 1985; Brannen et al. 1986). Access to the ureteropelvic junction is facilitated by percutaneous entry through a mid-calix. A supracostal approach above the 12th or 11th rib with entry through an upper calix may provide mechanical advantage in some cases. However, this approach may have the increased risk of hydrothorax or pneumothorax.

Access to the collecting system is facilitated by initial cystoscopically directed passage of a retrograde ureteral catheter into the renal pelvis. Injected contrast then distends and opacifies the renal pelvis and calices; the ureteropelvic junction is also identified for subsequent fluoroscopically directed antegrade passage of a safety guide wire in the initial stages of percutaneous dilation.

If the retrograde ureteral catheter cannot be advanced into the renal pelvis, the angiographic catheters (Rösch inferior mesenteric, RIM; cobra-head shape) and straight or large C-curve guide wire are maneuvered through the ureteropelvic junction with fluoroscopic guidance. This can also be done nephroscopically, which, however, would necessitate full nephrostomy tract dilation before placing safety guide wires in the ureter. A guide wire through the ureteropelvic junction stenosis and into the ureter is essential before making an endopyelotomy incision.

Once the guide wires are positioned in the

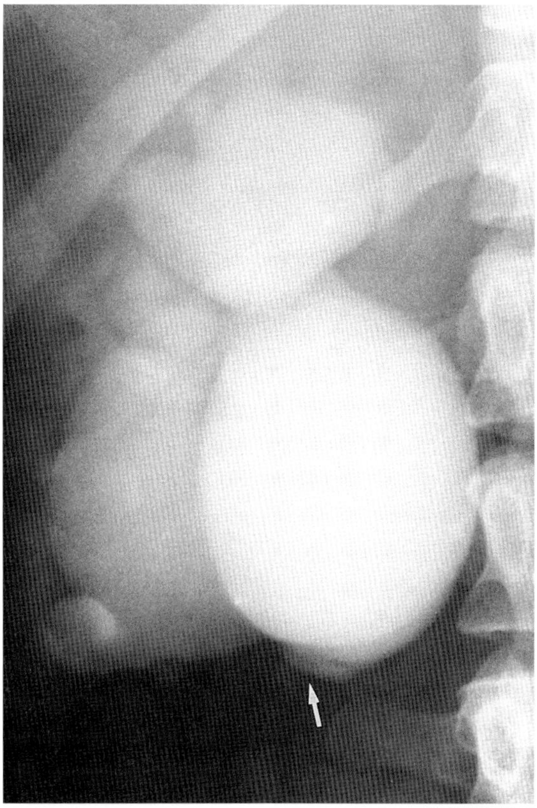

17–1 Excretory urogram shows distention of renal pelvis and calices with minimal filling of ureter – findings typical of ureteropelvic junction obstruction. Smooth contour of obstructed area suggests possibility of extrinsic compression (arrow).

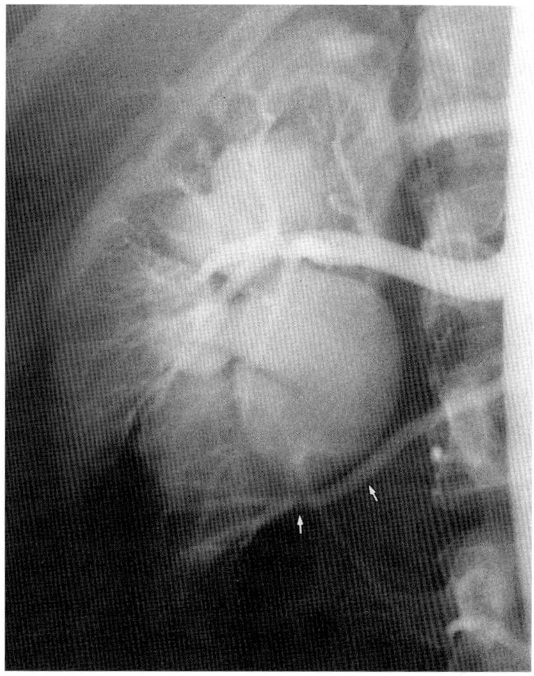

17–2 Angiographic demonstration of lower pole artery (arrows) crossing obstructed ureteropelvic junction.

ureter and the nephrostomy tract is dilated, the nephroscope is advanced fluoroscopically over a guide wire into the renal pelvis. A suction probe, such as the ultrasonic sonotrode, is advanced through the working portal to evacuate small blood clots. Following inspection of the renal pelvis and the ureteropelvic junction, the cold hook-blade endopyelotome (Wolf and Storz, Fig. 17–3) is advanced through the working portal in the nephroscope (Fig. 17–4). The endopyelotome is advanced beside the ureteral guide wire through the ureteropelvic junction with the hook-blade positioned posterolaterally. As the nephroscope is torqued posterolaterally, the blade is withdrawn through the ureteropelvic junction, creating a full-thickness incision (Fig. 17–5). Repeat incisions are often necessary; when yellow fat appears, the incision is complete.

After the full-thickness endopyelotomy is accomplished, a 8-mm diameter high-pressure angiographic balloon dilating catheter is placed over a guide wire through the ureteropelvic junction. The 4-cm-long polyethylene nondeforming balloon is pressure-filled with diluted radiographic contrast material, dilating the previously strictured area to 24 F (Kadir et al. 1982). Uniform distention of the balloon without a "waist" confirms that the full thickness incision extends into the upper ureter and more than 1 cm below the previously stenotic ureteropelvic junction.

The entire ureter, as well as the incised ureteropelvic junction, is stented (Fig. 17–6) using 8-F to 10-F stents (Smith Universal nephrostomy stent, Mentor; Uropass nephrostent, Surgitek) (Fig. 17–7). The stent is advanced over a guide wire into the bladder. Side-holes for urinary drainage are in the portion of the stent located in the renal pelvis and in the bladder (Fig. 17–8). The stent exits through the percutaneous nephrostomy tract and is initially connected to a drainage bag for several days. A nephrostogram 5–7 days after the endopyelotomy is done to confirm absence of extravasation. The external portion of the stent providing nephrostomy drainage may then be capped and coiled under a small dressing. The patient may expect to pursue normal activity for the remaining 6–8 weeks prior to stent removal.

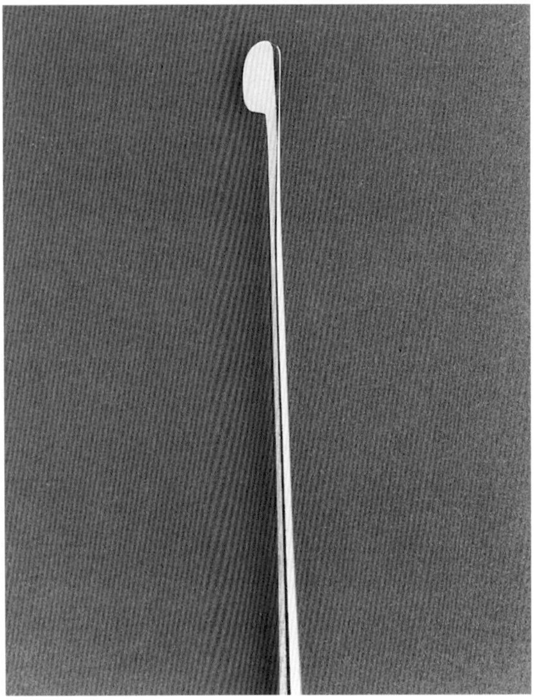

17–3 Endopyelotome (Wolf) used for making full-thickness incision through stenotic ureteropelvic junction.

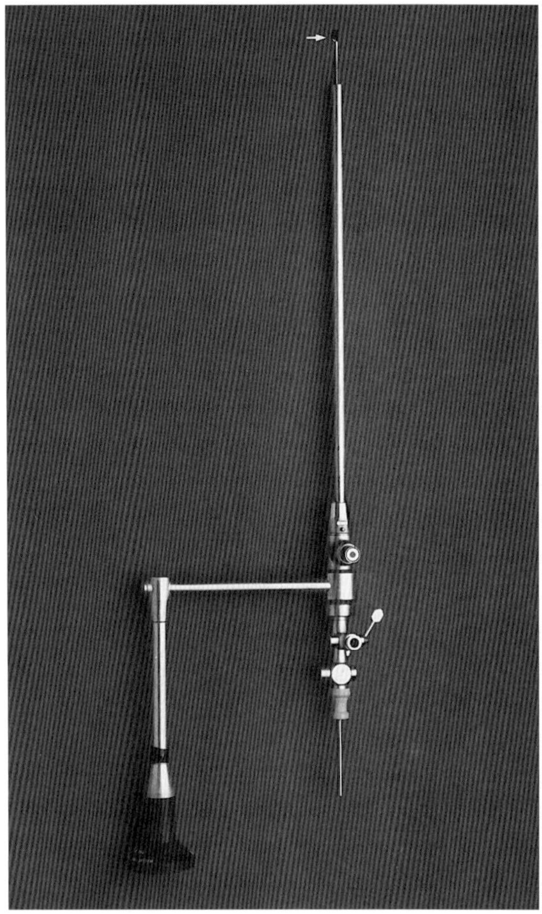

17–4 Endopyelotome (arrow) advanced through nephroscope. ▶

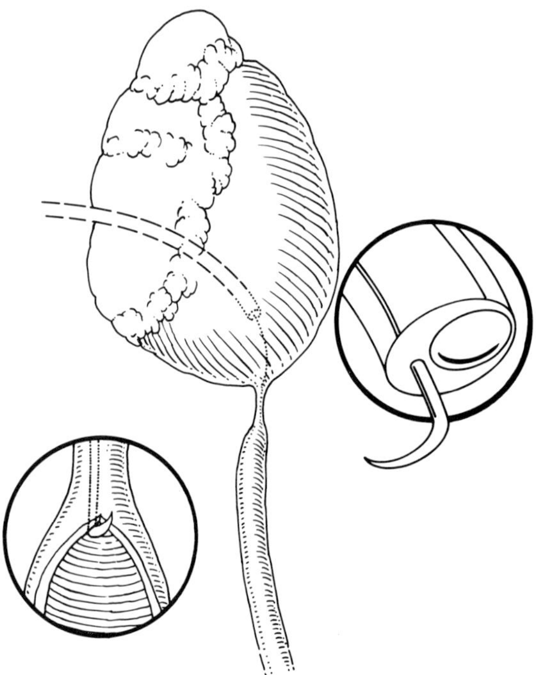

17–5 Diagrammatic illustration of endopyelotomy.

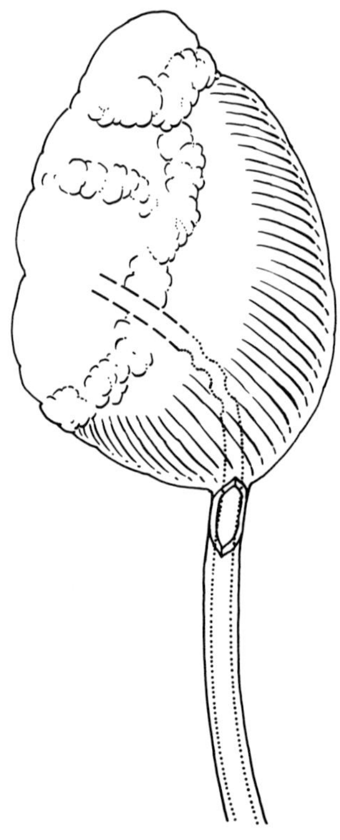

17–6 Incised ureter is stented for 6–8 weeks.

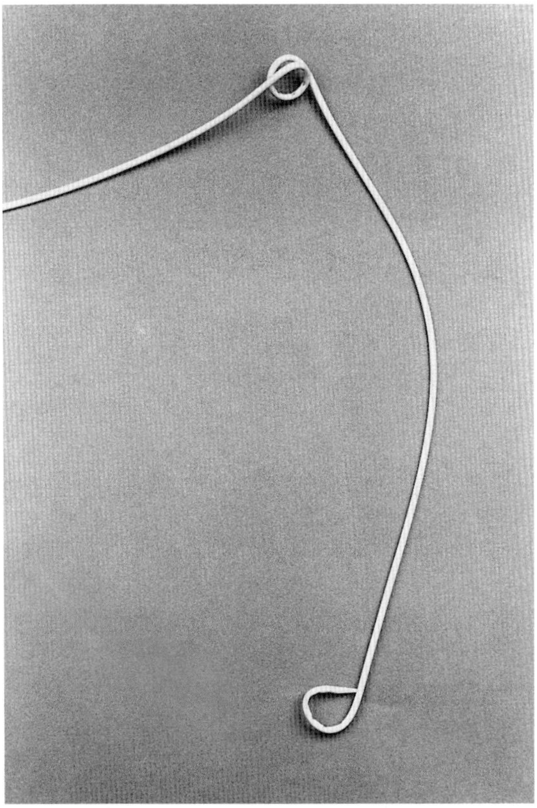

17–7 Nephrostent (Surgitek): "J" portion secures inferior portion in the bladder, while coiled portion remains in the renal pelvis. Side-holes in portion occupying renal pelvis and bladder ensure drainage through nephrostomy portion or into the bladder, as required during convalescence.

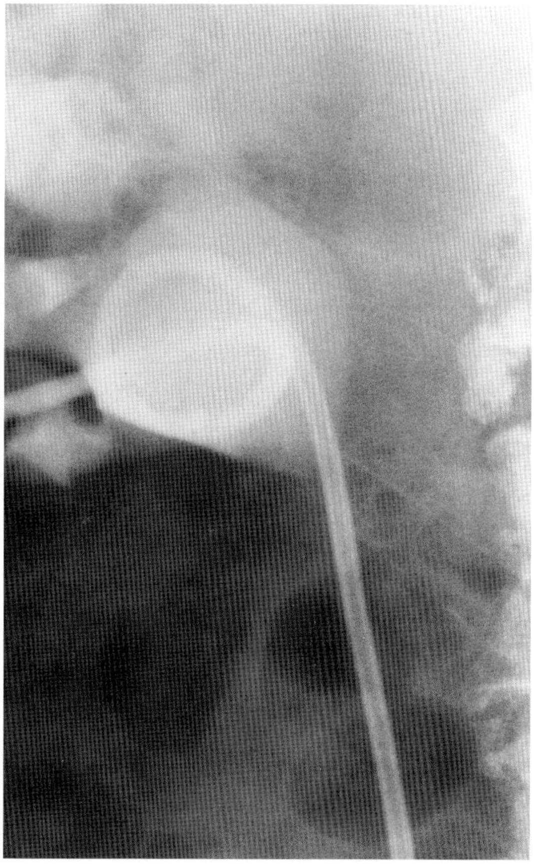

17–8 Radiographic demonstration of nephrostent in position.

Case Example

A 22-year-old woman presented with a 6-month history of right flank pain when taking in fluids. An excretory urogram demonstrated right hydronephrosis with caliectasis and a redundant renal pelvis (Fig. 17–9). Retrograde pyelogram confirmed that the hydronephrosis was secondary to stenosis of the ureteropelvic junction. She underwent percutaneous right endopyelotomy and required only 4 days' hospitalization; the ureteral stent was left in place for 8 weeks. Excretory urogram at 8 months confirmed absence of obstruction, with resolution of caliectasis and reduction in size of the previously redundant renal pelvis (Fig. 17–10). She has remained clinically well with minimal discomfort.

Discussion

Approximately 80% of adolescent and adult patients presenting with ureteropelvic junction obstruction may be candidates for endopyelotomy (Brannen et al. 1987). Early experience suggests clinical success of the procedure to be excellent (Karlin et al. 1988). In the series by Badlani and colleagues (1986), patients were successfully treated by endopyelotomy for congenital obstruction of the ureteropelvic junction as well as for recurrent stenosis following conventional surgical repair. In the current author and colleagues' series of 20 patients, 18 have shown radiographic improvement at follow-up several months after procedure.

On a study by Badlani et al. (1988), complications were negligible; patients did not require

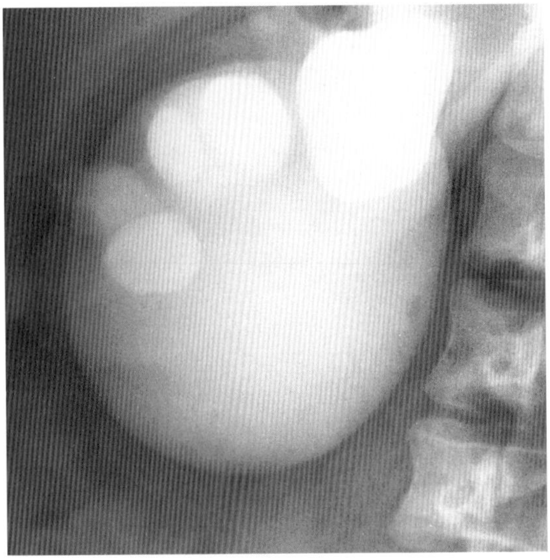

17–9 Case 1: Excretory urogram showing obstructed ureteropelvic junction.

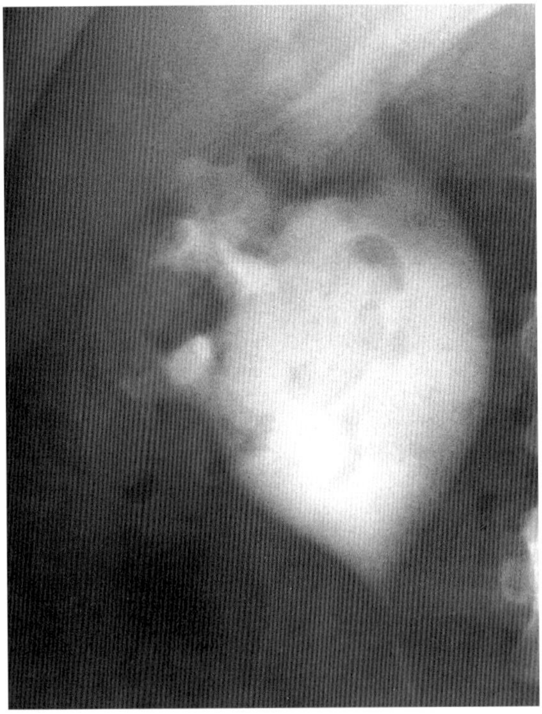

17–10 Case 1: Eight months after endopyelotomy, excretory urogram shows resolution of ureteropelvic junction obstruction.

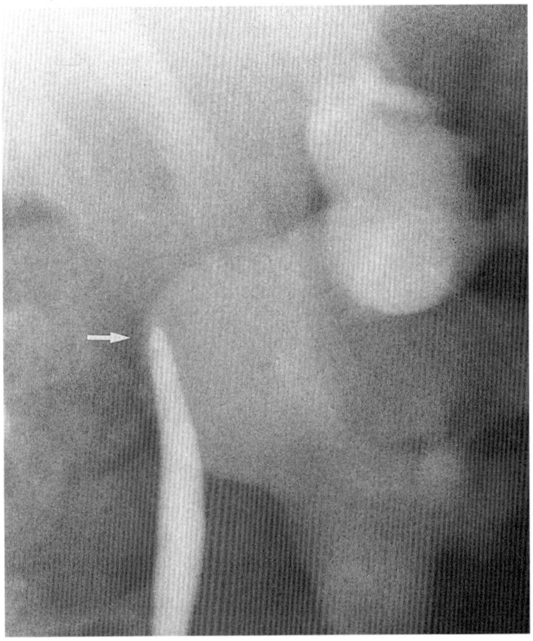

A

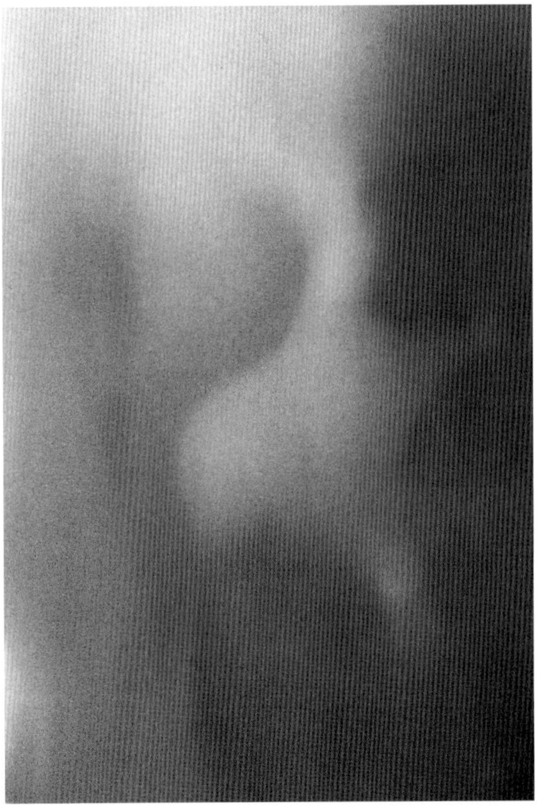

B

17–11 **(A)** Retrograde pyelogram demonstration of ureteropelvic junction obstruction in association with high insertion (arrow) of ureter. **(B)** Excretory urogram 3 months after endopyelotomy; obstruction has resolved.

prolonged hospitalization or surgical management of complications. Hospital stay and narcotic medications were considerably reduced compared to surgical pyeloplasty. A rapid recovery with diminished pain permits the endopyelotomy patient to return early to preoperative activity.

The urologic principles on which endopyelotomy is based are not new (Davis et al. 1948; Malcolm, Dorsey 1958; Oppenheimer, Hinman 1955). Repair of ureteral obstruction using a full-thickness ureterotomy incision followed by several (4–6) weeks of ureteral intubation was introduced in 1943 (Davis). Recent advancements in endourological instrumentation and lens optics now permit the "Davis intubated ureterotomy" to be performed percutaneously.

Successful outcome depends on a number of factors. First, an intact longitudinal strip of urothelium and ureter must remain to permit ureteral regeneration (Hinman, Oppenheimer 1956). Second, adequate urinary diversion must be provided during the early phases of ureteral regeneration to prevent formation of periureteral scar tissue with subsequent obstruction (Hinman, Oppenheimer 1957). Third, the stent must be 8–10 F to permit the formation of an adequate ureteral lumen (Smart 1961). Too large a stent may cause pressure necrosis of the ureteral wall with subsequent scarring obstruction. Fourth, the ureteral incision must be full-thickness through the ureteral wall and extend well beyond (≥1 cm proximal and distal) the area of stenosis. Fifth, the incision should be in the posterolateral region of the ureteropelvic junction to ensure an intact medial blood supply for adequate healing and regeneration. Finally, covering the affected area with perirenal fat prevents the incised ureter from adhering to adjacent structures with subsequent angulation and obstruction. The procedure is most effective when the ureter is not disturbed from its natural sheath (Hamm, Weinberg 1956).

Certain anatomic situations may represent relative contraindications to endopyelotomy. One is the association of an aberrant lower pole artery with stenosis of the ureteropelvic junction (Fig. 17–2). Although there may be little risk of vascular injury due to the posterolateral incision, the persistent extrinsic compression of the artery at the ureteropelvic junction may cause recurrent obstruction.

In cases of extreme redundancy of the renal pelvis over a band or narrowing, a reduction pyeloplasty may be done to remove a portion of the renal pelvis. However, the previously discussed case study illustrates a remarkable reduction in size of a redundant renal pelvis 8 months after release of the ureteropelvic junction obstruction (Figs. 17–9 and 17–10). Such observations suggest that an impressively redundant renal pelvis may undergo adequate reduction simply by correcting the obstruction. Nevertheless, if, in the surgeon's judgment, excision of a portion of the renal pelvis is indicated, repair through a flank incision is necessary. A surgical approach may also be required for repair of long segments of stenotic ureter and associated massive retroperitoneal fibrosis, and for correcting obstruction in children. Initially, high insertion of the ureter into the renal pelvis was thought to be a contraindication to endopyelotomy (Badlani et al. 1986); subsequent experience has demonstrated favorable results (Fig. 17–11). The most obvious major consequence of failed endopyelotomy would be restenosis of the ureteropelvic junction, requiring subsequent surgical reconstruction.

Patients who have undergone percutaneous endopyelotomy as the primary approach to correct ureteropelvic junction stenosis have done well clinically and have demonstrated radiographic improvement. Most patients with ureteropelvic junction stenosis may be offered endopyelotomy as an alternative to surgical reconstruction.

References

Anderson JC, Hynes W: Retrocaval ureter: Case diagnosed preoperatively and treated successfully by plastic operation. *Br. J. Urol.* 21:209–211, 1949.

Badlani G, Eshghi M, Smith AD: Percutaneous surgery for ureteropelvic junction obstruction (endopyelotomy): Technique and early results. *J. Urol.* 135:26–28, 1986.

Badlani GH, Karlin GS, Smith AD: Complications of endopyelotomy: Analysis in series of 64 patients. *J. Urol.* 140:473–475, 1988.

Brannen GE, Bush WH: Ultrasonic destruction of kidney stones. *West. J. Med.* 140(2):227–232, 1984.

Brannen GE, Bush WH, Correa RJ, Gibbons RP, Elder JS: Kidney stone removal: Percutaneous versus surgical lithotomy. *J. Urol.* 133:6–12, 1985.

Brannen GE, Bush WH, Lewis GP: Caliceal calculi. *J. Urol.* 135:1142–1145, 1986.

Brannen GE, Bush WH, Lewis GP: Endopyelotomy for primary repair of ureteropelvic junction obstruction. *J. Urol.* 1987.

Culp OS, DeWeerd JH: A pelvic flap operation for certain types of ureteropelvic obstruction: Preliminary report. *Mayo Clin. Proc.* 26:483–488, 1951.

Davis DM: Intubated ureterotomy: A new operation for ureteral and ureteropelvic strictures. *Surg. Gynecol. Obstet.* 76:513–518, 1943.

Davis DM, Strong GH, Drake WM: Intubated ureterotomy: Experimental work and clinical results. *J. Urol.* 59:851–856, 1948.

Foley FEB: New plastic operation for stricture at ureteropelvic junction: Report of 20 operations. *J. Urol.* 38:643–647, 1937.

Hamm FC, Weinberg SR: Experimental studies of regeneration of the ureter without intubation. *J. Urol.* 75:43–47, 1956.

Hinman F, Jr., Oppenheimer R: Ureteral regeneration. IV. Fascial covering compared to fatty connective tissues. *J. Urol.* 76:729–733, 1956.

Hinman F, Jr., Oppenheimer R: Ureteral regeneration. VI. Delayed urinary flow in the healing of unsplinted ureteral defects. *J. Urol.* 78:138–142, 1957.

Kadir S, White RI, Jr., Engel R: Balloon dilatation of a ureteropelvic junction obstruction. *Radiology* 143: 263–266, 1982.

Karlin GS, Badlani GH, Smith AD: Endopyelotomy versus open pyeloplasty: Comparison in 88 patients. *J. Urol.* 140:476–478, 1988.

Malcom DC, Dorsey JW: Reoperative correction of previous pelviureteral plastic surgery. *J. Urol.* 80:436–439, 1958.

Oppenheimer R, Hinman F, Jr.: Ureteral regeneration: Contracture vs. hyperplasia of smooth muscle. *J. Urol.* 74:476–480, 1955.

Scardino PL, Prince CL: Vertical flap ureteropelvioplasty: Preliminary report. *South. Med. J.* 46:325–329, 1953.

Smart WR: An evaluation of intubation ureterotomy with a description of surgical technique. *J. Urol.* 85:512–516, 1961.

Whitfield HN, Mills V, Miller RA, Wickham JEA: Percutaneous pyelolysis: An alternative to pyeloplasty. *Br. J. Urol.* (Suppl.), 93–96, 1983.

CHAPTER

18

Percutaneous Techniques for Renal Calculus Disease

George E. Brannen and William H. Bush

A combination of percutaneous access to the renal collecting system with ultrasonic fragmentation and evacuation of the calculus (percutaneous ultrasonic lithotripsy) is a joint urologic-radiologic procedure that has been used to remove kidney stones from thousands of patients since its inception in 1982. Subsequent refinements in flexible optics and in techniques of stone grasping and fragmentation have permitted successful percutaneous stone retrieval efforts in special situations.

Percutaneous access to the renal collecting system was first reported in the mid-1950s (Goodwin et al. 1955). Refinements of the technique that were introduced in the mid 1970s (Burnett et al. 1976) led to the widespread use of percutaneous nephrostomy procedures (Stables et al. 1978). Dilation of a nephrostomy tract permits placement of a nephroscope and direct inspection of the renal pelvis and calices. Radiologic involvement with multidirectional fluoroscopy and steerable catheters permits the percutaneous manipulation and removal of selected renal calculi under combined endoscopic and fluoroscopic control (Clayman, Castaneda-Zuniga 1984). Fragmentation of renal calculi by ultrasonic energy was pioneered in Germany (Alken et al. 1981; Alken 1982), and clinical application of percutaneous ultrasonic lithotripsy proliferated rapidly both in Europe (Marberger et al. 1982, Wickham et al. 1983) and in the United States (Segura et al. 1983).

Procedure

Urinary calculi targeted for complete removal include stones obstructing the urinary system and calculi in the renal pelvis and calices. Parenchymal stones or small punctate calcifications, as in diffuse nephrocalcinosis, are not targeted for removal. Only 16% of patients have had stones small enough to remove directly by grasping or basket extraction; the remainder require ultrasonic fragmentation before removal (Brannen et al. 1985). The procedure requires the combined efforts of a urologist and an interventional radiologist (Bush, Brannen et al. 1984). Use of a C-arm multidirectional fluoroscopy unit is critical for intermittent guidance throughout the procedure (Fig. 18–1).

General anesthesia is usually given, and the patient is placed in the lithotomy position; cystoscopy is performed to advance a 5-F or 6-F ureteral catheter into the renal pelvis. The patient is then placed in a prone oblique position. Radiographic contrast solution, 20% diatrizoate sodium, injected through the ureteral catheter, distends and opacifies the collecting system, aiding initial percutaneous needle placement under fluoroscopic guidance. A 15-cm long, 18-gauge needle is placed transcutaneously beneath the twelfth rib posterolaterally and is advanced into the selected calix or infundibulum. Free return of urine or contrast medium confirms position of the needle tip in the renal collecting system. A J-tipped movable-core guide wire, 0.89 mm (0.035 in.) or 0.97 mm (0.038 in.), is inserted through the needle and coiled in the renal pelvis.

Anatomy

Knowledge of renal anatomy aids in percutaneous access (Kaye, Goldberg 1982). The posterior row of calices generally form a 20° angle with the frontal plane of the kidney. Since the psoas

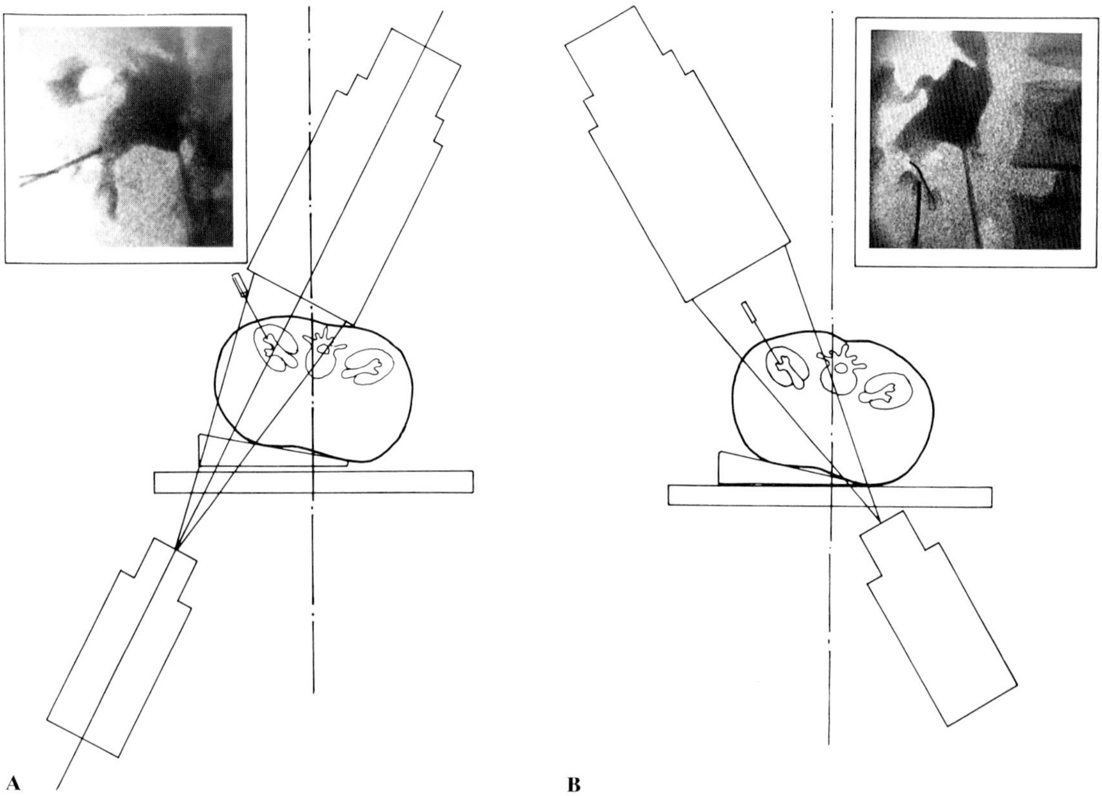

18–1 Illustration of multidirectional C-arm fluoroscopy and X-ray images obtained during percutaneous access of calculus removal. (Reprinted from *Appl. Radiol.* 14(6):87, 1985, with the permission of Macmillan Professional Journals, Santa Monica, CA.) **(A)** C-arm fluoroscope rotated so X-ray beam is perpendicular to needles. Cephalocaudal direction and depth of needles are defined. **(B)** C-arm fluoroscope rotated so X-ray beam is parallel to needle. Anteroposterior orientation of needles is defined.

muscle rotates the renal hilum 30°–50° to the anterior, the posterior row of calices are 50° to 70° off the body's frontal plane. Thus, they appear medial to the anterior calices in excretory urography (Fig. 18–2). With the patient prone and the side of entry elevated 30°, the posterior calices are 80° to 100°, or nearly perpendicular, to the table; this permits the posterior calix to lie in line with the vertical X-ray beam and allows a stable entry through renal parenchyma. The posterior calix is generally located beneath the "avascular" line of Broedel.

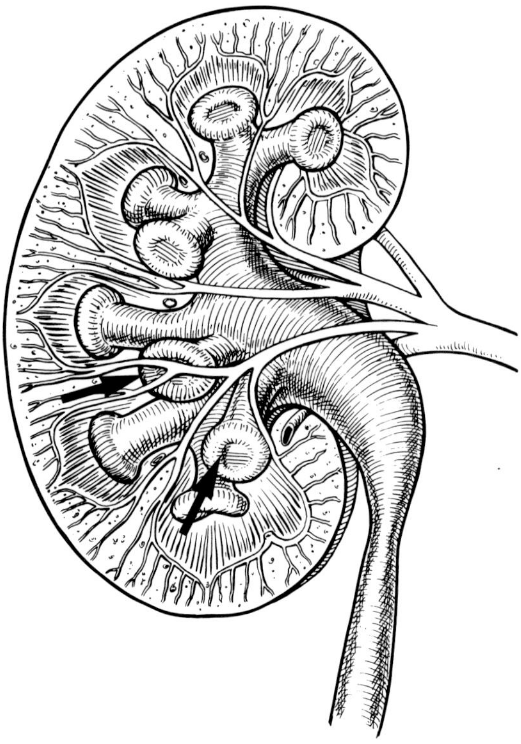

18–2 Illustration of caliceal anatomy renal vascularity. Posteriorly directed calices project medial to anterior calices in frontal view of kidney. Major vessel injury can be avoided by peripheral transrenal nephrostomy insertion (arrows). (After Melloni BJ: *Melloni's Illustrated Medical Dictionary.* Baltimore, Williams & Wilkins, 1979.)

Access

Antegrade Percutaneous

Stone location determines the route of percutaneous access (Fig. 18–3). A calculus located in the renal pelvis can be removed through either a lateral, inferolateral, or inferior calix. A calculus at the ureteropelvic junction or upper ureter is more readily retrieved with access through a lateral calix or supracostally through an upper calix. Stones located in a posterior, lateral, or inferior calix are approached through the calix containing the stone (Bush, Brannen et al. 1985). The rigid nephroscope usually may be manipulated into the superior calices after initial access through an inferior calix, although in some cases supracostal access may be necessary.

With the guide wire in position and the needle removed, initial 6-F, 8-F, and 10-F dilators are advanced. A second guide wire, most commonly a 0.89-mm (0.035-in.) or 0.97-mm (0.038-in.) 3-cm tapered straight wire, is advanced through the 10-F dilator, which is then removed; the straight guide wire is directed down the ureter with the aid of the small C-curved or inferior mesenteric (RIM) angiographic catheter (Cook Company). The catheter is advanced over the guide wire down the ureter until the coiled tip rests in the bladder. This antegrade angiographic ureteral catheter is partially occlusive, which prevents small fragments from falling into the ureter, and the catheter also provides orientation to the ureteropelvic junction during nephroscopy (Fig. 18–4). Also, a guide wire reinserted through this ureteral catheter can provide access to the kidney following inadvertent dislodgement of the nephroscope. The tract is dilated further over the original guide wire to approximately 30 F, using either the Amplatz fascial dilating system or one of the high-pressure 10-mm balloon catheters (Fig. 18–4). The dilating balloon catheter is suggested for those doing these procedures infrequently. A subcostal access approach is recommended for most cases, although other options are available.

Supracostal

Percutaneous access above the twelfth rib, for upper caliceal calculi, is associated with a 5% incidence of hydrothorax and a small incidence of pneumothorax; this risk may be minimized by making the skin entry puncture more laterally near

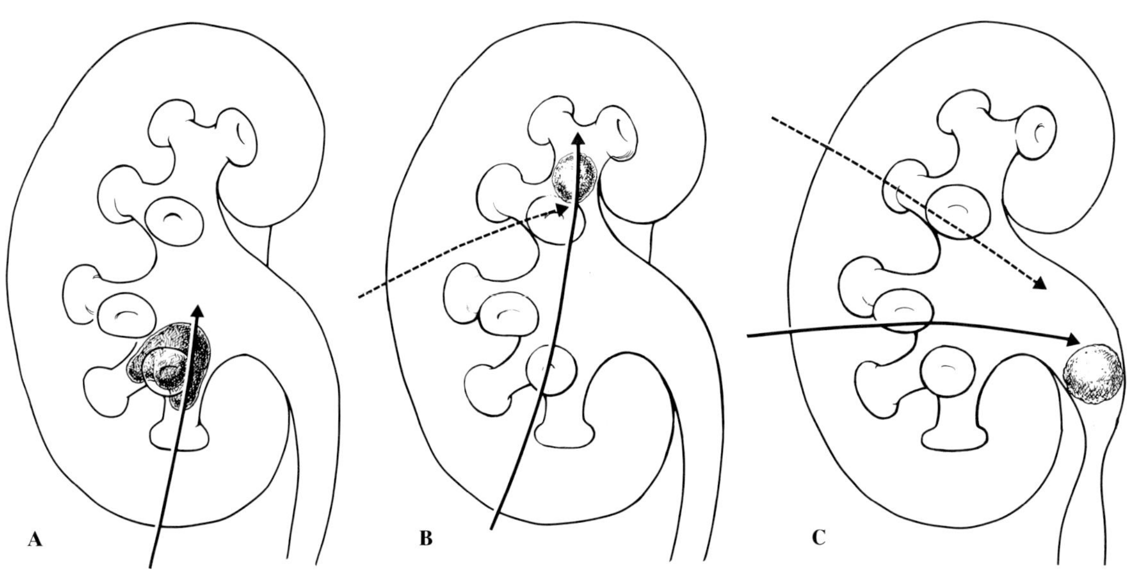

18–3 Location of stone determines entrance site for percutaneous nephrostolithotomy. **(A)** Calculus in lower caliceal area is approached directly with nephroscope inserted into calculus-containing calix. **(B)** An upper calix calculus is approached usually through an inferior calix and subcostal insertion (solid arrow). It may be necessary to approach calix directly through an intercostal insertion (dotted arrow). **(C)** Calculus in ureteropelvic junction is approached through a lateral calix; an upper ureter calculus is approached either through a lateral calix (solid arrow) or, if necessary, intercostally through an upper calix, intercostal approach (dotted arrow). (Reprinted from *Appl. Radiol.* 14(6):91, 1985, with the permission of Macmillan Professional Journals, Santa Monica, CA.)

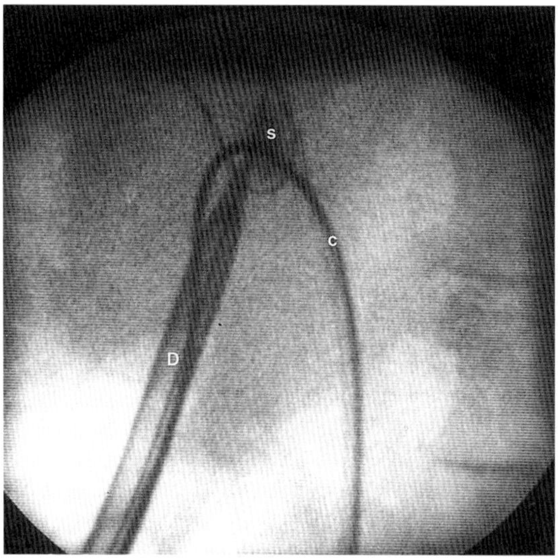

18–4 Dilation of tract. A 30-F fascial dilator (D) has been inserted over guide wire down to the stone (S). Antegrade ureteral catheter (C) and safety guide wire.

the tip of the twelfth rib, although colon or spleen position must then be recognized (Forsythe, Fuchs 1987; Young et al. 1985).

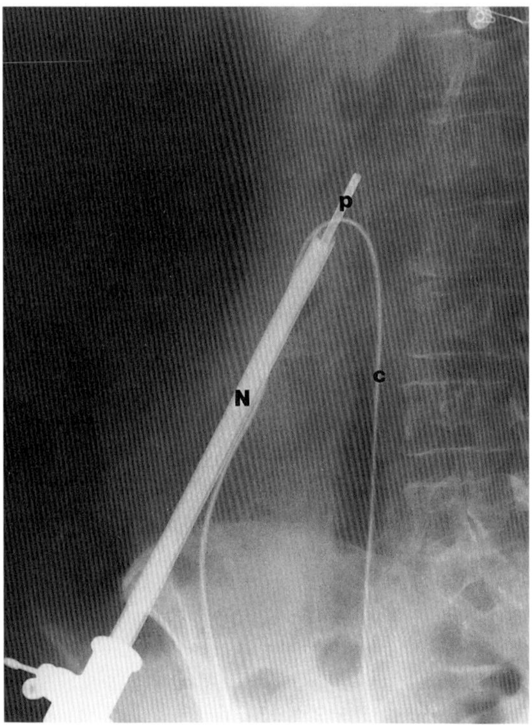

18–5 Radiograph of nephroscope (N) and ultrasonic probe (P) during PUL. C = antegrade safety ureteral catheter. (Reprinted, by permission, from Bush WH: Percutaneous stone therapy. *In* Putman CE, Ravin CE (eds.): *Textbook of Diagnostic Imaging,* pp. 1269–1279, © 1988 by W. B. Saunders Co., Philadelphia.)

Retrograde

A technique of retrograde nephrostomy tract entry has been published (Finlayson 1985). A 5-F Teflon ureteral catheter over a torque guide wire (Cook, Bloomington, IN) is advanced retrograde up the ureter. The malleable torque wire maintains a fixed flexion directed by the endoscopist. Consequently, the tip of the wire may be directed into a specific calix even in a nondilated system. A 9-F Teflon sheath is advanced over the 5-F sheath and guide wire; the 9-F Teflon catheter is left in position; the guide wire and 5-F catheter are removed, and the moderately stiff "rocket wire" with a needle on the end is advanced up the 9-F catheter and pushed out the renal calix toward the skin. Complete access from the urethra through the nephrostomy tract is obtained with a single wire.

Conventional antegrade percutaneous access is preferred for the majority of cases. Regardless of the method used for percutaneous access to the renal collecting system, successful access is generally achieved in over 95% of properly selected patients.

Stone Removal

The rigid 24-F Wolf or Storz nephroscope is advanced over the guide wire and positioned in the renal pelvis. The obturator and guide wire are removed and the lens system inserted. The long hollow metal sonotrode is inserted through the entry portal of the lens system (Fig. 18–5). Irrigation through the nephroscope using normal saline and outflow through the sonotrode suction are quantitated during the procedure. If an unaccounted difference of more than 1 L is identified, consideration should be given to placement of a nephrostomy tube and early termination of the procedure; a delayed procedure may be performed through the same nephrostomy tract. Clots are aspirated through the hollow sonotrode, and the renal pelvis is distended with saline irrigation, permitting visualization of the renal pelvis and calculi. Small calculi may be grasped with forceps or engaged in a Dormia basket and removed intact through the nephroscope.

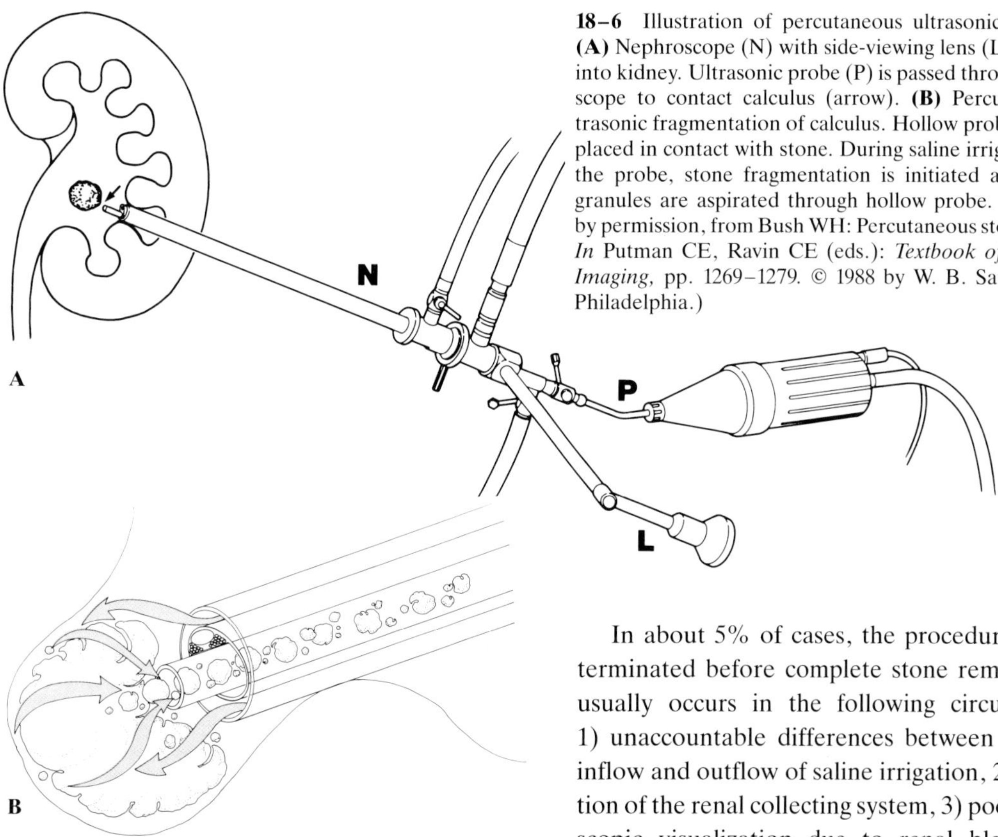

18–6 Illustration of percutaneous ultrasonic lithotriper. **(A)** Nephroscope (N) with side-viewing lens (L) is inserted into kidney. Ultrasonic probe (P) is passed through nephroscope to contact calculus (arrow). **(B)** Percutaneous ultrasonic fragmentation of calculus. Hollow probe is visually placed in contact with stone. During saline irrigation about the probe, stone fragmentation is initiated and sandlike granules are aspirated through hollow probe. (Reprinted, by permission, from Bush WH: Percutaneous stone therapy. *In* Putman CE, Ravin CE (eds.): *Textbook of Diagnostic Imaging*, pp. 1269–1279. © 1988 by W. B. Saunders Co., Philadelphia.)

Ultrasonic Lithotripsy

The sonotrode is generally advanced under direct vision through the nephroscope and placed in contact with the stone (Fig. 18–6). Upon electric activation (about 100 W) of the piezoceramic crystal, high-frequency sound waves in the range of 23–27 MHz are generated and transmitted down the metal probe. Vibrations from the end of the probe pulverize the stone. The particles are then evacuated by simultaneous irrigation through the nephroscope and suction through the hollow sonotrode (Figs. 18–6, 18–7).

By exchanging the sonotrode for a right angle lens, the renal pelvis may then be inspected. Following removal of the nephroscope over a guide wire, a 22-F radiopaque Councill nephrostomy catheter is inserted. It and the adjacent antegrade angiographic ureteral catheter are sutured to the skin. A final injection of contrast medium into the nephrostomy catheter confirms proper position and identifies areas of potential urinary extravasation. The tissue surrounding the nephrostomy tract and the subcostal nerve are infiltrated generously with as much as 50 ml of 0.25% bupivacaine hydrochloride (Marcaine).

In about 5% of cases, the procedure must be terminated before complete stone removal. This usually occurs in the following circumstances: 1) unaccountable differences between measured inflow and outflow of saline irrigation, 2) perforation of the renal collecting system, 3) poor nephroscopic visualization due to renal bleeding, or 4) prolonged procedure. In these patients, targeted calculi may be removed at a later time through the existing nephrostomy tract.

The day after percutaneous ultrasonic lithotripsy, plain film renal tomograms are taken. If there are no fragments, the antegrade angiographic ureteral catheter is removed and a nephrostogram is performed (Fig. 18–8). The nephrostogram confirms not only the absence of potential urinary extravasation and proper tube position but also assesses the degree of ureteral drainage. If the nephrostogram shows flow to the bladder and no extravasation, the nephrostomy tube may be clamped. If there is no fever, pain, or excessive urinary leakage around the tube after 12 hours, the tube may be removed and the patient discharged from the hospital. Patients commonly require additional days of inpatient or outpatient nephrostomy drainage to permit resolution of ureteral or ureteropelvic junction edema.

Additional retrieval efforts are necessary in 10%–15% of patients. Remaining fragments may often be removed successfully during the postoperative period through the existing nephrostomy tract under local anesthesia. In about 5% of total patients, repeat nephroscopy under general

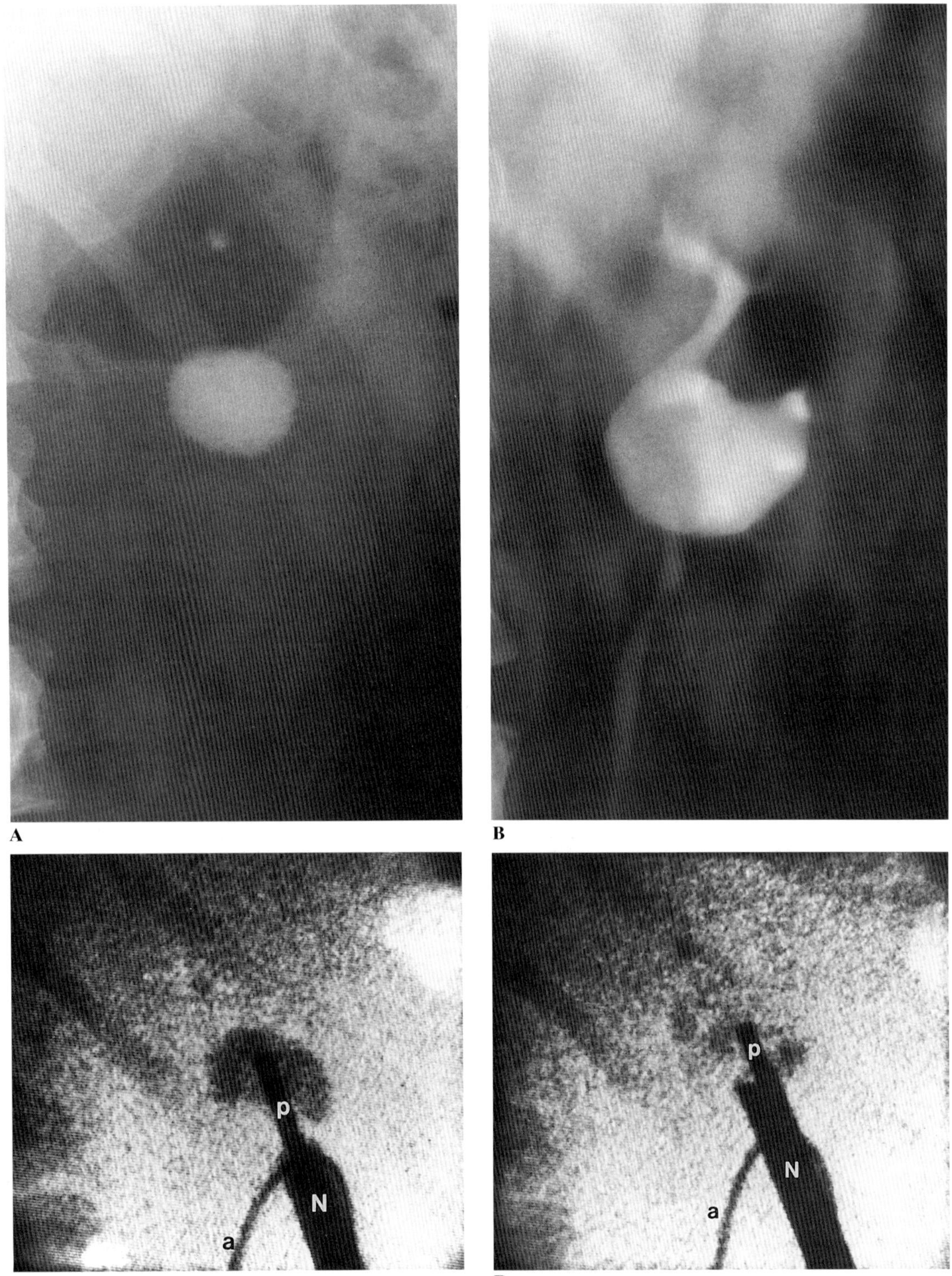

18–7 Percutaneous ultrasonic lithotripsy of renal pelvic and calix calculus. **(A)** Large 2.5-cm renal pelvic calculus and small upper calix calculus. **(B)** Excretory urography; tomogram of left kidney. **(C)** Nephroscope (N) has been inserted, and ultrasonic probe (P) has partially fragmented the calculus. a = antegrade ureteral catheter. **(D)** Further ultrasonic lithotripsy, and calculus is now in numerous fragments. N = nephroscope; P = ultrasonic probe; a = antegrade ureteral catheter.

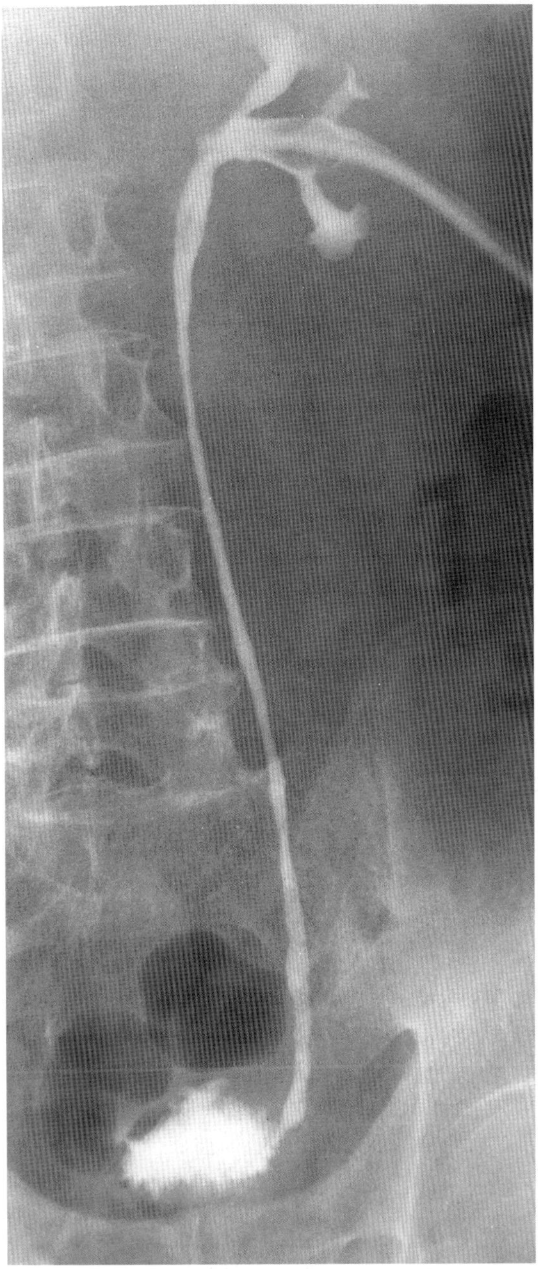

18–8 Nephrostogram done 1 day after percutaneous removal of large renal calculus. Councill catheter with partially inflated balloon is in a proper position; contrast flows freely to bladder, and there is no extravasation.

anesthesia is required to complete the removal of targeted calculi. Some patients undergo hemiacidrin irrigation after percutaneous ultrasonic lithotripsy to dissolve identifiable or potential residual struvite stone fragments.

Electrohydraulic Lithotripsy

Electrohydraulic lithotripsy (Clayman et al. 1984, Preminger et al. 1985) is performed using a flexible probe, placed nearly in contact with the urinary calculus through a nephroscope. The procedure was first used in the mid-70s for fragmentation and evacuation of renal calculi (Raney, Handler 1975), and became generally available in the early 80s (Clayman et al. 1983).

The electrohydraulic probe (ACMI, Wolf, Pentax) consists of a flexible central metal core surrounded by a layer of insulation and a concentric metal layer. A second layer of insulation covers the entire probe. An electrical discharge, up to 120 V, transmits a spark at the tip of the probe across the gap from the central metal core to the concentric metal ring. This intense heat vaporizes a small amount of water, and rapid expansion of the air bubble causes a shock wave, propagated at a rate slightly less than 5,000 ft/sec. Repeated impacts of the shock waves are sufficient to fracture most urinary calculi and are most effective on stones with irregular surfaces. A smoother stone surface often requires more discharges for fragmentation.

The goal of this electrohydraulic procedure is to produce fragments that may be removed by grasping. A fluid interface is required between the probe and the stone. Ideally, the probe should be about 1 mm from the stone surface, as the power of the shock wave decreases by the square of the distance. Consequently the impact of the shock wave at 2 mm is 25% of its impact at 1 mm. The probe should be ≥ 5 mm from both the lens and the urothelial surface to prevent thermal injury to the lens or perforation of the renal pelvis. Continuous flow of irrigation fluid dissipates heat, minimizing risk of injury. Probes are as small as 5 F and may be used through a 15-F flexible choledochonephroscope. Larger 7-F or 9-F probes may be used only through the rigid nephroscope.

The major advantage of electrohydraulic lithotripsy is the ability to dependably fragment calculi approachable only by flexible nephroscopy. Disadvantages include the tedious efforts required to grasp and remove each fragment and the possibility of small fragments imbedding in urothelium. Fourteen percent of patients have retained stone fragments following this procedure (Clayman et al. 1984).

Laser Lithotripsy

Laser fragmentation permits a flexible probe to be placed in contact with the urinary calculus via a ureteroscope or nephroscope (Dretler et al. 1987). Dye laser fragmentation (Candela Corporation, Natwick, MA) permits shock wave disruption of calculi with more control and less explosive impact compared to electrohydraulic lithotripsy. The energy source is a coumarin green dye laser excited by a pulsed tunable flashlamp. The energy is focused into a flexible quartz fiber with peak current generally at 5,000 A and 20 kV. The flexible 250 μ diameter quartz fiber (silica coated) is advanced through the endoscope and placed in direct contact with the stone. Pulses are delivered at a rate of 5/sec (5 Hz).

The laser is activated at the rate of ≤60 mJ/pulse. Wavelength may be varied from 450 nm to 510 nm to control the size of the fragments. A yellow glass filter is fitted to the eyepiece of the nephroscope to prevent retinal injury. Since the laser energy is delivered in brief pulses and a small diameter fiber is used, high laser power (106 W) may be used and power density increased. Brief pulse durations result in low heat and therefore minimal thermal tissue injury.

The advantages of dye laser fragmentation are: the quartz fiber may be placed through small flexible instruments; stone fragmentation is controlled; and the potential for urothelial injury is limited. Disadvantages are that only calculi ≤2 cm can be dependably fragmented, and additional efforts are required to retrieve stone fragments, as they may not evacuate spontaneously.

The ultrasonic probe can only be placed through the rigid nephroscope, while the electrohydraulic and laser probes may be used through

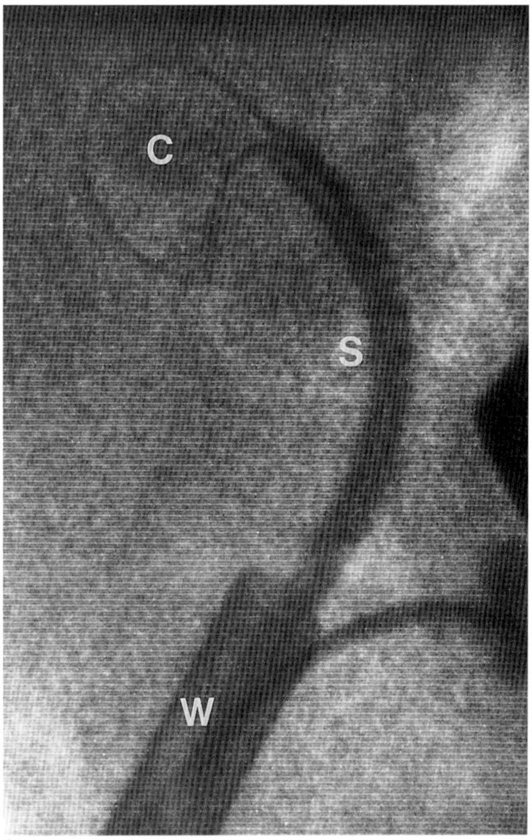

A

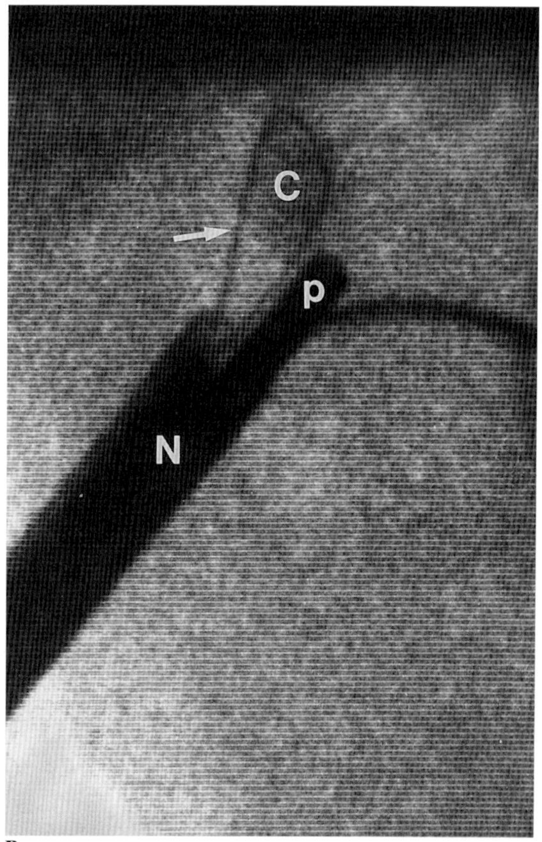

B

18–9 Use of steerable loop snare to retrieve calculus during initial percutaneous nephrostolithotomy. A 15-mm pelvic calculus migrated into upper infundibulum during percutaneous ultrasonic lithotripsy and could not be engaged with nephroscopic instruments. **(A)** Fluoroscopic image showing steerable catheter (S) inserted through Teflon working sheath of fascial dilator system (W). Single guide wire loop has engaged upper infundibulum calculus (C). **(B)** Calculus has been withdrawn back into renal pelvis; steerable catheter was removed and the nephroscope (N) was placed through sheath. Ultrasonic probe (P) has been inserted to fragment calculus (C) as it was held in place by the loop snare (arrow). (Reprinted, by permission, from Bush WH, Brannen GE: Percutaneous removal of caliceal calculi. *Am. J. Roentgenol.* 144:139–142, © 1985, American Roentgen Ray Society.)

either flexible or rigid nephroscopes. The flexibility is an advantage, but it limits irrigation and suction capabilities compared to the rigid scopes. This is especially a problem in an acute nephrostomy tract in which mild oozing of blood may impede vision. Stone particles must be retrieved in a separate effort after electrohydraulic or laser fragmentation.

Special Techniques

Specialized techniques for removal of calculi or remaining stone fragments have been introduced (Brannen et al. 1986). The steerable loop snare technique (Bush, Crane et al. 1984) combines use of the Medi-Tech steerable catheter with a guide wire loop snare to retrieve calculi (Fig. 18–9). One or two 0.71-mm (0.028-in.), fixed-core 145-cm-long guide wires are folded at the midportion. The folded ends of these wires are advanced through the side port of the handle of a 13-F Medi-Tech steerable catheter. The free ends of the guide wires can be advanced or withdrawn, resulting in side-to-side expansion of the loop snare for control of the steerable catheter. All four parts of two guide wires fit easily through the side port of the Medi-Tech handle. For increased maneuverability, a 10-F Medi-Tech steerable catheter may be used with two 0.64-mm (0.025-in.) guide wires.

The system is passed through an Amplatz Teflon working sheath or directly through a matured nephrostomy tract and is fluoroscopically guided to the calculus. The wire loops are expanded and maneuvered over the calculus. When the loops are tightened, the stone is trapped against the end of the steerable catheter, and the entire catheter loop system is withdrawn.

The parallel-tract push technique (Bush, Brannen 1984) is used to retrieve calculi not accessible to the usual nephroscopic route or not treatable by extracorporeal shock wave lithotripsy (ESWL) (Fig. 18–10). The small parallel tract is placed between the eleventh and twelfth ribs. An 18-gauge needle is inserted while the collecting system is distended with irrigating fluid from the nephroscope. The needle is guided into contact with the calix stone under fluoroscopic guidance. When fluid flows out of the needle, a 0.89-mm (0.035-in.) movable-core, J guide wire is inserted through the needle so that it freely coils in the renal pelvis.

Over this wire, small dilators are inserted. Initial advancement of the small dilators develops the nephrostomy tract and can dilate a narrow infundibulum; then, the 8-F Teflon catheter of the Amplatz fascial dilator system (Cook) is placed over the guide wire. The 12-F fascial dilator is inserted over the 8-F Teflon catheter down to the calculus. The inner-core 8-F catheter is removed, leaving a blunt "pusher" dilator against the stone (Fig. 18–10D). The guide wire remains through the hollow core of the "pusher" dilator during its advancement through the infundibulum into the renal pelvis. Once in the renal pelvis, the stone is removed using conventional percutaneous technology.

Additional manipulations may be needed under direct vision or fluoroscopic guidance through a 24-F, 26-F, or 28-F Teflon working sheath (Miller, Wickham 1984). Rigid grasping instruments include cable forceps, the Storz grasper, and the Wolf grasper and are easily used through a nephroscope. A stone basket or three-pronged flexible grasper may be maneuvered through a steerable catheter fluoroscopically. The Mazzariello-Caprini grasping forceps have the advantage of a long, twisting, nonexpansile shaft segment and are used to remove calculi from the renal pelvis or nephrostomy tract.

Many endourologists pursue the removal of caliceal calculi under direct vision with the use of flexible nephroscopy (Lange et al. 1984). Flexible nephroscopes generally are 15 F, permit 180° flexion in a single plane, and have a 5-F working port, but permit only a maximal irrigation of 20–25 ml/min (Olympus, Pentax, ACMI). Instruments that may be used through the flexible working port include stone baskets, alligator forceps, three- and four-pronged graspers, "W" graspers, electrocautery probes, electrohydraulic lithotriptor probes, and a fiber-light guide to deliver laser energy. Passage of the instruments through the working port decreases the flexibility by 30° to 50°.

The flexible nephroscope provides access to 90% of the calices through any nephrostomy tract. The nephroscopic flexibility permits antegrade passage down the ureter so that ureteral calculi may be manipulated under direct vision. Access for flexible nephroscopy must be through an existing nephrostomy tract or working sheath, because mild bleeding and diminished flow of irrigant may limit visualization. The endoscopist must become accustomed to the grid pattern produced by the

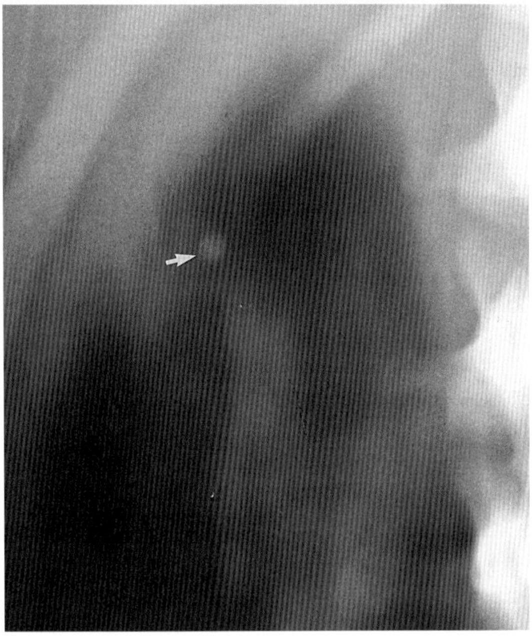

A

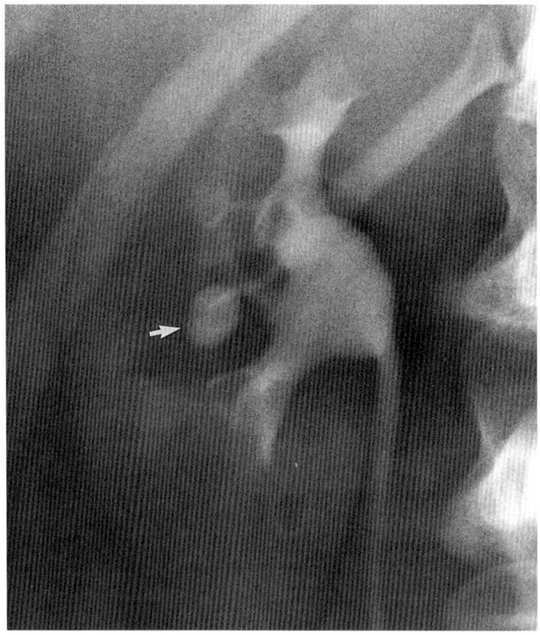

B

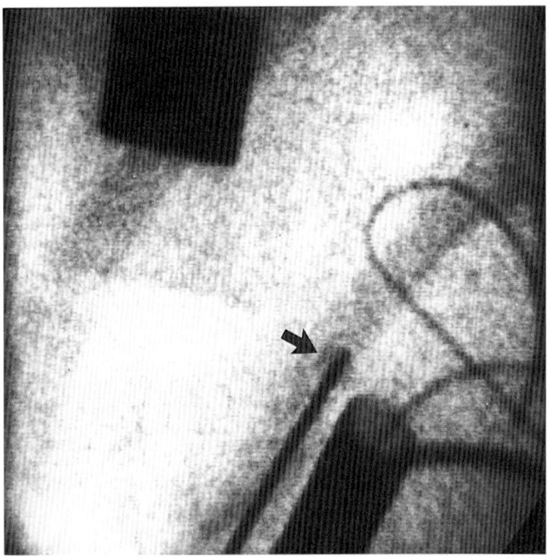

C

18–10 Parallel tract push technique for calix calculus dislodgement. **(A)** Twenty-two-year-old woman with recurrent urinary tract infection. Scout tomogram shows 5-mm calix calculus (arrow). **(B)** Film from excretory urogram. Calculus is located in deformed lateral calix with small infundibulum (arrow). **(C)** Fluoroscopic image during percutaneous nephrostolithotomy. Calculus (arrow) lies in calix adjacent to entrance tract and was inaccessible to instruments. An 18-gauge needle is inserted parallel to nephrostomy tract and directly into calix containing calculus (arrow). Guide wire is inserted past calculus into renal pelvis, as is 8-F catheter of Amplatz fascial dilator system. **(D)** Initial 12-F fascial dilator (D) of Amplatz fascial dilator set has been inserted until it is against calculus (arrow); 8-F catheter has been withdrawn. N = nephroscope. **(E)** Calculus (arrow) has been "pushed" by blunt end of dilator (D) along guide wire into renal pelvis; it was removed through nephroscope (N). (Reprinted, by permission, from Bush WH, Brannen GE: Parallel tract push: Adjuvant technique for percutaneous removal of renal calix calculi. *Am. J. Roentgenol.* 143:295–297, © 1984, American Roentgen Ray Society.)

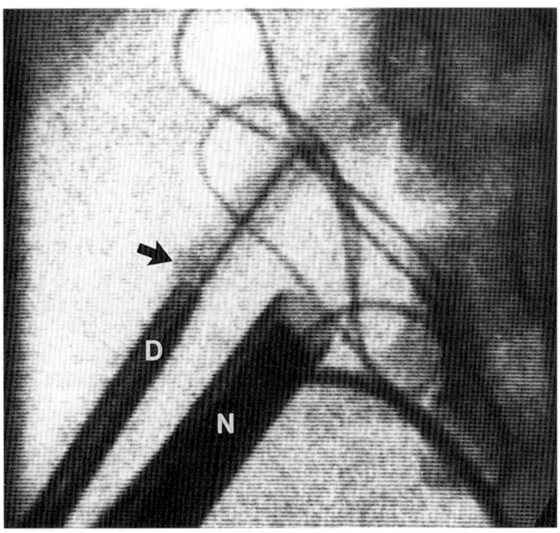

D

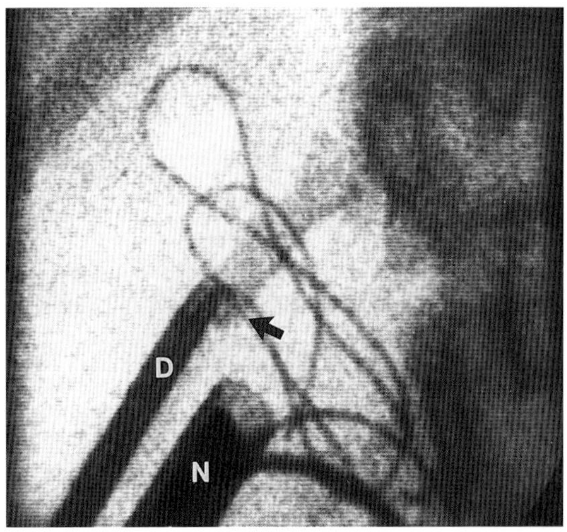

E

glass fiber bundles of the flexible system. The flexible nephroscope may be sterilized by gas or soaking; it may not be placed in the autoclave.

Results

Percutaneous removal of upper urinary tract calculi has been successful in over 90% of cases at large medical centers (Brannen, Bush 1985; Clayman, Castaneda-Zuniga 1984; Segura et al. 1986). Three hundred consecutive patients who underwent percutaneous lithotomy were compared with 100 consecutive patients who underwent surgical lithotomy; targeted upper urinary tract calculi were successfully removed from 97% of the percutaneous group (Brannen, Bush 1985). Removal was completed at the initial session in 243 (81%). In 36 patients (12%), stone removal required additional procedures through the existing nephrostomy tract under local anesthesia. Twenty-one patients (7%) required repeat nephroscopy under anesthesia. Targeted calculi were incompletely removed by percutaneous techniques in 9 patients (3%). However, only 1 patient required surgical lithotomy to remove a calculus impacted at the ureteropelvic junction. Eight additional patients remained asymptomatic with retained caliceal fragments. In the 100 surgical patients, targeted calculi were successfully removed from the upper portion of the urinary collecting system in 96. Four patients were asymptomatic with retained nonobstructing caliceal stone fragments. No patients required additional surgical procedures.

Need for perioperative blood transfusion was comparable in both the surgical and percutaneous groups. Postoperative fever, >38°C for 3 days, was considerably more common in the surgical group. There were no complications from extravasated stone fragments in either group. Contrast extravasation was identified at the conclusion of the percutaneous procedure in 31% of the patients, but extravasation was rarely seen by nephrostogram the day after the procedure. Five of the surgical patients had pneumothorax and responded promptly to aspiration or chest tube placement (Brannen, Bush 1985).

The anesthesia time and need for postoperative urinary drainage are similar for both groups. However, time of hospitalization and associated costs were significantly less for the percutaneous group ($p < 0.01$). Fewer narcotic pain medications were administered in the percutaneous group ($p < 0.01$) (Table 18–1) (Brannen, Bush 1985).

Patients in the percutaneous group returned to full activity an average of 2 (±0.16) weeks after stone removal. Less than 5% required more than 3 weeks before feeling completely recovered. Patients who previously had surgical lithotomy reported a postsurgical recovery period averaging 6 (±1.4) weeks ($p < 0.01$). No patient reported a surgical recovery period of less than 3 weeks (Brannen, Bush 1985).

Complications

Complications associated with percutaneous efforts to remove upper tract urinary calculi have been minimal, using surgical lithotomy as a standard for comparison (Brannen, Bush 1985; Dunnick et al. 1985). Percutaneous entry for nephrostomy tube placement has been associated with a 4% complication rate, including two deaths in a multicenter study (Stables 1982; Stables et al. 1978).

Urothelial Injury and Extravasation

Urothelial disruption is a common result of percutaneous entry and nephroscopic manipulation. In a series of 300 patients, 31% had extravasation of contrast from the collecting system at conclusion of the operative procedure, but it usually resolved in a day. Even major extravasation generally resolves within a few days with adequate nephrostomy drainage (Brannen, Bush 1985).

Disruptions of the urothelium may result in extrarenal fluid accumulations. Persistent retroperitoneal collections of urine or irrigant would likely be manageable by percutaneous drainage. Although increased risk of infectious complications may be expected with percutaneous removal of infected renal calculi, perinephric or retroperitoneal abscess or urinoma is possible but rare (even with infected calculi). The authors are aware of only one such abscess, and it resolved with percutaneous drainage. To continue stone removal in the presence of a large tear in the renal pelvis can be life-threatening. Extravasation of excessive irrigant may cause a fluid overload resulting in congestive heart failure, renal failure, electrolyte imbalances, hypothermia, mechanical effects of compression on major organs, and even death.

Intraperitoneal extravasation of irrigant is suspected if there is an expanding abdomen and drop in blood pressure. This happened in 2% of one series undergoing percutaneous stone removal. Further complications were avoided by termination of the procedure and proper placement of a nephrostomy tube. In addition, prompt placement of a peritoneal dialysis catheter allowed the removal of accumulated peritoneal fluid. The authors are aware of at least one death related to excessive extravasation of irrigant. Therefore, stone removal is terminated if large tears are present in the collecting system.

Manipulations of the nephroscope may result in tissue disruption and extravasation of stone fragments into the perirenal retroperitoneal tissue. In the authors' series of 300 patients, 8 patients with extravasation of stone fragments recovered without sequelae. This experience is confirmed in other centers (Kerlan et al. 1984; Pollack, Banner 1984).

Ureteral Injury

Extraluminal placement of ureteral instruments can occur. Optimally, the injury can be bridged using an internal double-J ureteral stent. Stent placement is often more easily achieved from the opposite direction; for example, if the injury occurred with retrograde ureteroscopy or manipulation, an antegrade approach via a nephrostomy may be successful. An internal ureteral stent left indwelling for 3 to 6 weeks minimizes the incidence of stricture formation. Ureteral avulsion may occur secondary to the extraction of ureteral calculi percutaneously. Methods of management include surgical reanastomosis and stent placement, nephrectomy, or permanent percutaneous nephrostomy. One reported case of ureteral ischemia following ureteroscopy required ureteral reimplantation with psoas hitch.

Excessive manipulation of the ureter or ureteropelvic junction may cause temporary obstruction. In 8 of 300 patients in the authors' series, persistent partial obstruction was recognized. Management consisted of placement of an internal double-J ureteral stent for 6 to 12 weeks.

If the patient requires removal of the nephrostomy tube while a ureteral stent is in place, a Foley catheter should be left in the bladder for 4–48 hr. This prevents reflux and possible pyelitis or nephrocutaneous fistula. Impacted ureteral stones removed by endoscopic or percutaneous methods require placement of an internal double-J ureteral stent for 6 to 12 weeks to prevent edema and stricture formation.

Bleeding

Some urinary tract bleeding occurs in all patients undergoing percutaneous procedures. Bleeding from the nephrostomy puncture site is usually controlled by tamponade with the dilators or nephroscope. A combination of irrigation through the nephroscope and suction through the sonotrode permits adequate vision despite persistent bleeding. If blood cannot be cleared sufficiently, the procedure must be terminated and reinitiated on another day.

Although nephrostomy tube placement generally provides adequate control, tamponade of the freshly dilated nephrostomy tract with an angioplasty balloon catheter is sometimes needed to control bleeding. Procedures requiring extensive manipulation of the rigid nephroscope are usually the cause of prolonged bleeding. Eight of the authors' 300 patients required blood transfusions, an incidence similar to that required for surgical lithotomy. None of the 300 required surgery for renal bleeding, but the authors know of at least 6 nephrectomies performed in association with efforts to control renal blood loss. Three of the authors' patients required transcatheter embolization of selected interlobar renal vessels (Fig. 18–11). Patients are cautioned to avoid prolonged motor vehicle travel or heavy lifting for 3 weeks to prevent delayed urinary bleeding. However, they may return to light activities as early as 2 weeks after percutaneous stone removal.

Retained Fragments

Removal of targeted calculi was achieved in 97% of the patients at Seattle's Virginia Mason Medical Center. This compares favorably with 96% complete stone removal experienced by 100 consecutive surgical patients. Eight patients remain asymptomatic with retained caliceal fragments, and 1 patient required surgical lithotomy for removal of a calculus impacted at the

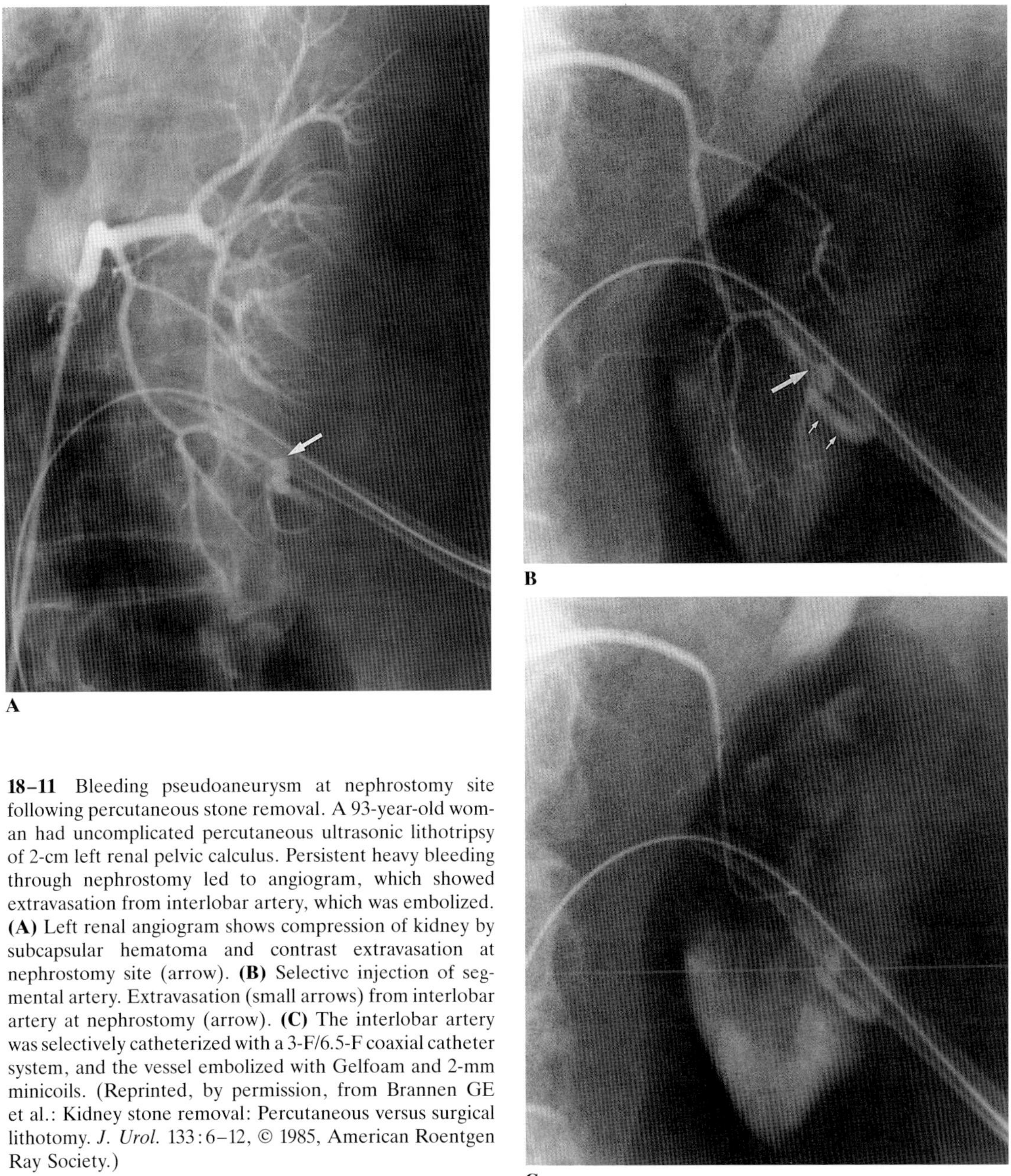

A

B

C

18–11 Bleeding pseudoaneurysm at nephrostomy site following percutaneous stone removal. A 93-year-old woman had uncomplicated percutaneous ultrasonic lithotripsy of 2-cm left renal pelvic calculus. Persistent heavy bleeding through nephrostomy led to angiogram, which showed extravasation from interlobar artery, which was embolized. **(A)** Left renal angiogram shows compression of kidney by subcapsular hematoma and contrast extravasation at nephrostomy site (arrow). **(B)** Selective injection of segmental artery. Extravasation (small arrows) from interlobar artery at nephrostomy (arrow). **(C)** The interlobar artery was selectively catheterized with a 3-F/6.5-F coaxial catheter system, and the vessel embolized with Gelfoam and 2-mm minicoils. (Reprinted, by permission, from Brannen GE et al.: Kidney stone removal: Percutaneous versus surgical lithotomy. *J. Urol.* 133:6–12, © 1985, American Roentgen Ray Society.)

ureteropelvic junction. However, only 81% of the patients undergoing percutaneous removal had fragments removed at the initial session; additional procedures in radiology or repeat nephroscopy under anesthesia were successful in 16%.

Infection and Pain

Sepsis has been occasionally associated with percutaneous removal of infected stones. A single case of perinephric or retroperitoneal abscess has been reported. Perioperative fever occurred in 7%, which compares favorably with the 26% incidence in 100 surgical lithotomy patients at Virginia Mason Medical Center. Antibiotic prophylaxis is administered perioperatively to all patients undergoing percutaneous lithotomy.

Less narcotic pain medication is required than with surgical lithotomy. Because postoperative discomfort is associated with twelfth-nerve irritation, it is advisable to make the percutaneous entry well below the twelfth rib. In addition, the entry tract from the renal cortex to the skin is infiltrated with 0.25% Marcaine at the termination of the procedure. Long-term flank discomfort has rarely been observed, whereas 21% of surgical lithotomy patients reported pain, bulging, or numbness of the flank 6 months following their surgery (Brannen et al. 1985).

Renal Injury

Kidney function was evaluated in 82 patients 3½ years after percutaneous stone removal. Studies using ^{131}I Hippuran clearance and ^{99m}technetium pertechnetate perfusion indicated no measurable loss of function. The incidence of hypertension, stone recurrence, and urinary infection was not increased over patients undergoing conventional surgical lithotomy (Marberger et al. 1985).

Bowel Injury

Perforation of the colon or duodenum has been reported in at least five cases (LeRoy et al. 1985). In the authors' only case (Fig. 18–12), urinary drainage was maintained by retrograde insertion of a JJ ureteral stent. The nephrostomy tube was then cautiously removed from the renal pelvis and permitted to remain as a drain next to the colon (Fig. 18–12B). Delayed removal (3–5 days) of the nephrostomy tube permitted resolution of the colon perforation without intervention or sequelae. The Hawkins-Hunter method of retrograde placement of a guide wire has been associated with a liver edge perforation. This was observed without sequelae. In cases of anatomic concern, a computed tomography (CT) scan of the abdomen may aid in avoiding initial aberrant tube placement.

Pleural Injury

Pleural injuries including pneumothorax, hydrothorax, and hemothorax seem to be associated exclusively with percutaneous entry above the twelfth rib. Using the retrograde transureteral method of access described by Hawkins and Hunter, 6 of 135 patients suffered pneumothorax. However, only 3 required treatment. Pneumothorax has not been observed at Virginia Mason Medical Center, where the authors use a standard subcostal approach. Percutaneous removal of renal calculi has been reported (Forsythe, Fuchs 1987; Young et al. 1985) using a supratwelfth rib approach; thoracic complications have been easily managed, although some require chest tube drainage. Small effusions are common; pneumothorax requiring a

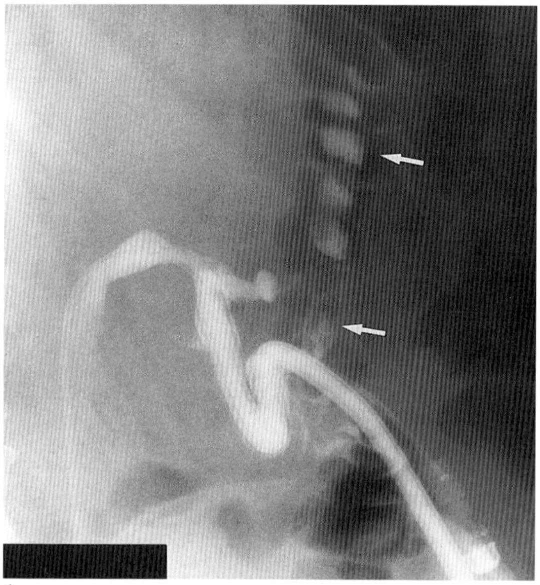

A

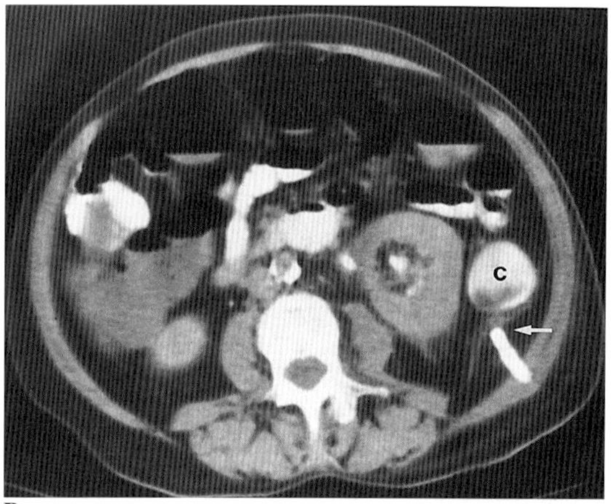

B

18–12 Colon perforation during percutaneous nephrostomy for stone removal. **(A)** Nephrostogram obtained on postprocedure day 1 shows nephrostomy tube in renal collecting system, but contrast along nephrostomy tract enters descending colon (arrows). A retrograde ureteral stent was placed to ensure kidney drainage; nephrostomy tube was withdrawn so that tip was out of the kidney and adjacent to colon perforation, so it could act as a drain (see **B**). **(B)** Transverse abdominal CT scan (oral and intravenous contrast) at kidney level shows nephrostomy tube tip (arrow) at site of colon perforation. Tube was left in place for 3 days and then gradually removed over 2 days; the fistula closed, and patient recovered without complication. C = opacified descending colon. (Reprinted, by permission, from Bush WH: Percutaneous stone therapy. *In* Putman CE, Ravin CE (eds.): *Textbook of Diagnostic Imaging,* pp. 1269–1279. © 1988 by W. B. Saunders Co., Philadelphia.)

Table 18–1 Comparison of Percutaneous Lithotripsy and Surgical Lithotomy

	PL (±S.E.M.[a])	SL (±S.E.M.)	P Value
Procedure time	155 ± 4 min	193 ± 8 min	>0.05
Fluoroscopy time	28 ± 1.5 min	–	–
Urinary drainage[b]	6.5 ± 0.48 days	7.7 ± 0.31 days	>0.05
Narcotic medications[c]	9.9 ± 0.7	16.8 ± 0.8	<0.01
Hospital days	5.7 ± 0.28 days	8.4 ± 0.46 days	<0.01
Associated costs[d]	$7,203 ± $255	$8,849 ± $660	<0.01

Note: PL = percutaneous lithotripsy; SL = surgical lithotomy.
[a] Standard error of the mean.
[b] Postoperative urinary drainage using nephrostomy tubes for percutaneous ultrasonic lithotripsy and Penrose drains for surgical lithotomy.
[c] Number of times narcotic medications administered during postoperative days 1 through 5.
[d] 1983 dollars.

chest tube is uncommon. In general, percutaneous entry should be guided below the twelfth rib except in selected circumstances.

Risk to Personnel

Audiograms of X-ray personnel remained unchanged from baseline (Marberger 1985). Radiation doses to patient, surgeon, and operating room personnel remain acceptable (Bush, Brannen, Gibbons et al. 1984; Bush, Jones et al. 1985).

Percutaneous Procedures and Extracorporeal Shock Wave Lithotripsy

The introduction of extracorporeal shock wave lithotripsy (ESWL) has demanded a reassessment of the role of percutaneous stone removal. ESWL has replaced percutaneous techniques for many uncomplicated stones (Bush et al. 1986). However, branched renal calculi with large stone bulk are still best managed by percutaneous techniques (Kahnoski et al. 1986; Schulze et al. 1986; Tegtmeyer et al. 1986). When branched calculi have large central pelvic stone bulk and branched portions located in calices, percutaneous ultrasonic lithotripsy is used for debulking the pelvic portion prior to ESWL of the caliceal components. The nephrostomy tube is left in position to aid in evacuation of stone material following ESWL. Further efforts to evacuate stone material may be carried out using Renacidin irrigation.

A combined percutaneous and ESWL approach to branched and staghorn calculi has been associated with an 85% stone-free status following treatment. Calculi located in a calix with a stenotic infundibulum require percutaneous removal with simultaneous dilation of the infundibulum (Brannen et al. 1986).

Renal calculi found in association with ureteropelvic junction (UPJ) obstruction are best removed percutaneously to ensure proper evacuation of fragments and possible endoscopic reconstruction of the UPJ obstruction (Brannen, Bush 1987). Relatively lucent renal calculi at times cannot be identified dependably on fluoroscopy to permit fragmentation by ESWL; consequently, percutaneous management is generally favored.

Percutaneous stone removal will continue to play an essential role in the management of properly selected cases of upper urinary tract calculi.

References

Alken P, Hutschenreiter B, Gunther R, Marberger M: Percutaneous stone manipulation. *J. Urol.* 125: 463–466, 1981.

Alken P: Percutaneous ultrasonic destruction of renal calculi. *Urol. Clin. North Am.* 9:145–150, 1982.

Brannen GE, Bush WH: Complications and morbidity of endourology. *AUA Update Series* 3:1–8, 1985.

Brannen GE, Bush WH: Percutaneous ultrasonic versus surgical removal of kidney stones. *Surg. Gynecol. Obstet.* 161:473–478, 1985.

Brannen GE, Bush WH, Correa RJ, Gibbons RP, Elder JS: Kidney stone removal: Percutaneous versus surgical lithotomy. *J. Urol.* 133:6–12, 1985.

Brannen GE, Bush WH, Lewis GP: Caliceal calculi. *J. Urol.* 135:1142–1145, 1986.

Brannen GE, Bush WH, Lewis GP: Endopyelotomy for primary repair of ureteropelvic junction obstruction. *J. Urol.* 139:29–32, 1988.

Burnett LL, Correa RJ, Bush WH: A new method for percutaneous nephrostomy. *Radiology* 120:557–561, 1976.

Bush WH, Brannen GE: Parallel-tract push: Adjuvant technique for percutaneous removal of renal calix calculi. *Am. J. Roentgenol.* 143:295–297, 1984.

Bush WH, Brannen GE: Percutaneous removal of caliceal calculi. *Am. J. Roentgenol.* 144:139–142, 1985.

Bush WH, Brannen GE, Burnett LL, Lewis GP: Access technique for successful percutaneous nephrostolithotomy. *Appl. Radiol.* 14:86–92, 1985.

Bush WH, Brannen GE, Burnett LL, Wales LR: Ultrasonic renal lithotripsy: Single-stage percutaneous technique and adjuvant radiologic procedures. *Radiology* 152:387, 1984.

Bush WH, Brannen GE, Gibbons RP, Correa RJ, Elder JS: Radiation exposure to patient and urologist during percutaneous nephrostolithotomy. *J. Urol.* 132: 1198–1152, 1984.

Bush WH, Crane RE, Brannen GE: Steerable loop snare for percutaneous retrieval of renal calix calculi. *Am. J. Roentgenol.* 142:367–368, 1984.

Bush WH, Gibbons RP, Lewis GP, Brannen GE: Impact of extracorporeal shock wave lithotripsy on percutaneous stone procedures. *Am. J. Roentgenol.* 147:89–98, 1986.

Bush WH, Jones D, Brannen GE: Radiation dose to personnel during percutaneous renal calculus removal. *Am. J. Roentgenol.* 145:1261–1264, 1985.

Clayman RV, Castaneda-Zuniga W: Nephrolithotomy: Percutaneous removal of renal calculi. *Urol. Radiol.* 6(2):113–123, 1984.

Clayman RV, Surya V, Miller RP: Percutaneous Nephrolithotomy: An approach to branched and staghorn renal calculi. *J.A.M.A.* 250:73–76, 1983.

Clayman RV, Vilanur S, Miller RP, et al.: Percutaneous nephrolithotomy: Extraction of renal and ureteral calculi from 100 patients. *J. Urol.* 132:868–871, 1984.

Dretler SP, Watson G, Parrish JA, Murray S: Pulsed dye laser fragmentation of ureteral calculi: Initial clinical experience. *J. Urol.* 137:386–389, 1987.

Dunnick NR, Carson CC, Braun SD, Miller GA, Cohan R, Degesys GE, Illescas FF, Newman GE, Weinerth JL: Complications of percutaneous nephrostolithotomy. *Radiology* 157:51–55, 1985.

Finlayson B: Retrograde nephrostomy and percutaneous stone removal. Paper presented at Third World Congress on Endourology, New York, NY, Sept. 20–22, 1985.

Forsythe MJ, Fuchs EF: The supracostal approach for percutaneous nephrostolithotomy. *J. Urol.* 137: 197–198, 1987.

Goodwin WE, Casey EC, Wolf W: Percutaneous trochar (needle) nephrostomy in hydronephrosis. *J.A.M.A.* 157:891–894, 1955.

Kahnoski RJ. Lingeman JE, Loury TA, Steele RE, Mosbaugh PG: Combined percutaneous and extracorporeal shock wave lithotripsy for staghorn calculi: Alternative to anatrophic nephrolithotomy. *J. Urol.* 135(4): 679–681, 1986.

Kaye KW, Goldberg ME: Applied anatomy of the kidney and ureter. *Urol. Clin. North Am.* 9:3–8, 1982.

Kerlan RK, Kahn RI, Ring EJ: Percutaneous renal and ureteral stone removal. *Urol. Radiol.* 113:123, 1984.

Lange P, Reddy P, Clayman R, et al.: Percutaneous removal of renal calyceal stones: Techniques and results. Paper presented at American Urological Association Annual Meeting, New Orleans, LA, May 10, 1984.

LeRoy AJ, Williams HJ, Bender CE, Segura JW, Patterson DE, Benson RC: Colon perforation following percutaneous nephrostomy and stone removal. *Radiology* 155:83–85, 1985.

Marberger M, Stack W, Hruby W: Percutaneous lithalopaxy of renal calculi with ultrasound. *Eur. Urol.* 8:236–240, 1982.

Marberger M, Stack W, Hruby W, Kroiss A: Late sequelae of ultrasonic lithotripsy. *J. Urol.* 133(2):170–173, 1985.

Miller RA, Wickham JEA: Percutaneous nephrolithotomy: Advances in equipment and endoscopic techniques. *Urology* 23:2–6, 1984.

Pollack HM, Banner MD: Percutaneous extraction of upper urinary tract calculi. *Urol. Radiol.* 6(2):124–137, 1984.

Preminger GM, Clayman RV, Hardeman SW, Franklin J, Curry T, Peters PC: Percutaneous nephrostolithotomy versus open surgery for renal calculi. *J.A.M.A.* 8:1054–1058, 1985.

Raney AM, Handler J: Electrohydraulic nephrolithotripsy. *Urology* 6:439–442, 1975.

Schulze H, Hertle L, Graff J, Funke J, Senge T: Combined treatment of branched calculi by percutaneous nephrolithotomy and extracorporeal shock wave lithotripsy. *J. Urol.* 135(6):1138–1141, 1986.

Segura JW, Patterson DE, LeRoy AJ, May GR, Smith LH: Percutaneous lithotripsy. *J. Urol.* 130:1051–1054, 1983.

Segura JW, Patterson DE, LeRoy AJ, Williams HJ, Jr., Barrett DM, Benson RC, Jr., May GR, Bender CE: Percutaneous removal of kidney stones: Review of 1,000 cases. *J. Urol.* 134:1077–1081, 1986.

Stables D: Percutaneous nephrostomy: Techniques, indications and results. *Urol. Clin. North Am.* 9:15–20, 1982.

Stables DP, Ginsberg NJ, Johnson ML: Percutaneous nephrostomy: A series and review of the literature. *Am. J. Roentgenol.* 130:75–82, 1978.

Tegtmeyer CJ, Kellum CD, Jenkins A, Gillenwater JY, Way WG, Barr J, Piros G, Springer R, Lippert MC, Wyker AW: Extracorporeal shock wave lithotripsy: Interventional radiologic solutions to associated problems. *Radiology* 161:587–592, 1986.

Wickham JEA, Kellett MJ, Miller RA: Elective percutaneous nephrolithotomy in 50 patients: An analysis of this technique, results, and complications. *J. Urol.* 129:904–906, 1983.

Young AT, Hunter DW, Castaneda-Zuniga WR, Hulbert JC, Lange P, Reddy P, Mercado S, Amplatz K: Percutaneous extraction of urinary calculi: Use of the intercostal approach. *Radiology* 154:633–638, 1985.

Suggested Reading

Bagley DH, Huffman JL, Lyon ES: *Urologic Endoscopy: A Manual and Atlas.* Boston, 1985.

Brannen GE: Endourology in perspective. *Urology* 28(3):161–172, Sept. 1986.

Bush WH: Percutaneous stone therapy. *In* Putman CE, Ravin CE (eds.): *Textbook of Diagnostic Imaging.* Philadelphia, W. B. Saunders Co., 1988, pp. 1269–1279.

Clayman RV, Castaneda-Zuniga WR: *Techniques in Endourology: A Guide to Percutaneous Removal of Renal and Ureteral Calculi.* Minneapolis, Univ. of Minn. Press, 1984.

Wickham JEA, Miller RA: *Percutaneous Renal Surgery.* New York, Churchill-Livingstone, 1983.

CHAPTER

19

Extracorporeal Shock Wave Lithotripsy for Renal and Ureteral Calculi

Robert P. Gibbons

In the usual patient population, 80% of symptomatic kidney stones will pass spontaneously; however, stones larger than 8 mm in diameter have less than a 50% chance of passing without intervention (Sandegard 1956; Wax, Frank 1965). Extracorporeal shock wave lithotripsy (ESWL®)[a], a noninvasive technique that uses high-energy pressure waves generated outside the body to pulverize stones, has become the method of choice for treating most of these patients. Approximately 90% can be treated with ESWL alone, or with ESWL combined with adjuvant percutaneous procedures with or without chemolysis. Most stones impacted in the ureter, with the exception of cystine stones, can be effectively fragmented with the pulsed dye laser delivered through a ureteroscope.

The rapid technical advances and significant changes in the management of patients with renal calculi will likely continue in the future, and it is clear that our traditional surgical operations will never again be common procedures.

Background

A shock wave is a high-energy pressure wave generated whenever the speed of an object in a medium (e.g., air or water) exceeds the speed of sound in that medium. The sonic boom generated by aircraft flying at supersonic speeds is a type of shock wave. In the lithotripter, a bubble of air is formed when water is vaporized by an electrode; the air expands faster than the speed of sound in water, creating a shock wave in the water bath. These shock waves generate a pressure of rapid onset and are unlike ultrasonic waves that have a specific frequency and are sinusoidal (Fig. 19–1). Shock (pressure) waves, like acoustical waves, can be focused by a reflector. They have little energy when randomly dispersed, but when focused to converge simultaneously at a specific point, can generate pressure up to 1,000 bar (14,700 psi). Stone disintegration is based on several effects that may occur individually or in combination. The stone will fragment by passage of the shock wave front if the pressure amplitude of the shock wave as it enters the stone is greater than the short-term pressure resistance of the stone. When the pressure wave exits the stone to surrounding higher impedance fluids, it is reflected back into the stone, causing increased destructive tensile stresses (Fig. 19–2). When repeated several hundred times, the passage of these to-and-fro pressure forces fractures and pulverizes the stone.

The first shock wave lithotripter was manufactured in West Germany by the Dornier Aircraft Company, the same company that made the world's largest seaplane in 1928. Their involve-

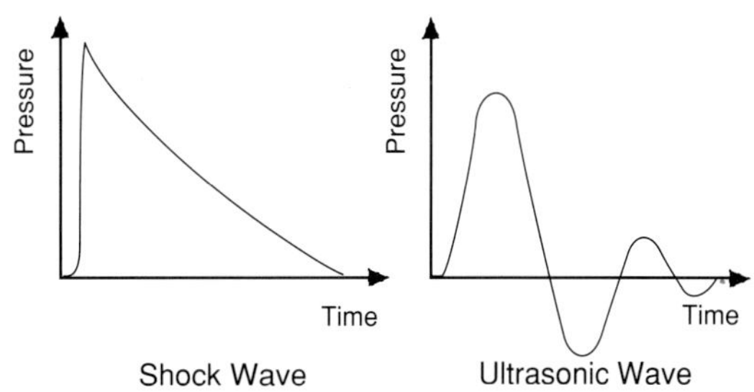

19–1 Graphs illustrating pressure curves for shock wave (left curve) and ultrasonic wave (right). Shock wave has high initial peak pressure with gradual decrease, whereas ultrasonic wave is a decreasing sinusoidal wave.

[a] ESWL is a registered trademark of Dornier Medical Systems, Marietta, GA.

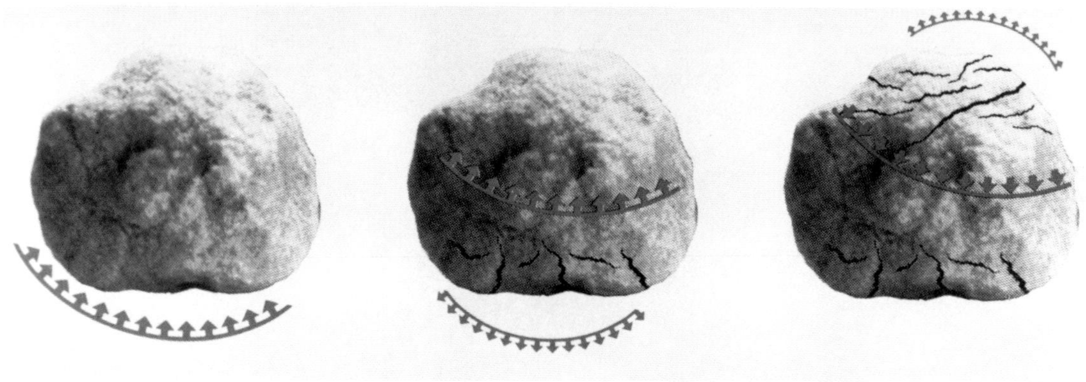

19–2 Stone disintegration by shock waves. When entering shock wave pressure amplitude exceeds tensile strength of the stone, fragmentation is initiated. A reversed tensile wave occurs at rear side of stone by reflection of exiting shock wave at interface between stone and fluid. Repetition of this phenomenon creates ultimate stone fragmentation. (Reproduced, by permission, from "Dornier Kidney Lithotripter," Dornier Medical Systems, Inc., Marietta, GA.)

ment in development of the lithotripter is an interesting combination of observation and perseverance. Dornier pilots observed pitting of aircraft wings and an occasional crack in a dial in the cockpit of planes when they flew at supersonic speeds through rainstorms (a consequence of randomly focused shock waves). The company, with government support, contacted universities in Germany that might be interested in pursuing the possible use of shock waves in medicine. Urology professor Egbert Schmiedt at the Ludwig Maximilian University in Munich and his resident, Christian Chaussy, took on the assignment in 1975. Their research with Dornier scientists encompassed studies of the physical properties of shock waves, the pressures associated with different voltages, and the effect of the waves on tissues of experimental animals (Chaussy et al. 1982).

Living bone is relatively unaffected by shock wave energy because of its resiliency, although bone does constitute acoustical interfaces and interferes with passage of the shock waves. Soft tissues, because of their similarity to water, sustain little effect. Blood cells *in vitro* are susceptible to hemolysis, but this has not proved a problem *in vivo* because the cells are constantly circulating and few are in the second focal point at any one time. Lung tissue, because of its many air-water interfaces, is highly susceptible to shock wave trauma.

The first human was treated in Germany with extracorporeal shock wave lithotripsy in 1980 (Chaussy et al. 1980). The Dornier HM-3 shock wave lithotripter was approved by the U.S. Food and Drug Administration in December 1984; worldwide, over 500,000 patients have been treated with ESWL. Several other manufacturers have developed shock wave lithotripters that vary in how the stone is imaged, how the shock wave is generated, how coupling to the patient and focusing occur, and other technical factors. Experience to date is limited with these models (Fuchs, Chaussy 1987).

ESWL Treatment

The Dornier HM-3 lithotripter consists of a large tub of warmed water with the underwater electrode (spark plug) in an ellipsoidal reflector at the base of the tub (Fig. 19–3). The water in the tub is degassed and demineralized. The patient is seated on a hydraulically driven support gantry capable of movement in three directions. The patient is positioned in the water so that the kidney stone is precisely at the focus of maximum energy. This precision is accomplished through the use of two fixed fluoroscopic X-ray units that create a three-dimensional X-ray system. Inflatable balloons over the underwater X-ray tubes displace the water and enhance the image. The superiorly located image intensifiers are positioned against the abdomen.

An 18-kV (voltage can be increased to 24 kV) electrical discharge across the spark gap of the electrode in the base of the ellipsoid creates the shock waves. The release of the electrical discharge is triggered by the r-wave peak of the electrocardiogram, which places the discharge in the cycle of the heart when it cannot be electrically

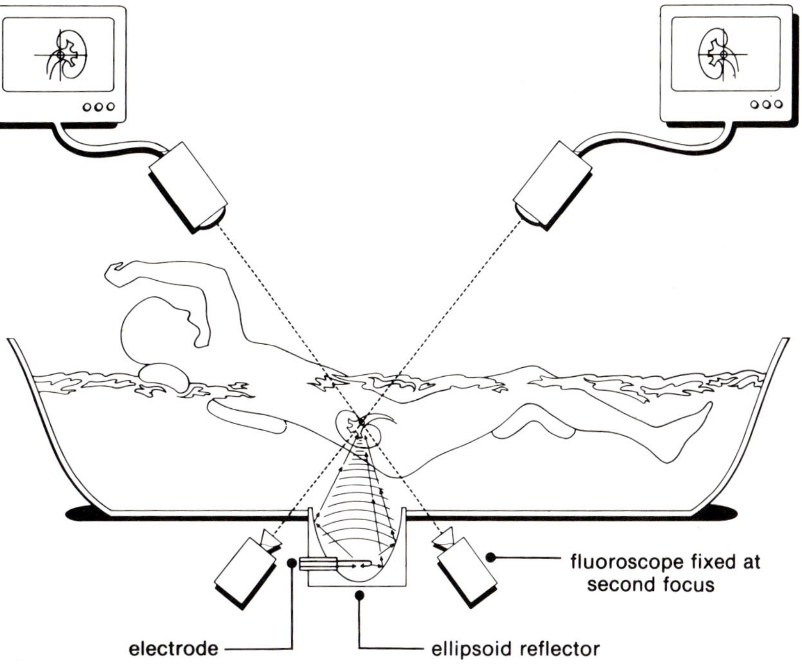

19–3 Illustration of Dornier HM-3 lithotripter with patient in water bath. Calculus is positioned at intersection of biplane fluoroscopes, which also denotes the point of maximal shock wave focus from underwater ellipsoidal reflector. Shock waves are generated at base of the ellipsoid reflector by the electrode.

stimulated. The spark gap of the electrode is also surrounded by a "Faraday cage", preventing electrical transmission through the water to the patient. The electrical discharge or spark vaporizes a small volume of water, and the rapid creation of the small bubble of air creates the shock wave, which is focused by the ellipsoidal reflector to converge at the second focal point where the kidney stone is fluoroscopically located. The stone will fragment, so long as the pressure wave has more energy than the tensile strength of the stone, which is the situation 99% of the time.

Water and living tissue have about the same composition, and the shock wave crosses the interface between the bath water and living tissue with little loss of energy.

Treatment consists of about 1,600 shocks average (range 300–2,400), after which the stone is reduced to 1- to 2-mm fragments that pass spontaneously down the ureter, usually within 90 days (Fig. 19–4). The shocks are generally given in series of 100–150 followed by fluoroscopic verification that the stone or large particles are in the "second focus".

The patient must remain immobile, and since after repeated shocks there is a prominent aching discomfort in the renal area, anesthesia is used. Anesthesia options include epidural, spinal, local, general, and high-frequency jet ventilation. With the patient immersed in water, the most common associated side effect during anesthesia is hypotension, occurring during 33% of anesthetic treatments (London et al. 1986). However, this has not been a significant clinical problem.

The newer lithotripter models use either a different energy source or a larger diameter ellipsoid so that the shock waves enter the body through a wider diameter. With these units, anesthesia will not always be required for ESWL, unless adjuvant manipulations are performed.

Patients who have an uneventful ESWL treatment are usually seen in 2 to 3 weeks, and a follow-up plain film is taken at that time to assess the passage of fragments. If the patient has more than the usual degree of pain immediately after ESWL, renal ultrasonography is performed to look for obstruction or evidence of perirenal urine or blood.

A renal function study (e.g., excretory urogram) should be performed at 3 months if residual fragments remain, since "silent" obstruction can result in loss of kidney function. Patients are informed of this possibility and of their responsibility for sharing in this follow-up.

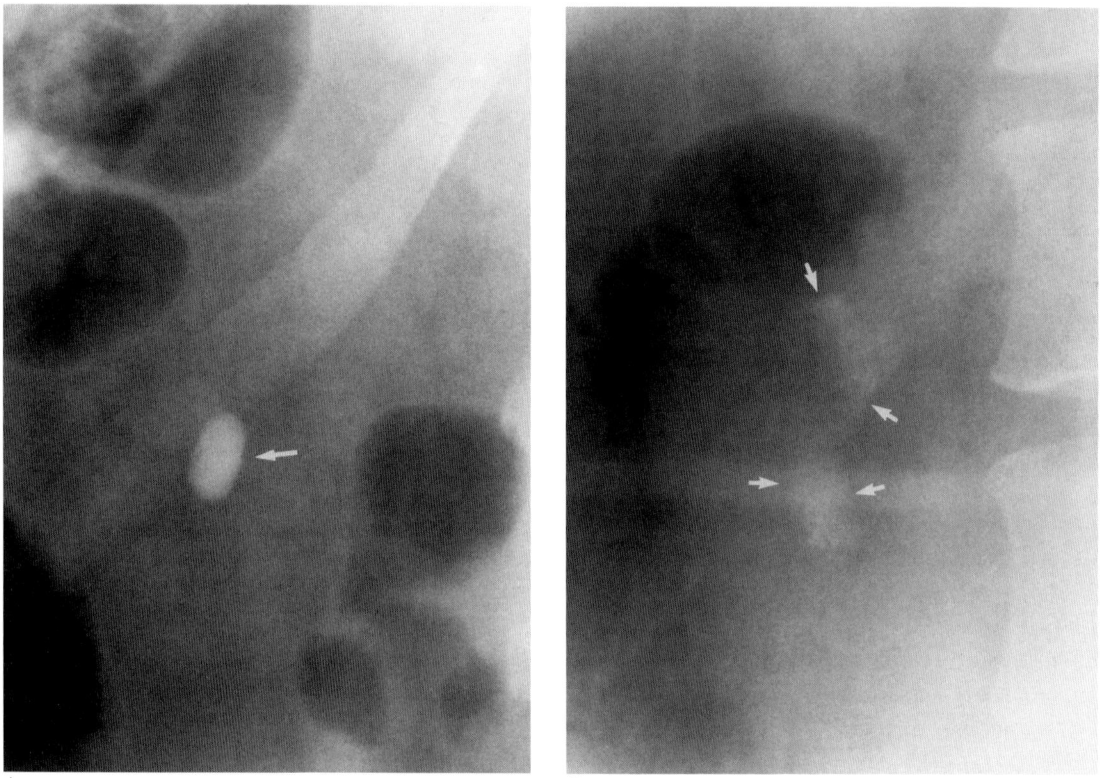

A

B

19–4 ESWL treatment of right renal pelvic calculus. **(A)** A 10- × 15-mm calculus (arrow) in lower right kidney, before ESWL. **(B)** In-bath radiograph after 800 shocks, showing excellent fragmentation of calculus with fine calculus debris filling lower infundibulum and calices (arrows).

Indications

Factors involved in the selection of ESWL for treatment include stone size, position, composition, and patient characteristics. The greater the level of patient activity and ability to maintain hydration, the more likely that the fragments will pass. Stones in the renal pelvis surrounded by urine will fragment more readily than a stone impacted in the ureter. Obstruction of the collecting system distal to the stone must be corrected prior to ESWL.

Calcium oxalate dihydrate, struvite, apatite, or uric acid stones disintegrate into small fragments more readily than do calcium oxalate monohydrate or pure calcium phosphate stones. Cystine stones disintegrate poorly and rarely into fragments less than 5 mm.

Ureteral stones above the bony pelvis can be treated *in situ* using ESWL; overall success is approximately 66%. If the ureteral stone can be pushed up into the renal pelvis or bypassed by a ureteral catheter or stent, success can approach 95% (Liong, Clayman 1987). Success of fragmentation with ureteral calculi is not always immediately apparent radiographically, because the pieces often remain together, unlike stones in the renal pelvis where the fragments can separate.

Stones in the distal ureter overlying the bony pelvis require that the patient be prone so that the shock wave can reach the stone without first going through the bony pelvis. Alternate positioning techniques for distal ureteral calculi or stones in pelvic kidneys have been described to allow the shock wave to pass through the sacrosciatic notch (Bush, Brannen 1987; Miller et al. 1987).

Some obese patients and others with congenital kidney variations have stones located in areas that cannot be positioned precisely in the shock wave focal point, but this does not preclude ESWL treatment. These stones can often be fragmented using the extended blast path field technique (Whelan, Finlayson 1987). The calculus receives a substantial pressure surge if located in the blast path, which extends 10 cm above and 10 cm below the converging shock wave focal point. An isobar pattern of energy exists in this area, with pressures capable of fragmentation of many stones, and has resulted in the successful treatment of urinary calculi that could not be directly placed into the shock wave focus.

Adjuvant Procedures

Stone burden (sum of the two largest diameters of the calculi), stone composition, stone location, and patient selection determine whether ESWL should be used alone or with an adjuvant procedure. Stone burden takes into account the volume of all calculi present in patients with multiple stones. Riehle et al. (1986) reported that 87% of patients were stone-free at 3 months following ESWL for solitary stones 2 cm or less in diameter (average stone burden 1.2 cm); however, the success rate was only 65% 3 months following ESWL monotherapy in patients with an average stone burden of 2.2 cm.

Newman found a direct relationship between the morbidity of ESWL monotherapy and stone size and an inverse relationship between stone size and ultimate result (in *Report of American Urological Association* 1986). Although 83% of patients with a stone burden between 2.1 and 3 cm had a "successful" result, only 39% were rendered stone-free. By comparison, 90% of patients with similar stone burdens treated by percutaneous nephrostolithotomy were stone-free at follow-up. Seventy-five percent of patients who had stone burdens greater than 3 cm required multiple treatments and ancillary procedures during the course of ESWL therapy; the majority of these patients returned with significant fragments 3 months following treatment.

Percutaneous Nephrostolithotomy

ESWL and percutaneous nephrostolithotomy are complementary technologies. Patients with stone burden greater than 2.5 cm or cystine stones are best treated using percutaneous surgery followed by ESWL. The majority of the stone can be percutaneously "debulked" followed by ESWL 2 to 3 days later while the nephrostomy tube is still in place. This assures adequate drainage and allows subsequent access if any fragments remain. It also allows chemolysis to be performed, which is recommended following treatment of any staghorn or partial staghorn calculus (Nemoy, Stamey 1971). Effective drainage also avoids the possibility of obstructive urosepsis. It is most important to eliminate all fragments before patients leave the hospital. This often requires more than one endoscopic or ESWL treatment.

Ureteral Catheter

Ureteral catheters are useful for localizing faint or small stones fluoroscopically in large patients. Radiopaque contrast media injected through the catheter can help localize radiolucent calculi. Ureteral catheters can also be used to manipulate ureteral stones back into the renal pelvis where fragmentation can be more successful. Spiral tip, flexible tip, or balloon occlusion catheters are available. They can be used to mechanically manipulate the stone; saline, or a combination of local anesthetic and saline, can be injected through the catheter to dislodge the stone back into the renal pelvis.

Ureteral Stents

Double-J silicone rubber ureteral stents can be passed following manipulation of a symptomatic ureteral calculus to keep the kidney decompressed until elective ESWL can be performed. They are also used when total stone burdens are greater than 1.5 cm, to reduce the incidence of renal colic or obstructive urosepsis as the fragments pass. These stents appear to produce peristaltic fatigue, resulting in dilation of the ureter, so that the fragments actually pass between the outer wall of the stent and the dilated ureter. Fragments as large as 5 mm pass painlessly around an indwelling stent.

The stents are usually left in place several weeks to 2 months and can be easily removed in the office if a 3–0 Prolene suture is attached to the distal end of the stent at the time it is placed and allowed to exit the urethral meatus. Intercourse is not impeded, and a higher incidence of urinary tract infection has not been associated with the procedure.

Occasionally, the stent irritates the bladder trigone in younger patients; this can be minimized by excising any excessive tubing lying within the bladder. Again, a suture attached to the lower end of the stent will allow its easy retrieval should upward migration occur.

Chemolysis

Because pure uric acid calculi are radiolucent, it is difficult to tell when adequate fragmentation has occurred. However, even partial fragmentation greatly increases the surface area of these stones, making them more amenable to oral alkalinization. Cystine calculi are best managed by primary percutaneous nephrostolithotomy; dissolution of residual fragments can be enhanced by the proper selection of solvents (Schmeller et al. 1984). Struvite stones in kidneys treated with combined percutaneous nephrostolithotomy and ESWL receive posttreatment intrarenal irrigation with 10% Renacidin.

Antibiotics

Urinary tract infections are treated with appropriate antibiotics beginning 24 hours before ESWL and continuing until the fragments have passed. These patients are also treated with a ureteral stent to reduce the possibility of post ESWL obstructive urosepsis. Approximately 5% of patients will develop urinary tract infection following ESWL; therefore, at Seattle's Virginia Mason Medical Center, prophylactic antibiotics are given patients for 5 days after ESWL treatment.

Treating Ureteral Stones

Laser photo-fragmentation lithotripsy is a valuable adjunct to ureteroscopy in the management of impacted ureteral stones (Dretler et al. 1987). The pulsed tunable dye laser generates laser energy in 1-μsec pulses at a wave length of 504 nm. The energy is selectively absorbed by the calculus but not by the surrounding tissue.

A small rigid or flexible diagnostic ureteroscope is placed to the impacted stone, through which the small (250 μ) flexible laser fiber is passed to touch the stone. Ten bursts/sec (10 Hz) of laser energy at 40–60 mJ/pulse are directed at the calculus until fragmentation occurs. The energy generated has been sufficient to fragment all except cystine stones.

In this author and colleagues' initial experience with the pulsed dye laser, 14 of 17 patients with impacted ureteral stones were successfully treated with laser alone. All patients were stone-free by 6 weeks; 12 of the 14 patients were treated as outpatients. An additional patient had the stone fragmented to sizes that could then be pushed back into the kidney and treated by ESWL, for an overall success rate of 88%. All patients had ureteral stents placed at the end of the procedure, which remained in place 4 to 60 days (average 18 days). Five patients sustained ureteral injury from the ureteroscopy (4 mucosal tears and 1 perforation), managed with indwelling double-J silicone rubber stents. No patient had tissue injury from the laser itself.

The technique is currently limited by the size and optics of available ureteroscopes, and it is ineffective with cystine stones.

Contraindications

Absolute contraindications to ESWL include obstructions of the urinary tract distal to the stone, a nonfunctioning kidney, and pregnancy.

Most obstructions that block passage of stone particles occur in the ureter and can be circumvented with the passage of a stent at the time of ESWL. If a stone is present in a dilated calix, significant infundibular stenosis is likely present. However, if delayed IVP films demonstrate ultimate draining of the calix, stone fragments will often pass satisfactorily. If collecting system obstructions cannot be corrected endourologically, open surgery is indicated as primary treatment for both the stone and correction of the obstruction.

Pregnancy is a contraindication because of the unknown effects of shock waves on the developing fetus and also because of the radiation associated with fluoroscopy.

Patients treated in the Dornier HM-3 lithotripter must weigh less than 135 kg (297 lbs) to avoid damage to the support gantry.

Relative Contraindications

Bleeding disorders need to be corrected prior to ESWL. Patients on anticoagulation for medical reasons can be managed as if they were undergoing an open surgical procedure. Aspirin or dipyridamole should be discontinued 1 week prior to therapy.

Children have tolerated ESWL quite well. If the child is less than 4 feet tall, modifications are necessary to support the child's back and protect the lungs. This can be done using plywood and lead or Styrofoam adapters to the Dornier gantry. There are no available data regarding possible damage to the epiphyses from repeated shocks or whether shock waves will impair renal growth.

Patients with pacemakers have been successfully treated. However, preoperative evaluation by a cardiologist is recommended so that a temporary transvenous pacemaker can be provided if the patient's pacemaker malfunctions. In an analysis of 22 different pacemaker pulse generators placed 5 cm lateral to the focal point of the Dornier ipter and subjected to synchronous and asynchronous shock waves, none were damaged or spuriously reprogrammed (Abber et al. 1987).

Results

At the Virginia Mason Medical Center, 1,977 patients with stones of all sizes, locations, and compositions have been treated since 1985. Three-month follow-up is available on 1,099 patients, and 70% are stone-free on abdominal radiograph. Eighty-two percent of patients with stones less than 2 cm in diameter located within the kidney were stone-free at 3 months, compared to 70% of patients with stones in a similar location but larger than 2 cm.

Average age was 48 years (range, 5–97 years), and the average number of shock waves per patient was 1,591. Multiple stones were present in 809 patients, and 287 patients had bilateral stones. A total of 3,638 stones were treated in these 1,977 patients.

Stone sizes were: less than 1 cm, 2,038; 1–2 cm, 1,356; and greater than 2 cm, 244. Fluoroscopy time averaged 5.07 min (range, 0.3–38.3 min). This compares to an average fluoroscopy time of 28 min for 300 consecutive percutaneous ultrasonic lithotripsies performed at the same institution prior to the availability of ESWL.

Adjuvant procedures were done before or at the time of ESWL in 58% of the patients. The majority of these procedures were for placement of a ureteral stent (27%) or a ureteral catheter for manipulation or visualization (27%). Two percent of patients had a percutaneous nephrostomy tube or percutaneous ultrasonic lithotripsy in conjunction with ESWL, and another 2% underwent ureteroscopy prior to ESWL.

One hundred forty-six patients (7.4%) required hospitalization and intervention following ESWL. Of these, 100 patients underwent a ureteral manipulation, 30 patients required a percutaneous endoscopic procedure, and 16 (0.8%) required an open surgical procedure.

In this author's series, 74% were treated as outpatients; that is, they arrived at the institution in the morning and were treated and left the hospital the same day. These patients were asked to spend the next 12–24 hr at a location within 1 hr of the medical center. The percentage of patients treated as short-stay patients increased as experience was gained; for example, 86% of the last 500 ESWL patients were treated as outpatients.

Complications

Media coverage and "marketing" efforts by various institutions throughout the United States have led patients to think that ESWL is a harmless, risk-free procedure. For most patients it is, but serious complications can and do occur, including death. Therefore, fully informed consent is important prior to ESWL.

An ad hoc committee of the American Urological Association evaluated the safety and clinical efficacy of current technology of percutaneous lithotripsy and noninvasive lithotripsy, based on data from 37 ESWL centers with a combined total of at least 10,000 patients treated. Major complications associated with the procedure are shown in Table 19–1.

The most frequent minor complication is obstruction of the ureter by an accumulation of calculus fragments, referred to as "Steinstrasse" (street of stones) (Fig. 19–5). In most cases, these fragments allow urine to pass, but occasionally they become impacted. These fragments are difficult to remove endoscopically. Usually attempts to pass a guide wire through the collection of fragments fail.

The problem usually resolves spontaneously within 48–72 hr, and the patient is managed with

Table 19–1 Major Complications in 10,000 Patients from 37 ESWL Centers

Complication	Patients
Perirenal hematoma[a]	27
Cardiovascular	
Myocardial infarction	8
Arrhythmia	13
Death	
Pulmonary embolus	2
Myocardial infarction	2
Hematoma	1
Renal hemorrhage	2
Subcapsular hematoma	5
Renal failure	1
Ureterolithotomy or pyelolithotomy	7
Pyelonephritis	4
Nephrectomy	2
Liver hematoma	1
Pancreatitis	
(elevated amylase)	2
(clinical)	3
Hyperthermia (tub too hot)	1
Pneumonitis	6
Pulmonary embolus	4
Hemoptysis (in children with myelodysplasia)	2
Cerebrovascular accident	3
Brachial palsy	4
Long thoracic nerve palsy	1
Falling off gantry	2
Retroperitoneal abscess	1
Strapped too tightly – could not be ventilated	1

Source: *Report of American Urological Association Ad Hoc Committee (1986).*
[a] *Excludes University of Florida data.*

adequate analgesia (Fig. 19–5B). If obstruction is accompanied with sepsis, percutaneous nephrostomy is recommended. The fragments will then, generally, pass spontaneously through the ureter over the next several days or few weeks. If endoscopic dislodgement is attempted, forceful intermittent irrigation through a ureteral catheter may be successful; a "water pik" can be useful in this situation. If a direct view ureteroscope can be placed, ultrasonic fragmentation combined with irrigation may resolve the problem. Successful treatment of "Steinstrasse" in the distal ureter has been reported using repeat ESWL, with the patient in a sitting position supported by a sling beneath the backrest and seat of the gantry (Miller et al. 1987). Sometimes a large single fragment obstructs the ureter distally, acting like a dam trapping other fragments. In this situation, extraction of the single obstructing stone is all that is necessary to allow the other fragments to pass spontaneously.

Prevention of "Steinstrasse" can usually be accomplished by the passage of a ureteral stent prior to ESWL. The stent allows adequate drainage of urine while producing relative dilation of the ureter through peristaltic fatigue, so that fragments pass down the ureter around the outside of the stent. The stent also assures access to the upper tract, should endoscopic manipulations be necessary. The incidence of "Steinstrasse" is directly related to the bulk of the initial stone treated, and can be reduced by percutaneous debulking of large stone burdens (>2.5 cm) prior to ESWL and by the pre-ESWL placement of a ureteral stent in patients with stone burdens greater than 1.5 cm.

The effects of ESWL on renal function and anatomy have been studied with MR imaging, renal scans, and renal function studies. Short-term abnormalities have been noted, but little long-term dysfunction has been found (Assimos et al. 1987). Lingeman and Kulb recently reported that new onset hypertension requiring pharmacologic therapy was present in 8.2% of 295 patients (average age 53 years) at least 1 year following ESWL. However, only one-third of surveyed patients responded, so the meaning of this percentage remains unknown. No identifiable explanation or difference in renal function was found, and the expected incidence of new onset hypertension in this group was not given (Lingeman, Kulb 1987).

The consequence of the residual debris in 20% of ESWL-treated patients and the incidence of recurrence of stones await further follow-up. Certainly, this new technology will not change the natural history of a disease that has an expected recurrence rate of 50%.

Radiation Exposure

Radiation dose to the patient during ESWL is primarily influenced by the opacity of the stones; the size of the patient, which affects the amount of radiation necessary for penetration and visualization of the stone; and the experience of the operator (Bush et al. 1987; Griffith et al. 1988).

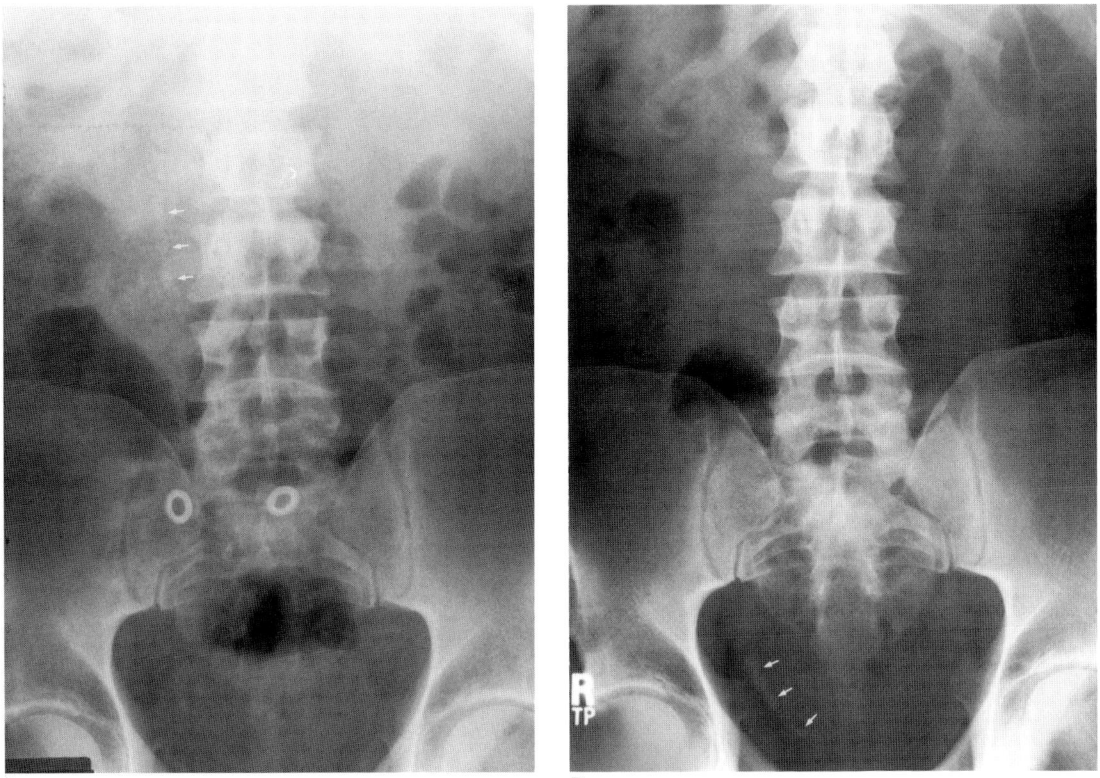

A B

19–5 Illustration of stone fragment passage down ureter after treatment of renal pelvic calculus by ESWL. **(A)** Column of granules and stone fragments ("Steinstrasse") is seen in upper ureter (arrows) 4 days after ESWL. **(B)** Further passage of "Steinstrasse" through ureter. One day later, column of granules and fragments is seen in lower ureter (arrows). Ureter was completely clear of fragments 2 weeks later.

Dose is less than for percutaneous procedures and is similar to that incurred during an upper gastrointestinal barium study. Exposure to personnel in the lithotripter suite is minimal. The urologist should be aware of the radiation being delivered to the patient and the steps that can be taken to minimize exposure. As a point of reference, the surface radiation dose to the patient for a plain abdominal film is 0.2–0.5 rad, and for 8-view excretory urography, 2–4 rad. During ESWL, using 90 kV, 3 mA on fluoroscopy, 3.0–3.5 rad/min are delivered.

The calculated radiation dose with each spot film ("quick pic") is about 0.44 rad per image using 60 kV, 160 mA setting (Bush et al. 1987; *Report of American Urological Association* 1986). Surface radiation dose to the patient during ESWL has averaged 10 rad per treatment in an institution where training about radiation has been emphasized (Bush et al. 1987). Familiarity with the fluoroscopy equipment and patient positioning system is best gained when there is no patient in the lithotripter. For small faint stones in obese patients, a ureteral catheter placed initially greatly aids in the localization, reducing radiation exposure. Localization can also be aided using the "in-bath" radiograph filming technique (Eusek et al. 1986).

It is imperative that an abdominal radiograph (KUB) be taken prior to placing the patient in the lithotripter, because it is common for stones to move. Once the patient is in the lithotripter gantry, the fluoroscopic collimators should be used to cone the radiation field as soon as possible; the fluoroscope should not be left on while the patient is being moved. "Quick pics" should be minimized. In difficult cases, the radiologist can offer considerable help as an imaging consultant and assist the urologist with stone localization (Bush et al. 1987).

References

Abber JC, Langberg J, Griffin JC: Cardiovascular pathology and ESWL. *J. Urol.* 137:142A, 1987 (abstract 156).

Assimos DG, Boyce WH, Furr EG, Espeland MA, Harrison LH, Kroovand RL: Urinary enzyme levels after extracorporeal shock wave lithotripsy (ESWL). *J. Urol.* 137:143A, 1987 (abstract 157).

Bush WH, Brannen GE: Extracorporeal shock wave lithotripsy (ESWL) of a pelvic kidney calculus: Use of C-arm fluoroscopy for correct position. *Urology* 29:352–361, 1987.

Bush WH, Jones D, Gibbons RP: Radiation dose to patient and personnel during extracorporeal shock wave lithotripsy (ESWL). *J. Urol.* 138:716–719, 1987.

Chaussy C, Brendel W, Schmiedt E: Extracorporeally induced destruction of kidney stones by shock waves. *Lancet* 2:1265–1268, 1980.

Chaussy C, Schmiedt E, Jocham D, Fuchs G, Brendel W: *Extracorporeal Shock Wave Lithotripsy: New Aspects in the Treatment of Kidney Stone Disease.* Basel, Karger, 1982.

Dretler SP, Watson G, Parrish JA, Murray S: Pulsed dye laser fragmentation of ureteral calculi: Initial clinical experience. *J. Urol.* 137:386–389, 1987.

Eusek JF, Bush WH, Burnett LL, Gibbons RP: In-bath filming during ESWL. *Radiology* 158:850–851, 1986.

Fuchs GJ, Chaussy CG: Extracorporeal shock-wave lithotripsy: An update. *Endourology* 2:1–8, 1987.

Griffith DP, Gleeson MJ, Politis G, Glaze S: Effectiveness of radiation control program for Dornier HM-3 Lithotripter. *Urology,* in press.

Lingeman JE, Kulb TB: Hypertension following extracorporeal shock wave lithotripsy. *J. Urol.* 137:142A, 1987 (abstract 154).

Liong ML, Clayman RV: Choice of treatment modalities for upper ureteral calculi: A multi-centered study. *J. Urol.* 137:160A, 1987 (abstract 225).

London RA, Kudlak T, Riehle RA: Immersion anesthesia for extracorporeal shock wave lithotripsy. *Urology* 28:86–94, 1986.

Miller K, Bubeck J, Hautmann R: Distal ureteral calculi: ESWL experience with more than 100 consecutive cases. *J. Urol.* 137:143A, 1987 (abstract 160).

Nemoy NJ, Stamey TA: Surgical bacteriological and biochemical management of "infection stones." *J.A.M.A.* 215:1470–1476, 1971.

Report of American Urological Association Ad Hoc Committee to Study the Safety and Clinical Efficacy of Current Technology of Percutaneous Lithotripsy and Noninvasive Lithotripsy. Baltimore, American Urological Association (1120 N. Charles St., Baltimore, MD 21201), May 22, 1986.

Riehle RA, Naslund EB, Fair WR, Vaughan ED: Impact of shock wave lithotripsy on upper urinary tract calculi. *Urology* 28:261–269, 1986.

Sandegard E: Prognosis of stone in the ureter. *Acta Chir. Scand.* 219(Suppl.):1–13, 1956.

Schmeller NT, Kersting H, Schuller J, Chaussy C, Schmiedt E: Combination of chemolysis and shock wave lithotripsy in the treatment of cystine renal calculi. *J. Urol.* 131:434–438, 1984.

Wax SH, Frank IN: A retrospective study of upper urinary tract calculi. *J. Urol.* 94:28–32, 1965.

Whelan JP, Finlayson B: Clinical application of blast-path kinetics. *Endourology* 2:13, 1987.

CHAPTER

20

ESWL: A Perspective

Egbert Schmiedt, Christian G. Chaussy, and Dieter Jocham

Extracorporeal shock wave lithotripsy (ESWL®)[a] is a registered U.S. trademark of Dornier Medical Systems, Marietta, GA. uses shock waves to disintegrate urinary calculi. This noninvasive method is used to treat over 95% of renal and ureteral calculi. By combining endourological procedures such as nephrolitholapaxy, ureterorenoscopy, and ureterorenotripsy with ESWL, difficult stones can be managed less invasively.

The idea of using shock waves to fragment urinary stones was conceived in 1969. From 1974 to 1980, experiments were carried out by the authors, with the first patient treated in Munich in February 1980 (Table 20–1). The clinical applications of ESWL were established at the Munich stone center of the Ludwig Maximilian University. This method has since been rapidly disseminated worldwide. Approximately 22 ESWL centers are located in the Federal Republic of Germany, and there are more than 250 centers internationally. At least 80% of upper urinary tract calculi are treated by ESWL alone. With the continuing improvements in lithotripter techniques, in a few years 90% of all urinary calculi will likely be treated successfully by ESWL alone.

Patient Selection

Experimental work plus extensive clinical experience show that ESWL is an especially low-risk technique. In principle, any stone that can be located in the focal area of maximal shock waves of the lithotripter can be successfully treated. Thus, in routine clinical practice, ESWL is indicated for kidney stones and ureteral stones positioned above the iliac crest, provided no contraindications to ESWL are present (Table 20–2). It is essential that there is no obstruction below the stone that could interfere with elimination of the disintegrated particles.

The mass or bulk of the stone is another major determinant of success. Small stones up to 2.5 cm in diameter – approximately 60% of all cases – are readily treatable by ESWL. With larger stones, particularly partial or total staghorn stones, percutaneous lithotripsy followed by ESWL is pre-

Table 20–1 Historical Development of Extracorporeal Shock Wave Lithotripsy

1966	Accidental discovery of shock wave effect on humans
1969	Emergence of the idea of stone disintegration
1969–71	Research program, "Interaction Between Shock Waves and Tissue in Animals," sponsored by the Ministry of Defense
1972	First in vitro experiments for stone disintegration
1972	Letter from Professors Schmiedt and Eisenberger stating, "It would be revolutionary to disintegrate kidney stones without surgery."
Jan 1974	Start of the ESWL research project sponsored by the Federal Ministry of Research and Development
1974–78	Various laboratory models of lithotripter with water bag and ultrasound system for stone location
1978	First water bath model with a two-axis X-ray system for animal experiments
1978–79	Animal experiments
1979	Lithotripter model HM-1
Feb 1980	Treatment of the first patient
1980–82	Treatment of 220 patients with HM-1
May 1982	Inauguration of the model HM-2 in Munich
Oct 1983	Inauguration of the first series model HM-3 in Stuttgart
1983–84	IDE procedure in U.S.
Dec 1984	Pre-market approval from the U.S. Food and Drug Administration
Nov 1985	Approval from the Japanese Ministry of Public Welfare
May 1987	257 Dornier lithotripters in operation worldwide
May 1987	350000 patients treated worldwide

Table 20–2 Contraindications to ESWL

Obstruction distal to the stone
Untreatable bleeding disorders
Aneurysms in the shock wave area
Pregnancy

[a] ESWL is a registered trademark of Dornier Medical Systems, Marietta, GA.

ferred over multisession ESWL therapy. After percutaneous lithotripsy, the remaining stone fragments are disintegrated by ESWL. Combination therapy is preferred in cases of large stone bulk. If only ESWL is used for large stones, extended hospitalization and multiple ESWL sessions are needed.

Furthermore, when much concrement material is present, the transport capacity of the urinary system may be exceeded, leading to transitory urinary obstruction and colic. The incidence of colic is surprisingly low (mean, 16% of all ESWL treatments). It is more of a problem with large stone masses; 35% of these patients experience pain with passage of fragments.

Contraindications

Untreatable bleeding disorders are contraindications for ESWL, since shock waves can induce bleeding. A patient history should be obtained regarding the use of salicylate or other medication that influences blood coagulation. Specific causes of a coagulation disorder should be researched and, in the case of high intake of analgesics such as acetylsalicylic acid, the prothrombin and plasma thrombin time, as well as the bleeding time, should be checked. ESWL can be performed in the case of hemophilia, provided that pathological blood coagulation values can be managed. In the authors' experience, patients with blood coagulation disturbances should be treated together with a hematologist.

Percutaneous nephrolitholapaxy and ureterorenoscopy have the same contraindications as open surgery, particularly regarding blood coagulation disorders. In addition, special anatomic circumstances blocking access to the stone, such as large adenomas of the prostate in ureterorenoscopy and splenomegaly for percutaneous nephrolitholapaxy, must be considered.

ESWL is contraindicated in pregnant women and in patients with aneurysms in the shock wave area because of insufficient clinical experience in those situations.

Anesthesia

Depending on the kind and extent of energy applied for stone disintegration, ESWL will cause pain. The use of general anesthesia allows control of ventilation frequency; accordingly, the proportion of shock waves that strikes the stone can be maximized. In addition, preparation time is shorter, although surveillance of the patient during recovery is required.

Peridural anesthesia is used in 70% of patients at the Munich center. Catheter peridural anesthesia permits anesthesia to be extended for longer treatments when required. Moreover, it requires less patient surveillance in the posttherapeutic phase. Covering the puncture site with a protective film prevents infection of the puncture channel. This applies particularly to patients who must remain in the water bath for an extended period of time, or when the catheter must be left in place in anticipation of an extended session. Peridural anesthesia is not recommended for anxious, nervous, or uncooperative patients; excessively deep or rapid respirations limit the effectiveness of ESWL treatment.

The authors have had limited experience with sedo-analgesia combining opioids and ketamine with a benzodiazepam sedative. Its importance can only be evaluated after more extensive clinical experience.

Diffuse infiltration of the flank with large amounts of local anesthesia reduces pain only for patients with a high pain threshold, who require minimal shock waves to disintegrate small stones. The use of a sedative during the session is often required. However, technical modifications on the Dornier lithotripter during 1987 have enabled the authors to treat approximately 90% of all patients without sedation or anesthesia.

Auxiliary Procedures

Techniques before ESWL

Techniques before ESWL include percutaneous nephrostomy, percutaneous ultrasonic lithotripsy, elimination of ureteral obstructions, balloon dilation or endourological slitting for ureteral strictures, manipulation of ureteral stones into the renal pelvis, transurethral resection of the prostate for adenomas, and urethrotomy for urethral strictures. Percutaneous nephrostomy is necessary for treatment of infected hydronephrosis and is important for treatment of radiotranslucent kidney and larger ureteral stones. Furthermore, a percutaneous nephrostomy channel is helpful after ESWL of radiotransparent stones. Sometimes, the stone passage can only be documented with the help of contrast medium and films taken at short intervals.

Techniques after ESWL

The authors find it necessary to establish a percutaneous nephrostomy channel after ESWL in 6% of cases, owing to hydronephrosis or complaints arising from delayed stone discharge. Placement of a percutaneous nephrostomy often results in rapid, spontaneous passage of the concrement particles in patients treated for multiple upper tract stones that caused urinary obstruction due to stone fragments. The patients frequently become stone-free within a short time. In the authors' opinion, this phenomenon is due to the restoration of ureteral peristaltic action.

Percutaneous nephrostomy therefore represents an effective alternative to ESWL retreatment, transurethral stone dislodgement, or stone extraction. A further indication for the placement of a percutaneous nephrostomy is local chemolitholysis of uric acid and especially cystine stones in conjunction with ESWL. The surface area of the stone mass can be considerably increased by ESWL, so that the chemolitholytic agent is more effective. Chemolitholysis is up to 50% faster when preceded by ESWL.

If multiple prevesical stones occur after ESWL, the dislodgement or extraction of the fragments with a ureterorenoscope is occasionally required (3.8%), sometimes in combination with ultrasound or laser lithotripsy, a ureteral loop, or a curved ureteral catheter.

Special Situations

Technical innovations such as the "blast path" technique, respiratory-controlled triggering of shock waves, and high-frequency or high-jet ventilation for decreased respiratory motion facilitate ESWL stone fragmentation. Modified strategies for ESWL are possible with these techniques, even in the case of large stone masses requiring multisession treatments. Basically, the urologist must determine the therapeutic concept for each individual case: ESWL monotherapy, a combination of ESWL and auxiliary techniques, or open surgery.

Strategic planning for stone treatment is directed at complete therapy and at avoiding tissue damage during treatment. According to clinical evidence, ESWL fulfills these requirements best. Even in cases where surgery would be useful in removing concurrent urinary obstruction, it is possible to refrain from a kidney-splitting incision for removal of caliceal stones when removing a central staghorn stone mass. After removal of the central staghorn segment by surgery or percutaneous lithotripsy, the part of the stone within the

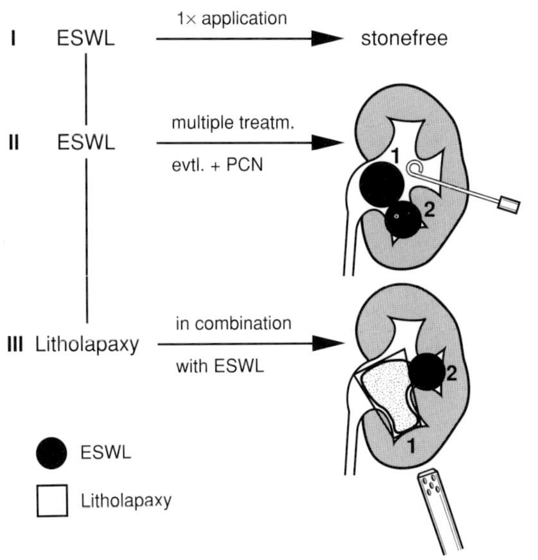

20–1 Modern treatment strategies in the case of partial staghorn stone.

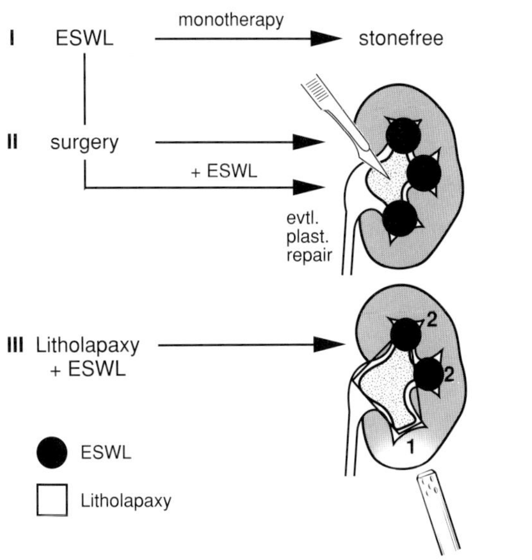

20–2 Modern treatment strategies in the case of total staghorn stone.

Table 20–3 Comparison of Various Treatment Modalities for Removal of Urinary Calculi

Open Surgery	ESWL	Percutaneous Lithotripsy	Local Chemolitholysis
Total staghorn stones Stone + surgical removal of ureteral obstruction Impacted ureteral stones	Small and medium size pelvic and caliceal stones with no obstruction in any location Partial staghorn stone Ureteral stones	Larger pelvic and partial staghorn stones in suitable location (perhaps combined therapy with ESWL) Stone + percutaneous removal of ureteral obstruction Stones in upper part of ureter Translucent stones	Adjunct to ESWL and litholapaxy in the case of cystine, uric acid, struvite, and apatite calculi

calices may be treated later using ESWL (Figs. 20–1, 20–2).

Broad clinical experience has shown that comprehensive and safe use of ESWL is possible only in the hands of a urologist who has mastered the alternative and auxiliary techniques, who can adapt these techniques to the individual case, and can integrate them in the therapeutic strategy (Table 20–3). The techniques for kidney stones also apply to ureteral stones, with some modifications.

Ureteral Stones

ESWL of ureteral stones, including some in the lower third of the ureter within the bony pelvis, can be carried out successfully (Fig. 20–3). In the authors' experience, more than 70% of all stones in all parts of the ureter can be successfully treated *in situ* with ESWL alone. In one-third of cases, treatment was successful only after displacing the stone up into the collecting system of the kidney. This so-called push-and-smash technique improves the success rate and reduces the shock wave energy required for stone disintegration. However, pushing the stone back into the renal collecting system requires more invasive techniques. The urologist must therefore decide on the best approach for each patient.

Auxiliary techniques prior to ESWL or alternative approaches are recommended for large ureteral stones at the ureteropelvic junction and stones that have been in the same position for more than 4 weeks. In such cases, it is important to flush or push the stone transureterally into the renal pelvis and then subject the "kidney stone" to ESWL.

Antegrade or retrograde ureteroscopy is required for stone extraction or destruction if ESWL therapy fails, if ESWL proves unsuccessful after initial ureteral stone manipulation, or if the stone

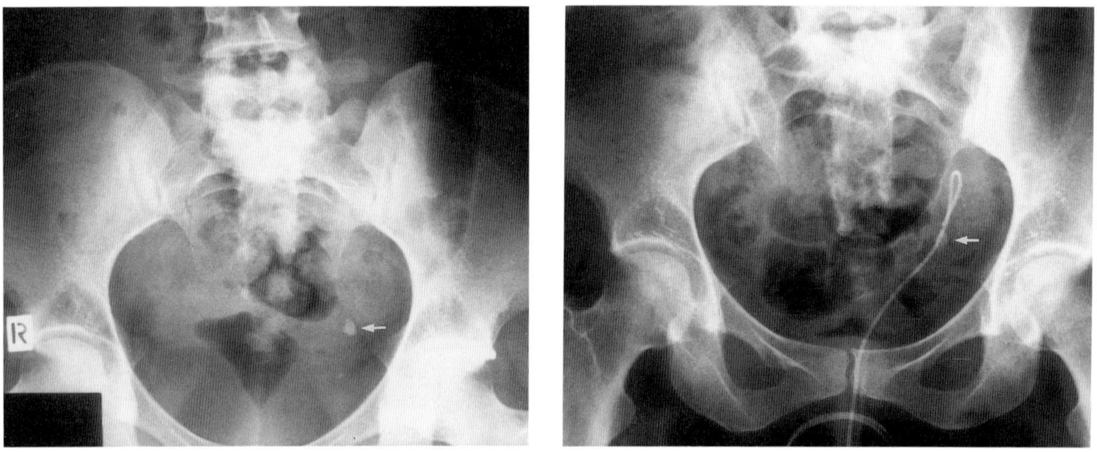

20–3 ESWL of ureteral stone located in lower part of ureter (arrow). Left, pre-ESWL; right, post-ESWL with stent placement.

is located in the iliosacral area of the ureter. ESWL or mildly invasive techniques such as loop, basket, ureteroscopy, and ureterolithotripsy can also replace open surgery for ureteral stones. Ureterolithotomy was unavoidable in only 2% of the authors' patients. The high success rate of ESWL for ureteral stones located outside the bony pelvis is only assured if X-ray fluoroscopy is used to localize the stone. Localization by sonography is not adequate for most ureteral calculi.

Infected Stones

ESWL can be safely performed, even in cases of urinary infection. In these cases, appropriate antibiotic treatment must be initiated. Urinary obstruction following ESWL must be relieved by, for example, the establishment of a percutaneous nephrostomy. In a patient with a history of infected stones, it is best to perform ESWL under antibiotic prophylaxis, even if the urine is primarily sterile.

Stones in Children

ESWL is safe in children, even babies, for all stone constellations in the upper urinary tract, including small caliceal stones, total staghorn stones, and ureteral stones. However, the application is somewhat limited because of children's small body size and the proximity of the treated area to lung tissue, which becomes severely contused by the shock waves. A prerequisite for the performance of ESWL is the ability to position the child appropriately on the patient support. By correctly shielding the child's lungs with a Styrofoam block, lung damage is avoided, as the air in the Styrofoam blocks the shock waves.

In addition, safety is assured by ECG-synchronized shock wave triggering in the absolute cardiac refractory period and by using respiratory-controlled high-frequency ventilation. Each single shock wave is transmitted to the body at the end of the expiratory phase.

Results of ESWL

More than 500,000 ESWL treatments have been performed throughout the world. Comparison of the authors' clinical results internationally proves their reproducibility and indirectly confirms the reliability of the ESWL procedure. On a follow-up plain film X ray 3 months after ESWL therapy, about 70%–85% of the patients were free of stones. In 16% of patients, residual concrements were found radiographically, usually in a dilated calix. Since the vast majority of these patients were free of complaints and infection, and the residual concrements were passable, further therapy was not indicated.

In only 20% of the authors' patients did residual concrements give rise to complaints, necessitating a second ESWL treatment 3 months after the first. In all cases, this resulted in complete stone clearance, so that, subsequently, 85% of the overall collective were radiographically free of stones 3 to 6 months after ESWL.

As a result of the increased range of indications, about 15% of the authors' patients underwent 2–6 ESWL sessions before they were completely free of stones. In cases of bilateral nephrolithiasis, stones on the contralateral side were treated in a later session. This approach avoids the risk of bilateral obstruction.

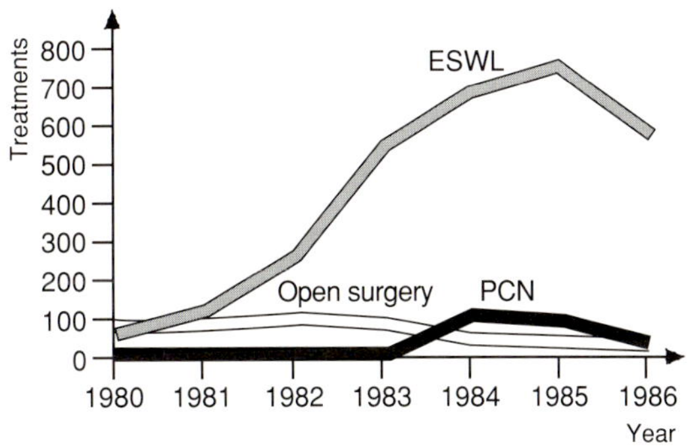

20–4 Change of treatment modalities of nephrolithiasis from 1980 to 1986.

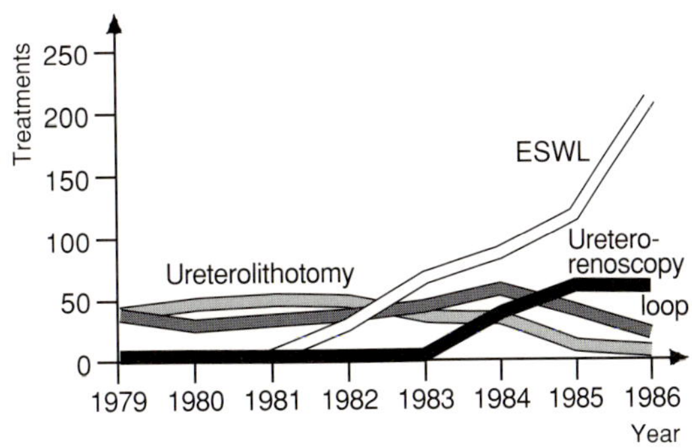

20–5 Change of treatment modalities for ureteral stones from 1979 to 1986.

Table 20–4 Comparative Clinical Results of ESWL Centers

Country	Successful Stone Disintegration (%)[a]	Stone-free after 3 Months (%)	Residual Concrements (%)[b]	Open Surgery (%)
Federal Republic of Germany:				
Munich	99	84	4.0	0.5
Stuttgart	97	75	5.0	0
Mainz	99	70	4.0	0
Hannover	99	78	3.0	0.5
Great Britain:				
London	97	76	3.0	<1
United States:				
Los Angeles	99	85	4.0	0
Indianapolis	90	84	8.5	<0.5
Houston	95	75	10.0	0
Charlottesville	99	70	1.0	0
Japan:				
Sapporo	99	77	3.0	0.2

[a] Stones ≤2 cm.

[b] Second treatment required after 3 months.

Table 20–5 Results of ESWL Monotherapy versus Percutaneous Lithotripsy for Staghorn Calculi

	ESWL Monotherapy		Percutaneous Lithotripsy Monotherapy	
	Partial Staghorn	Complete Staghorn	Partial Staghorn	Complete Staghorn
No. calculi	42	6	16	7
No. sessions	1.6	1.8	2.2	3.8
No. accesses	–	–	1.5	2.1
Duration of treatment (hr)	1.6	2.0	5.6	9.2
Blood transfusions	–	–	1.6	2.6
Auxiliary procedures (%)	48	67	–	–
Residual concrements (%)	39	39	14	14

Especially encouraging is the long-term observation that no more than 0.6% of ESWL patients subsequently require surgery for stone extraction (Table 20–4). On the basis of these experiences, it is not surprising that open surgery as well as the less invasive procedures of percutaneous ultrasonic lithotripsy and ureterorenoscopy are infrequently required (Figs. 20–4, 20–5). Percutaneous lithotripsy treatment offers advantages over ESWL only in the case of large stone masses (Table 20–5).

Complications

The results of thousands of treatments have shown that ESWL is a nontraumatic and low-risk technique. Foremost among the rare complications are ESWL-induced intrarenal edema and intra- and perirenal hematomas. The authors' own investigations have shown that the incidence of complications increases with the number of shock waves applied during the session and with the total shock wave energy delivered. Evaluation of patients with sonography, magnetic resonance imaging, and computed tomography revealed that all patients who had been treated with 2,000 pulses exhibited at least small intrarenal hematomas.

Results in Children

At the Munich center of the Ludwig Maximilian University, the authors treated 37 children, ages 2–14, with ESWL from March 1983 to April 1987. The following stones were treated: 3 ureter stones, 22 caliceal stones, 13 renal pelvic stones, 5 partial staghorn stones, and 5 total staghorn stones. Nine children were treated in two sessions and one child in four sessions. Excellent stone disintegration was achieved in all cases, with the exception of a single case of a cystine stone in an 8-year-old boy; the stone was subsequently cleared by chemolitholysis.

Ureteral colic and stone fragment discharge were similar to that observed with adults. Placement of a percutaneous nephrostomy was necessary in three cases, due to infected hydronephrosis caused by a so-called ureter Steinstrasse (street of stone). Disintegrated stone material usually passed spontaneously, even in the case of long Steinstrassen.

Only one case required stone material to be removed transurethrally with surgery. A nephrectomy following ESWL treatment became necessary in a 9-year-old girl with a total staghorn stone, hydronephrosis, and severely impaired renal function. Overall, hospitalization following ESWL treatment averaged 10 days and, at the time of discharge, 63% of children were stone-free. The others revealed spontaneously dischargeable stone fragments.

Percutaneous treatment procedures are possible in young children, but are more difficult than in adults. Transurethral manipulations often fail, owing to anatomic circumstances and relatively large instruments.

Future Perspectives

ESWL has contributed impressively toward an almost complete change in the strategy of urinary tract calculi therapy. Technical advances involving a piezoelectrical shock wave source and use of electrodes in conjunction with modified types of the shock wave ellipsoid and generator capacity are now resulting in anesthesia-free treatment.

Patients treated today with the internationally distributed Dornier lithotripter still require general or regional anesthesia or extensive local infiltration. Technical upgrading of these lithotripters for a pain-free ESWL treatment is available. For certain stones and anatomic configurations, percutaneous lithotripsy and ureterorenoscopy are necessary in combination with ESWL; consequently, the ESWL user, or a colleague, must master these urologic procedures.

The availability of lithotripters has reduced the necessity for open surgery to less than 10%. In some clinics, including the authors', less than 1% of patients required surgery for stone extraction in 1985. Of course, open surgical intervention will never be completely abandoned, especially when an anatomical deformity is present, such as an obstruction distal to the stone that cannot be endourologically cleared. Such an obstruction would prevent spontaneous discharge of the stone fragments, could possibly impair renal function, and could promote recurrent stones.

Today, shock wave application combined with the semi-invasive auxiliary methods spare the patient surgical therapeutic methods that are associated with considerably greater trauma, possible complications, or side effects. In the future, the patient might be referred to a nearby stone center for prompt, noninvasive treatment of urinary calculi. Postoperative care, if required, will be predominantly provided near the patient's home by a urologist who has the patient's special confidence.

In a few years, it will be possible to treat 90% of all upper urinary tract calculi with ESWL alone, but the urologist must also maintain the necessary skills for the rare open surgical interventions. In addition, restructuring the training of urologists to emphasize endourological procedures is needed.

In the authors' opinion, ESWL and endourologic treatment procedures are the methods of choice for urolithiasis.

References

Chaussy C, Brendel W, Schmiedt E: Extracorporeally induced destruction of kidney stones by shock waves. *Lancet* 2:1265, 1980.

Chaussy C, Schmiedt E, Jocham D, et al.: First clinical experience with extracorporeally induced destruction of kidney stones by shock waves. *J. Urol.* 127:417, 1982.

Drach GW, Dretler S, Fair W: Report of the United States cooperative study of extracorporeal shock wave lithotripsy. *J. Urol.* 135:1127, 1986.

Eisenberger F, Rassweiler J: The modern treatment of complicated renal stone disease. *Dornier Medizintechnik GmbH-News, User-Letter* 1 (September 1986).

Fuchs G, Chaussy C: *Worldwide experience with extracorporeal shock wave lithotripsy (ESWL). In* Dornier Medizintechnik GmbH-News, User-Letter, Premier Issue, September 1986.

Gravenstein JS, Peter K: *Extracorporeal shock wave lithotripsy for renal stone disease. Technical and clinical aspects.* London, Butterworth, 1985.

Jocham D, Chaussy C, Schmiedt E: Extracorporeal shock wave lithotripsy. *Urol. Int.* (Karger, Basel), 357–368, 1986.

Miller K, Bubeck JR, Hautmann R: Extracorporeal shockwave lithotripsy of distal ureteral calculi. *Dornier Medizintechnik GmbH-News, User-Letter* 1 (September 1986).

Riehle RA, Jr. (ed.): *Principles of extracorporeal shockwave lithotripsy.* New York, Churchill Livingstone, 1987.

Weber W, Hugler P, Lehmann, et al.: *ECG-synchronized procedures at the 1st International Symposium on Anesthesia and ESWL.* Springer Verlag, in press.

CHAPTER
21
Medical Management after Stone Removal

Edward A. Benson

Certain predisposing factors are known to be important in the development of the five major types of kidney stones (Table 21–1). Uncorrected, these factors will generally lead to continued stone formation and recurrent morbidity. The risk of recurrent stones after an initial episode of renal colic is between 20% and 50% over the subsequent 10 years. In most cases, however, the causative metabolic disorder, once identified, can be corrected with a substantial reduction in the risk of further stone formation. This chapter reviews the metabolic basis of urolithiasis and presents an approach to prevention of recurring stones.

Predisposing Factors

Stones Containing Calcium

Over 80% of kidney stones contain calcium in some form. Calcium oxalate stones most often develop owing to four causes: excess of urinary calcium, excess of urinary uric acid, excess of urinary oxalate, or deficiency of citrate in urine. The first two causes are the most common.

Approximately one-half of individuals with recurrent calcium stones have hypercalciuria, usually as an isolated metabolic disorder. Hypercalciuria is defined as a 24-hr urine calcium excretion of greater than 250 mg/day for women, 300 mg/day for men, or 4 mg/kg per day for either sex. In about 10% of cases, the hypercalciuria is secondary to conditions such as hyperparathyroidism, hyperthyroidism, Paget's disease, sarcoidosis, malignant neoplasm, immobilization, glucocorticoid treatment, or excessive vitamin D or calcium intake.

Hyperuricosuria, defined as a 24-hr urine uric acid level of greater than 750 mg in women or 800 mg in men, also predisposes to calcium oxalate stone formation. Although the mechanism is unclear, sodium urate crystals may provide a nidus for calcium oxalate precipitation. The cause of hyperuricosuria in many patients is a diet rich in red meat, a major source of purines (Coe 1978).

Hyperoxaluria most commonly occurs in patients with small bowel disease, intestinal bypass for obesity, chronic biliary or pancreatic disease, or other conditions associated with fat malabsorption. Free fatty acids bind calcium ions, allowing more free oxalate to reach the colon, the major site of oxalate absorption. In addition, in a diseased or shortened small bowel, the bile salts that are normally absorbed in the small bowel reach the colon, increasing the permeability of the colon to oxalate. The increased absorption of dietary oxalate leads to a rise in urinary oxalate excretion. Due to the relative insolubility of calcium oxalate in urine, a small increase in urinary oxalate concentration will result in a markedly increased risk of calcium oxalate stone formation.

Hypocitraturia has recently been identified as an important factor in the pathogenesis of calcium stones (Pak, Fuller 1986). Hypocitraturia occurs in a setting of systemic acidosis or as an isolated defect, and is defined by most laboratories as a urinary citrate excretion of less than 320 mg per day. Citrate competes with oxalate for binding to the calcium ion. Whereas calcium oxalate is relatively insoluble, calcium citrate remains in solution and is easily excreted in urine. A deficiency of urinary citrate therefore favors the formation of calcium oxalate crystals.

Pure calcium phosphate stones are most commonly found in patients with persistently alkaline urine, caused, for example, by renal tubular acidosis, urinary infection with urea splitting bac-

Table 21–1 Types of Kidney Stones

Stone Composition	Frequency[a] (%)	X-ray Appearance	Predisposing Factors
Calcium oxalate with or without calcium phosphate	75	Opaque; stippled serrated margins	Hypercalciuria Hyperuricosuria Hyperoxaluria Hypocitraturia
Pure calcium phosphate	9	Opaque; uniform opacity	Hyperparathyroidism Renal tubular acidosis Medications: Diamox, vitamin D
Magnesium ammonium calcium phosphate (struvite-apatite) (triple phosphate stone)	8	Opaque; laminated	Urea-splitting bacteria
Uric acid	6	Lucent	Hyperuricosuria Acid urine
Cystine	2	Mildly opaque	Cystinuria

[a] Data on 100 consecutive patients treated at Virginia Mason Clinic, Seattle.

teria, and treatment with certain antacids or acetazolamide (Diamox®).

Struvite Stones

The formation of struvite stones results from the precipitation of phosphates with magnesium and ammonium at a urine pH of 7 or greater. Necessary conditions for the formation of such stones is urine infected with urease-producing bacteria, such as *Proteus* species and some strains of *Pseudomonas, Serratia, Klebsiella*, and *Enterococcus*. Struvite stones may grow rapidly, take on the branched forms of staghorn calculi, and destroy renal parenchyma.

Uric Acid Stones

Low urine volume, hyperuricosuria, and persistently acid urine all contribute to the formation of uric acid stones. As previously stated, hyperuricosuria is often caused by excessive intake of purine-rich foods, primarily red meat. Approximately half of patients with uric acid stones have gout or hyperuricemia. Pure uric acid stones are radiolucent; however, these calculi often contain both calcium and uric acid and are moderately opaque.

Cystine Stones

Cystine stones develop only in patients with cystinuria, a rare congenital defect in the tubular reabsorption of the amino acids cystine, ornithine, lysine, and arginine. Cystine stones comprise about 2% of all kidney stones, and these calculi are moderately opaque. Urolithiasis is the only clinical consequence of cystinuria.

Metabolic Evaluation

If the chemical composition of the kidney stone is known, one can focus on the factors predisposing to the formation of that specific type of stone (Table 21–1). Even if the stone composition is unknown, the underlying metabolic disorder can usually be identified through a systematic approach.

The screening tests outlined in Table 21–2 will identify a metabolic disorder in the majority of

Table 21–2 Metabolic Evaluation of Recurrent Urolithiasis

Screening tests:	
Blood	Electrolytes, Ca^{++}, $PO_4^{=}$, uric acid, creatinine
Urine	pH, culture, cystine screen, 24-hr collection for: creatinine, calcium, uric acid
Special tests:	
If serum Ca^{++} >10.0	Parathyroid hormone
If pure $CaPO_4$ stone	Evaluate for renal tubular acidosis
If GI malabsorption	24-hr urine oxalate and citrate
If no metabolic abnormality detected with screening tests	24-hr urine citrate

patients with recurrent kidney stones. In addition, special circumstances may dictate more in-depth evaluation. For example, patients with recurrent calcium stones and a high normal serum calcium concentration (above 10 mg/dl) should be evaluated for hyperparathyroidism, since a substantial number will have mild or "eucalcemic" hyperparathyroidism as a cause of their stones. Measurement of parathyroid hormone is appropriate in patients with calcium kidney stones and a serum calcium above 10 mg/dl.

Individuals with pure calcium phosphate stones are more likely to have a systemic metabolic abnormality, such as renal tubular acidosis or hyperparathyroidism. In addition, about 10% of patients taking acetazolamide (Diamox®) will form stones of pure calcium phosphate. Renal tubular acidosis should be suspected in individuals with systemic acidosis, a urine pH persistently above 5.5, or in whom pure calcium phosphate stones have been identified.

Reduced levels of urinary citrate may be associated with systemic acidosis (renal tubular acidosis, chronic diarrhea, or treatment with Diamox®). These patients and patients with recurrent stones, but no metabolic abnormality identified by the screening tests, should have 24-hr urine citrate excretion measured.

Conditions associated with gastrointestinal malabsorption, such as Crohn's disease or jejunoileal bypass surgery, may be accompanied by hyperoxaluria and the formation of calcium oxalate stones. The contribution of intestinal disease to stone formation can be assessed by measuring 24-hr urine oxalate excretion.

Table 21–3 Metabolic Assessment of Recurrent Kidney Stones[a]

Metabolic Disorder	Number
Hypercalciuria	35
Hyperuricosuria	22
Hypercalciuria and hyperuricosuria	14
Hypocitraturia	5
Hyperparathyroidism	5
Incomplete renal tubular acidosis	2
Malabsorption with hyperoxaluria	2
Cystinuria	2
Infection due to urease-producing bacteria	5
Subtotal	92[a]
No metabolic disorder identified	8
Total	100

[a] Medicines (prednisone, Lasix, vitamin C, calcium, Benemid) were a potential contributing factor in 15 patients.

Medicines may contribute to the formation of kidney stones by increasing urine calcium (prednisone, Lasix, calcium, vitamin D); by increasing urinary uric acid (probenecid); by increasing urinary oxalate (vitamin C); and by raising urine pH (Diamox®, antacids).

By applying the diagnostic approach outlined in Table 21–2, a specific underlying metabolic disorder was identified in 92 of 100 consecutive patients (Table 21–3). The average cost of a metabolic diagnosis was $95 at Seattle's Virginia Mason Medical Center in 1986.

Preventing Stone Recurrence

The choice of treatment for patients with recurring stones depends on factors such as age, chemical composition of kidney stone, underlying metabolic disorder, and frequency of occurrence. All patients should be advised to increase their fluid intake and modify their diet if dietary excesses are identified.

Low urine volume is an important risk factor for urolithiasis (Robertson 1979). Patients with renal stones should be advised to increase their fluid intake to ensure adequate urine volume and the resultant dilution of urinary stone substrates. Attempting to increase urine volume to 2–3 L per day is a logical first step in any patient with kidney stones (Pak et al. 1980). This should include a glass of water taken some time during the night.

Medical therapy should be reserved for patients in whom a specific metabolic disorder has been identified. Medical treatment directed at correcting the metabolic abnormality is generally effective in preventing recurrence. Most therapeutic programs result in a 90% reduction in the rate of new stone formation.

Stones Containing Calcium

Many patients eliminate milk and dairy products when they learn they have passed a calcium-containing kidney stone. Reducing calcium intake alone leads to an increase in intestinal absorption of dietary oxalate. This increased oxalate absorption and the rise in urinary oxalate excretion that follows may negate any benefit of a low calcium diet (Bataille et al. 1983). Therefore, reducing dietary calcium should always be accompanied by efforts to reduce dietary oxalate as well (Table

Table 21–4 High-Oxalate Foods and Beverages

Beets
Chocolate
Cocoa
Instant coffee
Nuts
Peanuts and peanut butter
Rhubarb
Spinach
Sweet potatoes
Tea

21–4). Calcium intake should be reduced only if it is excessive. This generally applies to patients taking calcium supplements or calcium-containing antacids, or drinking more than two glasses of milk a day.

A variety of specific treatments are available, depending on which of the four metabolic abnormalities led to the calcium stone formation.

Hypercalciuria

For the patient with primary hypercalciuria, thiazide diuretics are an ideal treatment. Thiazides increase calcium reabsorption in the distal tubule and reduce urinary calcium excretion by approximately 40%. The overall effect is a reduction of calcium oxalate stone formation to 10% of pretreatment occurrence (Coe 1977). A combination of hydrochlorothiazide (25 mg) and amiloride (2.5 mg) twice a day (Moduretic® ½ tablet bid) is slightly more effective in reducing urinary calcium excretion than hydrochlorothiazide alone (Leppla et al. 1983).

Conversely, combinations of hydrochlorothiazide and triamterene (Diazide®, Maxzide®) should not be used in the treatment of hypercalciuria, as stones containing triamterene have been observed in patients on these drugs. The efficacy of thiazides depends on inducing mild sodium depletion. Since a high-sodium intake can defeat this treatment, patients must maintain a salt-restricted diet. About 10% of patients cannot tolerate thiazides, usually because of side effects of fatigue or impotence.

Hyperuricosuria

Reducing urinary uric acid with allopurinol significantly lowers recurrence rates in patients with calcium oxalate stones and hyperuricosuria (Coe 1977). The usual dose of allopurinol is 200–300 mg per day, but should be titrated to maintain urinary uric acid in the normal range.

Hyperoxaluria

Treatment of enteric hyperoxaluria consists of limiting dietary oxalate and fats. In addition, oral calcium, 1–4 g per day given in divided doses as calcium carbonate, reduces oxalate absorption by binding oxalate in the gut. Although this can result in increased urinary calcium excretion, the drop in urinary oxalate excretion is of greater significance. Cholestyramine can also be used to block bile acid and oxalate absorption.

Hypocitraturia

In renal tubular acidosis and chronic diarrheal syndromes, urinary citrate is often very low, and treatment with citrate or other forms of alkali is essential to correct the predilection to calcium stone formation. Citrate is also an effective treatment for recurrent calcium oxalate stones and mild idiopathic hypocitraturia (Pak, Fuller 1986). Currently available forms of citrate include Polycitra®, K-Lyte DS®, Urocit-K® tablets, and Citracal® (calcium citrate) (Table 21–5).

Table 21–5 Therapeutic Forms of Citrate

	Usual Dosage	Ca^{++} (mg)	K^+ (mEq)	Na^+ (mEq)	Citrate (g)	Approximate Daily Cost ($)
Polycitra (liquid)	3 tsp tid	–	45	45	12	0.45
K-Lyte DS (effervescent tabs)	1 bid	–	100	–	9	1.20
Urocit-K (tabs)	4 tid	–	60	–	5.6	1.06
Citracal (tabs)	2 tid	1,200	–	–	4.5	0.36

Stones with No Detectable Cause

Approximately 10% of patients with recurrent calcium stones have no identifiable metabolic abnormality. Phosphates have been advocated for the treatment of calcium oxalate stones in patients who do not have hypercalciuria or hyperuricosuria (Thomas 1978). Phosphates increase urinary excretion of pyrophosphate, an inhibitor of calcium oxalate crystal formation. Oral phosphorus is administered as 1,500–2,000 mg of elemental phosphorus daily in three or four divided doses (e.g., 500 mg of Neutra-Phos three or four times daily). However, the cathartic effect of phosphates may limit their use in some patients. Thiazide diuretics are also effective in patients with recurrent calcium stones and no specific metabolic disturbance (Cohanim, Yendt 1978).

Struvite Stones

Removal is the primary treatment for struvite stones. Chronic, long-term, culture-specific antibiotic therapy may help to suppress infection and stone growth. Complete eradication of the infection is rarely possible, however. In cases where stone removal is impossible and where stone growth persists despite antibiotics, acetohydroxamic acid (Lithostat®), an inhibitor bacterial urease, may be a helpful adjunctive treatment (Williams et al. 1984).

Uric Acid Stones

Reducing a primary source of purines – red meat – will often correct hyperuricosuria. In some patients, however, hyperuricosuria is the result of endogenous overproduction of uric acid. In patients whose hyperuricosuria persists despite purine restriction, 200–300 mg of allopurinol per day is effective in lowering urinary uric acid excretion. For patients with normal urinary uric acid excretion but persistently acid urine, alkalinization of the urine is the most effective approach to preventing uric acid stones. Alkalinization of urine with sodium bicarbonate ($NaHCO_3$ 0.6–1.2 g four times per day) or potassium citrate (K-Lyte DS® twice a day) is usually effective.

Cystine Stones

Although cystine stones account for only 2% of kidney stones, they are one of the most difficult to treat. At physiologic pH, cystine crystallizes at a concentration of 300 mg/L or greater. Thus, efforts to maintain urinary cystine concentration below this level are usually effective in preventing cystine stone formation. If the patient's daily cystine excretion is moderate (less than 1,000 mg/day), maintaining urinary cystine concentration below 300 mg/L can often be achieved by reducing protein in the diet and increasing fluid intake. The solubility of cystine increases with increasing pH, so that alkalinization of the urine is effective in preventing cystine stones. However, urine pH must be kept at 7.5 or higher to be effective.

If increased fluids and alkalinization are unsuccessful in controlling cystine stone growth, enicillamine can be tried to increase cystine solubility. Penicillamine forms a complex with cystine that is 50 times more soluble in aqueous solution than cystine itself. Administered in four divided doses totaling 1–3 g daily, penicillamine reduces excretion of free cystine to the range of 100–200 mg/day (Dahlberg et al. 1977). Nearly half of the patients taking penicillamine develop side effects, most commonly fever and rash and less commonly bone marrow depression and proteinuria.

Follow-up Treatment

The medical treatment for urolithiasis is undertaken with the goal of preventing future stone formation. A yearly abdominal film with or without renal tomograms will detect growth of opaque stones and is useful in assessing efficacy of medical treatment. Ultrasound or computed tomography can be used to follow patients with pure uric acid stones. The effect of treatment on urine chemistry should also be monitored by, for example, measurement of urine calcium excretion in patients taking thiazides or measurement of uric acid excretion in patients on allopurinol.

Measures to prevent recurrence of kidney stones should be continued indefinitely. Patients who have experienced renal colic are usually highly motivated and cooperative. Fortunately, medications used to prevent kidney stones are generally well-tolerated, inexpensive, and effective.

References

Bataille P, Charransol G, Gregoire I, Daigre JL, Coevoet B, Makdassi R, Pruna A, Locquet P, Sueur JP, Fournier A: Effect of calcium restriction on renal excretion of oxalate and the probability of stones in the various pathophysiological groups with calcium stones. *J. Urol.* 130:218–223, 1983.

Coe FL: Treated and untreated recurrent calcium nephrolithiasis in patients with idiopathic hypercalciuria, hyperuricosuria, or no metabolic abnormality. *Ann. Intern. Med.* 87:404–410, 1977.

Coe FL: *Nephrolithiasis.* Chicago, Yearbook Medical Publishers, 1978.

Cohanim M, Yendt ER: Prevention of calcium stones with thiazides. *Kidney Int.* 13:397–400, 1978.

Dahlberg PJ, Van Den Berg CJ, Kurtz SB, Wilson DM, Smith LH: Clinical features and management of cystinuria. *Mayo Clin. Proc.* 52:533–540, 1977.

Leppla D, Browne R, Hill K: Effect of amiloride with or without hydrochlorothiazide on urinary calcium and saturation of calcium salts. *J. Clin. Endocrinol. Metab.* 57:920–924, 1983.

Pak CYC, Fuller C: Idiopathic hypocitraturic calcium-oxalate nephrolithiasis successfully treated with potassium citrate. *Ann. Intern. Med.* 104:33–37, 1986.

Pak CYC, Peters P, Hurt G, et al.: Is selective therapy of recurrent nephrolithiasis possible? *Am. J. Med.* 71:615–618, 1981.

Pak CYC, Sakhaee K, Crowther C: Evidence justifying a high fluid intake in treatment of nephrolithiasis. *Ann. Intern. Med.* 93:36–39, 1980.

Robertson WG: Risk factors in calcium stone disease. *In* Brockis G, Findlayson B (eds.): *International Urinary Stone Conference.* Littleton, MA, PSG Publishing Co., 1979.

Thomas WC, Jr.: Use of phosphates in patients with calcareous renal calculi. *Kidney Int.* 13:390–396, 1978.

Williams JJ, Rodman JS, Peterson CW: A randomized double-blind study of acetohydroxamic acid in struvite nephrolithiasis. *N. Engl. J. Med.* 311:760–764, 1984.

Suggested Reading

Coe FL: Uric acid and calcium oxalate nephrolithiasis. *Kidney Int.* 24:392–403, 1983.

Coe FL, Parks JH, Moore ES: Familial idiopathic hypercalciuria. *N. Engl. J. Med.* 300:337–340, 1979.

Earnest DL: Enteric hyperoxaluria. *Adv. Intern. Med.* 24:407–411, 1979.

Gill WB: Renal calculus disease. *Semin. Urol.* 2:1–11, 1984.

Griffith DP: Infection-induced renal calculi. *Kidney Int.* 21:422–430, 1982.

Johnson CM, Wilson DM, O'Fallon WM, Malek RS, Kurland LT: Renal stone epidemiology: A 25-year study in Rochester, Minnesota. *Kidney Int.* 16:624–630, 1979.

Pak CYC, Smith LH, Resnick MI, Weinerth JL: Dietary management of idiopathic calcium urolithiasis. *J. Urol.* 131:850–852, 1984.

Preminger GM, Peterson R, Peters PC, Pak CYC: The current role of medical treatment of nephrolithiasis: The impact of improved techniques of stone removal. *J. Urol.* 134:6–10, 1985.

Their SO, Segal S: Cystinuria. *In* Stanbury JB, Wyngaarden JB, Frederickson DS (eds.): *The Metabolic Basis of Inherited Diseases.* New York, McGraw-Hill Book Co., 1978.

Thomas WC, Jr.: *Renal Calculi: A Guide to Management.* Springfield, IL, Charles C Thomas, Publisher, 1976.

Williams RE: Long-term survey of 538 patients with upper urinary tract stones. *Br. J. Urol.* 35:416–420, 1963.

CHAPTER

22

Renovascular Hypertension

Robert L. Wilburn

Renovascular hypertension is high blood pressure caused by occlusive disease of the aorta or renal arteries. It causes renal ischemia and results in a concatenation of hemodynamic and hormonal aberrations producing sustained systemic hypertension. In the absence of other concurrent causes of the hypertension, correcting the arterial narrowing will normalize blood pressure. Renovascular hypertension is, therefore, one cause of high blood pressure that is curable; thus, it seems appropriate to identify all cases of renovascular hypertension and treat them surgically.

Approximately 35 million people in the United States have sustained hypertension. Screening studies performed in the United States and Great Britain suggest that the prevalence of renovascular hypertension is about 4% of the hypertensive population (Kaufman 1979; Luke et al. 1968). In the United States alone there are over 1 million potentially curable cases of renovascular hypertension. The risk-benefit ratio of the diagnostic tests to screen the 35 million hypertensive patients to find the 4% must be considered. Once the 4% have been identified, decisions must be made among surgical treatment, percutaneous transluminal renal angioplasty, or medical therapy, all of which are becoming increasingly effective.

The clinician must decide who should be screened and what criteria must be met before recommending surgical or renal artery angioplasty intervention. The true cost-benefit ratio is the total cost of screening all potential cases plus the cost of treating those with renovascular hypertension, divided by the number of cases cured. Considering only the cost per individual case with successfully treated renovascular hypertension is not a true cost-benefit ratio. The cumulative risks of diagnostic studies and therapeutic intervention must also be compared to the risks of treating medically without first seeking a possible diagnosis of renovascular hypertension.

Pathophysiology

Of the many etiologies of renovascular hypertension, 60% are caused by atherosclerosis and 35% by fibromuscular dysplasia. The atherosclerotic lesions primarily involve the ostium and proximal one-third of the main renal artery. The left artery is more frequently involved than the right, and these changes are present bilaterally in one-third of the patients. Patients with atherosclerotic lesions are older, and the changes are usually not confined to the renal arteries.

Fibromuscular dysplasia usually involves the middle and distal third of the renal artery and may extend into the primary branches within the kidney. The right side is more frequently affected and the lesions may be bilateral. Fibromuscular dysplasia may be anatomically present in other visceral vessels, but is seldom functionally significant in these sites.

The first physiologic consequence in all cases of renovascular hypertension is an increased release of renin from the ischemic kidney. Renin acts on renin substrate to produce angiotensin I. Angiotensin converting enzyme (ACE) then converts angiotensin I to angiotensin II, a potent vasoconstrictor. Angiotensin II also stimulates the adrenal gland to secrete aldosterone, which causes the kidney to retain sodium, expand the extracellular volume, and increase urinary potassium loss. The expanded extracellular volume may suppress further renin release.

There are two types of renovascular hypertension. In the more common two-kidney model, only one kidney is ischemic and secretes an excess of renin, leading to elevated angiotensin-II levels and hypertension. In this case, the opposite nonischemic kidney responds to the systemic hypertension by diuresing sodium, water, and potassium. There is a net negative sodium balance, slightly contracted extracellular volume, persistent elevation of plasma renin activity, and angiotensin II.

The hypertension is caused by the vasoconstrictive action of angiotensin II, and remains responsive to medications that inhibit the renin-angiotensin system. These medications include: beta-adrenergic blockers that suppress renal renin release; agents such as saralasin that block the action of angiotensin II; and agents that inhibit the action of angiotensin-converting enzyme (ACE inhibitors), thereby reducing the conversion of physiologically inactive angiotensin I to angiotensin II. Diuretics will further aggravate the natriuresis and kaliuresis and further stimulate renin release. Diuretics are, therefore, not successful in controlling hypertension in this condition. Clinical variations of the two-kidney model of renovascular hypertension are unilateral main or segmental renal artery stenosis with a normal contralateral kidney; or a solitary kidney with segmental renal artery stenosis.

The second type of renovascular hypertension is the one-kidney model in which the only functioning kidney is ischemic or in which both kidneys are ischemic. The absence of a nonischemic kidney prevents sodium loss and leads to an expansion of extracellular volume, which then suppresses further renin release. Hypertension persists but is now primarily due to expanded extracellular volume rather than to persistent elevation of angiotensin II. The hypertension may not respond to inhibitors of the renin angiotensin system. Diuretics may contract the extracellular volume, but the hypertension may persist because extracellular volume depletion triggers renin release, leading to production of excessive angiotensin II. The hypertension merely changes from volume dependent to angiotensin dependent.

Clinical variations of the one-kidney model are: bilateral, high-grade main renal artery stenoses; main renal artery stenosis of a solitary kidney; and main renal artery stenosis of one kidney, but with a contralateral kidney unable to respond normally, owing to hypertensive nephrosclerosis or other primary renal parenchymal disease.

Clinical Features

Several clinical features help in diagnosing the 4% of hypertensive patients who have renovascular hypertension. Table 18–1 compares the clinical characteristics of patients with essential hypertension, fibromuscular dysplasia, and atherosclerotic lesions. Typically, the patient with renovascular hypertension due to fibromuscular dysplasia is a young or middle-aged woman with moderate to severe hypertension of recent onset, an epigastric or flank bruit, and minimal evidence of end organ damage. The bruit is holosystolic or may extend into diastole. Short, midsystolic epigastric bruits in a slim person have little clinical significance.

The typical atherosclerotic renovascular hypertensive patient is an older man with a history of mild to moderate hypertension that accelerates to severe levels. End organ damage including hypertensive retinopathy, cardiomegaly, and reduced

Table 22–1 Clinical Characteristics of Renovascular Hypertension Compared to Essential Hypertension

	Essential Hypertension	Fibromuscular Dysplasia	Atherosclerotic RVH
Age at onset (mean)	40	37	53
Duration < 1 year	+	++	++
Family history of hypertension	+++	++	++
Onset >50 years old	–	+	+++
Grade III or IV hypertensive retinopathy	+	–	++
Abdominal bruit	+	+++	++
Reduced GFR (BUN >20 mg/dl; serum creatinine >1.2 mg/dl)	–	–	+
Sex:			
Male	+++	+	+++
Female	++	+++	++

Source: Reproduced, by permission, from Smith MC, Dunn MJ: Renovascular and renal parenchymal hypertension. *In* Brenner BM, Rector FC (eds.): *The Kidney*, 3d. ed. © 1986, W. B. Saunders Co., Philadelphia.

renal function is typical. An abdominal bruit may be present and is often accompanied by carotid and femoral bruits and other clinical evidence of diffuse atherosclerotic disease.

A patient with severe, hard-to-control hypertension, especially if it is associated with decreasing renal function, should be studied. The onset of hypertension before puberty or after the age of 50 suggests renovascular hypertension, especially if it progresses quickly to severe levels and is associated with an abdominal bruit.

Diagnostic Studies

Although renovascular hypertension may be clinically suspected, it cannot be confirmed without specific diagnostic tests. If demonstration of a renal artery stenosis in a patient with hypertension established a diagnosis of surgically curable renovascular hypertension, then the only test required would be a renal angiogram. Unfortunately, finding a renal artery stenosis does not prove a causal relationship with the hypertension nor accurately predict that correcting the stenosis will normalize the blood pressure. Moderate and severe renal artery stenoses have been found in 32% and 17%, respectively, of unselected autopsy series without premortem hypertension (Holley et al. 1964). To prove the stenosis is causing the hypertension, tests must be done that demonstrate the functional state of the kidneys as well as the anatomy.

The clinician needs screening tests to evaluate those hypertensive patients in whom renovascular hypertension is highly suspected. If the screening tests are positive, confirming tests are necessary before selecting therapy.

Excretory Urogram (IVP)

Although the rapid-sequence IVP is a widely used screening test for renovascular hypertension, there is controversy regarding its usefulness. The Cooperative Study of Renovascular Hypertension evaluated the IVP in 2,442 patients, 179 of whom were surgically proven to have renovascular hypertension. The IVP gave an 11.4% false-positive rate in essential hypertension and a 16.7% false-negative rate in renovascular hypertension (Bookstein et al. 1972; Thornbury et al. 1982). Other studies have found false-positive results as high as 45% and false-negative results as high as 42%.

The IVP is an unreliable predictor of surgical result; only 60% to 75% of patients with a positive IVP will benefit from surgery. IVP interpretation depends in part on comparison between ischemic and normal kidney, which can be misleading in bilateral disease. Therefore, many clinicians no longer use the IVP for hypertensive screening; a positive result does not justify surgery without an angiogram, nor is a negative result evidence to discontinue testing if clinical circumstances are highly suggestive of renovascular hypertension.

The conventional radionuclide renogram approximates the IVP results and offers no significant advantage over it either as a screening test or as a predictor of surgical result.

Peripheral Plasma Renin Activity

Although it seems that peripheral plasma renin activity (PRA) would be elevated in the two-kidney model and in the one-kidney model, provided the patient was extracellular volume depleted, clinical experience has not shown peripheral PRA to be a reliable test for either screening or predicting surgical response. To maximize the usefulness of peripheral PRA, the patient should be free of all antihypertensive medication, and the PRA results must be indexed with 24-hr urinary sodium excretion in a stable state. Even so, the results are discouraging. In Kaufman's experience at the University of California at Los Angeles, the peripheral PRA was increased in only 56% of patients with renovascular hypertension and gave false positive results in 15% of those with essential hypertension (Kaufman 1979). The false-negative rate for peripheral PRA was greater than that for renal venous renin ratio, rapid sequence IVP, or saralasin testing. This undoubtedly reflects the influence of multiple factors controlling renin release.

Renal Vein Renins

A normal nonischemic kidney secretes renin, and the plasma renin activity of the renal vein will normally be about 25% greater than the renin activity of the renal artery. Plasma renin activity of the inferior vena cava below the renal veins will be equal to the plasma renin activity of the renal artery, because there is no significant renin addition or subtraction in the lower extremities. Therefore, by measuring renin activity in the inferior vena cava below the renal veins and from both renal veins, one can assess the relative contribution of renin from both kidneys. It is important to sample from near the iliac vein confluence to avoid an accessory circumaortic left renal vein joining the inferior vena cava.

Normally, renal vein renin activity would be about 25% greater than the inferior vena cava sample and equal in both renal veins. With the two-kidney model, one kidney is ischemic and has increased renin secretion while the other kidney is suppressed and may secrete no renin. This will result in a renin activity from the ischemic kidney that is 50% greater than that from the inferior vena cava, and a renin activity from the contralateral kidney equal to that from the inferior vena cava. The ratio of renin activity from the ischemic kidney to the contralateral nonischemic kidney will therefore be 1.5 or greater.

Virtually all studies have confirmed that a renin activity ratio of 1.5 or greater comparing the kidney with the renal artery stenosis to the normal contralateral kidney will predict response to surgical or renal artery angioplasty relief of the stenosis in over 90% of patients. A nonlateralizing ratio (less than 1.5), however, does not always preclude surgical cure. False-negative rates range from 30% to 80%. The false-negative rate may be minimized by careful attention to the conditions under which the test is performed.

The sensitivity of the test may be increased by: stimulating renin secretion with passive tilting of the patient to the semi-upright position to create mild relative hypotension at the time the samples are obtained; reducing blood pressure with diazoxide or hydralazine; or by inducing acute extracellular volume depletion by diuretic administration. The patient should not be studied while extracellular volume is expanded or while taking antihypertensive medications that suppress renal renin release. Ideally, sampling of venous blood for renin levels should be performed while the patient is hypertensive, taking no medications except those specifically given acutely to stimulate renin release and in a slightly depleted volume state. However, it is not always possible or safe to create ideal circumstances, and the clinician must take these factors into consideration when interpreting the results.

In the case of segmental renal artery stenosis, increased renin release from the ischemic segment of the kidney may be offset by suppression of renin release from the nonischemic segment of the same kidney; thus, renin activity measured in the main renal vein may fail to detect any lateralization. If the arteriogram shows segmental lesions, then venous samples must be obtained from the suspected ischemic segment and the nonischemic segment as well as the main renal veins on both sides and the inferior vena cava below the renal veins.

Angiography

Demonstration of the renal artery stenosis remains a requirement in all cases for definitive diagnosis. Given the problems with screening tests, many clinicians have suggested that angiography should be the first test for patients in whom renovascular hypertension is suspected clinically. If no renal artery stenosis is found, further evaluation is unnecessary. If a stenosis is found, a clinical decision must be made as to whether further testing is needed.

Not all renal artery stenoses cause renovascular hypertension. The best confirming test remains the renal vein renin test. This is especially true in cases of the two-kidney model where one renal artery is stenotic and the artery to the other kidney is normal. Even in bilateral renal artery stenosis, renal vein renins are useful to assess the relative ischemia of each side, and serve as a guide to which side should be corrected first. If a sequence of renal films, as well as delayed films, is taken in conjunction with the angiogram, additional information – such as renal size, time until visualization of the caliceal system, and evidence of delayed hyperconcentration – is available. These observations give indirect assessment of the functional state of the kidneys.

Angiography is required to demonstrate not only the renal artery stenosis but the location, extent of the disease, and degree of obstruction, as well as to distinguish fibromuscular dysplasia from atherosclerotic disease. If atherosclerotic disease is found, then the angiographer must obtain oblique views to assess the extent the disease involves the aorta and aorto-iliac system. The clinician, vascular surgeon, and interventional radiologist can then plan appropriate therapy.

When the patient undergoes angiography, certain factors need to be considered in advance. The clinician must have done a complete medical evaluation not only concerning the hypertension but of all cardiovascular disease and general health. Treatment of certain lesions such as carotid artery stenosis and coronary artery disease takes precedence over normalizing blood pressure. If unstable angina is present, it must be medically controlled or surgically treated before angiography is attempted. If high-grade carotid stenosis is present, it may be necessary to correct it before lowering the blood pressure.

The patient must have been advised of the problem and of all therapy options. The clinician and radiologist must have agreed whether the arteriogram is to be diagnostic only or, if a suitable lesion is found, whether to proceed at once to renal angioplasty. If angioplasty is contemplated, then the patient must be prepared for surgical intervention in the event of complications. If a lesion is found that is to be treated surgically, the surgeon should be available to review the case with the clinician and radiologist while the procedure is in progress.

Therapy

Renovascular hypertension may be treated with antihypertensive medications or by correcting the renal artery stenosis either by percutaneous transluminal angioplasty or by surgery. The treatment for each patient must take into account the following factors: 1) etiology of the stenosis; 2) location and severity of the lesion; 3) other cardiovascular risk factors and lesions; 4) general health and life expectancy; 5) renal function; 6) severity of hypertension and response to medical therapy, including not only ability to control blood pressure but to preserve renal function.

Medical therapy using combinations of diuretics, beta-blockers, angiotensin converting enzyme inhibitors, and arteriolar dilators can control the blood pressure in 75% to 80% of patients with renovascular hypertension. Normalizing blood pressure with antihypertensive medication may not preserve renal function, however, because lowering renal perfusion pressure across a remaining stenosis may compromise renal function and even precipitate complete thrombosis of the renal artery. Angiotensin converting enzyme inhibition may further compromise intraglomerular hemodynamics and reduce filtration fraction and glomerular filtration rate, particularly with bilateral renal artery stenosis.

Surgical therapy of renovascular hypertension has progressed during the past decades from simple nephrectomy, to in situ revascularization procedures, to the use of ex vivo microsurgical techniques performed under hypothermic conditions. In a review of six published series from 1975 to 1981, which included 885 patients treated by current surgical and anesthetic techniques, 52% were cured and 32% were improved (Smith, Dunn 1986). Fifteen percent failed to improve, and a 2% mortality occurred. These series included patients with both atherosclerotic and fibromuscular lesions. The cure rate for fibromuscular hyperplasia is better than for atherosclerosis.

Renal angioplasty offers the opportunity to ablate renal artery stenosis with less expense, risk, pain, hospitalization, and recovery time than surgical treatment in selected patients, particularly those with fibromuscular dysplasia.

Conclusion

We now have the technical ability to diagnose all cases of renovascular hypertension. Treatment options include surgery or percutaneous transluminal angioplasty to correct the stenosis and cure the hypertension or antihypertensive drugs to control it. The challenge is to use this ability in the most cost-effective manner and to minimize the risk-to-benefit ratio.

References

Bookstein JJ, Abrams HL, Buenger RE, et al.: Radiologic aspects of renovascular hypertension. Part 2. The role of urography in unilateral renovascular disease. *J.A.M.A.* 220:1225–1230, 1972.

Holley KE, Hunt JC, Brown AL, et al.: Renal artery stenosis: A clinical-pathologic study in normotensive and hypertensive patients. *Am. J. Med.* 37:14–22, 1964.

Kaufman JJ: Renovascular hypertension: The UCLA experience. *J. Urol.* 121:139–144, 1979.

Luke RG, Kennedy AC, Briggs JD, et al.: Results of surgery in hypertension due to renal artery stenosis. *Br. Med. J.* 2:76–80, 1968.

Smith MC, Dunn MJ: Renovascular and renal parenchymal hypertension. *In* Brenner BM, Rector FC (eds.): *The Kidney,* 3d. ed. Philadelphia, W. B. Saunders Co., 1986, pp. 1221–1251.

Thornbury JR, Stanley JC, Fryback DC: Hypertensive urogram: A nondiscriminatory test for renovascular hypertension. *Am. J. Roentgenol.* 138:43–49, 1982.

Suggested Reading

Franklin S: Renovascular hypertension. *In* Massrey SA, Glassock RJ (eds.): *Textbook of Nephrology,* vol. 2. Baltimore, Williams & Wilkins, 1983, pp. 6383–6388.

Franklin SF: Renovascular hypertension. *In* Glassock RJ (ed.): *Current Therapy in Nephrology and Hypertension, 1984–1985.* Philadelphia, B. C. Decker, 1984.

Hunt JC, Strong CG: Renovascular hypertension. Mechanisms, natural history and treatment. *In* Laragh JH (ed.): *Hypertension Manual,* 1st ed. New York, Yorke Medical Books. Dun-Donnelley Publishing Co., 1974.

Simon N, Franklin SS, Bleifer KH, et al.: Clinical characteristics of renovascular hypertension. *J.A.M.A.* 220:1209–1218, 1972.

Tuck M, Stern N, Sowers J: Hypertension. *In* Gonick HC (ed.): *Current Nephrology,* vol. 9. Chicago, Yearbook Medical Publishers, 1986, pp. 272–275.

CHAPTER
23
Percutaneous Transluminal Renal Angioplasty

Thomas J. Kofler and Charles J. Tegtmeyer

Approximately 40–50 million people in the United States have hypertension. Of this group, 2 million have potentially correctable renovascular hypertension. These patients are also susceptible to progressive renal ischemia.

Treatment with long-term medical therapy or surgical revascularization has significant shortcomings. Drugs may only partially control blood pressure, and the side-effects may deter patients from using them (Dollery, Bulpitt 1977; Genest et al. 1977; Youngberg 1977). If the renal artery is severely stenosed, lowering the blood pressure with medication will further reduce renal blood flow to the kidney and may cause ischemic atrophy or renal infarction. Many patients are poor risks for surgical revascularization because of severe diffuse atherosclerotic disease or renal insufficiency. The mortality rate for surgery is currently 1%–2% (Smith, Dunn 1986).

As an alternative to these traditional modes of treatment, percutaneous transluminal renal angioplasty (PTRA) was first introduced by Gruentzig et al. in 1978. Since that time, the procedure has been a highly successful treatment for renovascular hypertension (Colapinto et al. 1982; Geyskes et al. 1983; Martin et al. 1985; Schwarten 1981; Sos et al. 1983; Tegtmeyer et al. 1980, 1984). In addition to the therapeutic benefits, angioplasty offers significant cost advantages over either a lifelong course of antihypertensive medications or renovascular surgery.

Dotter and Judkins (1964), in their original work, attributed the effectiveness of angioplasty to the redistribution and compressibility of the atheromatous plaque. More recent studies, however, have shown that the atherosclerotically altered intima is relatively incompressible (Block et al. 1980; Castaneda-Zuniga et al. 1980). Examination of cadaver and animal models demonstrates that angioplasty produces a controlled injury in the vessel wall (Wellons et al. 1981).

When the balloon is inflated across an atherosclerotic stenosis, fracturing or splitting of the plaque occurs first. After the plaque is fractured, there may be fissuring of the atherosclerotic intima and stretching or splitting of the media. This is seen as an intramural linear collection of contrast material at the dilatation site. The immediate effect of angioplasty is a mechanical increase in the vessel diameter, which is maintained by the patient's blood pressure and blood flow.

Following the controlled injury to the vessel wall, smooth muscle cells within the media begin to disintegrate. Macrophages clear damaged cells from the area and fibroblasts begin repair of the damaged artery; a neointima is formed. These changes are similar to the healing process following surgical endarterectomy. Most of the healing occurs during the first few days after dilatation; however, complete repair of the vessel usually requires 4 to 6 weeks.

Technique

Since Gruentzig et al. 1978 introduction of percutaneous transluminal renal angioplasty, the technique has been refined (Tegtmeyer et al. 1981; Tegtmeyer et al. 1980). However, it remains more complex than peripheral angioplasty, and should only be performed by angiographers who have had considerable experience dilating peripheral vessels. Martin and colleagues (1986) had a significant increase in success rate and a decrease in complications with their second 100 renal angioplasties as

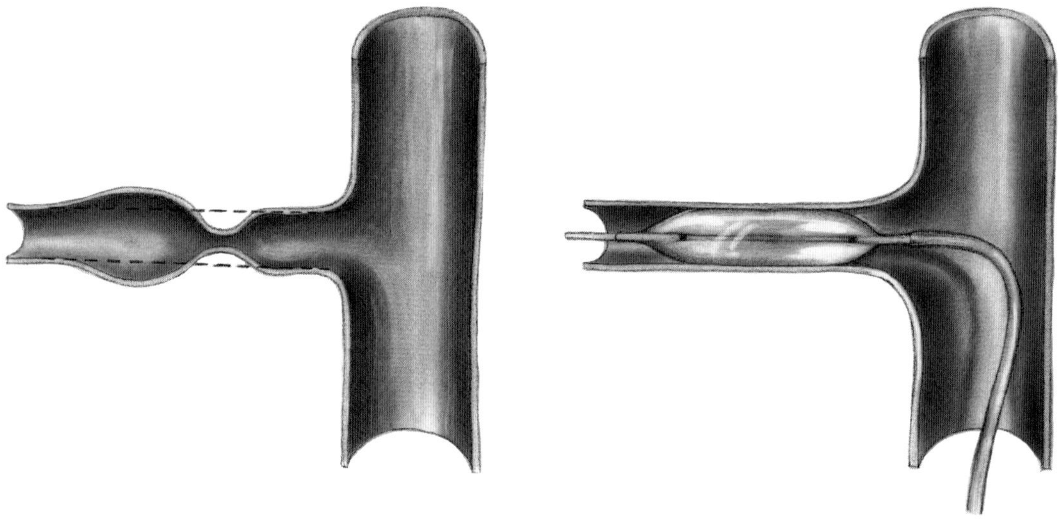

23–1 Determining the size of balloon catheter. Balloon catheter is selected to correspond to original diameter of renal artery. Poststenotic dilatation must be taken into account. Renal arteries are magnified by 15%–20% on standard angiograms; therefore, arteries will be overdilated intentionally by approximately 1 mm.

compared to their first 100 cases.

Before performing angioplasty, a high-quality midstream cut-film aortogram is necessary to evaluate the patient's vascular anatomy (Tegtmeyer, Sos 1986). Digital subtraction arteriography may be helpful prior to the midstream aortogram to determine proper obliquity for demonstrating the origins of the renal arteries, but at least one standard film series is necessary. The newer low-osmolar contrast material should probably be used in patients with renal insufficiency. If an abdominal aortogram has been done previously, but more than a month has elapsed, a repeat arteriogram should always be obtained because significant changes in the vessels may occur.

Balloon Selection

Inflation of the balloon across a stenosis provides almost a pure radial force. Since there is no axial component of force once the balloon is in place, the chance of distal embolization is reduced. The artery to be dilated and the balloon catheter are thin-walled, somewhat elastic cylinders. Forces on a thin-walled cylinder are governed by the Law of Laplace, which states that all tension (T) is equal to the internal pressure (P) multiplied by the internal radius (R): $T = P \times R$. Therefore, increasing the radius of the balloon increases the tension on the lesion. If the balloon is undersized for the stenosis, very little force will be applied to the lesion, no matter how much pressure is applied to the balloon.

Balloon size is determined by the original size of the artery in the area of the stenosis. This is obtained by measuring the diameter of the artery proximal and distal to the stenosis, and correcting for poststenotic enlargement or dilatation. If the estimated original diameter at the stenosis is 5 mm, a 5-mm diameter balloon is used (Fig. 23–1). Intentionally, this does not take into account the magnification factor created during the radiography; therefore, the artery will be overdilated by approximately 20%.

Patients normally experience flank or abdominal pain during balloon inflation. However, the pain diminishes almost immediately following balloon deflation and usually disappears completely within a minute. If the patient experiences severe pain during inflation, the balloon should be deflated immediately; if the pain disappears rapidly, it is safe to reinflate the balloon or use a smaller one. Intense pain continuing after balloon deflation is often associated with severe renal artery injury such as rupture or occlusion.

On the other hand, if the patient does not feel any discomfort during inflation and a plaque indentation on the balloon persists, the angioplasty balloon was too small. If the plaque indentation on the balloon reappears during deflation, or a residual stenosis is seen with a test injection of contrast material, a repeat dilatation with a larger balloon should be performed. Renal artery

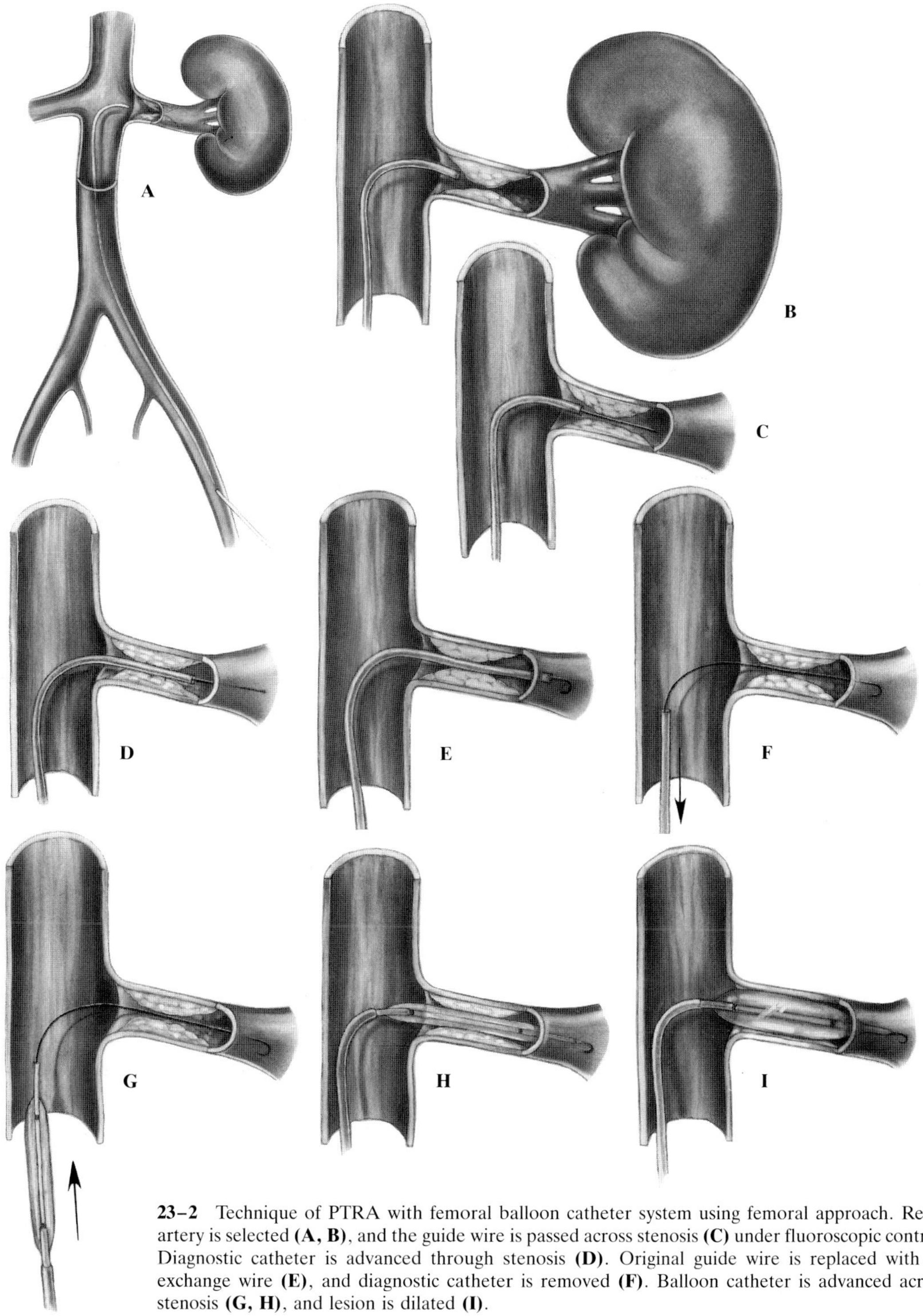

23–2 Technique of PTRA with femoral balloon catheter system using femoral approach. Renal artery is selected **(A, B)**, and the guide wire is passed across stenosis **(C)** under fluoroscopic control. Diagnostic catheter is advanced through stenosis **(D)**. Original guide wire is replaced with an exchange wire **(E)**, and diagnostic catheter is removed **(F)**. Balloon catheter is advanced across stenosis **(G, H)**, and lesion is dilated **(I)**.

stenosis is more likely to recur when a 30% residual stenosis remains after dilatation (Sos et al. 1983; Tegtmeyer et al. 1981; Tegtmeyer et al. 1984).

Crossing the Stenosis

The guide wire and catheter must remain intraluminal when crossing the lesion. This requires careful technique and high-resolution fluoroscopy. Digital subtraction angiography and magnification fluoroscopy are also helpful.

The initial crossing of the lesion should be performed with as little trauma as possible (Fig. 23–2). With the tip of the catheter in the renal artery proximal to the stenosis, a 0.89-mm

(0.035-in.) diameter long-tapered, tight-curved (2-mm) J guide wire is advanced beyond the stenosis into the renal artery. When using a J guide wire, it is important to form the J tip before the wire is in contact with the lesion. If the stenosis is too tight to allow the J wire to pass easily, align the catheter tip so that it approximates the center of the stenosis; this can be checked with small injections of contrast media. A straight Bentson wire or the Terumo Glidewire® with a flexible tip can then be negotiated through the stenosis. When a slight curve is needed at the tip, the wire can be shaped by drawing it between the tip of the index finger and the thumbnail. If the Bentson wire fails to cross the lesion, other guide wires may be tried. The 0.36-mm to 0.46-mm (0.014-in. to 0.018-in.) floppy platinum-tipped steerable guide wire, as is used for tibial and coronary angioplasty, can be tried by itself or in a coaxial combination with a 0.89-mm (0.035-in.) injectable guide wire.

Another helpful technique is to gently advance an appropriate-shaped 5-F diagnostic catheter across the stenosis while simultaneously injecting contrast material. The steady flow of contrast material keeps the tip away from the wall and delineates the lumen of the vessel. If the catheter is advanced slowly, difficult lesions can often be crossed. Patients can vary their depth of inspiration and expiration to alter the craniocaudal direction of the renal artery, or can be asked to cough, which may help advance the guide wire through difficult stenoses. A combination of these maneuvers is often necessary to cross long fibromuscular lesions.

Dilatation

Once the diagnostic catheter has crossed the stenosis, 2,000–5,000 U of heparin and 2.5 mg of the calcium-channel blocker verapamil are injected intra-arterially through the catheter. Verapamil is used to prevent vessel spasm induced by the guide wire or catheter. It is not used, however, if the patient has cardiac contraindications. A guide wire is then selected so that the diagnostic catheter can be exchanged for an appropriate balloon catheter. To avoid injuring the vessel wall during the exchange, a guide wire with a flexible tip is used. The guide wire should be stiff enough throughout most of its length to facilitate passing the balloon catheter through the lesion.

Two basic exchange wires are used: a 0.89-mm (0.035-in.) heavy-duty movable-core 1.5-mm J wire with the core withdrawn 1–2 cm, or a 0.89-mm (0.035 in.) 1.5-mm J-tipped Rosen wire. If the 7-F balloon catheter cannot be passed through the lesion owing to the tightness of the stenosis, initial dilatation with a smaller 4.5-F or 5-F shaft catheter having a 2–4 mm diameter balloon may be helpful. These smaller balloons have a low profile and are ideal for crossing tight or resistant stenoses. The stenosis is then partially dilated by inflating the balloon; the smaller balloon catheter is exchanged for a 7-F catheter with a larger balloon.

After the balloon tip has been placed beyond the stenosis, a Y-adapter is connected to the catheter hub and a 0.64-mm (0.025-in.) 1.5-mm J guide wire is inserted through the catheter, allowing the guide wire to remain in place. Contrast media can be injected through the Y-adapter to monitor progress of the dilatation while the guide wire remains in position across the lesion.

The balloon catheter is placed across the lesion and inflated with a device designed for that catheter or a syringe with a pressure gauge attached. Initially, the balloon is partially inflated to 2 atm of pressure to determine the position of the balloon relative to the stenosis. Once the balloon has been properly positioned, it is inflated with 4–6 atm of pressure. It may be necessary to inflate the balloon several times for 30–60 sec each time. The amount of indentation of the plaque on the balloon during the inflation and deflation is an indication of the progress of the dilatation. When there is little or no indentation of the balloon by the lesion, the balloon is carefully withdrawn over the 0.64-mm (0.025-in.) wire, and contrast material is injected to assess the results of the angioplasty. If further dilatation is necessary, the balloon catheter can be advanced over the wire again. The results are immediately documented with a midstream aortogram using a pigtail catheter.

Specific Catheter Approaches

Five different percutaneous angiographic approaches can be used to treat stenoses or occlusions of the renal artery:

1. Femoral balloon catheter system – femoral approach
2. Femoral balloon catheter system – axillary approach

3. Femoral balloon catheter system – femoral sidewinder approach
4. Guided coaxial balloon catheter system
5. Kissing balloon technique

Femoral Balloon Catheter System – Femoral Approach

The femoral approach uses a 5-F or 7-F double lumen balloon catheter originally designed by Gruentzig for peripheral angioplasty (Fig. 23–2). These catheters are available with balloons having 4-mm, 5-mm, 6-mm, 7-mm, and 8-mm diameters and several balloon lengths. The 2-cm-long balloon is used in renal angioplasty, since it is usually long enough to straddle the lesion without causing unnecessary damage to the adjacent normal portions of the vessel. In pediatric cases or in patients with small renal arteries, the 4.5-F or 5-F balloon catheter system should be used.

The femoral artery is punctured and the appropriate 5-F diagnostic catheter is advanced into the abdominal aorta using the Seldinger technique. The orifice of the renal artery is carefully selected, and the lesion is crossed and dilated according to the techniques described earlier.

Only catheters with a tightly wrapped, low-profile balloon located close to the tip of the catheter should be used in the renal arteries. To facilitate passage of the balloon through a tight stenosis, the balloon should not be test inflated first. A primary advantage of this technique is that only a 5-F or 7-F puncture in the femoral artery is necessary. If the severity of the stenosis permits easy passage of the 5-F diagnostic catheter, this is the simplest approach. However, if the stenosis is tight or if the renal artery branches from the aorta at an acute angle, it is often difficult to cross the stenosis, and the catheter has a tendency to buckle in the aorta when axial force is applied. If predilatation with the 5-F diagnostic catheter, tapered Van Andel catheter, or mini-balloon catheter does not permit successful crossing of the stenosis, the axillary or femoral sidewinder approach may be necessary.

Femoral Balloon Catheter System – Axillary Approach

The axillary approach may also be used to dilate the renal arteries (Tegtmeyer et al. 1980) (Fig. 23–3). When the renal arteries originate from the aorta at a sharp caudal angle, the axillary approach simplifies the procedure. The stenotic renal artery is easily entered via the axillary approach with either a multipurpose or a cobra-shaped catheter. Once the guide wire is in place across the lesion, the dilatation catheter has a natural tendency to follow the gentle downward curve of the guide wire across the stenosis. The patient facilitates passage of the guide wire and the catheter across the stenosis by taking a deep breath. The axillary approach is also useful when severe atherosclerotic disease or bypass grafts are present in the pelvic or abdominal vessels.

This technique also uses the 5-F or 7-F double-lumen balloon catheter designed by Gruentzig for superficial femoral artery angioplasty. A left axillary approach is selected, because this is the straightest approach to the descending thoracic aorta. When the right axillary approach is attempted, the balloon catheter tends to buckle in the ascending thoracic aorta.

There is an increased risk of damage to the smaller axillary artery; however, this can be minimized by deflating the balloon and rotating it carefully during insertion and removal. The possibility of brachial plexus injury from hematoma in the axillary sheath can be decreased by using the high brachial approach in which the brachial artery is entered just below the axillary crease. Bleeding from the artery is easier to control in this area because it can be compressed against the humerus, thereby decreasing the chances of hematoma formation and brachial plexus injury. The serious complication of dislodging atherosclerotic plaque material from the subclavian artery into the left vertebral artery during catheter manipulations must be considered in patients with severe generalized atherosclerotic disease; in these patients the axillary approach should be avoided if possible.

Femoral Balloon Catheter System – Femoral Sidewinder Approach

The femoral sidewinder approach combines the advantages of the femoral and axillary approaches and is the technique the authors use in the majority of cases (Fig. 23–4). The femoral artery is used for catheter insertion, and the renal artery is approached in a manner that takes advantage of the

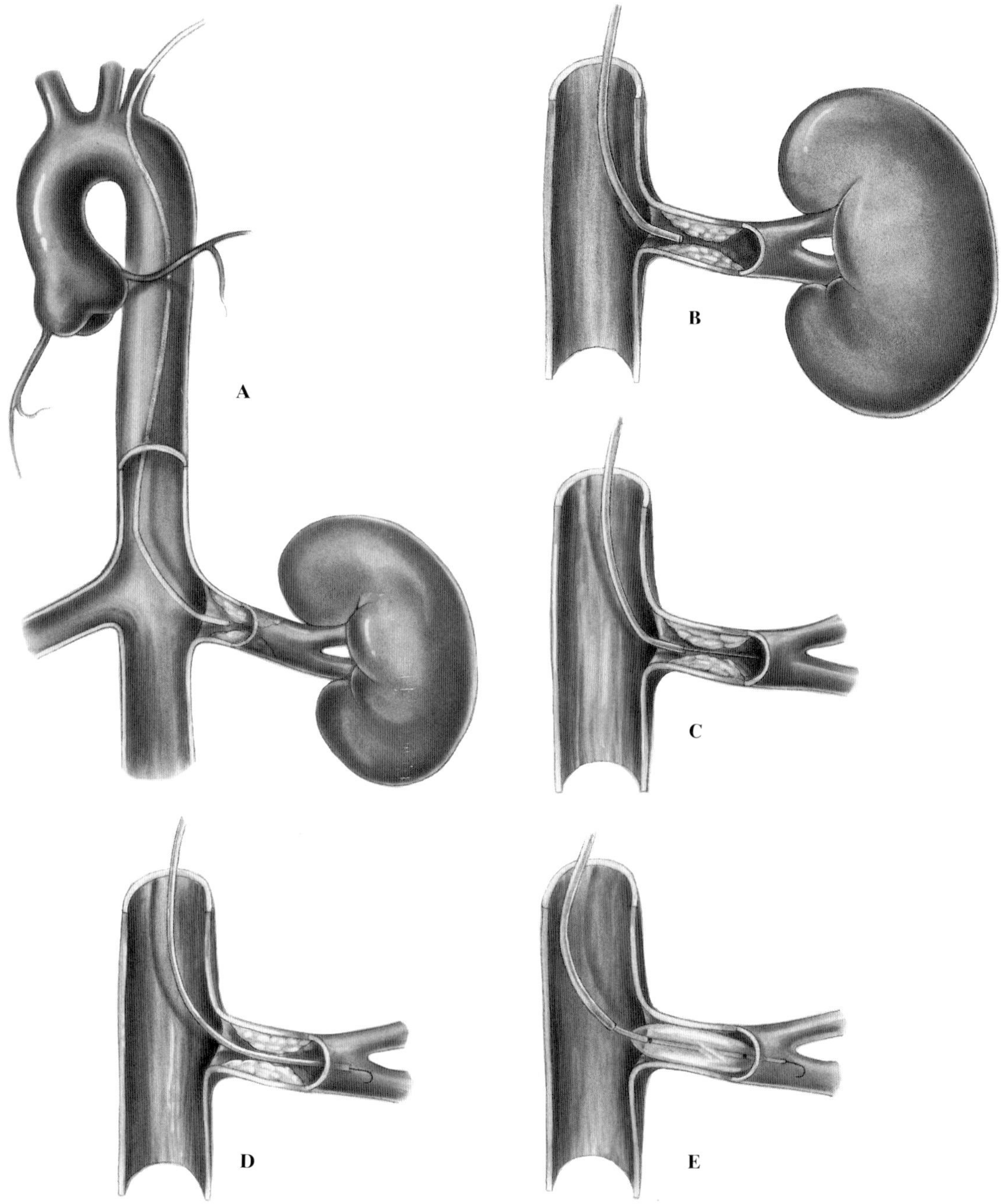

23–3 Technique of PTRA with femoral balloon catheter system using axillary approach. Renal artery is selected **(A, B)** and guide wire is carefully passed across stenosis **(C)**. Diagnostic catheter is advanced across lesion and guide wire is replaced with an exchange wire **(D)**. Diagnostic catheter is exchanged for balloon catheter and lesion is dilated **(E)**.

natural downward curve of the renal artery by using a 5-F shepherd's crook catheter or a sidewinder catheter (Grable, Smith 1980; Sos 1981; Tegtmeyer 1977; Tegtmeyer et al. 1984). The catheter is carefully advanced across the lesion under fluoroscopic control as contrast material is injected to keep the tip within the lumen of the artery; or a flexible tip guide wire is advanced across the stenosis followed by the catheter.

The major advantage of this technique is that the shepherd's crook catheter tip is advanced across the stenosis by withdrawing the catheter at the femoral puncture site. Considerable downward force at the catheter tip can be generated by

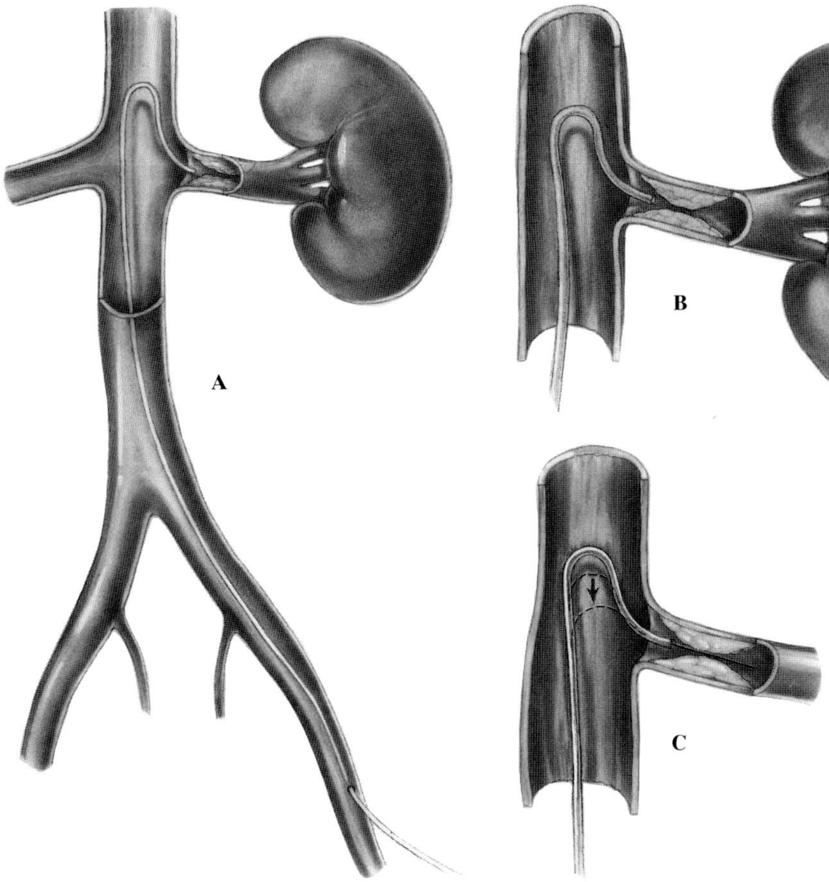

23–4 Technique of PTRA with femoral balloon catheter system using sidewinder approach. Renal artery is selected **(A, B)**. Guide wire is passed across lesion and catheter is advanced over guide wire by withdrawing the catheter at the puncture site **(C)**. Guide wire is replaced with an exchange wire. Catheter is exchanged for a balloon catheter and lesion is dilated.

this mechanism, and this technique helps traverse tight stenoses or complete occlusions. However, because large forces can be generated at the catheter tip; great care must be taken to keep the catheter tip intraluminal.

Once the catheter has crossed the stenosis, the dilatation is performed as described earlier, using an exchange wire with a 5-F or 7-F Gruentzig balloon-type catheter.

Guided Coaxial Balloon Catheter System

The guided coaxial balloon catheter system uses an 8-F or 9-F renal guiding catheter and a 4.3-F or 4.5-F coaxial balloon catheter (Fig. 23–5). The large guiding catheter is inserted through the femoral approach, and the tip is positioned at the orifice of the renal artery. The small coaxial catheter is then passed through the guiding catheter and across the stenosis. The small balloon catheter will accept a 0.36-mm or 0.46-mm (0.014-in. or 0.018-in.) platinum-tipped steerable guide wire that is highly visible at fluoroscopy; it is passed across the stenosis prior to advancing the balloon catheter. This fine steerable guide wire greatly facilitates passage of the balloon catheter in the presence of a tortuous renal vessel, a tight stenosis, or a stenosis in a branch. If the stenosis is not too tight, the smaller coaxial catheter can be advanced across the stenosis without the guide wire while a small amount of contrast material is being injected.

Advantages of this technique are that the small coaxial balloon catheter passes through a tight stenosis more readily than the usual 7-F balloon catheter, and it is easier to steer this catheter into the branches of the renal artery. Therefore, this catheter system is usually used in the renal arteries in the presence of a very tight stenosis that cannot be passed by other techniques, or in the treatment of distal or branch stenoses.

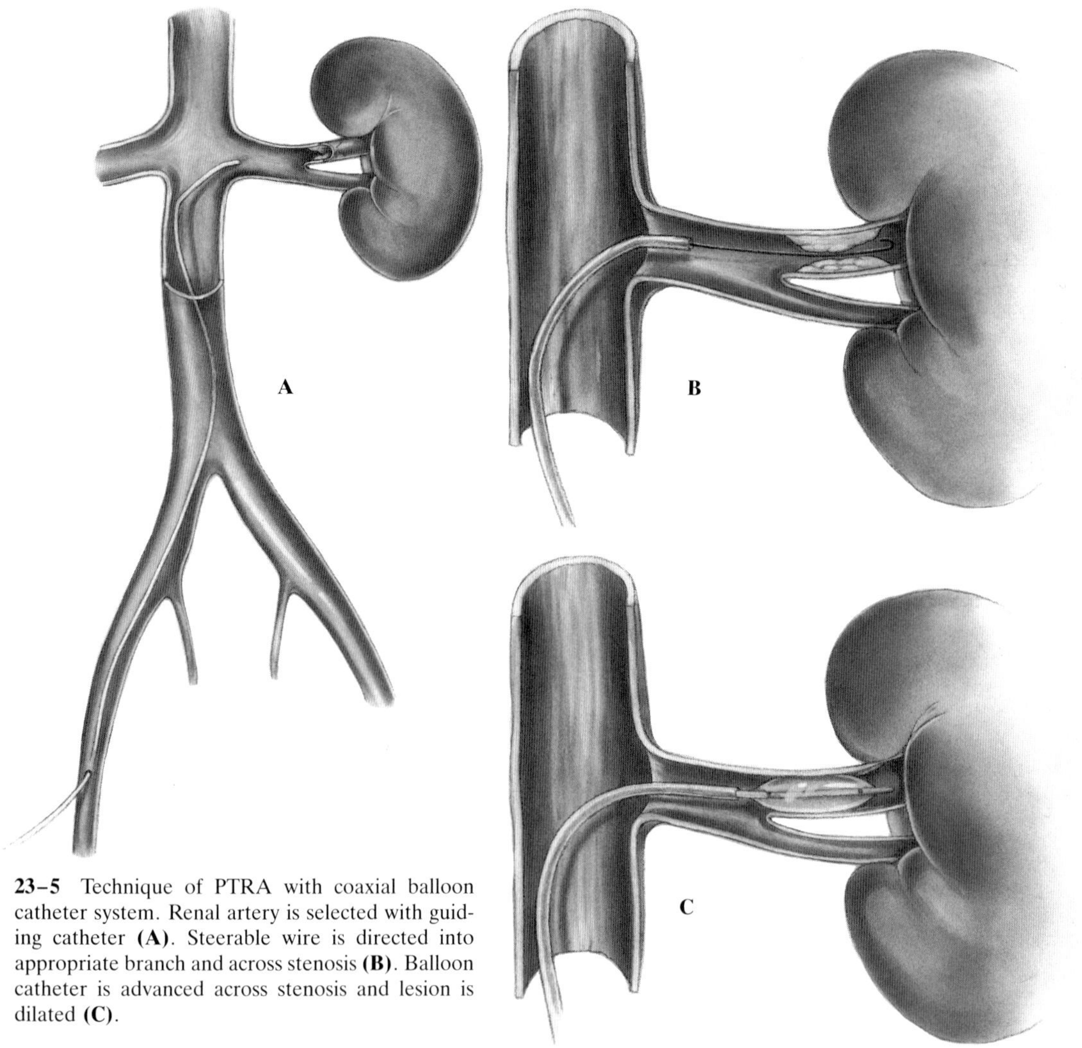

23–5 Technique of PTRA with coaxial balloon catheter system. Renal artery is selected with guiding catheter **(A)**. Steerable wire is directed into appropriate branch and across stenosis **(B)**. Balloon catheter is advanced across stenosis and lesion is dilated **(C)**.

The disadvantages to this technique are that it is necessary to make an 8-F or 9-F puncture wound in the femoral artery; and the stiff guiding catheter is inserted over a 1.60-mm (0.063-in.) guide wire, both of which may injure the aortic wall. Balloon sizes are available from 2 mm to 4.2 mm. However, if an 8-F guiding catheter system is used, the balloon diameter is limited to less than 3 mm.

The technique is also more complex than with the standard femoral balloon catheter approach, thereby increasing the risk of complication. The common femoral artery is punctured and a two-part sheath is introduced over a 0.92-mm (0.038-in.) guide wire. The sheath is advanced into the distal abdominal aorta. Once the sheath is in place, the inner cannula is removed and the 1.60-mm (0.063-in.) guide wire is advanced into the abdominal aorta to the level of the diaphragm. The guiding catheter is then advanced over the guide wire through this sheath and into the abdominal aorta. The guide wire is removed, and the guiding catheter is used to select the renal artery orifice. The smaller balloon catheter is then advanced coaxially through the guiding catheter and across the stenosis. Progress can be monitored by injecting contrast material through the guiding catheter, which at times is advantageous, but caution should be exercised when injecting contrast material in the area of the dilatation because of the injury to the intima.

An alternative technique for dilatation of smaller vessels or tight stenoses uses a 4.5-F balloon catheter in a way similar to the femoral balloon catheter system. A 5-F arterial sheath is placed in the femoral artery, and a 5-F selective catheter is then used to enter the proximal renal artery. A 0.36-mm to 0.46-mm (0.014-in. to 0.018-in.) heavy-duty rigid guide wire with a 4-cm long floppy steerable platinum tip can be used to cross the stenosis initially. The 5-F diagnostic catheter is then removed and exchanged for a 4.5-F angioplasty balloon catheter, which is advanced into the renal artery over the guide wire. The advantage of this technique is that only a 5-F puncture is necessary in the femoral artery, and manipulation of the 8-F or 9-F rigid guiding catheter is avoided. The major disadvantage is that relatively little axial force can be generated to advance the small catheters over the small guide wire through the lesion.

Kissing Balloon Technique

This technique, which was originally described for dilating lesions at the bifurcation of the abdominal aorta, has application in selected cases in the renal arteries (Baker et al. 1986; Tegtmeyer et al. 1985). If two renal arteries originate from the aorta in close proximity, or if the lesion involves a major bifurcation of the renal artery (Fig. 23–6A), dilating only one vessel or using only a single dilating catheter may occlude the adjacent vessel. In this situation, a catheter is inserted through each femoral artery; one catheter is passed across one artery or branch to protect it while the stenotic lesion is dilated with the balloon catheter (Fig. 23–6B). The origin of the uninvolved branch is usually protected by the diagnostic catheter (Fig. 23–6C). If the origin of this vessel is also involved by the lesion or compromised by the procedure, a second balloon catheter is used for it and this lesion is dilated also.

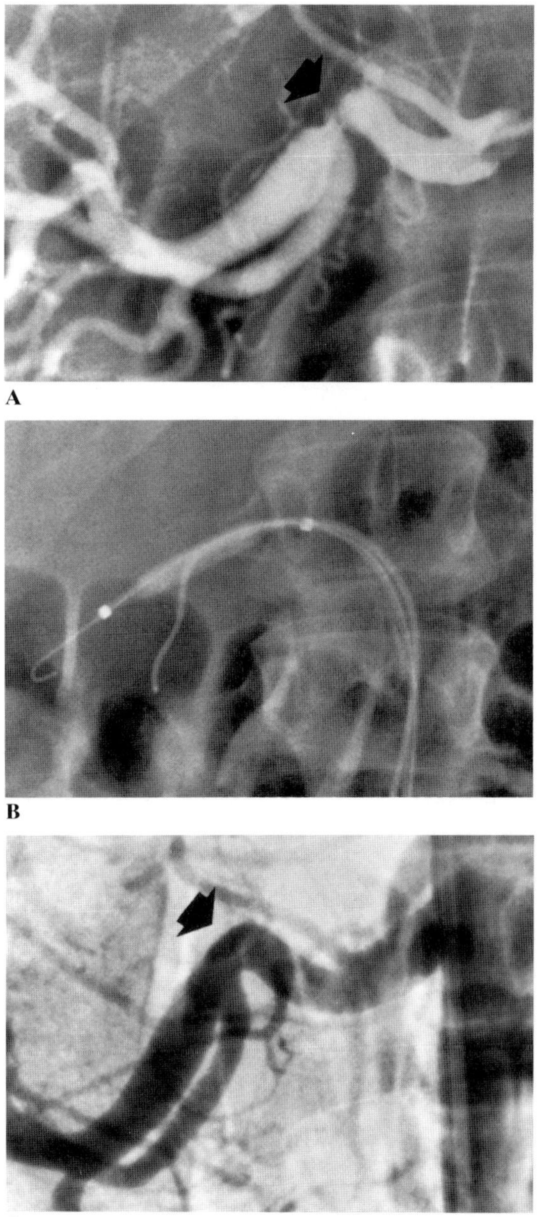

A

B

C

23–6 Kissing balloon technique in renal arteries. Twenty-eight-year-old woman presented with 2-year history of hypertension. **(A)** Selective arteriogram demonstrates tight stenosis at junction of dorsal and ventral branches of renal artery (arrow). **(B)** One-hundred-millimeter spot radiograph shows balloon inflated in upper branch, dilating lesion, and catheter in lower artery protecting orifice of the artery. **(C)** Immediately after PTRA, renal artery and both branches are widely patent (arrow).

Patient Management

Proper management of patients undergoing renal angioplasty requires a team approach. Selection of patients and management of the patient's blood pressure require close cooperation of a hypertension specialist. Inadvertent occlusion or rupture of the renal artery may create a surgical emergency. Although this complication is uncommon, renal angioplasty should only be performed when a skilled vascular surgeon is available.

Before renal angioplasty, the patient's blood pressure should be controlled by angiotensin-converting enzyme inhibitors such as captopril or enalapril, whenever possible. These agents inhibit the production of angiotensin-II, the active hypertensive substance in renin-mediated renovascular hypertension. The pharmacologic action of these agents is physiologically the same as that of a successful renal angioplasty. For this reason, sudden drops of blood pressure after renal angioplasty due to removal of the renin-angiotensin-aldosterone effect following successful dilatation are not seen when patients are being treated with these drugs. The patient's blood pressure must be monitored during the first 24–48 hr following angioplasty because profound changes may, nevertheless, occur. If the diastolic pressure rises above 110 mm Hg, the blood pressure should be controlled by a repeat dose of captopril or with rapid- and short-acting antihypertensive drugs such as phentolamine (Regitine) or a nitroprusside infusion. A drop in blood pressure can usually be controlled by the rapid intravenous infusion of normal saline. Therefore, an intravenous line should be in place prior to the procedure.

If it is not contraindicated, the patient receives 2,000 U of heparin subcutaneously or intravenously every 6 hr, beginning 8 hr after the procedure and continuing for 2 days. The patient also receives 75 mg dipyridamole (Persantine; Boehringer Ingelheim, Ridgefield, CT) orally twice a day and 325 mg of aspirin once a day beginning the day of angioplasty and continuing for at least 6 months. Patients are strongly encouraged to stop smoking. After angioplasty, the patient should be followed by a physician who specializes in the control of high blood pressure. Such a specialist should participate in the selection of patients for renal angioplasty and should follow them after the dilatation procedure, because blood pressure medication usually needs adjusting at that time. If the blood pressure rises in the ensuing months, a repeat arteriogram or digital subtraction angiography should be performed to evaluate for a recurrent or new stenosis.

Complications

The complication rate following renal angioplasty varies between 5% and 10%. Most of the complications are minor, but major complications may occur, the most common of which is transient renal insufficiency due to the injected contrast media. Severity of this complication in patients with renal insufficiency can be reduced by: 1) performing the diagnostic arteriogram several days prior to the therapeutic procedure; 2) using digital subtraction techniques to reduce the amount of contrast media; 3) ensuring that the patient receives adequate intravenous fluids during and after the procedure; 4) using a low osmolar contrast media, although this is currently unproven.

Subintimal dissection with the guide wire or the diagnostic catheter may occur when attempting to cross the stenosis. A small intimal flap will usually heal; however, in the presence of such an intimal dissection, angioplasty should be postponed for 4 to 6 weeks to allow healing. Infrequently, thrombosis of the renal artery may occur immediately following balloon angioplasty; this may be treated by the infusion of urokinase directly into the renal artery following the dilatation. However, it is important that sufficient collateral renal vessels are apparent so that prolonged renal ischemia does not develop during the urokinase infusion.

A renal artery rarely ruptures during balloon dilatation. If it does occur, this complication may result from dilating a weakened arterial wall, from overdilatation, or from subintimal placement of the balloon catheter. If rupture of the renal artery is noted immediately following deflation of the balloon, the balloon should be reinflated, occluding the proximal renal artery, and the patient should be taken immediately to the operating room. Distal embolization is an infrequent complication; however, a recently occluded renal artery should be approached carefuly. Thrombi may be dislodged by the catheter, occluding one or more of the segmental renal branches.

Spasm of the main renal artery or of a major arterial branch is the most frequent minor complication encountered during angioplasty. This is usually caused by mechanical stimulation of the vessel wall by the guide wire or catheter and may occur locally or more distally in the kidney. To help avoid spasm, the guide wire should not be placed within the segmental branches of the renal artery. Focal spasm caused by the angioplasty may occur in the area immediately adjacent to the dilatation site or even in distal small branches. Calcium channel blockers effectively prevent and reverse spasm in the renal arteries. The only calcium channel blocker available in a liquid parenteral form is verapamil. Sublingually administered nifedipine, on the other hand, is the most potent vasodilator of the calcium channel blockers available. As soon as the lesion is crossed, the patient is given 2.5 mg verapamil intra-arterially through the diagnostic catheter. If spasm is still encountered, another 2.5 mg of intra-arterial verapamil is given.

If spasm occurs in spite of the calcium channel blockers, intra-arterial nitroglycerine in a dose of

100–200 μg is given. Nitroglycerine effectively relieves spasm, but its mechanism of action is different from that of the calcium channel antagonists. It has an additive effect when given with calcium channel blockers, so it is effective when spasm is encountered after the blocker has previously been administered. The calcium channel blockers should be used initially because their duration of action is longer than that of nitroglycerine.

Calcium channel blockers, however, may induce hypotension, and they should be used with caution in patients who have known cardiac conduction defects. It is important to remember that the guide wire is the major cause of spasm and that continued stimulation of the vessel will cause spasm to recur. All catheter and guide wire manipulation should be kept to a minimum, and the most effective treatment of spasm is to remove the catheter and guide wire.

Results

In experienced hands, renal angioplasty is a highly effective method for correcting renal artery lesions. An initial success rate greater than 90% should be achieved when dilating renal artery stenoses (Table 23–1).

Long-term results can be assessed in three ways: the effect of the procedure on vessel patency, the effect of angioplasty on the blood pressure, and the effect of angioplasty on renal function. The effect of the procedure on vessel patency is related to the etiology of the lesion and characteristics of the lesion. The patients can be divided into five groups: atherosclerotic renal artery stenoses or occlusions; fibromuscular dysplasia of the renal artery; transplants; saphenous vein bypass grafts; and renal insufficiency.

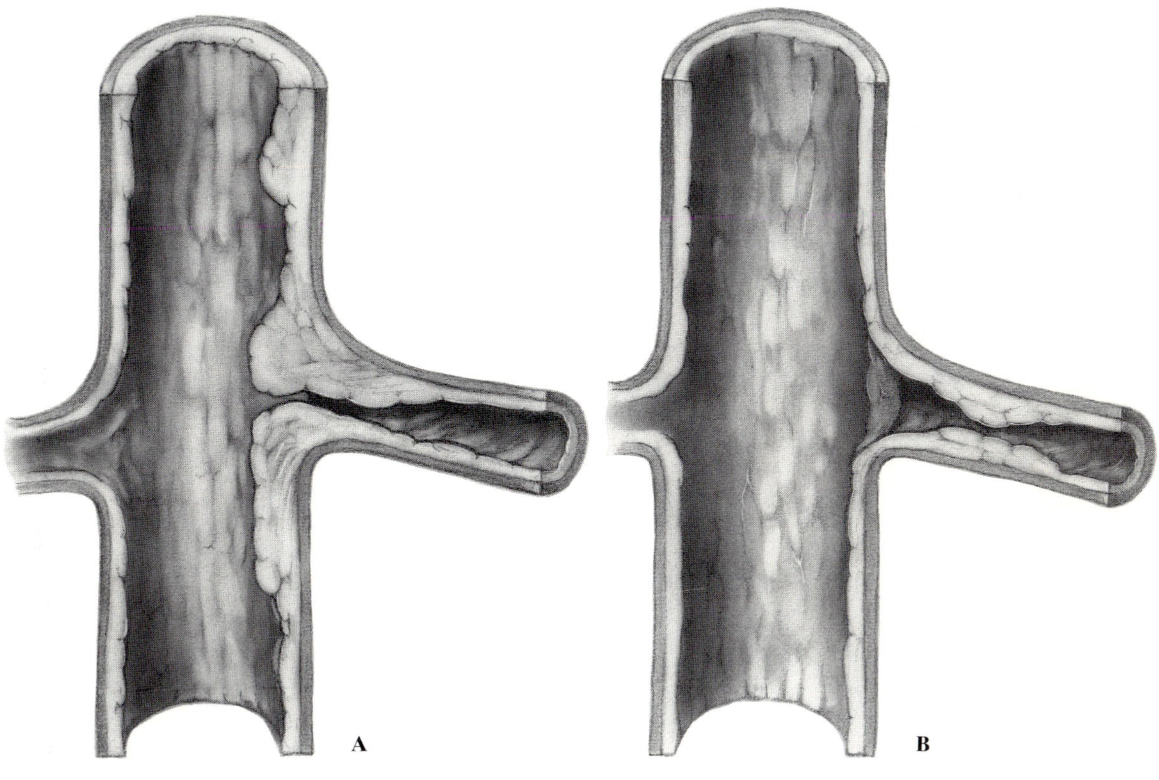

23–7 Types of atherosclerotic lesions. **(A)** A diminished response to balloon dilatation can be anticipated; lesion is caused by atherosclerotic plaque in abdominal aorta that engulfs orifice of the renal artery. Occasionally a good result is obtained, but usually results are poor when compared with results in other types of lesions. **(B)** A good response can be anticipated in short stenoses within renal artery.

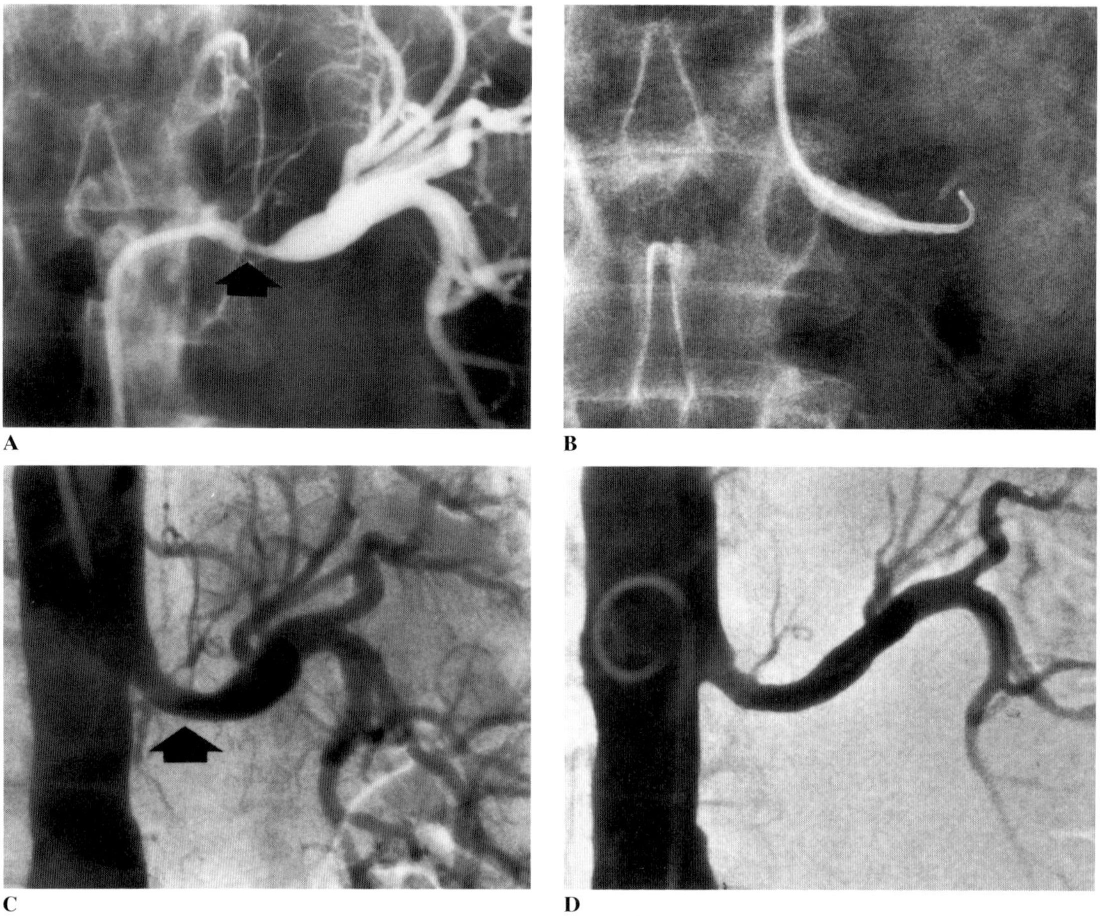

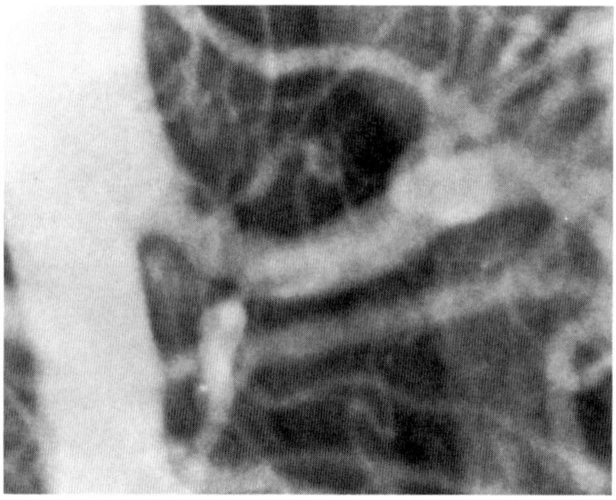

E

23–8 Long-term results of angioplasty in an atherosclerotic lesion are illustrated in 60-year-old man with solitary kidney and hypertension. **(A)** Selective arteriogram reveals tight stenosis (arrow) in the renal artery. **(B)** One-hundred-millimeter spot radiograph shows 5-mm balloon in place. **(C)** Immediately after PTRA, the stenosis ablated (arrow). **(D)** Repeat arteriogram, obtained 3 months after PTRA, demonstrates the widely patent vessel. **(E)** Repeat arteriogram, obtained 4½ years after angioplasty, shows continued patency of the artery.

Atherosclerotic Lesions

Atherosclerotic disease is the most frequent cause of stenosis treated by renal dilatation. In the University of Virginia series, 94% of the 65 hypertensive patients with atherosclerotic lesions were helped by the procedure. Of these patients, 23% were cured and 71% were improved with PTRA. Analysis of the results in the patients with atherosclerotic lesions revealed several other factors that are important when selecting patients for angioplasty. Better results are achieved in patients with unilateral renal artery stenoses than in patients with bilateral artery stenoses. The restenosis rate is higher in patients with bilateral renal artery stenosis (Tegtmeyer et al. 1984).

Sos et al. (1983) and Martin et al. (1985) also showed that success was more frequent with patients with unilateral lesions than in patients with bilateral disease. Furthermore, it is becoming increasingly clear that certain lesions are more amenable to balloon dilatation than others. A good result can be anticipated in short isolated atherosclerotic lesions (Fig. 23–7); however, when the renal artery stenosis is caused by a large

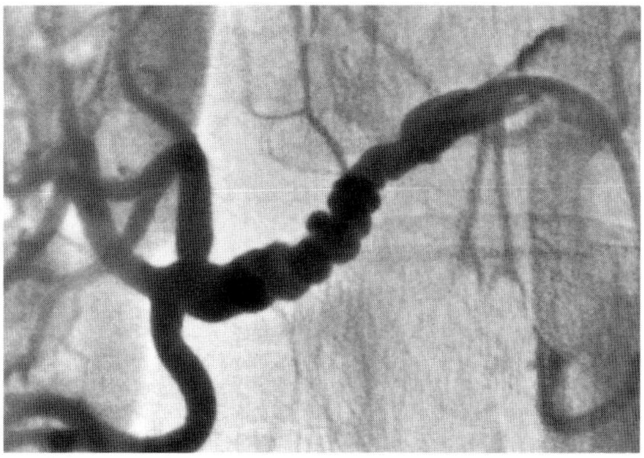

A

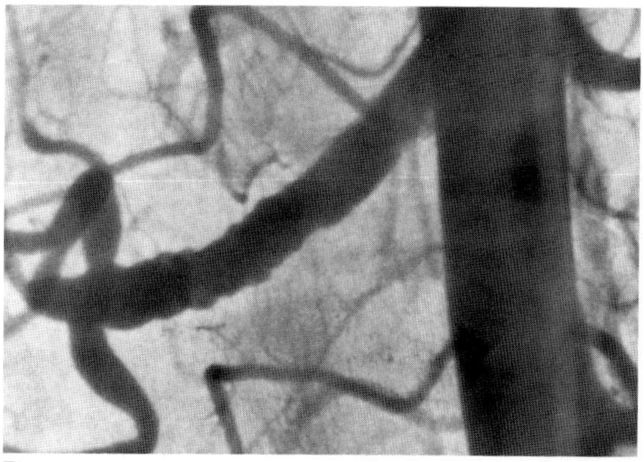

B

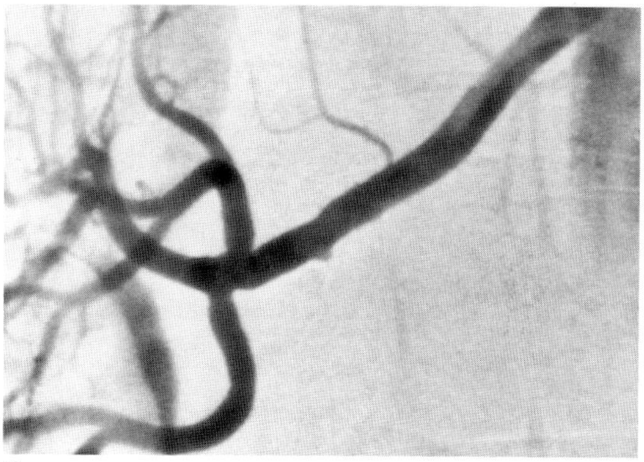

C

23–9 Long-term results in renal angioplasty in fibromuscular dysplasia are illustrated in 51-year-old woman with hypertension. **(A)** Renal arteriogram reveals extensive fibromuscular dysplasia of right renal artery. **(B)** Immediately after dilatation with a 5-mm balloon, vessel appears irregular, but there is good flow through it. This appearance is typical immediately after PTRA of fibromuscular dysplasia. **(C)** Arteriogram obtained 12½ months later shows no evidence of former lesion. This is the usual long-term appearance after dilatation of fibromuscular lesions.

plaque in the abdominal aorta that engulfs the origin of the renal artery, chances of success are diminished (Fig. 23–8) (Cicuto et al. 1981; Schwarten 1984; Sos et al. 1983). In the University of Virginia series, one-third of the redilated lesions were due to stenoses caused by aortic plaques that engulfed the origin of the renal artery (Tegtmeyer et al. 1984).

Complete blocks are more difficult to dilate than renal artery stenoses, and complete blocks that are not perfectly straight should not be dilated. Also, recanalization should be attempted only if the renal artery proximal and distal to the occlusion is clearly identified and the size of the kidney warrants salvage (Sniderman, Sos 1982; Tegtmeyer et al. 1984).

Fibromuscular Dysplasia

The best results in renal angioplasty are achieved in patients with fibromuscular lesions (Fig. 23–9). These lesions respond well to balloon dilatation, usually at pressures of 4 atm or less. If the lesion can be crossed, a good result can be anticipated (Tegtmeyer 1983; Tegtmeyer et al. 1984). In the University of Virginia series, there were 31 hypertensive patients with 37 lesions due

Table 23–1 Results of Renal Angioplasty

Study	No. Patients	Initial Success Rate (% Patients)	Patency Rate after Initial Success (% Patients)	Length of Follow-up
Katzen et al., 1979	17	94% lesions	75% lesions	1 yr
Puijlaert et al., 1981	54	96%	70%	
Schwarten, 1981	70	93% lesions	71%	6 mo.
Colapinto et al., 1982	68	85%	81%	3 yr
Sos et al., 1982	101	79%		
Tegtmeyer et al., 1984	109	95%	93%[a]	5 yr
Martin et al., 1986	100	88%	70%	3 yr
Total	519			
Range		79%–96%	70%–93%	½–5 yr

[a] Includes successful redilatations.

to fibromuscular dysplasia (Tegtmeyer et al. 1984). All of the patients benefited from renal angioplasty. Only one patient with fibromuscular dysplasia required repeat dilatation. Similar results have been achieved in several other series. Geyskes et al. (1983) dilated 21 patients for fibromuscular dysplasia, and 95% of them were cured or improved; there was only 1 failure. Sos et al. (1983) achieved a technical success when dilating lesions due to fibromuscular dysplasia in 27 of 31 patients.

Stenoses in Renal Transplants

Renal transplant arteries are anastomosed either end-to-end to the hypogastric artery or end-to-side to the external iliac artery. Stenoses may be proximal to, at, or distal to the anastomosis. Proximal stenoses in the hypogastric arteries are usually atherosclerotic in origin, and they respond well to PTRA. Anastomotic stenoses are largely due to surgical technique, perfusion injury, or local reaction to the suture material. Hypogastric anastomoses are best approached with a retrograde contralateral femoral artery puncture or from the axilla. End-to-side transplant renal artery to external iliac artery anastomoses, on the other hand, are best approached from the retrograde ipsilateral femoral artery. Stenoses at end-to-side anastomoses are usually focal elastic fibrotic bands and often require multiple vigorous inflations to achieve a permanent dilatation. Distal stenosis is common and may result from altered hemodynamics, vessel trauma, immunologic factors, and arterial kinking or extrinsic compression. Arterial kinking does not respond to dilatation as well as does intimal hyperplasia, which is often seen in this area.

In the University of Virginia series, seven patients with arterial stenoses in renal transplants were dilated (Fig. 23–10) (Tegtmeyer et al. 1984). Five patients were improved, and there were two failures. One failure resulted from the inability to dilate the lesion initially, probably because a polyvinyl chloride balloon was used. Since polyethelene balloons are now available, better results should be achievable.

In another patient, a tight stenosis at the anastomosis of the transplant to the hypogastric artery failed after 7 months despite three attempts at dilatation. Pressures as high as 14 atm were used. Sniderman et al. (1983) attempted to dilate 15 patients with stenoses in the arteries to their renal transplants. Three patients underwent repeat dilatations. The procedure was technically successful in 15 of the 18 attempts and in 13 of 15 patients. Gerlock et al. (1983) successfully dilated all 7 patients with renal transplant stenoses in their series. Since there are no collateral vessels to the kidney, dilating lesions in patients with renal transplants must be done carefully. If the vessel is occluded, surgery must be undertaken immediately. Therefore, in cases of renal transplant dilatation, a surgeon should be readily available.

Stenoses in Saphenous Bypass Grafts

In the University of Virginia series, three patients underwent successful dilatation of stenoses in their renal saphenous bypass grafts (Tegtmeyer et al. 1984).

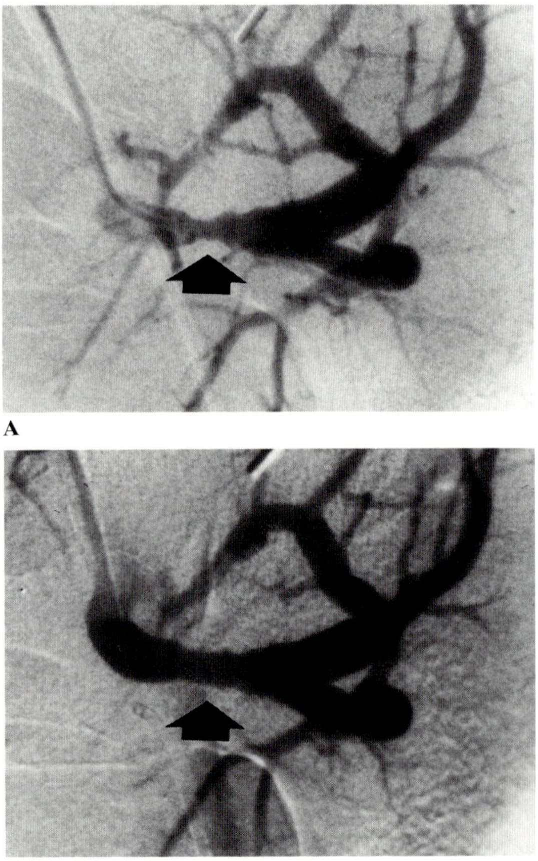

A

B

23–10 PTRA of stenosis in transplant artery in 26-year-old woman. **(A)** Selective arteriogram demonstrates severe stenosis (arrow) in vicinity of anastomosis in artery supplying renal transplant. **(B)** Vessel is widely patent (arrow) after balloon dilatation from the axillary approach.

Renal Insufficiency

Under certain circumstances, alleviation of renal artery stenosis preserves renal function. This is useful in unilateral disease if the kidney size indicates potentially significant preservation of renal mass or if bilateral renal artery stenoses are present. In the latter case, an attempt to alleviate stenosis to the largest kidney should be given priority even though the small kidney is secreting all the renin.

The results in patients treated primarily for renal insufficiency are not as dramatic as in patients treated primarily for hypertension. Nevertheless, the results are encouraging. In the University of Virginia series, 10 patients were treated primarily for renal insufficiency (Tegtmeyer et al. 1984). They all had atherosclerotic lesions. The mean serum creatinine level was 5.2 mg/dl before dilatation; after PTRA this decreased to 2.3 mg/dl for the group. Five of the patients had a positive response to dilatation; 5 have not been helped. Twenty-nine of the patients treated primarily for hypertension also had accompanying renal insufficiency; 9 of these patients had improved renal function following the procedure, and 4 have normal BUN and creatinine values. In some of the patients, the improvement was gradual after angioplasty, with full benefit of the procedure not apparent for several months.

Blood Pressure Response

Percutaneous transluminal renal angioplasty is a clinically effective means of treating renovascular hypertension. In the University of Virginia series, the blood pressure response has been analyzed in the 92 hypertensive patients whose initial dilatation was successful (Tegtmeyer et al. 1984). The patients have been followed from 1 to 60 months (mean, 23.7 months; median, 23.0 months). The mean systolic pressure of the patients (mmHg) was 199.74 before renal angioplasty and 140.4 after angioplasty, a difference of 59.34; the mean diastolic pressure was 117.05 before renal angioplasty and 93.74 afterward, a difference of 23.31.

Analysis of the long-term clinical results in the 98 hypertensive patients who underwent renal angioplasty to control their blood pressure reveals that 26% were classified as cured, defined by the Cooperative Study of Renovascular Hypertension as having an average diastolic pressure of less than or equal to 90 mmHg with at least a 10-mmHg decrease from the predilatation level (Simon et al. 1972). Sixty-seven percent were classified as improved, and their blood pressure was easier to control on medication as a result of the angioplasty procedure. Only 7% were nonresponders, although 1 patient was helped for several months.

Recurrence

A review of several large series in the world literature (Table 23–1) shows that if the initial dilatation is successful, the vessels can be expected to remain patent in 70% to 90% of the patients. If the vessel remains patent for at least 8 months, it is likely to remain patent for at least 5 years. The recurrence rate after PTRA has been variously reported at between 12.9% (Tegtmeyer et al. 1984) and 22.5% (Schwarten 1984). The recurrence rate is clearly higher in the atherosclerotic stenoses than in other types of stenoses.

A major factor in determining the recurrence rate is the success of the initial dilatation. Lesions that exhibit 30% or greater residual stenosis on the immediate postdilatation films are more likely to recur than lesions in which a better result has been obtained (Tegtmeyer et al. 1981, 1984). Therefore, it is essential that a good initial result be obtained. Restenoses, however, are usually successfully redilated, and the procedure is often easier than the initial procedure.

Conclusion

Renal angioplasty is considered the treatment of choice in patients with angiotensinogenic hypertension and renal artery stenosis due to fibromuscular dysplasia or short isolated atherosclerotic lesions. Recurrences are rare in fibromuscular lesions and are easily redilated. Atherosclerotic lesions of the renal artery orifice can be dilated; however, if the stenosis is caused primarily by a large plaque in the abdominal aorta, the chances of long-term success are diminished (Fig. 23–8). Good results can also be obtained in renal transplant artery stenosis and in stenosis of a bypass graft to the kidney.

Angioplasty often provides a better treatment option than surgery or long-term medical therapy.

Excellent results can be obtained if the patients are selected appropriately. In addition, the procedure has the potential for improving renal function in patients with renal insufficiency due to renal artery stenoses. In experienced hands, the results of renal angioplasty compare favorably with surgical results, and the duration of hospital stay is reduced (Doubilet, Abrams 1984).

References

Baker KS, Sawyer RW, Tisando J, et al.: Percutaneous transluminal angioplasty of the renal arteries: Double catheter technique. *Radiology* 159:554–555, 1986.

Block PC, Fallon JT, Elmer D: Experimental angioplasty: Lessons from the laboratory. *Am. J. Roentgenol.* 135:907–912, 1980.

Castaneda-Zuniga WR, Formanck A, Tadavarthy M, et al.: The mechanism of balloon angioplasty. *Radiology* 135:565–571, 1980.

Cicuto KP, McLean GK, Oleaga JA, et al.: Renal artery stenosis: Anatomic classification for percutaneous transluminal angioplasty. *Am. J. Roentgenol.* 137:599–601, 1981.

Colapinto RF, Stronell RD, Harries-Jones EP, et al.: Percutaneous transluminal dilatation of the renal artery: Follow-up studies on renovascular hypertension. *Am. J. Roentgenol.* 139:727–732, 1982.

Dollery CT, Bulpitt CJ: Management of hypertension. *In* Genest J, Koiw E, Kuchel O, et al. (eds.): *Hypertension: Physiopathology and Treatment.* New York, McGraw-Hill Book Co., 1977.

Dotter CT, Judkins MP: Transluminal treatment of arteriosclerotic obstruction: Description of a new technique and a preliminary report of its application. *Circulation* 30:654–670, 1964.

Doubilet P, Abrams H: The cost of underutilization. Percutaneous transluminal angioplasty for peripheral vascular disease. *N. Engl. J. Med.* 310:95–102, 1984.

Genest J, Boucher R, Rogo-Ortega JM, et al.: Renovascular hypertension. *In* Genest J, Koiw E, Kuchel O, et al. (eds.): *Hypertension: Physiopathology and Treatment.* New York, McGraw-Hill Book Co., 1977.

Gerlock AJ, Jr, MacDonnell RC, Jr, Smith CW, et al.: Renal transplant arterial stenoses: Percutaneous transluminal angioplasty. *Am. J. Roentgenol.* 140:325–331, 1983.

Geyskes CG, Puylaert CBAJ, Oei HY, et al.: Follow-up study of 70 patients with renal artery stenosis treated by percutaneous transluminal dilatation. *Br. Med. J.* 287:333–336, 1983.

Grable GS, Smith DC: The use of Simmons' "sidewinder" catheter in percutaneous transluminal angioplasty of the renal arteries. *Radiology* 137:541–543, 1980.

Gruentzig A, Kuhlmann U, Vetter W, et al.: Treatment of renovascular hypertension with percutaneous transluminal dilation of a renal-artery stenosis. *Lancet* 1:801–802, 1978.

Martin LG, Casarella WJ, Alspaugh JP, et al.: Renal artery angioplasty: Increased technical success and decreased complications in the second 100 patients. *Radiology* 159:631–634, 1986.

Martin LG, Price RB, Casarella WJ, et al.: Percutaneous angioplasty in clinical management of renovascular hypertension: Initial and long-term results. *Radiology* 155:629–633, 1985.

Schwarten DE: Percutaneous transluminal renal angioplasty. *Urol. Radiol.* 2:193–200, 1981.

Schwarten DE: Percutaneous transluminal angioplasty of the renal arteries: Intravenous digital subtraction angiography for follow-up. *Radiology* 150:369–375, 1984.

Simon N, Franklin SS, Bleifer KH, et al.: Clinical characteristics of renovascular hypertension. *J.A.M.A.* 220:1209–1218, 1972.

Smith MC, Dunn MJ: Renovascular and renal parenchymal hypertension. *In* Brenner BM, Rector FC (eds.): *The Kidney,* 3d ed. Philadelphia, W. B. Saunders Co., 1986, pp. 1221–1251.

Sniderman KW, Sos TA: Percutaneous transluminal recanalization and dilatation of totally occluded renal arteries. *Radiology* 142:607–610, 1982.

Sniderman KW, Sos TA, Sprayregen S: Post renal transplantation. *In* Castaneda-Zuniga W. (ed.): *Transluminal Angioplasty.* New York, Thieme-Stratton, 1983, pp. 80–89.

Sos TA, Pickering TG, Phil D, et al.: Percutaneous transluminal renal angioplasty in renovascular hypertension due to atheroma or fibromuscular dysplasia. *New Engl. J. Med.* 309:274–279, 1983.

Sos TA, Sniderman KW: Percutaneous transluminal angioplasty. *Semin. Roentgenol.* 16:26–40, 1981.

Tegtmeyer CJ: A simplified technique for selective and superselective abdominal angiography: Technical note. *J. Can. Assoc. Radiol.* 28:224–226, 1977.

Tegtmeyer CJ, Ayers CA, Wellons HA: The axillary approach to percutaneous renal artery dilatation. *Radiology* 135:775–776, 1980.

Tegtmeyer CJ, Dyer R, Teates CD, et al.: Percutaneous transluminal dilatation of the renal arteries: Techniques and results. *Radiology* 135:589–599, 1980.

Tegtmeyer CJ, Elson J, Glass TA, et al.: Percutaneous transluminal angioplasty: The treatment of choice for renovascular hypertension due to fibromuscular dysplasia. *Radiology* 143:631–637, 1982.

Tegtmeyer CJ, Kellum CD, Ayers C: Percutaneous transluminal angioplasty of the renal artery: Results and long-term follow-up. *Radiology* 153:77–84, 1984.

Tegtmeyer CJ, Kellum CD, Kron IL, et al.: Percutaneous transluminal angioplasty in the region of the aortic bifurcation: The two-balloon technique with results and long-term follow-up study. *Radiology* 157:661–665, 1985.

Tegtmeyer CJ, Sos T: Techniques of renal angioplasty. *Radiology* 161:577–586, 1986.

Tegtmeyer CJ, Teates CD, Crigler N, et al.: Percutaneous transluminal angioplasty in patients with renal artery stenosis: Follow-up studies. *Radiology* 140:323–330, 1981.

Tegtmeyer CJ, Tegtmeyer VL, Kellum CD, et al.: Percutaneous transluminal angioplasty: The treatment of choice for vascular lesions caused by fibromuscular dysplasia. *Semin. Intervent. Radiol.* 1:289–300, 1984.

Wellons HA, Jr, Tegtmeyer CJ, Crosby IK: Balloon catheterization of the iliac artery: Results in 34 patients. *Virginia Medical* 108:598–602, 1981.

CHAPTER

24

Shunt Failure in Hemodialysis: Diagnosis and Percutaneous Therapy

Robert D. Crane

When hemodialysis access sites fail, the cause can usually be determined angiographically. The puncture site should be chosen in such a way that percutaneous therapy, usually balloon angioplasty, can be accomplished without a second puncture. With a combination of urokinase infusion and balloon angioplasty, many thrombosed shunts can be reopened.

Types of Vascular Access for Hemodialysis

Direct Venous Catheter

The Scribner-Quinton external arteriovenous shunt was the first popular method of vascular access suitable for short-term dialysis. It has now been replaced by a large-bore central venous catheter for dialysis via a subclavian or femoral vein (Table 24–1).

Autogenous Shunts

Internal fistulas are favored for chronic dialysis because of their longevity and relatively low incidence of complications. The favored vascular access is the Brescia-Cimino distal forearm radial artery-to-cephalic vein shunt. This is usually created as an end-of-vein to side-of-artery anastomosis or side-of-vein to side-of-artery anastomosis. Distal fistula sites on the nondominant arm are generally selected. If the fistula fails, a new site can be created proximally.

The Brescia-Cimino fistula is preferred for chronic dialysis because of its patency rate and resistance to infection; however, some patients do not have suitable vessels for its creation. Moreover, the Brescia-Cimino fistula requires a 6- to 12-week wait for venous enlargement adequate to permit hemodialysis. Other patients in whom Brescia-Cimino fistulae have failed may not have suitable anatomy for reconstructing a second primary arteriovenous fistula. Because of these limitations, nonautogenous graft conduits are often necessary.

Nonautogenous Grafts

Expanded polytetrafluoroethylene (PTFE, Gore-Tex®) is the preferred graft material. Patency rates are slightly less than for primary arteriovenous fistulae: 70% versus 84% at 3 years

Table 24–1 Types of Hemodialysis Vascular Access

Access	Advantage	Disadvantages
Direct venous catheter	Easily established	Risk of infection with time
Brescia-Cimino arteriovenous fistula	High patency rate; infection rare	Needs time to mature; veins may be inadequate
PTFE (Gore-Tex®)	Does not need to mature	Intimal hyperplasia; venous stenosis; infection
Bovine carotid artery heterograft	Does not need to mature	Intimal hyperplasia; venous stenosis; infection; aneurysm formation

(Winsett, Wolma 1982); and 50% versus 64% at 3 years (Kherlakian et al. 1986).

The modified bovine graft, a beef carotid artery that has undergone a modification process to create a nonantigenic collagen tube, was commonly used prior to the availability of PTFE. The bovine graft has a lower patency rate and a higher complication rate, particularly aneurysm formation and infection (Winsett, Wolma 1982). Even so, a moderate number of these grafts are in use. Saphenous vein and umbilical vein graft materials are no longer used.

Arteriovenous grafts are created in either a straight or loop configuration. The straight graft usually extends from the radial artery to the basilic or median antecubital vein below the antecubital crease of the elbow. Straight forearm grafts provide a long segment that is technically easy to puncture for dialysis.

With the loop graft, arterial and venous anastomoses are at approximately the same level. These are usually created from the proximal radial artery to an antecubital vein. Other graft sites include brachial artery, axillary artery, and superficial femoral artery. However, upper extremity access is preferred, since these vessels are typically less involved with atherosclerosis. The artery selected for inflow must be 3 mm or greater to support blood flow of at least 300 ml/min.

Angiographic Technique

Angiographic methods for evaluating failing hemodialysis access fistulae include direct graft injection, venous injection, or arterial injection.

Both the venous and graft injection methods avoid potential damage to the arterial system of the arm or hand and are less complicated than an arterial approach. The majority of the patients at Virginia Mason Medical Center in Seattle are being evaluated for high venous pressure or decreased venous outflow. Venous or graft puncture generally permits the best visualization of the stenosis and provides access for subsequent angioplasty. A method of venous approach for fistula angiography with serial filming and subtraction capability has been outlined by Gilula and colleagues (1975) (Table 24–2). The author finds this more complex technique unnecessary.

For direct graft injection, a blood pressure cuff is applied to the upper arm and briefly inflated to higher than arterial pressure (e.g., 250 mm Hg) during contrast injection. A single film is obtained at the end of injection, with good opacification of both venous and arterial anatomy. Additional views are obtained in different projections as needed. Serial filming or digital subtraction techniques can also be used to clarify findings. The site

Table 24–2 Angiographic Technique

	Direct Graft Injection		Arterial Injection
	Single film	Serial film	
Approach	18-g standard angiographic needle; or butterfly needle; or hemodialysis needle; or 5-F dilator	18-g standard angiographic needle; or butterfly needle; or hemodialysis needle; or 5-F dilator	Retrograde femoral with 5-F catheter (i. e., Head Hunter 1); or direct puncture antecubital or midhumerus area
Contrast	10–15 ml Contrast media[a]	15–20 ml Contrast media[a]	20–25 ml Contrast media[a]
Injection	Rapid hand injection, upper arm BP cuff inflated to 250 mm Hg	Mechanical injection over 4–5 sec	20–25 ml at 5–7 ml/sec
Filming	1 exposure at immediate end of hand injection	BP cuff inflated; preliminary subtraction film just prior to injection; filming begins 0.5–1 sec before end of injection; BP cuff released 1 sec later; film at 2/sec for 4 sec; or 1 film/sec for 10 sec, deflating BP cuff halfway through run	1 or 2 films/sec for 6–8 sec

[a] Newer low-osmolar contrast agents cause much less discomfort.

Table 24–3 Presenting Clinical Problems of Patients with Chronic Dialysis Access Sites

Problem	Possible Etiology
Increased venous pressure during dialysis	Venous stenosis downstream from needle site
Difficulty establishing needle placement	Intimal hyperplasia of graft; deep or small veins; partial thrombosis of primary fistula; arterial stenosis; multiple or proximal graft stenosis
Decreased graft thrill or fullness	Arterial or proximal graft stenosis
Inadequate inflow on dialysis run	Arterial stenosis or venous/graft stenosis upstream from puncture
Local swelling	Aneurysm formation at puncture site (often associated with downstream venous stenosis)
Painful hand (especially with exercise)	Distal steal syndrome with ischemia
Venous insufficiency	Venous hypertension (often in side-to-side fistula)
Painful swelling	Infection or aneurysm
Congestive heart failure	Fistula flow too great
Lack of thrill	Thrombosis

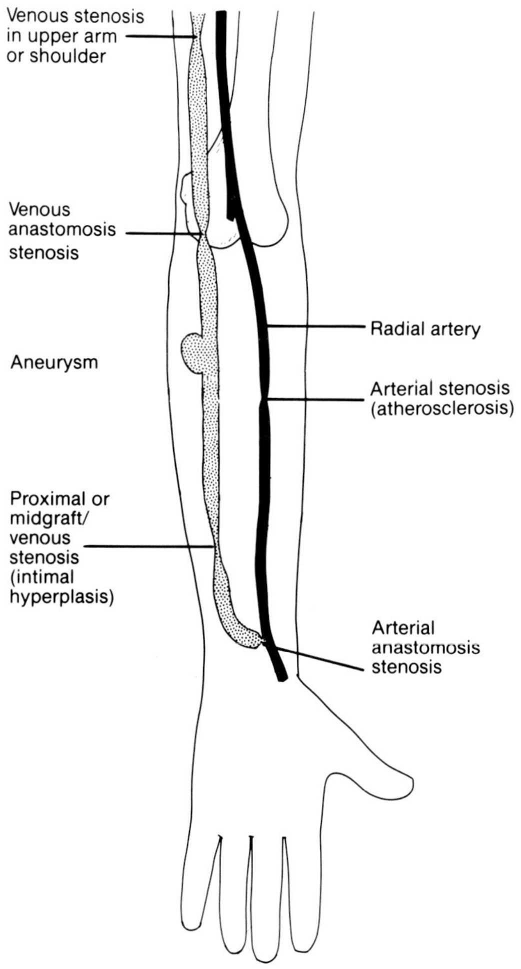

24–1 Chronic vascular access problems. Stenoses in artery, at proximal anastomosis, and in proximal graft will cause decreased arterial pressures; stenoses in upper graft or in upper arm vein will cause increased venous pressures.

of needle insertion for the venous or graft technique should be proximal (upstream) to allow enough vessel for insertion and inflation of an angioplasty balloon.

The arterial injection technique is reserved for evaluating decreased arterial inflow or ischemia of the extremities. This can be done via a retrograde femoral artery approach (Table 24–2) or through an antegrade midbrachial artery direct puncture. The latter allows access for angioplasty. Rapid filming by either arterial or retrograde venous routes provides information on flow dynamics not possible by the single film approach.

Venous Stenosis

Evaluation

Fistula angiography is indicated for graft venous hypertension when the measured pressure in the dialysis outflow line increases to 100–150 mm Hg. Venous hypertension is most frequently due to stenosis at the venous anastomoses of a graft, but may be due to stenosis in the arm or shoulder veins or within the graft itself caused by intimal hyperplasia (Table 24–3).

Normally, the palpable graft pulsation decreases progressively toward the venous end. When a significant venous stenosis is present, a prominent pulsation is felt throughout the graft up to the stenosis, at which point the pulsation diminishes abruptly. Knowing the likely site and cause of graft malfunction allows one to choose a level for initial needle puncture that can be used for subsequent angioplasty.

Usually the needle is directed toward the elbow from a site in the proximal (upstream) or midportion of the graft. The site should be adequately away from the arterial anastomosis to avoid damaging it, yet still sufficiently upstream from any palpable potential stenoses so that an angioplasty balloon can be fully inserted and inflated. Occasionally, if the history and palpation of the graft suggest only a mid-to-upstream graft stenosis, the needle puncture must be in the proximal forearm (downstream) and directed toward the hand.

For patient comfort, diluted medicine for analgesia or sedation can be administered through a needle or catheter in the graft before angioplasty. A 1- to 2-ml dose (50–100 μg) of fentanyl (Sublimaze®) acts quickly, lasts for about 30–45 min, is well tolerated, and eases the discomfort of the subsequent contrast injection or dilation.

Prior to balloon insertion and inflation, it is helpful to indicate the site of stenosis either by bony landmarks or by placing a marker on the skin surface during fluoroscopic observation while injecting contrast. The diameter of the normal lumen is measured just proximal and distal to the stenosis. That measurement, generally between 6 mm and 10 mm, is used as the choice of diameter for a high-pressure angioplasty balloon catheter. The degree of angiographic magnification of the forearm is considerably less than at other sites commonly evaluated for angioplasty; hence, the graft or venous stenosis is distended to a lesser degree than elsewhere in the body.

Balloon Dilation

A 0.89-mm (0.035-in.) 3-cm tapered standard straight angiographic wire is introduced through the diagnostic needle if the approach is appropriate for the lesion. Occasionally a J wire is used to avoid perforation of cul-de-sacs. The guide wire will usually slide through the stenosis, with the end positioned in the upper arm. If any resistance to initial passage of guide wire through the stenosis is encountered, the wire is left proximal to the stenosis until after the introduction of a 5-F dilator. Through this dilator, a contrast study defines anatomy, and the 3,000-unit dose of heparin is then administered.

To negotiate irregular, angled, or tight stenoses, torque control catheters or specialized guide wires may be needed. Helpful ones are: the Bentson wire with a loose floppy atraumatic end; the 1-mm J wire; and a torque control wire with a soft malleable end such as Wholey Wire (Advanced Cardiovascular Systems) or the Glidewire® (Medi-Tech). Subsequently, a 7-F dilator and a 7-F angioplasty balloon are introduced.

Diluted contrast (1:2) is used for balloon inflation. As the balloon is distended, an initial constriction or hourglass deformity occurs at the stenosis. With further inflation, this waist disappears. The balloon is fully inflated for 15–30 sec, then deflated. Higher-pressure angioplasty balloons tolerate 17 atm as compared to 5 atm of the earlier polyvinylchloride Gruentzig balloons. These newer balloon catheters are almost always successful in achieving good dilation on the first or second inflation, although sometimes multiple, longer inflations are necessary.

Patients will often feel discomfort at the angioplasty site, but the procedure is usually well tolerated. Once good dilation has been achieved, evidenced by the absence of hourglass balloon deformity, the angioplasty catheter is pulled away from the stenosis. Contrast is injected through the catheter for angiographic confirmation of success, either by single film technique, rapid sequence camera, or digital subtraction technique.

Incompletely dilated stenoses are apt to recur soon, particularly if the residual stenosis exceeds 30% of normal lumen. For these cases, additional dilation with a larger balloon is recommended. A dissection plane in the vein (although not in a graft) after dilation is occasionally encountered. This is part of the trauma of angioplasty and will resolve over several weeks.

If recrossing of the stenosis after creation of an intimal flap or dissection plane becomes necessary, it is best to carefully lead with a J wire so that it stays in the true lumen. Optimally, however, redilation of such a lesion should be postponed or avoided. This author rarely measures pressures across stenotic lesions, since the angiographic anatomy usually correlates well with the clinical presentation.

Occasionally, the initial angiographic evaluation can be misleading, since a tight stenosis may

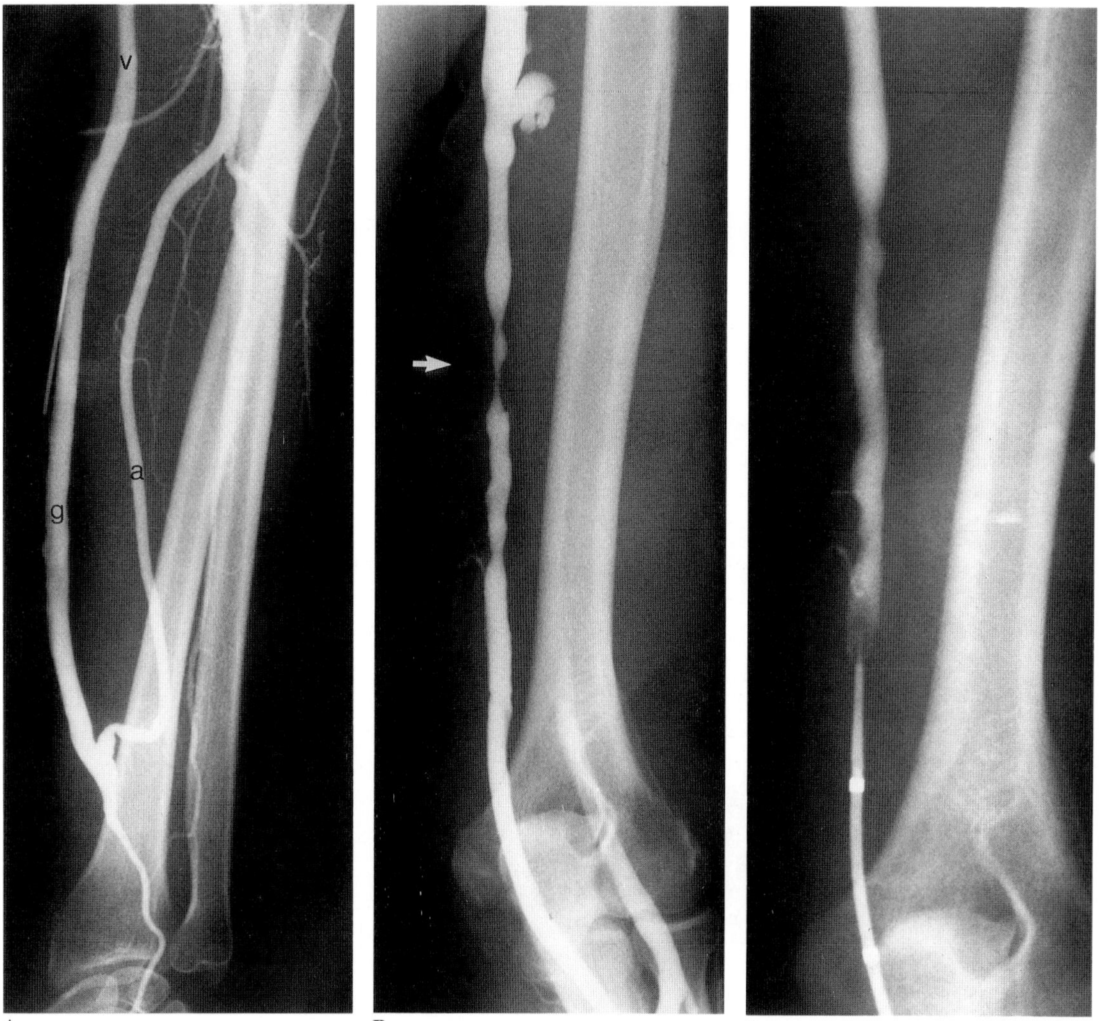

A B C
24–2 **(A)** Fistulogram of forearm shows no obvious reason for elevated venous pressures. a = radial artery; g = graft; v = antecubital vein. **(B)** Venogram of basilic vein shows high-grade stenosis at midhumerus level (arrow). **(C)** Venogram following balloon angioplasty showing substantial resolution of stenosis.

appear as a venous outflow occlusion (Fig. 24–2). Injection immediately proximal to the lesion can reveal the pseudo-occlusion and lead to successful angioplasty.

Venous spasm is sometimes encountered above the elbow. Removing the guide wire from the region and waiting 5 min usually allows the spasm to resolve. If the spasm is severe enough to occlude flow and does not resolve with simple measures, direct injection of antispasmodic agents (100 μg of nitroglycerine diluted in 10 ml saline; 2.5 mg of verapamil) may be necessary. Pretreatment with the calcium channel blocker nifedipine (10–20 mg sublingually) is recommended if any arterial manipulation is planned. It takes effect within 15 min and lasts 3–4 hr.

Glanz and colleagues (1984) reported on 56 balloon dilation procedures of upper extremity access fistulas and grafts. With a 70% initial success rate, 80% of those remained patent at 3 months and 55% were patent at 1 year. Three complications occurred: two graft thromboses and one pseudoaneurysm at the dilation site. Saeed and colleagues (1987) performed angioplasty on 25 dialysis access fistulas with a success rate of 80% and a 6-month patency rate of 76%. Results have been similar at Virginia Mason Medical Center.

Graft Occlusion

Evaluation

Graft occlusion is usually obvious by absence of previously present pulsation and thrill. Initially, angiography can be performed by direct puncture of the graft with a 21-gauge or 19-gauge butterfly needle. If clotted blood cannot be withdrawn, 1 ml of sterile saline is injected and aspirated, which almost always yields clotted blood and confirms position of the needle within the shunt (Zeit 1986). Contrast media is then carefully injected to evaluate the shunt. Manual compression of one end of the graft with a leaded glove, while injecting contrast, can be used to help demonstrate the proximal or distal anastomosis. Thrombosis of the graft is confirmed, and the underlying cause can often be identified.

Fibrinolytic Therapy

Results using transcatheter fibrinolytic therapy with streptokinase or urokinase for graft thrombosis have been variable. Radkin and colleagues (1983) achieved lysis with streptokinase (40,000 U bolus, 7,500 U/hr) via catheter injection in 8 of 9 clotted access fistulas. Zeit (1986) had successful lysis of 54 of 79 shunts (68%) using direct injection of streptokinase (100,000 U over 60–90 min) into the clot, followed by massage of the clot. Embolization of clot fragments was demonstrated angiographically in 6 of 79 cases (7.6%); all patients remained asymptomatic. There were no general hemorrhagic complications or local hemorrhaging that required blood transfusion.

To Hunter and colleagues (1984), early fistula failure implied a surgical or anatomic complication not amenable to percutaneous therapy. They recommended surgical revision for any such patient. In this author's experience, local transcatheter infusion of streptokinase 5,000 U/hr has had only limited success.

Davis and colleagues (1987) had a high success rate administering high-concentration urokinase directly into Gore-Tex® grafts. In this technique, two 5-F catheters with 30-degree distal curves are introduced from opposite ends of the graft, and the catheter tips are placed at opposing ends of the graft (crisscrossed). The clot is macerated as the catheters are spun helically and partially withdrawn, during which time the clot is laced with 100,000 U urokinase diluted in 4 ml saline and injected into each catheter. Infusion of 2,000 U/min (5,000 U/ml concentration) urokinase into each catheter is then begun immediately with crisscrossed catheters positioned with tips at the midgraft and arterial anastomosis levels. After return of pulsation, a contrast study is performed to determine the best position of the catheter tip for final clot lysis.

Lysis was achieved in 37 of 41 cases (90%). Average thrombolysis time was 86 min (range: 15 min to 4 hr), and the average urokinase dose was 389,000 U. Angioplasty was performed in appropriate cases with administration of 5,000 U heparin prior to balloon dilation. Sixty-two percent had a useful graft at 6 months. No uncontrolled hemorrhage was encountered (Davis et al. 1987). Initial experience at Virginia Mason Medical Center with this technique has been favorable, and the method is now used for treating thrombosed fistulas (Table 24–4).

This author and colleagues do not monitor blood clotting parameters when using urokinase infusion. Similar to Davis et al. (1987), there have been no problems with hemorrhage. Judging from experience using urokinase to dissolve thrombus

Table 24–4 Urokinase Therapy of Thrombosed Grafts

1. Two 5-F catheters with distal 30° curves introduced from opposite ends of graft.
2. Catheter tips placed at opposing ends of graft ("crisscrossed").
3. Macerate clot as catheters spun helically and partially withdrawn, injecting 100,000 U of urokinase in 4 ml into each catheter.
4. Position catheter tips at midgraft and arterial anastomosis levels and begin urokinase infusion of 2,000 U/min (5,000 U/ml concentration) into each catheter.
5. Contrast study at 2 hr and 4 hr or whenever graft pulsation returns, to determine best position of catheters for final clot lysis (average 1.5 hr).
6. Balloon angioplasty of stenosis after 5,000 U heparin.

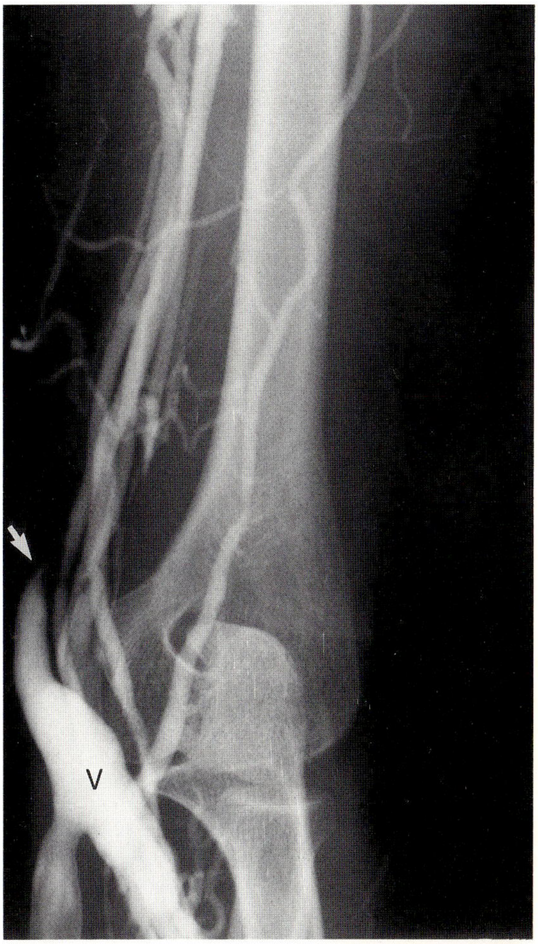

A

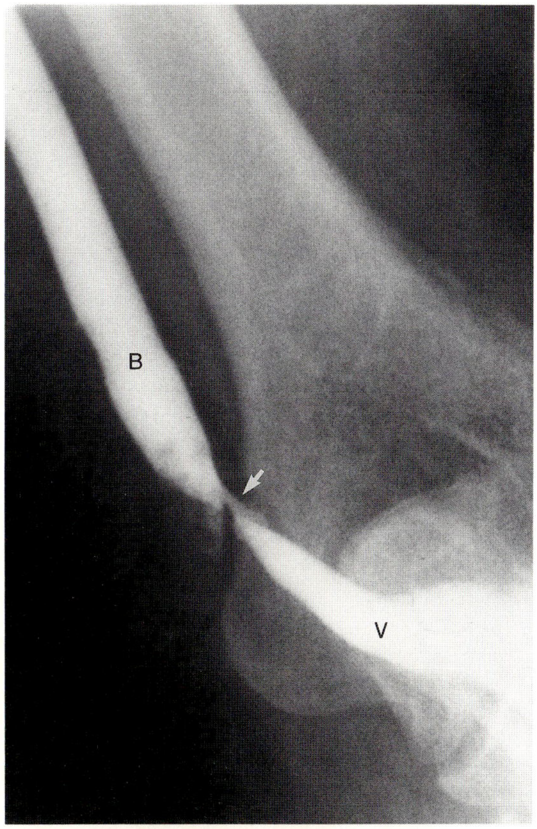

B

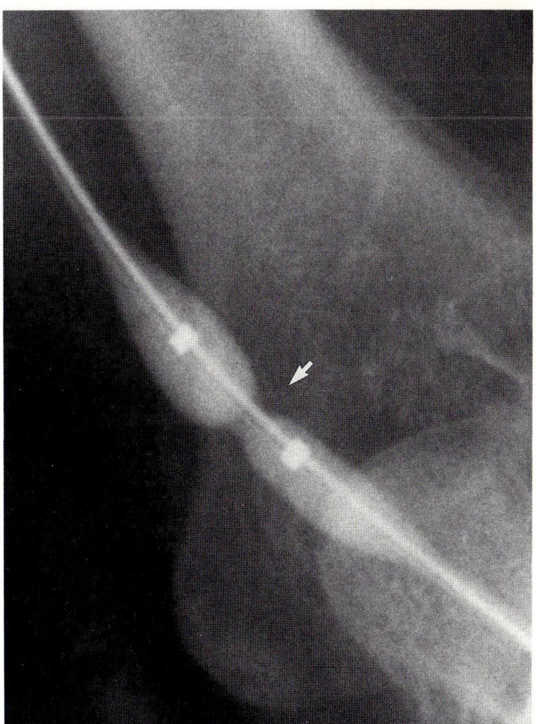

C

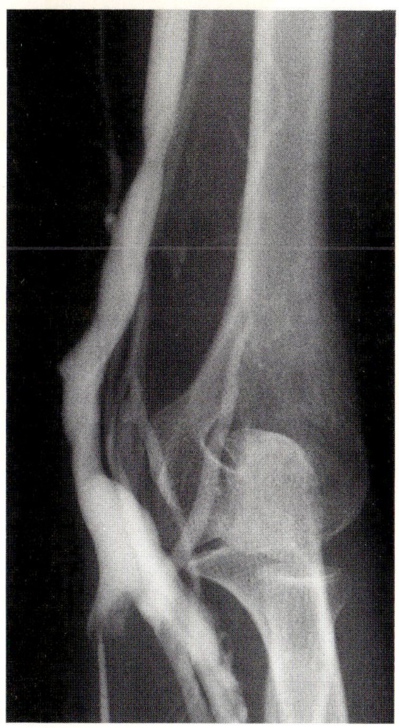

D

24–3 (A) Fistulogram showing apparent occlusion (arrow) of major venous outflow channel. V = antecubital vein. **(B)** Injection with catheter tip at stenosis reveals pseudo-occlusion with high-grade stenosis (arrow). V = antecubital vein; B = basilic vein. **(C)** Hourglass configuration (arrow) of balloon early in angioplasty prior to full stretching. **(D)** Resolution of stenosis postangioplasty.

elsewhere in the body, bleeding problems are most likely to occur when the fibrinogen level falls below 70–100 mg/dl (normal 190–430 mg/dl) after 24 hr of infusion. However, patients with intracranial mass lesions or hemorrhage, recent gastrointestinal bleeding, recent retinal hemorrhage, surgery within 3–4 weeks, or other bleeding conditions that might cause significant morbidity if aggravated are not candidates for urokinase therapy.

The cost of 250,000 U of urokinase at Virginia Mason Medical Center is $165 versus $35 for 250,000 U of streptokinase. Nevertheless, urokinase is preferred because of its success rate and reduced incidence of allergic reaction. Hospital time is decreased, which reduces overall cost.

References

Connolly JE, Brownell DA, Levine EF, McCart PM: Complications of renal dialysis access procedures. *Arch. Surg.* 119:1325–1328, 1984.

Davis GB, Dowd CF, Bookstein JJ, Maroney TP, Lang EV, Halasz N: Thrombosed dialysis grafts: Efficacy of intrathrombotic deposition of concentrated urokinase, clot maceration, and angioplasty. *Am. J. Roentgenol.* 149:177–181, 1987.

Gilula LA, Staple TW, Anderson CB, Anderson LS: Venous angiography of hemodialysis fistulas. *Radiology* 115:555–562, 1975.

Glanz S, Gordon D, Butt KMH, Hong J, Adamson R, Sclafani SJA: Dialysis access fistulas: Treatment of stenoses by transluminal angioplasty. *Radiology* 152:637–642, 1984.

Graor RA, Bisius B, Young JR, Geisinger MA, Zelch MG, Smith JAM, Ruschhaupt WF: Low-dose streptokinase for selective thrombolysis: Systemic effects and complications. *Radiology* 152:35–39, 1984.

Hunter DW, Castaneda-Zuniga WR, Coleman CD, Young AT, Salomonowitz E, Mercado S, Amplatz K: Failing arteriovenous dialysis fistulas. Evaluation and treatment. *Radiology* 152:631–635, 1984.

Kherlakian GM, Roedersheimer LR, Arbaugh JJ, Newmark KJ, King LR: Comparison of autogenous fistula versus expanded polytetrafluoroethylene graft fistula for angioaccess in hemodialysis. *Am. J. Surg.* 152:238–243, 1986.

Mangiarotti G, Canavese C, Thea A, Segoloni GP, Stratta P, Salomone M, Vercellone A: Urokinase treatment for arteriovenous fistulae declotting in dialyzed patients. *Nephron* 36:60–44, 1984.

O'Reilly RJ, Hansen CC, Rosental JJ: Angiography of chronic hemodialysis arteriovenous grafts. *Am. J. Roentgenol.* 130:1105–1113, 1978.

Palder SB, Kirkman RL, Whittenmore AD, Hakim RM, Lazarus JM, Tilney NL: Vascular access for hemodialysis. *Ann. Surg.* 235–239, 1985.

Porter JA, Sharp WV, Walsh EJ: Complications of vascular access in a dialysis population. *Curr. Surg.* 42(4):298–300, 1985.

Radkin RS, Bookstein JJ, Heeney DJ, Davis GB: Streptokinase and transluminal angioplasty in the treatment of acutely thrombosed hemodialysis access fistulas. *Radiology* 149:425–428, 1983.

Saeed M, Newman GE, McCann RL, Sussman SK, Braun SD, Dunnick NR: Stenosis in dialysis fistulas: Treatment with percutaneous angioplasty. *Radiology* 164:693–697, 1987.

Tortolani EC, Tan AHS, Butchart S: Percutaneous transluminal angioplasty: An ineffective approach to the failing vascular access. *Arch. Surg.* 119:221–223, 1984.

Winsett OE, Wolma FJ: Complications of vascular access for hemodialysis. *South Med. J.* 78:513–517, 1985.

Young AT, Hunter DW, Castaneda-Zuniga WR, So SKS, Mercado S, Cardella JF, Amplatz K: Thrombosed synthetic hemodialysis access fistulas: Failure of fibrinolytic therapy. *Radiology* 154:639–642, 1985.

Zeit RM: Arterial and venous embolization: Declotting of dialysis shunts by direct injection of streptokinase. *Radiology* 159:639–641, 1986.

CHAPTER

25

Embolotherapy for the Genitourinary System

Robert K. Feldman and Timothy P. Maroney

Transcatheter embolization is a relatively new procedure that may be used as an alternative or adjuvant to surgical therapy in the genitourinary system. Although embolization of surgically exposed carotid-cavernous fistulas was first performed in the 1930s, application to the genitourinary system was not common until after 1969 when Lalli et al. (1969) reported on the percutaneous embolization of renal carcinomas.

Various types of occlusive agents have been used, including (a) particles, such as autologous clot, Gelfoam, and Ivalon; (b) mechanical devices, such as the Gianturco-Anderson-Wallace steel coil and detachable balloons; (c) ethanol; and (d) tissue adhesives, like isobutyl 2-cyanoacrylate (Bucrylate). Each of these agents has advantages and disadvantages. Applying the agents requires an understanding of the pathophysiology of the disease, the vascular anatomy, the size of the vessel to be embolized, and whether temporary or permanent occlusion is desired.

Occlusive Agents and Devices

Gelfoam

Gelfoam, a slowly absorbed gelatin sponge, is the best known and easiest to use embolic agent (Bookstein et al. 1978; Katzen et al. 1976). The principal application of Gelfoam has been in the management of hemorrhage. It is available in two forms: a sheetlike sponge, about 12 cm^2 by 7 mm thick, which may be cut or torn into fragments of appropriate size; and a sterile powder most typically used as a hemostatic agent in the operating room. One advantage of Gelfoam is that it can be cut into pledgets equal to the size of the vessel. Although the pledgets are compressed when inserted, they regain most of their original size and shape after extrusion from the catheter.

Because Gelfoam lasts only 3 to 4 weeks, it sometimes needs to be used with other agents if a more durable occlusion is desired. Jander has demonstrated that dense packing of a vessel with Gelfoam can cause permanent occlusion (Jander, Russinovich 1980). Since Gelfoam is easily contaminated (Greenfield 1982), strict sterile technique must be observed during embolization. All members of the angiography team wear surgical hats, masks, and gowns. Care should be taken to prevent prolonged exposure of Gelfoam to air.

The authors' preferred method of using Gelfoam is to load a single compressed pledget into the tip of a tuberculin syringe, remove the stopcock from the catheter, inject directly into the catheter, and flush with small aliquots of contrast medium or saline. Steady injection helps keep the catheter in proper position. The effectiveness of embolization must be carefully monitored during the procedure; small amounts of contrast medium are injected using a small syringe to assess blood flow. When the flow has been diminished significantly, the embolization is stopped to avoid reflux of pledgets into other vessels and to allow the resulting thrombus to extend proximally over time.

Ivalon

A polyvinyl alcohol foam, Ivalon (Pacific Medical Industries), serves as a permanent agent for distal embolization. Sterile, nonradiopaque Ivalon particles are available in seven sizes ranging from 200–300 μ to 2,000–2,500 μ in either a dry or wet (normal saline suspension) form. Saline and contrast medium are mixed with the Ivalon particles to create a slurry, and injections are made using the method described by Kerber to keep the particles uniformly suspended (Kerber et al. 1978; Tadavarthy et al. 1975). When flow has been slowed, Gelfoam particles are injected to cleanse the catheter of further Ivalon particles so as to prevent peripheral embolization during catheter removal. Ivalon's ease of application makes it a widely used material.

Steel Coils

The steel coil has undergone several modifications since being developed in 1975 by Gianturco (Gianturco et al. 1975). Originally attached to a wool strand to enhance thrombogenicity, the coil now consists of pieces of tightly wrapped guide wire with Dacron strands attached. The occluding spring coil emboli are preformed and available in 2-mm, 3-mm, 5-mm, 8-mm, and larger-diameter sizes. Coil size should be matched to vessel size to prevent distal migration or aortic reflux and peripheral embolization. The advantages of the steel coil are its permanence and ease of use (Wallace et al. 1976).

An end-hole polyethylene catheter is used to facilitate passage. The coil is inserted by removing the stopcock from the catheter and placing the introducer tip of the coil cartridge into the catheter. The coil is pushed into the catheter using the stiff end of a guide wire, and is then appropriately positioned using the floppy end of the guide wire. If catheter migration occurs during placement, the catheter is removed through a sheath without extruding the coil.

Like surgical ligatures, coils stop flow in one direction while allowing retrograde filling or collateralization to the site of embolization. For this reason, coils are often used in conjunction with Gelfoam to ensure occlusion of the entire vascular bed. Pretreatment of the coil with Thrombin (Parke, Davis & Co.) is an effective means of occluding large vessels in cases where coagulopathies or high-flow states inhibit the formation of thrombus (McLean et al. 1986).

Detachable Balloons

The silicone detachable balloon (B-D Mini-Balloon; Bectin-Dickinson) is designed to provide proximal occlusion of larger vessels. Unlike other embolization agents, silicone balloons can be repositioned prior to detachment to optimize vessel occlusion. In the genitourinary system, they are ideally suited for embolization of the internal spermatic vein as treatment for a varicocele causing pain or contributing to infertility.

A 1-mm miniballoon for occlusion of vessels less than 4 mm and a 2-mm miniballoon for vessels less than 9 mm are most commonly used. Any venous spasm must be allowed to resolve prior to balloon detachment to avoid subsequent migration and pulmonary embolization. Selection of the position for balloon detachment is important to minimize the development of collateral veins and recurrence of the varicocele. Because detachable balloons are expensive and require a 9-F coaxial delivery system, their use has been limited.

Ethanol

Absolute ethanol (dehydrated alcohol injection, USP; Abbott Laboratories) is an excellent permanent intravascular necrosing agent. It should be applied only in end organs where shunting is not a possible complication. It is ideally suited for performing *in situ* nephrectomies.

While alcohol provides the advantage of rapid, permanent necrosis, these features also make it dangerous. Complications can be avoided by using a balloon occlusion catheter placed in the main renal artery. The balloon, inflated until it conforms to the arterial shape, stops all blood flow. The authors' technique is as follows: the arteries of the kidney or tumor are filled with a known volume of contrast medium; the balloon is deflated and blood flow is allowed to return; the balloon is reinflated; using a glass syringe, the same measured volume of alcohol is injected and allowed to remain for 10 min; the alcohol is aspirated; then the balloon is deflated and the fluoroscopic results examined. If more alcohol is required for embolization, the entire procedure is repeated. Concentration of ethanol in the renal vein during renal ablation remains sufficiently low to be harmless when using the proper technique (Haapanen, Dean 1986).

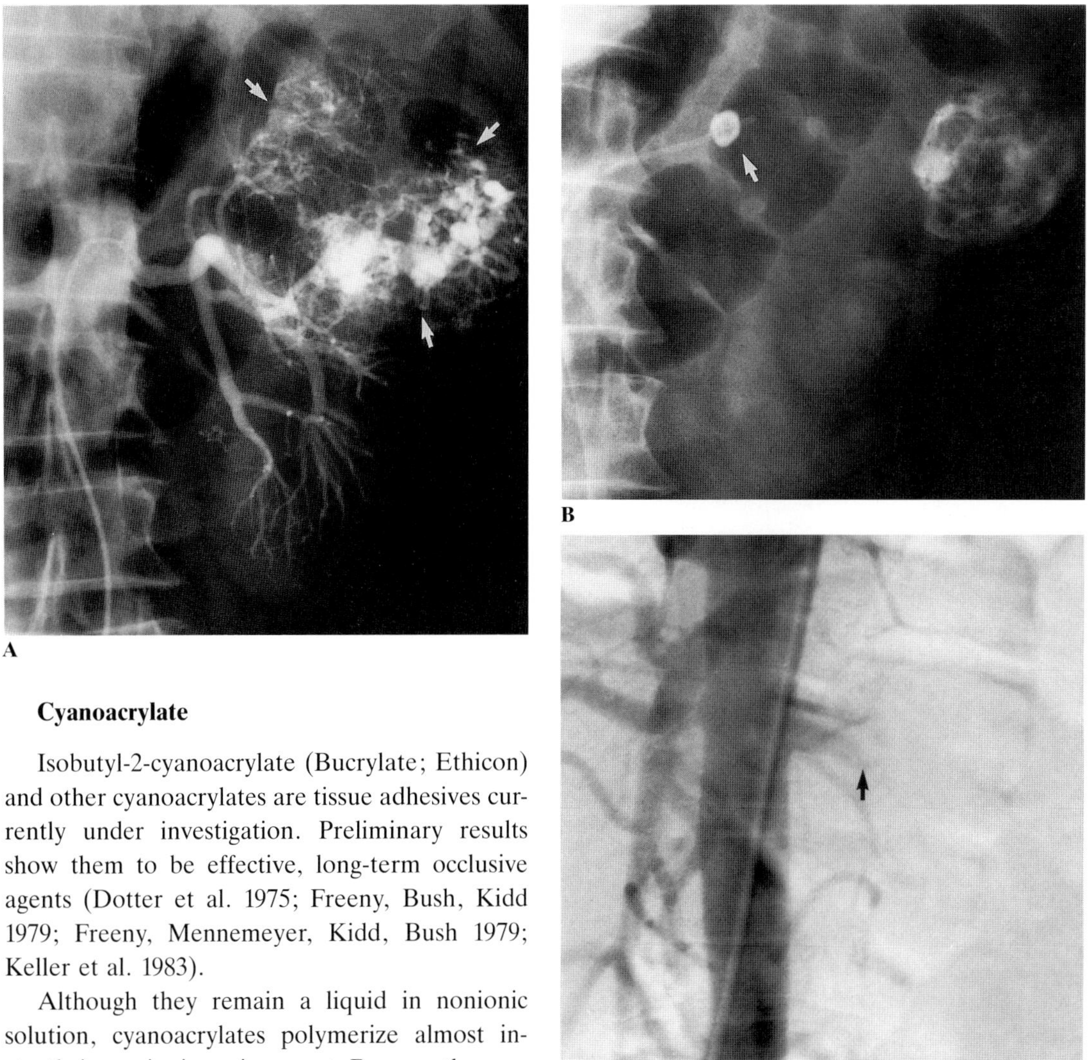

A B C

25–1 Left renal carcinoma, preoperative embolization. **(A)** Arteriogram shows large hypervascular neoplasm (arrows). **(B)** Contrast-opacified occlusion balloon (arrow) inflated in main renal artery. **(C)** Postembolization aortogram demonstrates stump of left main renal artery (arrow) and no filling at tumor site.

Cyanoacrylate

Isobutyl-2-cyanoacrylate (Bucrylate; Ethicon) and other cyanoacrylates are tissue adhesives currently under investigation. Preliminary results show them to be effective, long-term occlusive agents (Dotter et al. 1975; Freeny, Bush, Kidd 1979; Freeny, Mennemeyer, Kidd, Bush 1979; Keller et al. 1983).

Although they remain a liquid in nonionic solution, cyanoacrylates polymerize almost instantly in any ionic environment. Because they are fast-acting, permanent, provide both main arterial and peripheral capillary occlusion, and can be made radiopaque with the addition of tantalum powder (Fansteel Metals) or Pantopaque (iophendylate, Pharmacol), cyanoacrylates are potentially ideal agents.

Safe injection of the adhesive requires a coaxial delivery system. Overinjection, reflux into major vessels, and inadvertent gluing of the catheter are potential complications. Cyanoacrylates should be used only by experienced angiographers.

Renal Embolization

Renal Carcinoma

The usefulness of transcatheter occlusive therapy for the management of renal cell carcinoma varies somewhat from hospital to hospital. Preoperative embolization can facilitate tumor resection by reducing operative blood loss, improving delineation of the tissue planes due to perirenal edema, and allowing transection of the renal vein early in the resection (Wallace et al. 1981).

Rapid vascular occlusion is the goal in this setting. Because alcohol produces rapid extensive coagulative necrosis of the kidney and is readily available and inexpensive, it is the agent of choice. Alcohol must be used with a balloon occlusion device to avoid aortic reflux (Fig. 25–1). Bowel infarction has been reported by Cox and others as a complication of the procedure (Cox et al. 1982; Mulligan, Espinosa 1983). This complication can be avoided if an occlusion balloon is used and the alcohol is aspirated from the vessel before the balloon is deflated.

Instant, permanent vascular occlusion of the kidney can also be achieved with cyanoacrylate infusion. Cyanoacrylates form a spongelike matrix in the renal artery that entraps red blood cells in its interstices and stops all blood flow. Particulate embolization with Gelfoam and Ivalon is effective, but substantially lengthens the embolization procedure. Steel coil embolization has been associated with coil extrusion into the aorta and distal embolization during intraoperative crossclamping of the renal artery.

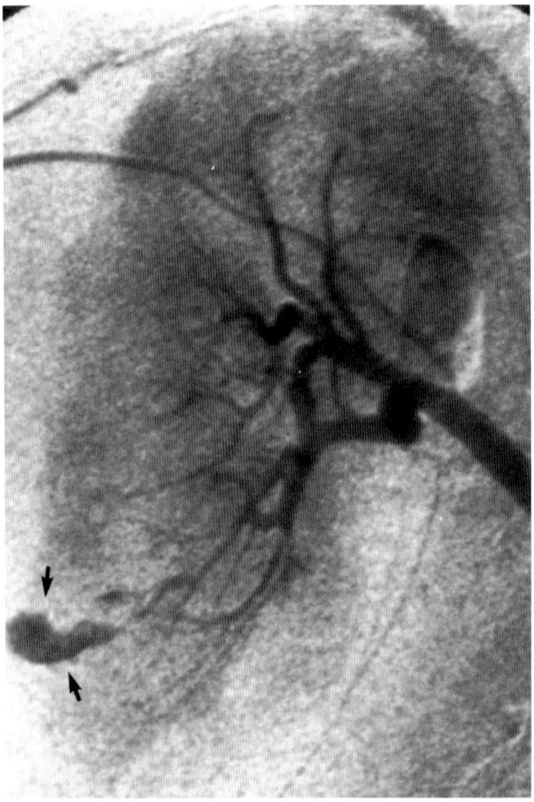

A

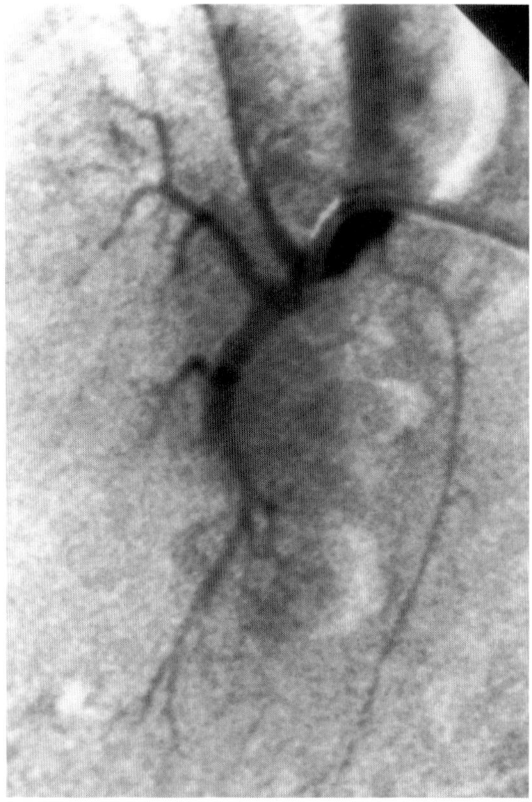

C

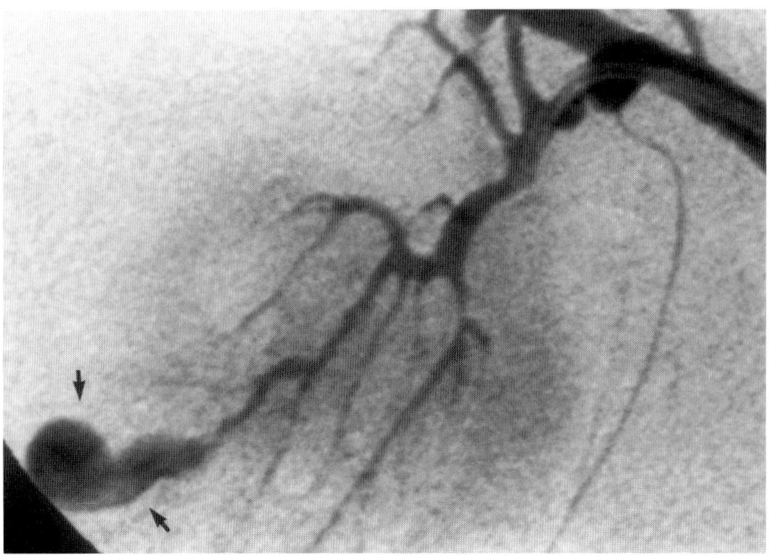

B

25–2 Palliative selective renal artery embolization for control of hemorrhage after renal biopsy. **(A)** Right renal arteriogram with lower pole bleeding (arrows). **(B)** Subselective arteriogram clearly demonstrates bleeding site (arrows). **(C)** Embolization was done subselectively with Gelfoam pledgets; arteriogram post-Gelfoam embolization demonstrates preservation of the adjacent interlobar arteries and no further bleeding.

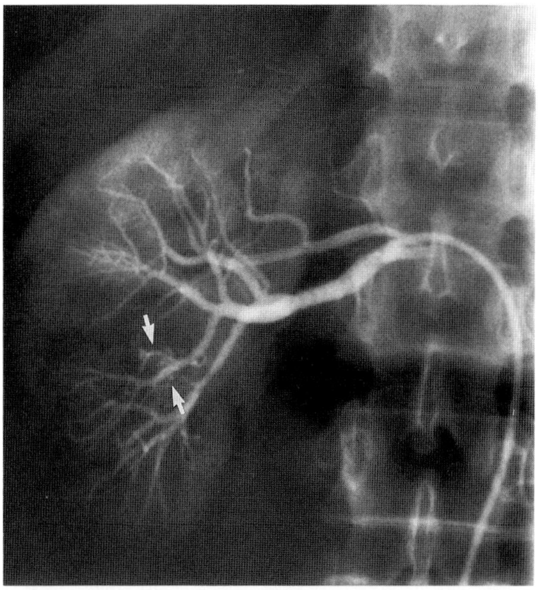

A

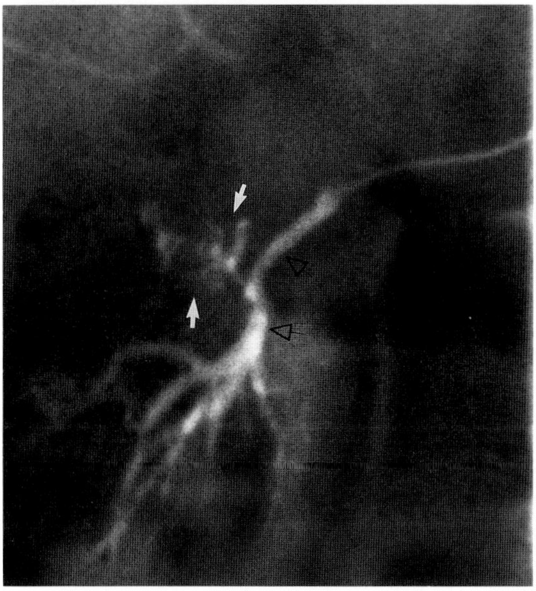

C

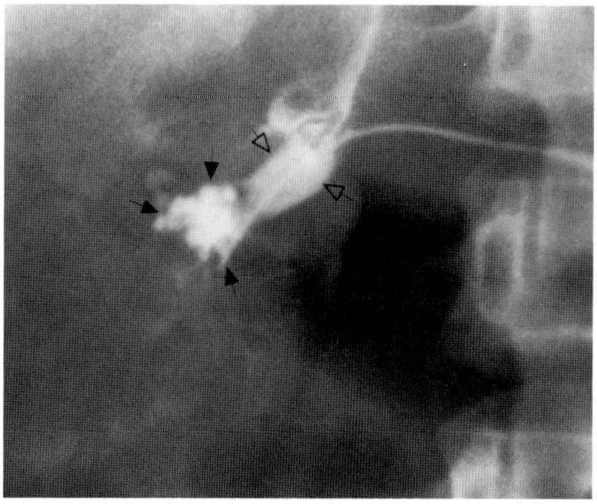

B

25–3 Palliative subselective renal artery occlusion for control of intermittent hematuria due to renal arteriovenous malformation (AVM). **(A)** Selective right renal arteriogram. Tangle of abnormal vasculature (arrows) representing AVM. **(B)** Subselective renal arteriogram. Arteriovenous malformation (closed arrows). Early draining renal vein (open arrows). **(C)** Subselective lower pole renal angiogram. Bucrylate-tantalum cast (white arrows) occluding AVM. Patent lower pole vasculature (open black arrows).

Immediate nephrectomy is recommended to minimize the effects of the postinfarction syndrome (nausea, vomiting, fever, moderate pain, elevated white blood cell count, elevated temperature and ileus) (Chuang et al. 1981; Hemingway, Allison 1988). Patients should be well sedated and analgesics should be used liberally to avoid the pain cycle, which is difficult to reverse.

Angiomyolipoma

Angiomyolipoma, a rare benign renal tumor, usually occurs sporadically as a solitary lesion. However, 80% of patients with tuberous sclerosis have multiple and bilateral renal tumors. Patients with angiomyolipomas often present with complications of hemorrhage. Embolization provides a nonsurgical treatment option (Webb et al. 1986).

Selective embolotherapy with ethanol, Ivalon, or cyanoacrylates is effective for achieving safe, permanent occlusion. As mentioned earlier, Gelfoam fragments last only 3 to 4 weeks and therefore should be combined with steel coils to produce permanent occlusion. Selective renal artery balloon occlusion would also be effective.

Unresectable Renal Tumor

Palliation of unresectable renal tumor is performed primarily to control hematuria and relieve flank pain. Unlike preoperative renal embolization, palliative embolization must be permanent. Alcohol, or if available, cyanoacrylates, are the agents of choice. They produce rapid permanent necrosis and are independent of systemic clotting factors. Combining Gelfoam with steel coils would be equally effective; however, this requires a more lengthy procedure.

Renal abscess has been reported as a complication of alcohol ablation (Tupper et al. 1986). Gram stain and culture of the urine are recommended before the procedure. The computed tomographic (CT) appearance of an infarcted kidney may resemble a renal abscess, making diagnosis difficult.

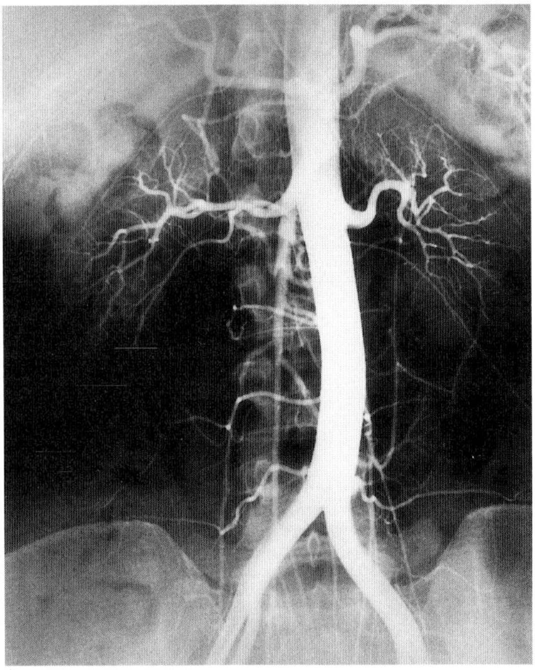

A

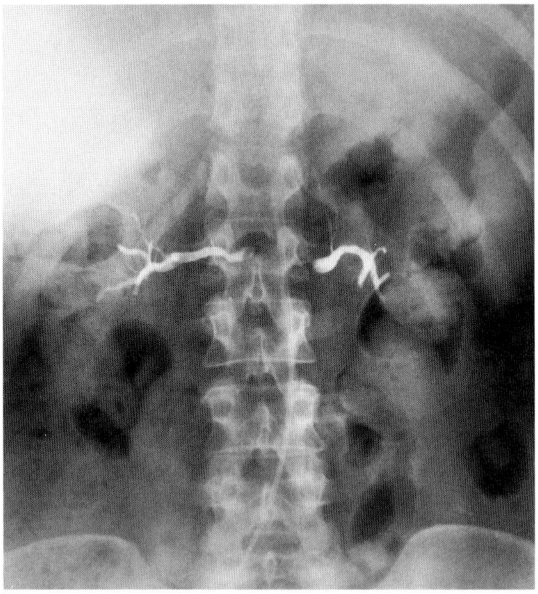

B

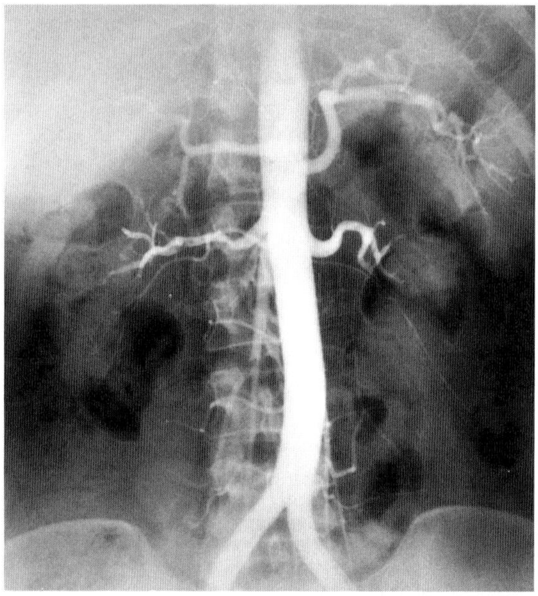

C

25–4 Palliative renal artery occlusion for control of hypertension due to renal disease. **(A)** Aortogram before occlusive procedure. Changes of bilateral arterionephrosclerosis. **(B)** Bucrylate-tantalum casts within renal vessels after occlusion. **(C)** Postocclusion aortogram confirming excellent obliteration of vessel lumina. (Reprinted, by permission of publisher and author, from Freeny PC, Bush WH, Kidd R: Transcatheter occlusive therapy of genitourinary abnormalities using isobutyl 2-cyanoacrylate (Bucrylate). *Am. J. Roentgenol.* 133:647–656, ©1979.)

Trauma

Gross hematuria following blunt or penetrating abdominal trauma, including percutaneous biopsy, can be effectively controlled with selective embolization (Fig. 25–2). Gelfoam embolization produces rapid hemostasis in the majority of cases. Selective embolization with cyanoacrylates, Ivalon, or detachable balloon would be equally effective but are more costly. Ethanol is not recommended, as it could prove dangerous because of potential retroperitoneal extravasation.

Arteriovenous Fistulas and Malformations

Renal arteriovenous fistulas following blunt or penetrating injury and arteriovenous malformations can be effectively managed with embolotherapy (Clark et al. 1983) (Fig. 25–3). Control of intermittent hematuria and hypertension is the goal. Arteriovenous fistulas can also occur following nephrectomy or renal artery aneurysm rupture, and with hypernephromas.

Precise definition of vascular anatomy is a prerequisite to embolotherapy. Subselective embolization of the feeding arteries permits maximum sparing of functional renal parenchyma. A large arteriovenous connection may predispose to pulmonary embolization if particulate embolization is used. Steel coils, detachable balloons, and cyanoacrylates can all be used successfully in this setting. Detachable balloons have the advantage of retrieval if inflation does not adequately occlude the fistula. However, in a large, high-flow fistula, care must be taken, as a balloon may accidentally

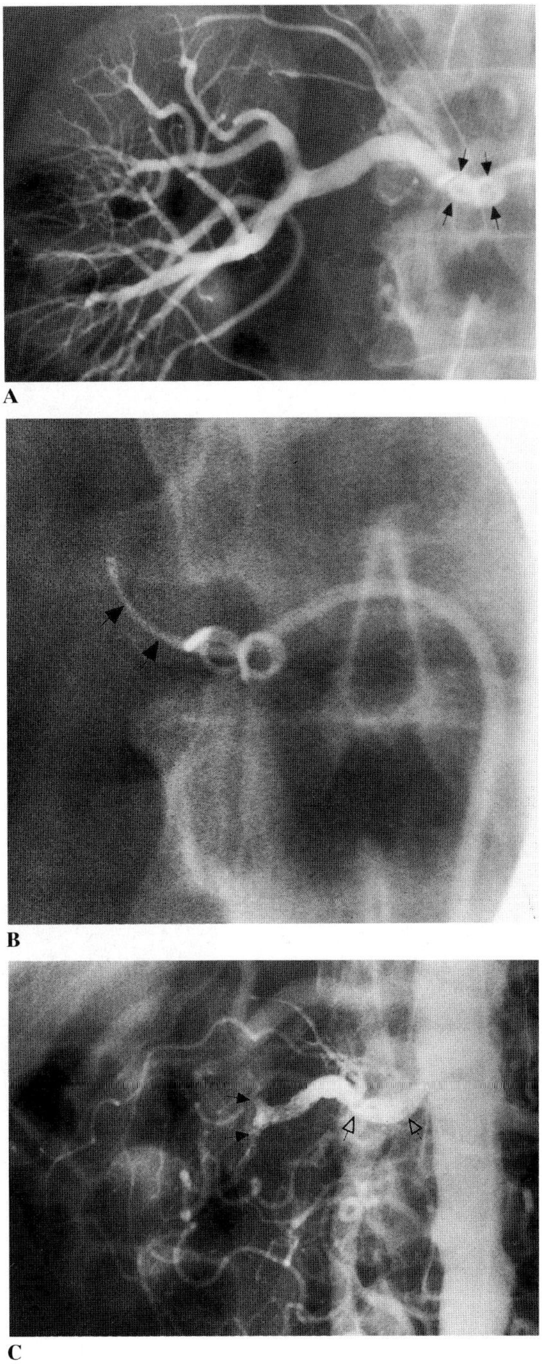

25–5 Palliative renal artery occlusion for control of hemorrhage due to diffuse intravascular coagulopathy. Failure of Gianturco coil. **(A)** Selective right renal arteriogram one day after placement of Gianturco coil (arrows). Patent renal artery with no thrombus within coil. **(B)** 3-French coaxial catheter (arrows) for Bucrylate injection passed through coil. **(C)** Postocclusion aortogram. Bucrylate-tantalum cast (closed arrows) occluding renal artery. Gianturco coil (between open arrows). (Reprinted, by permission of publisher and author, from Freeny PC, Bush WH, Kidd R: Transcatheter occlusive therapy of genitourinary abnormalities using isobutyl 2-cyanoacrylate (Bucrylate). *Am. J. Roentgenol.* 133:647–656, ©1979.)

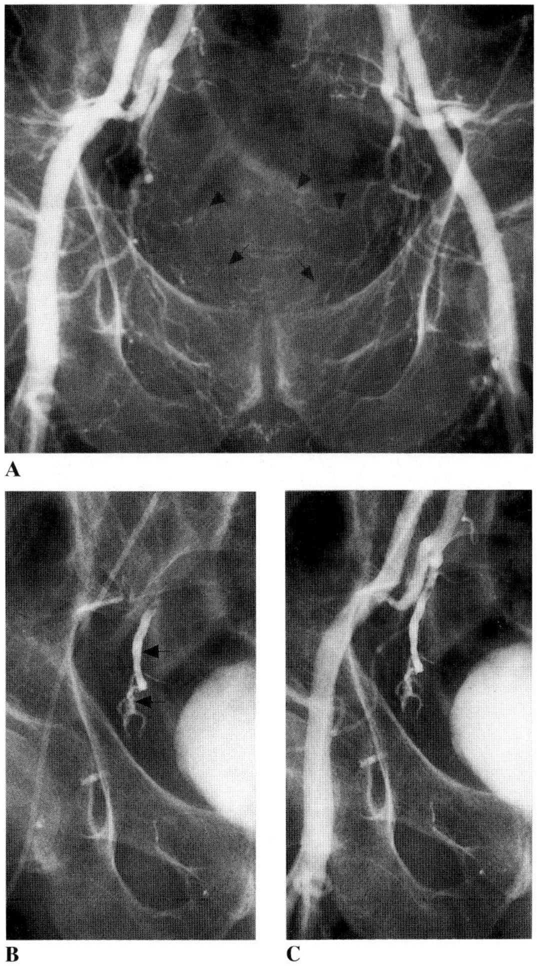

25–6 Palliative pelvic artery occlusion for control of recurrent hemorrhage from unresectable bladder carcinoma. **(A)** Pelvic arteriogram. Numerous small, irregular vessels surround bladder (arrows). Specific bleeding site not identified. **(B)** Pudendal and gluteal arteries subselectively catheterized bilaterally and occluded with Bucrylate-tantalum. Bucrylate casts in vessels on right (arrows). **(C)** Postocclusion right iliac arteriogram confirms obliteration of vessel lumina. Similar findings were seen on left (not shown). (Reprinted, by permission of publisher and author, from Freeny PC, Bush WH, Kidd R: Transcatheter occlusive therapy of genitourinary abnormalities using isobutyl 2-cyanoacrylate (Bucrylate). *Am. J. Roentgenol.* 133: 647–656, ©1979.)

detach during inflation but before occlusion of the vessel has been achieved. With smaller fistulas, particulate embolization with Gelfoam or Ivalon can be performed. Ethanol would be less desirable in high-flow states, owing to its ability to cause rapid coagulation necrosis.

Unlike arteriovenous fistulas, arteriovenous malformations are frequently associated with multiple feeding vessels and can recruit additional vessels after incomplete embolization. The success of embolotherapy depends on successful elimination of the "nidus" of the malformation. This can be effectively achieved with either cyanoacrylate or Ivalon.

Function Ablation for End-Stage Disease

Percutaneous renal embolization can be an effective alternative to surgical removal in patients with end-stage renal disease (Keller et al. 1986). Embolotherapy can be used for control of hypertension from renin production, for control of massive proteinuria from the nephrotic syndrome (Fig. 25–4), and for control of renal bleeding occurring with a systemic coagulopathy (Fig. 25–5).

Ethanol, cyanoacrylates, Gelfoam combined with steel coils, and detachable balloons are equally effective. Ethanol and Gelfoam with steel coils are the agents of choice, due to cost and availability.

Bladder Embolization

Carcinoma of the bladder, direct tumor invasion from cervical, uterine, or prostatic carcinoma, and radiation cystitis can be associated with persistent hematuria. Selective, subselective, or main hypogastric arterial embolization with Gelfoam and proximal steel coil (Fig. 25–6), cyanoacrylate infusion (Fig. 25–7), or detachable silicone balloons can be used to control hemorrhage. Bilateral embolization is frequently necessary to prevent rebleeding from the development of crosspelvic collaterals. Pretreatment of the steel coils with thrombin may be necessary to control bleeding in patients with coagulopathies. Ethanol is contraindicated because of its propensity to produce rapid coagulation necrosis. Gelfoam combined with steel coils is most commonly used in this clinical setting.

Varicocele Embolization

Embolotherapy is indicated in the treatment of subfertility and for pain and swelling that can accompany varicoceles (White et al. 1981). Selective catheterization of the internal spermatic vein is done through a transbrachial, transfemoral, or transjugular approach. The authors prefer the transfemoral approach and have achieved catheterization of the desired vein in over 90% of patients.

A recurrence rate of 15% has been reported (Formanek et al. 1981), primarily related to incomplete embolization or development of collaterals; numerous accessory channels can potentially recollateralize an embolized internal spermatic vein. Therefore, anatomic assessment to locate and successfully eliminate these potential collateral pathways is critical prior to embolization.

The silicone balloon allows test occlusions to be performed prior to detachment. Potential collateral channels can be identified and proper balloon positioning can be performed to occlude them (Fig. 25–8). Alternatively, steel coils can be selectively placed to occlude the internal spermatic vein and collateral channels.

Although the majority of varicoceles are located on the left, an 80% incidence of subclinical right varicoceles has been reported (Formanek et al. 1981). Evaluation of the right internal spermatic vein during left embolotherapy may improve the management of subfertility.

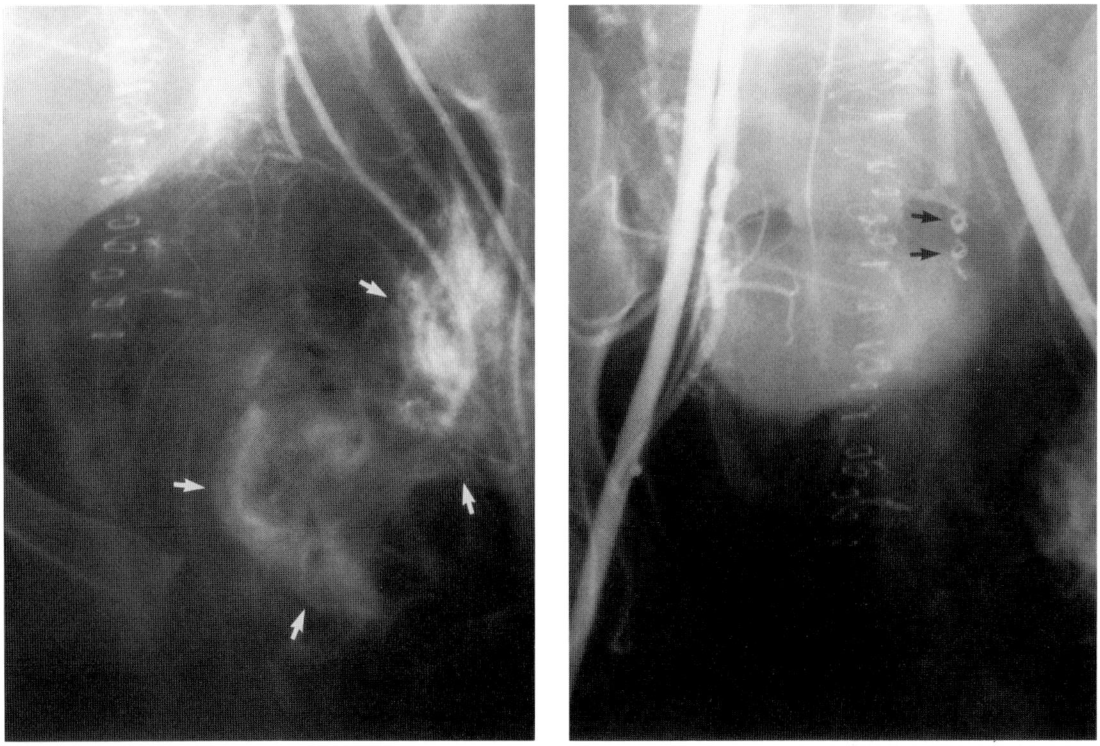

A

B

25–7 Pelvic embolization for control of massive pelvic hemorrhage following motor vehicle accident. **(A)** Catheter placed in left pudendal artery demonstrates gross extravasation into perineum (arrows). **(B)** Post-Gelfoam and steel coil (arrows) embolization demonstrates no further bleeding. (Reprinted, with permission, from Maroney TP: Transcatheter embolization thrives despite controversy. *Diagn. Imaging* (Basel), (July), 102–106, ©1986.)

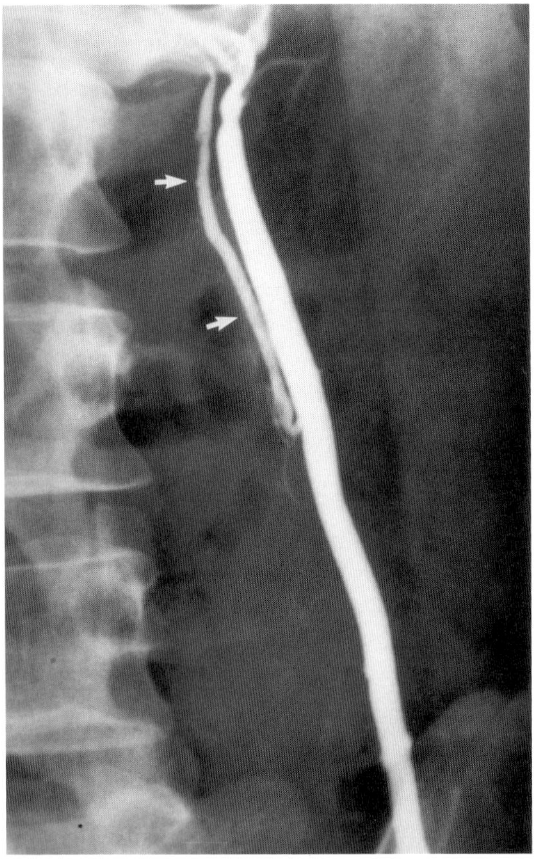

A

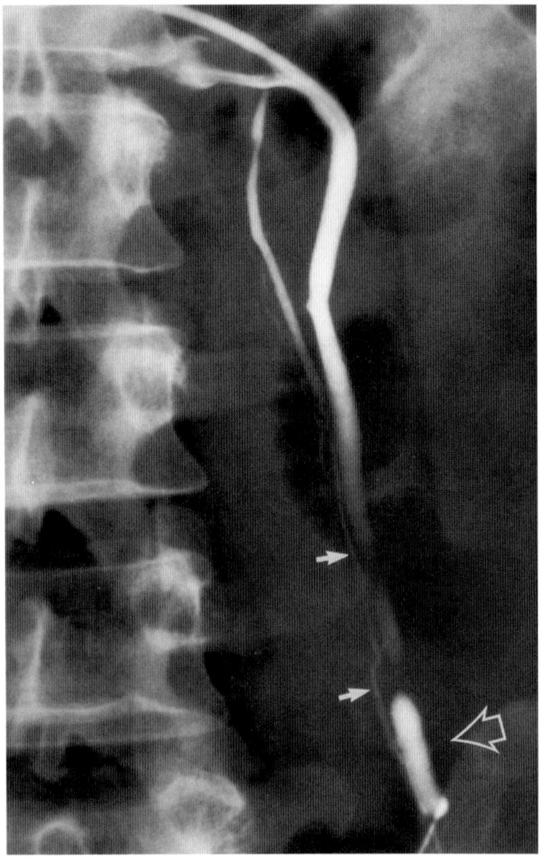

B

25–8 Varicocele embolization. Palliative left internal spermatic vein (ISV) occlusion for reversal of subfertility due to varicocele. **(A)** Selective left gonadal venogram. Parallel accessory channel (arrows) capable of reconstituting an occluded ISV. Varicocele not pictured. **(B)** Left gonadal venogram performed after contrast-opacified inflatable silicone balloon (open arrow) positioned via catheter; balloon inflated but not detached. A major paralleling accessory vein (arrows) fills, permitting continued opacification of the varicocele. **(C)** Left gonadal venogram performed after balloon was repositioned to occlude this accessory channel. The silicone balloon (open arrows) was detached, successfully occluding the main ISV (black arrow). Gianturco steel coil (minicoil) embolization of an additional accessory vein was then done (small white arrows), completing the vein occlusion.

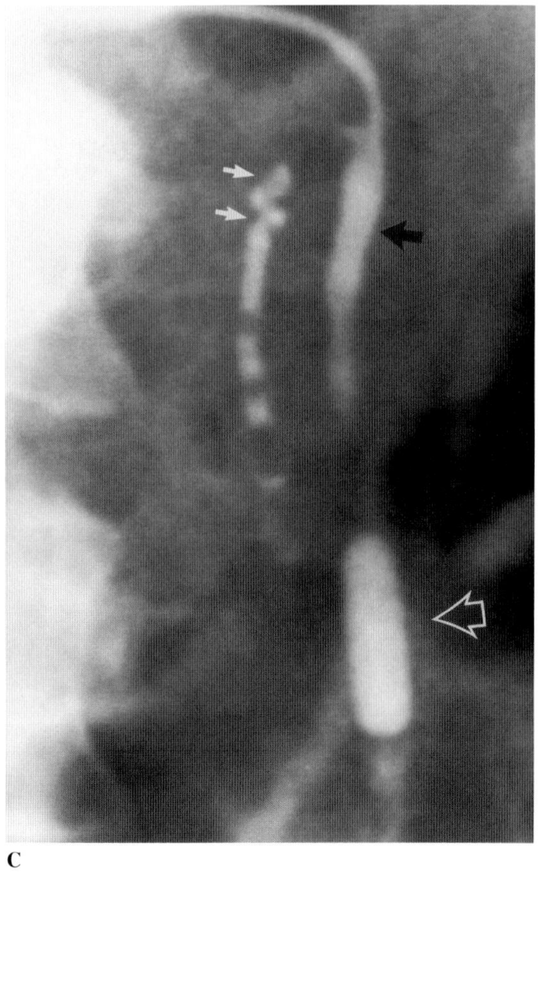

C

References

Bookstein JJ, Naderi MJ, Walter JF: Transcatheter embolization for lower gastrointestinal bleeding. *Radiology* 127:345–349, 1978.

Chuang VP, Wallace S, Swanson DA: Technique and complications of renal carcinoma infarction. *Urol. Radiol.* 2:223–228, 1981.

Clark RA, Gallant TE, Alexander ES: Angiographic management of traumatic arteriovenous fistulas: Clinical results. *Radiology* 147:9–13, 1983.

Cox GG, Lee KR, Price HE, et al.: Colonic infarction following ethanol embolization of renal cell carcinoma. *Radiology* 145:343–345, 1982.

Dotter CT, Goldman ML, Rosch J: Instant selective arterial occlusion with isobutyl 2-cyanoacrylate. *Radiology* 114:227–230, 1975.

Formanek A, Rusnak B, Zollikofer C, Castaneda-Zuniga WR, Narayan P, Gonzalez R, Amplatz K: Embolization of the spermatic vein for treatment of infertility: A new approach. *Radiology* 139:315–321, 1981.

Freeny PC, Bush WH, Kidd R: Transcatheter occlusive therapy of genitourinary abnormalities using isobutyl 2-cyanoacrylate (Bucrylate). *Am. J. Roentgenol.* 133: 647–656, 1979.

Freeny PC, Mennemeyer R, Kidd R, Bush WH: Long-term radiologic-pathologic follow-up of patients treated with visceral transcatheter occlusion using isobutyl 2-cyanoacrylate (Bucrylate). *Radiology* 132:51–60, 1979.

Gianturco C, Anderson JH, Wallace S: Mechanical devices for arterial occlusion. *Am. J. Roentgenol.* 124:428, 1975.

Greenfield AJ: Transcatheter vessel occlusion: Methods and materials. *In* Athanasoulis C, Pfister R (eds.): *Interventional Radiology.* W. B. Saunders Co., Philadelphia, 1982.

Haapanen AA, Dean PB: Renal vein ethanol concentration during ablation of renal cell carcinoma. *Cardiovasc. Intervent. Radiol.* 9:205–208, 1986.

Hemingway AP, Allison DJ: Complications of embolization: Analysis of 410 procedures. *Radiology* 166:669–672, 1988.

Jander HP, Russinovich NAE: Transcatheter Gelfoam embolization in abdominal, retroperitoneal, and pelvic hemorrhage. *Radiology* 136:337–344, 1980.

Katzen BT, Rossi P, Passariello R, et al.: Transcatheter therapeutic arterial embolization. *Radiology* 120:523–531, 1976.

Keller FS, Coyle M, Rösch J, Dotter CT: Percutaneous renal ablation in patients with end-stage renal disease: Alternative to surgical nephrectomy. *Radiology* 159:447–451, 1986.

Keller FS, Rösch J, Bird CB: Percutaneous embolization of bony pelvic neoplasms with tissue adhesive. *Radiology* 147:21–27, 1983.

Kerber CW, Bank WO, Horton JA: Polyvinyl alcohol foam: Prepackaged emboli for therapeutic embolization. *Am. J. Roentgenol.* 130:1193–1194, 1978.

Lalli AF, Peterson N, Bookstein JJ: Roentgen-guided infarctions of kidneys and lungs: A potential therapeutic technique. *Radiology* 93:434, 1969.

McLean GK, Stein EJ, Burke DR, Meranze SG: Steel occlusion coils: Pretreatment with thrombin. *Radiology* 158:549–550, 1986.

Mulligan BD, Espinosa GA: Bowel infarction: Complication of ethanol ablation of a renal tumor. *Cardiovasc. Intervent. Radiol.* 6:55–57, 1983.

Tadavarthy SM, Moller JH, Amplatz K: Polyvinyl alcohol (Ivalon) – A new embolic material. *Am. J. Roentgenol.* 125:609–616, 1975.

Tupper TB, Cronan JJ, Wald LM, Dorfman GS: Renal abscess: A complication of ethanol embolization. *Radiology* 161:35–36, 1986.

Wallace S, Chuang VP, Swanson D, et al.: Embolization of renal carcinoma. *Radiology* 138:563–570, 1981.

Wallace S, Gianturco C, Anderson JN, et al.: Therapeutic vascular occlusion utilizing steel coil technique: Clinical applications. *Am. J. Roentgenol.* 127:381–387, 1976.

Webb JE, Mazer MJ, Winfield AC: Angiomyolipomas in tuberous sclerosis: Subselective embolotherapy with alcohol with long-term follow-up study. *Radiology* 160:437–441, 1986.

White RI, Kaufman SL, Barth KH, et al.: Occlusion of varicoceles with detachable balloons. *Radiology* 139:327–334, 1981.

INDEX

Page numbers in *italics* indicate figures; those followed by "t" indicate tables.

D

E

R